HEALTH AND HUMAN DEVELOPMENT SERIES

ADOLESCENCE AND CHRONIC ILLNESS: A PUBLIC HEALTH CONCERN

HEALTH AND HUMAN DEVELOPMENT SERIES

JOAV MERRICK, EDITOR

Adolescent Behavior Research: International Perspectives
Joav Merrick and Hatim A. Omar
2007. ISBN: 1-60021-649-8

Complementary Medicine Systems: Comparison and Integration
Karl W. Kratky
2008. ISBN: 978-1-60456-475-4

Pain in Children and Youth
Patricia Schofield and Joav Merrick
2008. ISBN: 978-1-60456-951-3

Obesity and Adolescence: A Public Health Concern
Hatim A. Omar, Donald E. Greydanus, Dilip R. Patel and Joav Merrick
2009. ISBN: 978-1-60456-821-9

**Health and Happiness from Meaningful Work:
Research in Quality of Working Life**
Søren Ventegodt and Joav Merrick
2009. ISBN: 978-1-60692-820-2

Behavioral Pediatrics 3rd Edition
Donald E. Greydanus, Dilip R. Patel, Helen D. Pratt and Joseph L. Calles, Jr.
2009. ISBN: 978-1-60692-702-1

Behavioral Pediatrics 3rd Edition
Donald E. Greydanus, Dilip R. Patel, Helen D. Pratt and Joseph L. Calles, Jr.
2009. ISBN: 978-1-60876-630-7 (Online Book)

Poverty and Children: A Public Health Concern
Alexis Lieberman and Joav Merrick
2009. ISBN: 978-1-60741-140-6

**Living on the Edge: The Mythical, Spiritual, and Philosophical
Roots of Social Marginality**
Joseph Goodbread
2009. ISBN: 978-1-60741-162-8

Alcohol-Related Cognitive Disorders: Research and Clinical Perspectives
Leo Sher, Isack Kandel and Joav Merrick
2009. ISBN: 978-1-60741-730-9

Alcohol-Related Cognitive Disorders: Research and Clinical Perspectives
Leo Sher, Isack Kandel and Joav Merrick
2009. ISBN: 978-1-60876-623-9 (Online Book)

Challenges in Adolescent Health: An Australian Perspective
David Bennett, Susan Towns, Elizabeth Elliott and Joav Merrick (Editors)
2009. ISBN: 978-1-60741-616-6

Children and Pain
Patricia Schofield and Joav Merrick (Editors)
2009. ISBN: 978-1-60876-020-6

Chance Action and Therapy. The Playful Way of Changing
Uri Wernik
2010. ISBN: 978-1-60876-393-1

Adolescence and Chronic Illness. A Public Health Concern
Hatim Omar, Donald E. Greydanus, Dilip R. Patel and Joav Merrick (Editors)
2010. ISBN: 978-1-60876-628-4

HEALTH AND HUMAN DEVELOPMENT SERIES

ADOLESCENCE AND CHRONIC ILLNESS: A PUBLIC HEALTH CONCERN

HATIM OMAR,
DONALD E. GREYDANUS,
DILIP R. PATEL AND
JOAV MERRICK
EDITORS

Nova Science Publishers, Inc.
New York

Copyright © 2010 by Nova Science Publishers, Inc.

All rights reserved. No part of this book may be reproduced, stored in a retrieval system or transmitted in any form or by any means: electronic, electrostatic, magnetic, tape, mechanical photocopying, recording or otherwise without the written permission of the Publisher.

For permission to use material from this book please contact us:
Telephone 631-231-7269; Fax 631-231-8175
 Web Site: http://www.novapublishers.com

NOTICE TO THE READER

The Publisher has taken reasonable care in the preparation of this book, but makes no expressed or implied warranty of any kind and assumes no responsibility for any errors or omissions. No liability is assumed for incidental or consequential damages in connection with or arising out of information contained in this book. The Publisher shall not be liable for any special, consequential, or exemplary damages resulting, in whole or in part, from the readers' use of, or reliance upon, this material.

Independent verification should be sought for any data, advice or recommendations contained in this book. In addition, no responsibility is assumed by the publisher for any injury and/or damage to persons or property arising from any methods, products, instructions, ideas or otherwise contained in this publication.

This publication is designed to provide accurate and authoritative information with regard to the subject matter covered herein. It is sold with the clear understanding that the Publisher is not engaged in rendering legal or any other professional services. If legal or any other expert assistance is required, the services of a competent person should be sought. FROM A DECLARATION OF PARTICIPANTS JOINTLY ADOPTED BY A COMMITTEE OF THE AMERICAN BAR ASSOCIATION AND A COMMITTEE OF PUBLISHERS.

LIBRARY OF CONGRESS CATALOGING-IN-PUBLICATION DATA

Adolescence and chronic illness : a public health concern / editors, Hatim Omar ... [et al.].
  p. ; cm.
 Includes bibliographical references and index.
 ISBN 978-1-60876-628-4 (hardcover)
 1. Adolescent medicine. 2. Chronic diseases in adolescence. I. Omar, Hatim A.
 [DNLM: 1. Chronic Disease. 2. Adolescent Behavior. 3. Adolescent Psychology. 4. Adolescent. WS 460 A23912 2009]
 RJ550.A315 2009
 616.00835--dc22
2009039015

Published by Nova Science Publishers, Inc. ✢ *New York*

CONTENTS

Preface		xi
Part I. Introduction		1
Introduction	Adolescents, Chronic Disease and Disability	3
Part II. Infectious Disease		11
Chapter 1	Infections in Adolescents with Disabilities *Stephen K. Obaro*	13
Part III. Neoplasms		21
Chapter 2	Adolescents with Cancer *Renuka Gera, Elna N. Saah, Ajovi B. Scott-Emuakpor and Roshni Kulkarni*	23
Part IV. Endocrine, Nutritional and Metabolic Diseases		33
Chapter 3	Endocrine Aspects of Chronic Disease *Manmohan K. Kamboj*	35
Chapter 4	Endocrinological Aspects of Intellectual Disability *Mohammed Morad, Efrat Merrick-Kenig and Joav Merrick*	51
Chapter 5	Metabolism and Disease *Efrat Merrick-Kenig, Mohammed Morad and Joav Merrick*	57
Part V. Diseases of the Blood		63
Chapter 6	Chronic Hematological Disorders *Elna N. Saah, Renuka Gera, Ajovi B. Scott-Emuakpor and Roshni Kulkarni*	65
Chapter 7	Severe Pain in Children with Sickle Cell Disease *Eufemia Jacob, Marilyn Hockenberry, Brigitta U. Mueller, Thomas D. Coates and Lonnie Zeltzer*	81

Part VI. Mental Disorders — 97

Chapter 8   Mental Health and Chronic Disease — 99
Marlene B. Huff, Kimberly K. McClanahan and Hatim A. Omar

Chapter 9   Psychiatric Issues in Chronically Ill Children, Adolescents and Young Adults — 109
Joseph L. Calles, Jr.

Chapter 10   Eating Disorders and Therapeutic Health Outcome — 123
Bruce Kirkcaldy, Marlies Pinnow and Georg R. Siefen

Chapter 11   Psychological Issues in Chronically Ill Adolescents — 151
Helen D. Pratt

Part VII. Nervous System — 165

Chapter 12   Neurological Impairment and Disability — 167
Dilip R. Patel and Donald E. Greydanus

Chapter 13   Youth with Chronic Pain — 173
Paula Forgeron and Patrick J. McGrath

VIII. Circulatory System — 187

Chapter 14   A Comprehensive Approach to Obesity, Hypertension, and Mental Health Evaluation — 189
Stefan G. Kiessling, Kimberly K. McClanahan and Hatim A. Omar

Part IX. Respiratory System — 201

Chapter 15   Pulmonary Disabilities in Adolescents — 203
Douglas N. Homnick

Chapter 16   Childhood Asthma Management and Control — 221
Frank Mo, Chris Robinson and Bernard C.K. Choi

Part X. Digestive System — 233

Chapter 17   Nutrition and Gastroenterology Issues — 235
Arthur N. Feinberg, Lisa A. Feinberg and Orhan K. Atay

Part XI. Genitourinary System — 245

Chapter 18   Chronic Kidney Disease — 247
Timothy E. Bunchman

Chapter 19   Chronic Kidney Disease and Quality of Life — 255
Jane Anne Smith and Stefan G. Kiessling

Part XII. Pregnancy and Sexuality — 271

Chapter 20   Pregnancy and Young Women with Disabilities — 273
Kathy Sheppard-Jones, Harold Kleinert, Cindy Paulding and Christina Espinosa

Chapter 21	Down Syndrome and Sexuality *Maria José Carvalho Sant'Anna, Bruna Marques Bononi,* *André Chao Vasconcellos de Oliveira, Tadeu Silveira Renattini,* *Carla Franchi Pinto, Maria Lúcia Passarelli, Veronica Coates and* *Hatim A. Omar*	283

Part XIII. Skin — 291

Chapter 22	Acne Vulgaris and Adolescence *Donald E. Greydanus and Dilip R. Patel*	293

Part XIV. Musculskeletal System — 305

Chapter 23	Acute Musculoskeletal Sports Injury and Topical NSAID *Amit M. Deokar, Shawn J. Smith and Hatim A. Omar*	307
Chapter 24	Chronic Disability from Hip Abnormalities in Adolescence *Avinash L. Jadhav and Dale E. Rowe*	311

Part XV. Genetics — 337

Chapter 25	Intellectual Disability and Genetics *Helga V. Toriello*	339
Chapter 26	Down Syndrome and Adolescence *Efrat Merrick-Kenig, Joav Merrick and Isack Kandel*	349
Chapter 27	Rett Syndrome and Snoezelen or Controlled Multi-Sensory Stimulation *Meir Lotan and Joav Merrick*	357

Part XVI. Physical Activity and Sports — 367

Chapter 28	Sports and Adolescents with Disability *Dilip R. Patel and Donald E. Greydanus*	369
Chapter 29	Sports Preparticipation Examination *Donald E. Greydanus and Dilip R. Patel*	375
Chapter 30	Adolescents with Intellectual Disability and Physical Activity *Meir Lotan and Joav Merrick*	383

Part XVII. Dental Aspects — 395

Chapter 31	Dental Care Needs *Joseph D'Ambrosio*	397

Part XVIII. Transition — 401

Chapter 32	Adolescents with Sickle Cell Disease and Transition to Adult Care *Joseph Telfair, John E. Ehiri, Penny S. Loosier and* *Monica L. Baskin*	403
Chapter 33	The Transition of Care for Young People with Chronic Disease *Katherine S. Steinbeck, Lynne Brodie and Susan J. Towns*	421

Part XIX. Acknowledgements	431
About the Editors	433
About the Division of Adolescent Medicine at the University of Kentucky, Lexngton, Kentucky, United States	435
About the Department of Pediatrics and Human Development, Michigan State University College of Human Medicine, MSU/Kalamazoo Center for Medical studies, Kalamazoo, Michigan, United States	437
About the National Institute of Child Health and Human Devlopment in Israel	441
Index	445

PREFACE

The prevalence of chronic illness or disability in adolescence has increased in recent years due to medical advances and adolescents are now more than ever able to lead a productive life even in spite of serious illness. In the past children with many diseases would not reach adolescence, but over the last decade or more the survival rate for children with cystic fibrosis, for spina bifida and congenital heart disease has increased. The old morbidity (infectious disease, poor housing, poverty, lack of immunisation) has been exchanged with the new morbidty of adolescence, where a longer life expectancy is followed by an increase in life long disability.

The concern in chronic illness include medical, psychological, physiological, biological, reproductive, cognitive and social aspects. Practitioners of the healing arts must become familiar with the most common disabilities likely to afflict children and adolescents so that appropriate evaluation, treatment, and management may occur.

This book will cover a broad area of chronic illness in adolescence written by leading experts in this field.

PART I. INTRODUCTION

In: Adolescence and Chronic Illness
Editors: H. Omar et al.

ISBN: 978-1-60876-628-4
© 2010 Nova Science Publishers, Inc.

INTRODUCTION

ADOLESCENTS, CHRONIC DISEASE AND DISABILITY

The prevalence of chronic illness or disability in adolescence has increased in recent years due to medical advances and adolescents are now more than ever able to lead a productive life even in spite of serious illness. In the past children with many diseases would not reach adolescence, but over the last decade or more the survival rate for children with cystic fibrosis has increased by 700%, for spina bifida with 200% and 300% for congenital heart disease [1]. The old morbidity (infectious disease, poor housing, poverty, lack of immunisation) has been exchanged with the new morbidty of adolescence, where a longer life expectancy is followed by an increase in life long disability.

Disability

Disabilty in childhood and adolescence suffers from the lack of a uniform definition or classification [2]. Ruth Stein and co-workers at the Department of Pediatrics, Albert Einstein College of Medicine in New York have worked on the development of a questionnaire and definition to identify children and adolescents with chronic conditions [3-5]. They have developed a non-categorical or generic approach by defining and measuring chronic health conditions instead of using a list of diagnoses. The framework [3] is based on three concepts, which must be present in a child or adolescent in order to be classified as having a chronic health condition or disability:

1. Disorder on a biological, psychological or cognitive basis
2. Duration or expected duration of at least 12 months
3. Produce one or more of the following sequelae:
   a. Limitation of function, activities or social role compared with healthy peers in the same age group in the general areas of physical, cognitive, emotional and social growth and development
   b. Dependency on one of the following to compensate for or minimize limitation of function, activities or social role: medications, special diet, medical technology, assistive device or personal assistance

c. Need for medical care or related services, psychological services or educational services over and above the usual for the child's age or for special ongoing treatments, interventions or accommodations at home or in school.

Others have used a definition with a shorter period of three or more months during the last year [6] or others with both a duration longer than three months in a year and hospitalization for more than one month in a year [7].

The Child Health Indicators of Life and Development (CHILD) project recently published its recommendations for use in Europe to monitor child and adolescent health [8,9] through 38 core national indicators.

Epidemiology

Data from the United Kingdom, United States, Scandinavia and Israel showed the prevalence of disability in adolescence (age 12-18 years) was the lowest in Denmark (6.5%) and highest in Finland (9.9%) [6].

The trend in prevalence of disability in childhood and adolescence has been studied extensively in the United States by Paul W Newacheck from the Institute for Health Policy Studies at the University of California in San Francisco. In a sample of 7,465 persons aged 10-17 years from the 1988 National Health Interview Survey on Child Health, where chronic conditions in adolescents was defined, if it was first noted more than three months before the interview or a condition that ordinarily would be of lengthy duration, such as arthritis or heart disease, an estimated 31.5% of US adolescents were reported to have one or more chronic conditions [10].

More and more adolescents have chronic health conditions, which cause disability [11]. This has been shown in several papers with data from the US National Health Interview Surveys (NHIS) [11-13] with a prevalence of 1.8% in 1960 that increased to 6.5% in 1998 for prevalence of chronic conditions among all children. The figure for adolescents (13-18 years) was 9.3% [6]. An extensive national survey of children with special health care needs (CSHCN) in the United States is conduted in order to produce uniform national and state data on the prevalence and also impact of special health care needs among children using the CSHCN screener [14].

In Israel the children and adolescents (aged 8-17 years) who received the disabled child benefit increased from 6.5% in 1996 to 8.4% in year 2000 [15].

CAUSES OF CHRONIC ILLNESS IN ADOLESCENCE

In the study with the sample of 7,465 persons aged 10 to 17 years from the 1988 National Health Interview Survey on Child Health [10] the most commonly reported chronic conditions included respiratory allergies, asthma, and frequent or severe headaches, which correspond with other studies where asthma is the most reported chronic illness [6]. In table 1 estimates for various childhood conditions are listed for American children [16].

Table 1. Estimated prevalence of representative childhood chronic conditions in United States Children [16]

Chronic conditions	Rates per 1,000
Asthma (moderate and severe)	15.00
Congenital heart disease	10.00
Seizure disorder	3.00
Arthritis	3.00
Diabetes mellitus	1.40
Cleft lip/palate	1.40
Sickle cell anemia	1.20
Down syndrome	1.00
Cystic fibrosis	0.20
Hemophilia	0.15
Acute lymphocytic leukemia	0.11
Muscular dystrophy	0.06

Disparities, Access and Expenditure of Health Care

Disparities between African American and white children have also been studied [17] using the US National Health Interview Surveys (NHIS) from 1979-2000. The results indicated that the prevalence of activity limitation had increased for both black and while during during 1979-2000. For black children the prevalence increased from 37.9/1,000 to 67.1/1,000 (a 77% increase), while for white children from 40.7/1,000 to 59.7/1,000 (47% increase). So from being equal in 1979 the difference in 2000 showed that black children were 13% more likely to have a reported limitation. With further multivariate analysis the racial effect disappeared and it seemed that the difference was attributed to difference in income.

In another study of 12,434 adolescents (10-18 years) without disability from the 1999 and 2000 NIHS it was found that adolescents in low-income families were at a disatvantage to receive health care [18].

Access to health is different in Europe and the United States, because of the lack of universal health insurance in the United States. Another study from the 1994-1995 NIHS [19] analyzed data on 57,553 children to examine special health care needs, insurance status and access to health care. 95% of the children had a usual source of care, but those who were uninsured were far more likely to be without a usual source of care. Publicly insured were again more likely than privately insured to be without a usual source of care. 12.2% of children were unable to get needed medical care, most prevalent unmet needs were dental care (8.1%), prescriptions and eyeglasses (4.1%) and medical care (3.2%). A low percentage of families reported unmet need for mental health care (1.2%).

The 1997 Medical Expenditure Panel Survey was analyzed to examine adolescent health expenditure [20]. Compared with adults health care expenditures for adolescents were low with an average of 799US$ per adolescent in 1997, but disabled and functionally impaired adolescents had an average expenditure of 1,960 US$. When covered by insurance that provided substantial financial protection for families with adolescents, those with public insurance paid 8%, those with private coverage paid 32% and those without paid 61% of their health care bills out of pocket.

Psychosocial and Family Aspects

Chronic illness can have significant psychological and social consequences and present many challenges for both the adolescent, but also for the family involved. A recent study from Australia [21] with in-depth interviews of 35 adolescents with chronic illness revealed five broad themes: control, emotional reactions, acceptance, coping strategies and a search for meaning. They found that many of these young people were relatively resilient in the face of adjustment challenges.

Another study [22] used data from the 1994-1995 NIHS to examine family stressors and psychosocial adjustment. This study included 5,089 children aged 6-17 years with disability and 24,820 without. Children with disabilities were more likely to be male, black and 11-14 years old. These children with disability were more likely to be in poor health, have activity limitattions and functional impairment in self care or mobility, communication and learning. A total of 11.1% of children with disabilities experienced poor psychological adjustment with the most common psychosocial problems being peer relations (16.9%) and hostility (12.6%). Mothers of children with disabilities were more likely to be divorced, separated or never married, lower levels of education and not employed. These mothers also had significantly higer rates of poor health, activity limitations, distress and depression. More than 21% of families with a disabled child experienced a work, sleep and a financial burden with work related burdens being most common (19.3%). Families with a disabled child were also more likely to be under the poverty line.

Table 2. Developmental tasks of adolescence [24]

1	Autonomy or independence from parents and other adults
2	Increasing role of peer relationships
3	Developing a realistic body image
4	Self-identity formation that is realistic, positive and stable
5	Sexual self-identity formation
6	Consolidation of a moral or value system (moral development)
7	Educational and vocational goal development

Promote Better Outcomes

The goals of the physician, family and the adolescent to promote better outcomes are not always the same [23]. The adolescent is interested in the developmental task set out for adolescence (see table 2)[24], whereas the physician and also the family are trying to achieve control (like blood glucose level in diabetes) and prevent or reduce further complications of the chronic illness.

In order to provide better outcomes for adolescents with disability or chronic illness there will be a need to focus on [23]:

1. Building the capacity of the adolescent
   It is very important for the physician and health team responsible for health and treatment of adolescents with disability and chronic illness to understand the developmental tasks of adolescence (see table 2) and the different coping

mechanisms [25]: insightful acceptance (unusual in adolescents), denial (common strategy), regression (common), projection, displacement, acting out, compensation or intellectualization. The adolescent can go through one or many of these and at different times, so it is important that the care giver is aware and act accordingly with insight and wisdom.

2. Building the capacity of the family

Parents often also go through psychological stages when confronted with diagnosis of a chronic illness and the worry about prognosis and survival [23], both when diagnosis is in adolescence or in childhood [26]. The health provider must be aware of the role of the family and both guide the parents through this period, but also provide them with information and a network to support them.

3. Building the capacity in schools

On average adolescents in the 1988 NHIS [10] experienced 3.4 bed days and 4.4 school absence days related to their chronic condition in the year before the interview. It was also estimated that 23% of those with disabling chronic coonditions were limited in their ability or unable to attend school on a longterm basis. The education system must take into account disabled adolescents and find ways to educate them even in case of hospitalization or having to stay home due to disease. Collaboration between the educational system, the health provider and parents is essential.

4. Building peer support programs

The peer group is very important for every adolescent and even more so for the one with chronic illness. Parents, school and health provider must do their utmost to facilitate peer interaction and participation in programs

5. Building suitable community health care

It is important that the adolescent and his family will have access to a permanent health provider (a pediatrician, a specialist in adolescent medicine or a family physician) that understands all the aspects of adolescence, the psychology involved and also the aspects of the specific disease or syndrome causing the chronic disability. This is important for continuity and optimal health care [16].

6. Building suitable in-patient units

Adolescent medicine does not exist as a specialty in every country, every pediatric department or medical center around the globe. Whatever the local situation it is important to build and arrange for suitable space and environment that can cater to the adolescent with chronic illness during hospitalization. This should include possibilities for educational and school programs also during hospitalizations.

7. Building a model for transition to adult care

With adolescence reaching adulthood also comes the responsibility for health care in the adult setting. Adolescents with disability often find this transition especially difficult [23,27,28]. To facilitate this transition the physician in care can help by providing a comprehensive case summary and explain its contents with the adolescent, perform a physical exam with the adolescent as partner, facilitate support groups and networks and continue care for a transition period or be available for both the adolescent and the new health provider.

CONCLUSIONS

More adolescents are found to have chronic illness and some of these will be with life long disability. Several studies, especially in the United States with the National Health Interview Surveys (NHIS), have over time showed an increase in the prevalence of disability among adolescents, focused on issues concerned with insurance, examined health utilization and school absence.

James M Perrin from Harvard Medical school in a review [11] reflected on the need for future research in the area of health service for adolescents with disabilities:

- In clinical and heatk serive epidemiology there is a need for better describtion of the changing numbers of adolescents with disabilities and how their functioning has been affected
- Research on how to minimize the effects of disability on ability to engage in age-appropriate activities
- What makes a good transition to adult health care
- Research on social and structural determinants of new epidemics of chronic conditions and what determines if the condition with bring disability
- Research on what treatment and management that works and the bost benefits
- The role of the family and the role of primary and subspecialty services
- Comprehensive studies of expenditures and utilization of services
- Research on appropriate measures of health status and quality of life

Professor Donald E Greydanus, MD
Pediatrics and Human Development, Michigan State University College of Human Medicine, Kalamazoo, Michigan, United States. E-mail: Greydanus@kcms.msu.edu

Professor Dilip R Patel, MD
Pediatrics and Human Development, Michigan State University College of Human Medicine, Kalamazoo, Michigan, United States. E-mail: patel@kcms.msu.edu

Professor Hatim Omar, MD, FAAP
Adolescent Medicine and Young Parent programs, Department of Pediatrics, Kentucky Children's Hospital, University of Kentucky College of Medicine, Lexington, United States. E-mail: haomar2@uky.edu

Professor Joav Merrick, MD, MMedSci, DMSc
National Institute of Child Health and Human Development, Office of the Medical Director, Division for Mental Retardation, Ministry of Social Affairs, Jerusalem and Kentucky Children's Hospital, University of Kentucky, Lexington, United States. E-Mail: jmerrick@zahav.net.il

REFERENCES

[1] Blum RW. Chronic illness and disability in adolescence. *J. Adolesc. Health.* 1992;13:364-8.
[2] Aron LY, Loprest PJ, Steuerle CE. Serving children with disabilities. *A systematic look at the programs.* Washington, DC: Urban Inst Press, 1996.
[3] Stein RE, Bauman LJ, Westbrook LE, Coupey SM, Ireys HT. Framework for identifying children who have chronic conditions: The case for a new definition. *J. Pediatr.* 1993;122(30:342-7.
[4] Stein RE, Westbrook LE, Bauman LJ. The questionnaire for identifying children with chronic conditions: A measure based on a noncategorical approach. *Pediatrics.* 1997;99(4):513-21.
[5] Stein RE, Silver EJ. Comparing different definitions of chronic conditions in a national data set. *Ambul. Pediatr.* 2002;2(1):63-70.
[6] Merrick J. Prevalence of disabilities in adolescence. *Int. J. Adolesc. Med. Health.* 2000;12(2-3):127-40.
[7] Pless IB, Pinkerton P. Chronic childhood disorder: *promoting patterns of adjustment.* Chicago: Year Book Med Publ., 1975.
[8] Rigby M, Kohler L, eds. Child health indicators of life and development (CHILD): *Report to the European Commission.* Keele, UK: Centre Health Plan Management, European Comm, 2002.
[9] Rigby MJ, Kohler L, Blair ME, Metchler R. Child health indicators for Europe. A priority for a caring society. *Eur. J. Public Health.* 2003;13(3 Suppl):38-46.
[10] Newacheck PW, McManus MA, Fox HB. Prevalence and impact of chronic illness among adolescents. *Am. J. Dis. Child.* 1991;145(12):1367-73.
[11] Perrin JM. Health services research for children with disabilities. *Milbank Quarterly.* 2002;80(2):303-24.
[12] Newacheck PW, Budetti PP, McManus P. Trends in childhood disability. *Am. J. Public Health.* 1984;74(3):232-6.
[13] Newacheck PW, Halfon N. Prevalence and impact of disabling chronic conditions in childhood. *Am. J. Public Health.* 1998;88(4):610-7.
[14] van Dyck PC, McPherson M, Strickland BB, Nesseler K, Blumberg SJ, Cynamon ML. The national survey of children with special health care needs. *Ambul. Pediatr.* 2002;2(1):29-37.
[15] Aburbeh M, Ozeri R, Gordon E, Stein N, Marciano E, Haklai Z, eds. *Health in Israel, 2001 selected data.* Jerusalem: Min. Health, 2001.
[16] Perrin JM. Chronic illness in childhood. In: Behrman RE, Kliegman RM, Jenson HB, eds. *Nelson textbook of pediatrics.* Philadelphia: WB Saunders, 2000:123-5.
[17] Newacheck PW, Stein REK, Bauman L, Hung Y. Disparities in the prevalence of disability between black and while children. *Arch. Pediatr. Adolesc. Med.* 2003;157:244-8.
[18] Newacheck PW, Hung YY, Park MJ, Brindis CD, Irwin CE. Disparities in adolescent health and health care: Does socioeconomic status matter? *Health Ser. Res.* 2003;38(5):1229-33.

[19] Newacheck PW, McManus M, Fox HB, Hung YY, Halfon N. Access to health care for children with special health care needs. *Pediatrics.* 2000;105(4Pt1):760-6.
[20] Newacheck PW, Wong ST, Galbraith AA, Hung YY. Adolescent health care expenditures: A descriptive profile. *J. Adolesc. Health.* 2003;32(6 Suppl):3-11.
[21] Olsson CA, Bond L, Johnson MW, Forer DL, Boyce MF. Adolescent chronic illness: A qialitative study of psychosocial adjustment. *Ann. Acad. Med. Singapore.* 2003:32:43-50.
[22] Witt WP, Riley AW, Coiro MJ. Childhood functional status, family stressors and psychosocial adjustment among school-aged children with disabilities in the United States. *Arch. Pediatr. Adolesc. Med.* 2003;157:687-95.
[23] Yeo M, Sawyer SM. Strategies to promote better outcomes in young people with chronic illnesses. *Ann. Acad. Med. Singapore.* 2003:32:36-42.
[24] Heaven P. Contemporary adolescence: *A social psychological approach.* Melbourne: Macmillan Education, 1994.
[25] Coupey SM, Neinstein LS, Zeltzer LK. Chronic illness in the adolescent. In: Neinstein LS, ed. *Adolescent health care.* A practical guide. Philadelphia: Lippincott Williams & Wilkins, 2002:1511-36.
[26] Kandel I, Merrick J. The birth of a child with disability. Coping by parents and siblings. *Scientific World Journal.* 2003;3(8):741-50.
[27] Blum RW. Introduction. Improving transition for adolescents with special health care needs from pediatric to adult centered care. *Pediatrics.* 2003;110(6Tt2):1301-3.
[28] Merrick J, Kandel I. Adolescents with special needs and the transition from adolescent to adult health care. *Int. J. Adolesc. Med. Health.* 2003;15(20:103.)

PART II. INFECTIOUS DISEASE

Chapter 1

INFECTIONS IN ADOLESCENTS WITH DISABILITIES

Stephen K. Obaro[*]
Department of Pediatrics and Human Development, B240 Life Sciences,
Michigan State University, Lansing, Michigan, United States of America.

ABSTRACT

As a result of advances in medicine, the prevalence of chronic illness or disability in adolescence has increased. This paradox has brought about prolongation of life for children with certain chronic diseases who in the past did not reach adolescence, but over the last decade the survival rate has increased significantly. This paradox has brought with it new challenges for the management of problems in adolescence with lifelong disability. This review discusses infectious disorders often associated with chronic disability in adolescence.

INTRODUCTION

Technical advances over the past few decades have increased significantly, survival for conditions which otherwise would have been fatal in early childhood. Consequently, there are a growing number of children with chronic disease and disability, who reach adolescence. It is in fact estimated that there are now more adolescents with special health care needs than children [1]. These conditions are diverse and include, for example, spina bifida, cerebral palsy, cystic fibrosis, myotonic dystrophy and congenital muscular dystrophy. Although the underlying defects vary in these conditions they are often characteristically associated with a number of infectious complications for various reasons often associated with the fundamental abnormalities in these conditions. These include recurrent episodes of one or more of the

---

[*] *Correspondence:* Stephen K Obaro, MD, FRCPH, PhD, Associate Professor of Pediatrics, Department of Pediatrics and Human Development, B240 Life Sciences, Michigan State University, Lansing MI 48824, United States. E-mail: Stephen.obaro@hc.msu.edu

following; aspiration pneumonia, pneumonia, urinary tract infection and pressure ulcers. All these conditions pose peculiar challenges for the adolescent and managing the complexity of these problems can be more challenging than in any other age groups.

In this chapter the underlying mechanism for these infectious complications and specific approach to management are discussed.

RECURRENT PNEUMONIA

The mechanisms underlying recurrent episodes of pneumonia are diverse in different conditions and may include any or a combination of the following:

- decreased airway sensation
- decreased airway clearance
- poor respiratory effort
- increased viscosity of respiratory secretion

Decrease in sensorium increases the risk of foreign body aspiration resulting in mechanical obstruction or asphyxiation. The cough, gag and swallowing reflexes protect the respiratory tract and conditions in which these protective reflexes are compromised predispose to aspiration as occurs for example when there is loss of consciousness following a prolonged seizure or impaired neuromuscular function.

Aspiration Pneumonia

Aspiration pneumonia results from the aspiration of colonized oropharyngeal or gastric contents, leading to an infectious process. A separate entity caused by aspiration of non-colonized gastric contents leading to chemical pneumonitis is termed aspiration pneumonitis (Mendelson's syndrome). Both diseases are included in the aspiration syndrome; however, they are distinctly different from one another with regards to their predisposing factors and clinical presentation.

Table 1. Bacteria pathogens often implicated in aspiration pneumonia

Gram-negative enteric bacteria	Aerobic Gram-positive	Anerobes
E.coli	Staphylococcus	Bacteroides
Klebsiella	Haemophilus	Prevotella
Serratia	Streptococcus	Fusobacterium
Proteus		Peptostreptococcus
Pseudomonas		

Aspiration pneumonitis is an inflammatory response caused by aspiration of gastric acid but may also occur with aspiration of milk products mineral oils, acids, fat or other fluids, with resulting damage to the bronchial and alveolar wall. The resulting inflammatory response induces a neutrophil response. The inflammatory response results in atelectasis.

There is in addition to this migration of polymorphonuclear cells, alveolar macrophages and alveolar-capillary membrane disruption. In animal models, the risk of pneumonia has been shown to increase following the inflammatory changes associated with aspiration. Oral hygiene is an important risk factor. The aspiration of oropharyngeal secretions, colonized in particular with Gram-negative bacteria, increases the risk of infection [2]. The presence of gastroesophageal reflux contributes to colonization of gastric fluid and increases the risk of aspiration pneumonia. Furthermore, numerous animal studies have suggested that acid aspiration primes the lung for an enhanced inflammatory response to various antigens [3,4].

Patients may be initially asymptomatic or present with acute onset of respiratory distress, fever, bilateral rales and pulmonary infiltrates on radiography. Chest radiography in aspiration pneumonia often shows characteristic but non-specific abnormalities. When solid metallic objects are involved and these are radio opaque, this is quite often obvious on radiography. However, as it is more often the case, aspiration episodes tend to be subtle. Aspiration pneumonia is diagnosed when patients with risk factors for oropharyngeal aspiration develop pneumonia [5].

The most characteristic radiographic finding consists of patchy bilateral airspace consolidation with perihilar of basilar distribution. The anatomy of the right main stem bronchus makes it more susceptible to aspiration. If the respiratory injury is severe, the clinical state can progress rapidly to non-cardiogenic pulmonary edema, hypoxemia and respiratory failure.

Management

Most episodes of aspiration involve aspiration of oral or upper gastrointestinal commensal flora, the alveolar get exposed to aerobic and anerobic bacteria (see table 1).

The antimicrobial commonly used include; ampicillin-sulbactam, piperacillin-tazobactam, clindamycin, metronidazole with a penicillin, imipenem for variable duration depending on the severity of clinical presentation. In addition to the use of antimicrobials, optimal management of the risk factors should involve multidisciplinary consultation with speech pathologist, nutritionist, and Physical therapist.

As a long-term preventive measure in patients with recurrent aspiration pneumonia, different tube feeding methods have been adopted but the benefit of tube feeding to prevent aspiration pneumonia in patients with impaired swallow or cough reflex remains unclear. In a report by Nakajoh and colleagues [6] the incidence of aspiration pneumonia in post-stroke patients who were fed orally showed significantly higher incidence of pneumonia as compared with tube-fed patients. An extensive review of articles in Medline between 1966 and March 1999 on the effects of tube feeding on the outcome of patients with dementia by Finucane and colleagues [7] concluded that tube feeding does not prevent aspiration pneumonia. They and other investigators found no data to support survival benefit with tube feeding [7,8]. Other tube feeding approaches which bypass the pylorus (nasogastric compared with gastrostomy or gastrostomy compared with postpyloric) have also been evaluated and do not seem to significantly impact the incidence of aspiration pneumonia [9,10]. Positional techniques such as upright or semi-recumbent positioning may also be helpful in reducing the risk of aspiration.

Poor respiratory effort or poor airway clearance are associated with increased risk of recurrent pneumonia and these are generally managed as community-acquired pneumonia in addition to supportive care and intensive chest physiotherapy. In special circumstances where oral secretion is copious and swallowing is compromised, anticholinergic agents may be helpful in drying the secretions.

CYSTIC FIBROSIS

Cystic fibrosis (CF) is the commonest, fatal, autosomal recessive disorder in the Caucasian population. It is caused by mutations in the CF transmembrane regulator, an adenosine triphosphate-dependent chloride channel that is expressed primarily in the lung and exocrine glands [11]. About six decades ago, most cases died in childhood, but now up to 80% reach adulthood and the predicted median survival for babies born in the 21st century is now more than 50 years [12]. This condition is characterized by chronic and recurrent pulmonary infections, poor growth secondary to exocrine pancreatic insufficiency and malabsorption. Sinusitis secondary to nasal polyposis and endocrine pancreatic insufficiency also contribute to significant morbidity. Of particular importance in adolescence are the pulmonary complications, which quite often result in end stage lung disease necessitating lung transplant and endocrine pancreatic insufficiency warranting life time insulin therapy.

Table 2. Age related appearance of respiratory pathogens in cystic fibrosis

Patient Age	Pathogens
Early Infancy	Staphyloccus aures
Early Childhood	Haemophilus influenzae
Adolescence	Pseudomonas aeruginosa
Late in Disease	Burkholderia cepacia
	Sternotrophomonas maltophilia
	Achromobacter(Alcaligenes) xyloxidans
	Aspergilus fumigatus

Although much is known about the abnormal physiology of pulmonary secretions in CF, it is not clear why the spectrum of organisms causing pulmonary infection vary by age [13,14]. The spectrum of pathogens by age is summarized in table 2. The basic pathophysiologic mechanisms responsible for promoting colonization by P.aeruginosa remain unclear. However, this association has been known to promote recurrent exacerbations of pulmonary infection and the main stay of management remains aggressive pulmonary toileting and short courses of antibiotics.

Daily treatment with human recombinant DNAse (rhDNase) reduces the number of pulmonary exacerbations, improves pulmonary function, is tolerated well and is safe in mild, moderate and severe CF cases [15,16].

There are a number of factors which make the management of CF a major clinical challenge in adolescents. Several problems are inherent in the selection and use of antibiotics in adolescent CF patients, because of repeated exposure to different class of antibiotics in early life; in adolescence most patients already harbor strains of bacteria that are resistance to multiple antibiotics. Chronic inflammation in the lungs and localization of infection in the airway lumen poses a challenge for achieving adequate antibiotic levels at the site of inflammation. The pharmacokinetics of the antibiotics is also a confounder since the clearance of many drugs is higher in these patients and they would generally require modification of drug dosing [17]. In addition, since bacterial pathogens are almost never completely eradicated, defining a bacteriologic end point for treatment is a challenge.

Recurrent Urinary Tract Infection

The primary predisposing factor to recurrent urinary tract infection in adolescents with chronic illness is secondary to inability to empty the bladder physiologically. This defect is often secondary to loss of bladder sensation or loss of sphincter control. In children with spina bifida there is a prevalence of about 60% with lack of bladder sphincter control and 80% have neurogenic bladder [18,19] and this condition seem to apply regardless of the level of spinal lesion or extent of paralysis.

The loss of bladder innervation or sphincter control often results in lack of co-ordination between relaxation of the urethral sphincter and contraction of the detrussor muscle of the bladder and this result in dysfunctional voiding. Dysfunctional voiding is the main risk factor for developing UTI although it could also occasionally be a complication of UTI.

The failure of the sphincter to relax causes an obstruction to the outflow of urine with consequent increase in intravesical pressure, bladder distention and often with residual urine in the bladder after voiding attempts.

Constipation is often associated with this condition as a result of the inability to relax the pelvic floor musculature. Constipation may result primarily from other causes associated with chronic illness, but has been know to interfere with urodynamics. The distended rectum in constipated children presses on the bladder wall and produces an outflow obstruction [20].

Another factor which is known to predispose to recurrent infection is catheterization, particularly in the hospital setting. In adult patients, bacteriuria develops in at least 10-15% of hospitalized patients with indwelling urethral catheter [21]. These infections are typically caused by multi drug resistant strains of E. coli, Klebsiella, Pseudomonas, Proteus and Serratia. While seldom associated with bacteremia, these episodes can result in gram negative sepsis.

Pressure Ulcers

Despite the advances of the twenty first century and our ability to provide treatment for immediately fatal conditions in previous times, the recent demise of Christopher Reeve [22], a famous actor after being salvaged from a C2 cervical injury from an infected pressure ulcer drives home the importance of this condition [23].

Often referred to as bedsore among English-speaking people, this condition has been variously referred to as decubitus ulcers or pressures sores. The connotation inferred by decubitus ulcers implies that these lesions are acquired from lying down in the "decubitus position" however, since this is not always the case, a more accurate terminology would be pressure ulcers. Paraplegic adolescents who spend long hours in their wheel chairs are clearly prone to pressure ulcers over the Ischia and other prominences [24].

These lesions are initiated by insidious physical trauma in soft tissues and have traditionally been associated with prolonged bed rest on ordinary mattresses with a consequent tissue pressure over bony prominence. The resulting tissue damage may extend from the epidermis through the underlying tissue, through to the bone and may be infected by different bacterial agents with the degree of infection varying from cellulitis to osteomyelitis or septicemia. When infected, these pressure ulcers may be associated with offensive odor and discharge.

The clinical appearance should be differentiated from a number of other conditions such as friction rub, arterial ulcers and ulcers associated with drug ingestion [25] or thermal injury.

These ulcers often are colonized by multiple bacteria frequently including, E.coli, S.aureus, Serratia, Klebsiella and bacteroides and it is often difficult to establish which of these agents are primarily causing infection versus colonizers. While some of these bacteria may originate from urine or feces contaminating the perineum, seeding of the necrotic tissue from another source of primary bacteremia is also possible.

Management

The approach to the management of pressure ulcers is often multidisciplinary and should involve Infectious Disease Specialists, Physical therapists and surgeons. Extensive tissue necrosis may require debridement to restore tissue vitalization and frequent repositioning to optimize healing. Detailed attention to wound care is crucial in ensuring healing. Septicemia is the most dreaded complication from infected pressure ulcers and may be the initial presenting problem in patients who may have ulcers that have not been previously identified. Selection of appropriate antimicrobial agents in such circumstance can be challenging, since prolonged use can be associated with multidrug resistant organisms and should involve infectious disease specialists. Whether treatment should be directed at selected bacterial isolated from the wound or at all pathogens isolated remains controversial [26] from the lesions and also from the blood stream when accompanied by bacteremia.

The use of maggots [27] and hyperbaric oxygen [28] has been proposed for management of pressure ulcers, but the effectiveness remains controversial.

CONCLUSIONS

The adolescent period remains a very challenging phase of development for the young adult who is transitioning from childhood into adulthood and this period is even more daunting for those who have to go through it with the additional challenge of a disability. However, technological developments in medicine have continued to provide new facilities for not just the prolongation of life but life with improved quality for several previously fatal conditions. Infectious complications in this population will continue to be a challenge, since they tend to be recurrent and repeated exposure to antibiotics increases the risk for multidrug resistance.

REFERENCES

[1] US Department of Health and Human Services, Health Resources and Services Administration, Maternal and Child Health Bureau. The National Survey of Children with Special Health Care Needs Chartbook 2001. Rockville, Md: *U.S. Dept. Health Hum. Serv.* 2004.

[2] Yamaya M, Yanai m, et al. Interventions to prevent pneumonia among older adults. *J. Am. Geriatr. Soc.* 2001;49(1):85-90.

[3] Mitsushima H, Oishi k, et al. Acid aspiration induces bacterial pneumonia by enhanced bacterial adherence in mice. *Microb. Pathog.* 2002;33(5):203-10.

[4] Rotta AT, Shiley KT, et al. Gastric acid and particulate aspiration injury inhibits pulmonary bacterial clearance." *Crit. Care Med.* 2004;32(3):747-54.

[5] Marik PE. Aspiration pneumonitis and aspiration pneumonia. *N. Engl. J. Med.* 2001;344(9):665-71.

[6] Nakajoh K, Nakagawa T, et al. Relation between incidence of pneumonia and protective reflexes in post-stroke patients with oral or tube feeding. *J. Intern. Med.* 2000;247(1):39-42.

[7] Finucane TE, Christmas C, et al. Tube feeding in patients with advanced dementia: a review of the evidence. *JAMA.* 1999;282(14): 1365-70.

[8] Mitchell SL, Kiely DK, et al. The risk factors and impact on survival of feeding tube placement in nursing home residents with severe cognitive impairment. *Arch. Intern. Med.* 1997;157(3): 327-32.

[9] Strong RM, Condon SC, et al. Equal aspiration rates from postpylorus and intragastric-placed small-bore nasoenteric feeding tubes: a randomized, prospective study. *JPEN J. Parenter Enteral. Nutr.* 1992;16(1):59-63.

[10] Ukleja A, Sanchez-Fermin M. Gastric versus post-pyloric feeding: relationship to tolerance, pneumonia risk, and successful delivery of enteral nutrition. *Curr. Gastroenterol. Rep.* 2007;9(4):309-16.

[11] Rommens JM, Iannuzzi MC, et al. Identification of the cystic fibrosis gene: chromosome walking and jumping. *Science.* 1989;245(4922):1059-65.

[12] Dodge JA, Lewis PA, et al. Cystic fibrosis mortality and survival in the UK: 1947-2003." *Eur. Respir. J.* 2007;29(3):522-6.

[13] Gilligan PH. Microbiology of airway disease in patients with cystic fibrosis. *Clin. Microbiol. Rev.* 1991;4(1):35-51.

[14] Rosenfeld M, Gibson RL, et al. Early pulmonary infection, inflammation, and clinical outcomes in infants with cystic fibrosis." *Pediatr. Pulmonol.* 2001;32(5):356-66.

[15] Quan JM, Tiddens HA, et al. A two-year randomized, placebo-controlled trial of dornase alfa in young patients with cystic fibrosis with mild lung function abnormalities. *J. Pediatr.* 2001;139(6):813-20.

[16] Hodson ME, McKenzie S, et al. Dornase alfa in the treatment of cystic fibrosis in Europe: a report from the Epidemiologic Registry of Cystic Fibrosis. *Pediatr. Pulmonol.* 2003;36(5):427-32.

[17] de Groot R, Smith AL. Antibiotic pharmacokinetics in cystic fibrosis. Differences and clinical significance. *Clin. Pharmacokinet.* 1987;13(4):228-53.

[18] Chauvel P. Spina bifida and hydrocephalus. In: Capute AJ, Acardo PJ eds. *Developmental disabilities in infancy and childhood.* Baltimore, MD: Paul H Brookes, 1991:383-93.

[19] Charney EB. Neural tube defects: Spina bifida and myelomenigocoele. In: Batshaw M, Perret Y, eds. *Children with disabilities: a medical primer.* Baltimore, MD: Paul H Brookes, 1993.

[20] Yazbeck S, Schick E, et al. Relevance of constipation to enuresis, urinary tract infection and reflux. *A review. Eur. Urol.* 1987;13(5): 318-21.

[21] Stamm WE. Catheter-associated urinary tract infections: epidemiology, pathogenesis, and prevention. *Am. J. Med.* 1991;91(3B):65S-71S.

[22] Christopher Reeve: Actor who made the perfect Superman. *Independent.* 12 Oct 2004:38

[23] Parish LC, Lowthian PT, et al. The infected decubitus ulcer: Superman's kryptonite. *Skinmed.* 2005;4(1):7-8.

[24] Garber SL, Krouskop TA. Wheelchair cushion modification and its effect on pressure. *Arch. Phys. Med. Rehabil.* 1984;65(10):579-83.

[25] Renwick AA, Chong DS, et al. Chronic non-healing anal ulceration and Nicorandil: further evidence of an emerging problem. *ANZ J. Surg.* 2004;74(12):1128-9.

[26] Stotts NA, Hunt TK. Pressure ulcers. Managing bacterial colonization and infection. *Clin. Geriatr. Med.* 1997;13(3):565-73.

[27] Sherman RA. Maggot versus conservative debridement therapy for the treatment of pressure ulcers. *Wound Repair Regen.* 2002;10(4): 208-14.

[28] Frantz RA. Adjuvant therapy for ulcer care. *Clin. Geriatr. Med.* 1997;13(3):553-64.

PART III. NEOPLASMS

Chapter 2

ADOLESCENTS WITH CANCER

Renuka Gera[*], Elna N. Saah,
Ajovi B. Scott-Emuakpor and Roshni Kulkarni*

Division of Pediatric and Adolescent Hematology/Oncology,
Pediatric and Adolescent Sickle Cell Program,
MSU Center for Bleeding and Clotting Disorders,
Department of Pediatrics/Human Development,
Michigan State University, East Lansing,
Michigan, United States of America.

ABSTRACT

Survival in adolescents and children with cancer has improved due to advances in medical treatment and ironically increased the number of adolescent survivors of cancer, who have disabilities resulting from their treatment. Long-term cancer survivorship for most cancers is defined as continuous remission at five years from diagnosis. Despite the low risk of relapse beyond five years, cancer continues to remain a major cause of mortality and morbidity in children and adolescents. In addition to a constant threat of relapse, long-term cancer survivors suffer from disabling late complications. Adolescents and children with cancer fall into this category. Although the literature evaluating the impact of cancer on the growth and development of adolescents is plentiful, the magnitude of impairment and disability caused by cancer has not been completely realized. This discussion considers some of these disabilities.

INTRODUCTION

Advances in medical treatment have resulted in improved survival in adolescents with cancer. Long-term cancer survivorship for most cancer is defined as continuous remission at

---

[*] Correspondence: Renuka Gera, MD, Professor and Associate Chair, Department of Pediatrics/Human Development, Division of Pediatric and Adolescent Hematology/Oncology, Michigan State University, B220

five years from diagnosis. Despite the low risk of relapse beyond five years, cancer continues to remain a major cause of mortality and morbidity in children and adolescents. In addition to a constant threat of relapse, long-term cancer survivors suffer from disabling late complications. Perrin [1] described disability as inability to perform age-appro-priate daily activities, whereas chronic conditions are health conditions that at the time of diagnosis are predicted to last longer than three months. Adolescents and children with cancer meet both criteria. Therefore, cancer may be considered as a chronic illness with a potential to cause disability in adolescents and children. Although the literature evaluating the impact of cancer on the growth and development of adolescents is plentiful, the magnitude of impairment and disability caused by cancer has not been completely realized.

The incidence of cancer in adolescents is higher and rising more rapidly than in children. The incidence of cancer in adolescents and young adults ages 15-29 in the United States (US) is 2.7 times higher than in children younger than 14 years [2]. The incidence of cancer in adolescents 15-19 years worldwide ranged from 95 to 255 per million person years. The highest rates were in Australia and among Jews in Israel, and the lowest in India and Japan [3]. The most common tumors in this age group are lymphomas (22%), sarcomas (16%), leukemia (12%), brain tumors (9%), testicular cancer (9%), female genital tumors (7%), thyroid cancer (8%), and melanoma (7%) [3]. Lymphomas are the most frequent cancers in Western industrialized countries of the northern hemisphere and in the Middle East, and occur in substantial numbers in all other regions. Most cancers in this age group are curable. The survival results from European and American data show that the 5-year overall survival among adolescents with cancer is approximately 73% to 78% [4]. This extraordinary improvement in survival ironically increases the number of adolescents and young adults with disabilities because survivors of pediatric and adolescent cancer are at much higher risk for complications when compared with their normal peers [5].

Cancer and therapeutic interventions may cause such patients to be more vulnerable to long-term physical, emotional, and social problems. Most cancers in this age group are treated with chemotherapy. Patients with solid tumors also undergo surgical resections and radiation. Side effects such as nausea, vomiting, infection, pain, and bleeding are common during treatment, causing the temporary disruption of normal activities, such as attending school, being with friends, and participation in sports events. This social isolation may cause depression in vulnerable patients. Most of these symptoms resolve after the treatment is completed and may not cause a long-term disability. However, some disabling side effects and toxicity that are due to radiation and chemotherapy may manifest years later. Understanding the delayed complications of cancer therapy and its impact on the quality of life has just begun to unfold, and the full magnitude of the disability caused by cancer and its treatment has yet to be appreciated.

Although it is encouraging that treatments are constantly being modified to attain cure with minimum toxicity, in the interim, there continues to be a large at-risk population of survivors who need care and support. Studies estimate that two-thirds of survivors have at least one chronic or late-occurring complication of their cancer therapy with one-third having serious or life threatening complications [6]. Preadolescent children who complete treatment in early childhood would remain at risk for treatment related problems in adolescence. This

---

Clinical Center, 138 Service Road, East Lansing, MI 48824-1313 United States. Tel: 517-355-5082; Fax: 517-355-8312; E-mail: Renuka.Gera@hc.msu.edu

morbidity may cause significant disruptions and could affect an adolescent's ability to conduct a normal life and to pursue his/her life goals. These challenges must be considered in the context of patient's age and stage of development. The knowledge of impairments and disability and its affect on age-appropriate activity, mobility, self-care, communication, cognition, and psychosocial function is imperative for the rehabilitation of this patient population.

This chapter provides an overview of the disability issues faced by adolescent survivors of cancer. For the reasons stated above, we have included all survivors of childhood and adolescent cancer. Knowledge and awareness of the potential problems and early diagnosis with timely interventions will facilitate independent function by minimizing impairment and maximizing participation in age- and development-appropriate physical, educational, vocational, and recreational activities. Cancer-related impairments and disability have been organized in four broad categories in this chapter:

1   Intellectual and cognitive impairment and disability
2   Psychosocial and emotional impairment and disability
3   Musculoskeletal problems resulting in impaired mobility
4   Major organ dysfunction

Intellectual and Cognitive Impairment and Disability

Intellectual decline and impairment in cognition either can result from direct insult to the brain caused by the malignant process or can occur as a result of therapeutic interventions for remote cancer. Primary brain tumors, head and neck tumors, and leukemia can affect higher brain function. Therapeutic interventions used for the treatment of these cancers include surgery and cranial or craniospinal radiation for brain tumors, and chemo-therapy, including intrathecal methotrexate and cytosine arabinoside, for the treatment of presymptomatic central nervous system (CNS) leukemia. The treatment of CNS leukemia and patients at high risk for relapse includes cranial radiation. Total-body radiation is an integral part of many bone marrow transplant regimens. These thera-peutic modalities can cause acute or delayed CNS toxicity, with the potential to affect normal intellectual and cognitive development. Cranial irradiation, intrathecal methotrexate, and high dose intravenous methotrexate have been associated with leukoencephalopathy as well as learning disabilities.

Cognitive functioning and the educational achieve-ments of cancer survivors have been extensively studied. Deficits have been found in various domains, including intelligence, learning and memory, attention, cognitive speed, academic achievement, and executive as well as visual-motor functioning. Kingma et al [7] evaluated 94 acute lymphoblastic leukemia (ALL) survivors at age 20 years, compared their academic performance with 134 of their siblings, and found that significantly more patients than siblings were placed in special educational programs. A significant difference was found for the level of secondary education. No effect of gender or irradiation dose was found, but younger age at diagnosis was significantly related to both referrals and school levels. Another study evaluated scholastic achievements of childhood ALL survivors by evaluating their school records [8]. At the time of diagnosis, 371 ALL survivors were younger than 16 years and in the ninth grade at the time of this study. Their performance was compared with five age-matched controls. The ALL survivors who received irradiation as part of their treatment had lower overall mark averages in all assessed school subjects compared with their controls [8]. Of the patients treated with chemotherapy alone, the females diagnosed before age 7 years had lower scores than their controls.

The use of special educational services and attainment of educational goal was retrospectively studied in the Childhood Cancer Survivor Study (CCSS) [9]. The CCSS is a cohort of cancer survivors who were diagnosed with a cancer in childhood and were alive and free of cancer at least five years post diagnosis and their healthy siblings. This study determined the use of special education services and attainment of educational goals of 12,430 childhood cancer survivors and compared them with their 3,410 full siblings. The study found that 23% survivors used the special education services, whereas only 8% of siblings used these services [9]. The differences were greatest in survivors who were younger than six years of age at the time of diagnosis. The reason for the use of special education was prolonged school absenteeism in children and adolescents with bone tumors and sarcoma. Problems with concentration, learning disability, and poor test scores were reasons for the use of special education services by patients treated with cranial radiation, either alone or in conjunction with chemotherapy. Survivors of leukemia, brain tumors, non-Hodgkin lymphoma, and neuroblastoma in this cohort were significantly less likely than their siblings to finish high school. Paulino et al. [10] reported intellectual and academic delays in 3/17 long-term survivors of head and neck sarcomas. Intellectual decline is more profound in patients with brain tumors. Cognitive impairment is most common with hemispheric and supratentorial midline tumors.

Both cognitive and motor impairment are associated with failure in securing and retaining employment. The CCSS study also evaluated the employment status of cancer survivors and reported that a significant number of survivors (5.5%) in this cohort reported unemploy-ment compared with 1.2% of their siblings [11]. Subtle deficits in intellectual and cognition may be difficult to diagnose and may need a thorough neuro-psychological evaluation. Neuropsychological testing therefore should be part of the evaluation of all patients with brain tumors and should be performed on cancer survivors who receive cranial radiation or CNS-directed therapies at an early age. The early diagnosis of deficit and the institution of appropriate educational interventions would maximize the chances of developing life skills. As they transition to adulthood, adolescents with cognitive and intellectual problems would benefit from vocational rehabilitation counseling.

Psychosocial and Emotional Impairment and Disability

Adolescence is the time of transition from childhood to adulthood, with important physical and emotional changes as well as challenges. This period can be the time of turmoil without any physical illness. A diagnosis of cancer during this time has a major impact on physical and psychological development [12]. The diagnosis of cancer affects an adolescent's pursuit of autonomy and independence while placing them at risk for psychosocial and emotional difficulties later on in life. Several studies have addressed survival-related concerns in this patient population. Elisabeth Maunsell et al [13] studied the effects of childhood and adolescent cancer on the quality of life in 1,334 adolescent and adult survivors and 1,477 age-matched controls.

The study subjects responded to a questionnaire that included the Short Form-36 (SF-36) and measures of self-esteem, optimism, and life satisfaction. Very few survivors compared with control subjects reported very good or excellent health. The survivors of CNS or bone tumors, the adolescents receiving more than one treatment series, or those having two or more organ dysfunction, reported poor physical quality of life. The survivors with two or more organ dysfunction reported poorer quality of life in both physical and psychological domains.

The psychological literature suggests that stress plays a role in risk behavior initiation and maintenance, including multiple behavioral risks. Psychosocial maladjustment of the survivors may lead to behaviors that could further jeopardize their physical health. To understand the adolescent survivors' attitude, 58 adolescents who participated in the Survivor Health and Resilience program were asked to complete a multiple risk behavior survey [14]. The survey addressed behaviors like cigarette smoking, insufficient physical activity, and non-adherence to exercise program. Of the participants, 28% reported at least one of the three risk behaviors, 12% reported two, and 7% reported all three risk behaviors. Older age and greater stress were associated with more health risk behaviors. The behavioral and social outcomes of adolescent cancer survivors [15] were evaluated in 2,979 adolescent cancer survivors and 649 siblings. The authors, using a parental report survey, evaluated difficulty in six behavioral and social domains of depression/anxiety, headstrong, attention deficit, peer conflict/social with-drawal, antisocial behaviors, and social competence. The mean ages of survivors and their siblings were 14.8 and 14.9 years of age. The survivors were 1.5 times more likely than siblings to have symptoms of anxiety and depression and were 1.7 times more likely to have antisocial behaviors. Psychosocial problems are prevalent in adolescent and young cancer survivors. Knowledge of the psychological risk factors and an appreciation of cancer survivor's attitudes may help in developing effective interventions.

Musculoskeletal Problems Resulting in Impaired Mobility

Mobility and musculoskeletal problems can be a direct consequence of cancer or its treatment. Sarcomas are the most common malignancy involving the musculo-skeletal system, and treatment involves wide excision and/or amputations. Although most surgical procedures currently used aim to preserve musculoskeletal function, such patients are often left with some impairment and disability. Amputation followed by prosthesis results in better mobility, and these adolescents may be able to participate in athletic activity. However, this modality is associated with higher emotional stress, is chosen by fewer patients, and is done only when because of anatomical location limb salvage is not an option.

Limb salvage procedures are more acceptable to adolescents [16]. Limb salvage procedures can be divided in two broad categories, orthodesis, and orthoplasty. Orthodesis involves using either an allograft or a vascular autograft. This type of procedure provides a durable stable reconstruction resistant to physical stress and activity and requires minimal follow-up [17]. The disadvantage of this procedure is loss of joint function with some limitation of activity. Orthoplasty preserves the joint function and may be done using an allograft or a metallic prosthesis. The complications associated with limb salvage procedures include nonunion, fractures, joint instability, higher infection rates, and inability to participate in athletic activities. Revision free survival rate of the prosthesis is 15% to 72%. A large number of patients will experience some loss of range of movement (ROM). Factors associated with decreased range of movement include lower-extremity or truncal lesions. Women with decreased ROM and strength are likely to have slow walk velocity, low exercise tolerance, and high risk for functional loss [18]. After many revisions, some patients may end up with an amputation.

Adolescents with tumors of the CNS, including both spinal cord and brain, can also experience loss of limb function and mobility. Although deficits resulting from tumor and surgery in these patients are apparent immediately, radiation-related damage may not manifest for years. Loss of function is usually permanent and the patients need assistance for the rest of their lives. Radiation and chemotherapy associated musculoskeletal impairment and disability may occur in patients with a variety of other cancers. Temporary and permanent impairments and disabilities caused by these therapeutic modalities are listed in Tables 1 and 2.

Table 1. Reversible/transient disability

Treatment	Mechanism	Symptoms	Disability
Corticosteroid	Preferential atrophy of type II muscle fibers	a. Myopathy b. Osteoporosis	a. Decreased mobility b. risk of fractures
Cyclophosphamide		Reversible neurotoxicity, lethargy, somnolence, disorientation, hallucination	Unable to perform age appropriate ADLs (activities of daily living)
Vincristine/vinblastine	Axonal sensorimotor polyneuropathy	Paresthesia, pain, weakness, foot drop, poor fine motor function	Need assistance with ADL (activities of daily living)

Table 2. Irreversible/permanent disability

Treatment	Mechanism	Symptom	Disability
Cranial radiation	Ischemic events	Functional deficit, decreased cognition	Stroke-like
Spinal irradiation	Irradiation myelitis	Spastic paraplegia or quadriplegia	Functional impairment in mobility and ADLs (activities of daily living) dependence dependent on extent of injury
Methotrexate	Neurotoxicity, leukoencephalopathy	Cognitive impairment, deficits in coordination and high level skills	School performance, age appropriate ADLs (activities of daily living), athletic activity, social competence May also result in loss of motor function
Cisplatinum	Injury to hair cells of organ of Corti	High frequency sensorineural hearing loss	Affects communication and social competence
Corticosteroid	Avascular necrosis of the joints, osteonecrosis	Chronic pain, deformity	Affects mobility, participation in athletic activities

Major Organ Dysfunction

Curative therapy for cancer also affects all growing and developing tissues. Because of this exposure, adolescents and children are at risk for developing major organ dysfunction. The toxicity often is dose-dependent and does not manifest immediately. Patients cured of cancer seek healthcare outside of oncology offices in variety of healthcare settings. The term risk-based health care refers to a conceptualization of lifelong health care that integrates cancer and survivor-ship experience in overall health care needs of an individual [19]. The knowledge of risk for organ dysfunction caused by cancer and its treatment is necessary to provide risk-based care. The risk of morbidity and mortality caused by cancer therapy is further modified by a survivor's genetics, life style, and other co-morbid conditions. Important organ dysfunction and offending agents are listed in table 3.

Table 3. Major organ toxicity and offending agent

Organ System involved	Therapeutic exposure
Growth hormone deficiency	Cranial radiation
Obesity	Cranial radiation
Pulmonary fibrosis	Chest radiation, Bleomycin, Carmustine, Busulfan
Cardiomyopathy and congestive heart failure	Anthracyclines
Myocardial infarction	Chest radiation
Renal Failure	Cisplatinum, carboplatinum
Osteopenia/ osteoporosis	Corticosteroid, gonadal radiation, craniospinal radiation
Dental abnormalities	Cranial, head and neck radiation
Cataract	Steroids, radiation
Hearing Loss	Cisplatinum/carboplatinum
Second malignancy (skin cancer, brain tumors, thyroid cancer, bone tumors)	Radiation to the organ of origin of the cancer
Myelodysplastic syndromes/leukemia	Alkylating agents, topoisomerase II inhibitors.

Survivors with pulmonary or cardiac toxicity would experience decreased exercise tolerance and may not be able to participate in vocations that require weight lifting and strenuous physical activity. Cisplatinum can cause high frequency hearing loss; symptomatic high frequency hearing loss was detected in 20% of the survivors of testicular cancer treated with cisplatinum [20]. At cumulative dose of 400mg/m2, hearing loss at lower frequency was seen in a significant number of patients. Hearing loss is more profound in children treated with cisplatinum at younger age [21]. Further studies are needed to evaluate the impact of hearing loss on patients' quality of life and employment.

Exposure to antineoplastic agents such as a high dose of cyclophosphamide or ifosfamide, or pelvic or brain radiation can result in decreased gonadal function and fertility. Male or female fertility can be temporarily or permanently compromised in patients with cancer. In female patients, the infertility may manifest as premature menopause. Gonadal dysfunction can affect an adolescent's self esteem and may put them at risk for psychosocial and emotional problems in life. Assisted reproductive procedures like the cryopreservation of gametes, embryo, or gonadal tissue fall into an experi-mental category and can only be done as part of an IRB-approved trial. It has been suggested that the consent for such procedures be done in two stages. The initial procedure, in addition to parental consent, would require either the patient's assent or consent. The decision about how to use the preserved tissue would be made by the patient at a later date [22].

CONCLUSIONS

Adolescents and children with cancer have an excellent chance of cure and long-term survival. Aggressive therapy to cure the cancer causes significant acute toxicity that interferes with normal age-related activities, such as school attendance, participation in athletic activities, and socialization. Unfortunately, many adolescents will experience some delayed toxicity many years after completing their treatment. Although the magnitude of these problems and the impact on normal physical, cognitive, and psychosocial functioning of adolescents have become apparent, the extent of the disability caused by cancer diagnosis in this population is not very clear. Studies conducted to understand delayed complications have evaluated specific aspects of function and have relied on parent or patient reports. As a result, the evaluation of impairment and disability is neither complete nor objective. Performance status scores using scales like the Karnofsky score, the Lansky score, and the Zubrod score are used to quantify patients' general well being before cancer treatment is started. Performance status is a good measure of the patients' functional abilities and is used for evaluating patients with other chronic illnesses. The evaluation of performance status of survivors may provide better appreciation of the impairment and disability caused by the diagnosis and treatment of cancer in adolescents.

REFERENCES

[1] Perrin JM. Health services research for children with disabilities. *Millbank Q.* 2002;80(2):303-24.
[2] Bleyer A, O'Leary M, Barr R, Ries LAG, eds. Cancer epidemiology in older adolescents and young adults 15 to 29 years of age, including SEER incidence and survival: 1975-2000. Bathesda, MD: *Nat. Cancer Inst,* NIH Pub 06-5767, 2006.
[3] Stiller CA. International pattern of cancer incidence in adolescents: *Cancer Treat. Rev.* 2007; 33:631-45.
[4] Desandes E. Survival from adolescent cancer. *Cancer Treat. Rev.* 2007;33:609-15.
[5] Pentheroudakis E, Pavlidis N. Juvenile Cancer: improving care for adolescent and young adults within the frame of medical oncology. *Ann. Oncol.* 2005;16(2):181-8
[6] Albritton K, Bleyer WA. The management of cancer in older adolescent. *Eur. J. cancer.* 2003;39: 2584-99.
[7] Kigma A, Rammeloo AJ,Does-van den Berg, Rekers-Mombarg L, Pstma A. Academic career after treatment for acute lymphoblastic leukemia. *Arch. Dis. Child.* 2000;82:353-7.
[8] Harila-Saari AH, Lähteenmäki PM, Pukkala E, Kyyrönen P, Lanning M, Sankila R. Scholastic achievements of childhood leukemia patients: a nationwide register-based study. *JCO.* 2007;25:3518–24.

[9] Robinson LL, Whitton JA, Zevon MA, Gibbs IC, Tersak JM, Meadows, et al. Utilization of special education services and special education attainment among long-term survivors of childhood cancer: A report from childhood cancer survivor study. *Cancer.* 2003;97:1115-26.

[10] Paulino AC, Simon JH, Zhen W, Wen BC. Long-term effects in children treated with radiotherapy for head and neck rhabdomyosarcoma. *Int. J. Radiat. Oncol. Biol. Phys.* 2000;48(5):1489-95.

[11] Pang JW, Friedman DL, Whitton JA, Stovall M, Mertens AC, Robinson LL, et al. Employment status among adult survivors in Childhood Cancer Survivor Study. *Pediatr. Blood Cancer.* 2008; 50(1): 104-10.

[12] Abrams AN, Hazen EP, Penson RT. Psychosocial issues in adolescent with cancer. *Cancer Treat. Rev.* 2007;33:622-30.

[13] Maunsell E, Maru P, Barrera A, Speechley KN. Quality of life among adolescent and adult Sur-vivors of childhood cancer. *JCO.* 2006;24:2527-35.

[14] Tercyak KP, Donze JR, Prahlad S. Mosher RB, Shad AT. Multiple behavioral risk factors among adolescent survivors of childhood cancer in the Survivor Health and Resilience Education (SHARE) program. *Pediatric Blood Cancer.* 2006;47(6):825-30.

[15] Schultz KA, Ness KK, Whitton J, Reklitis C, Zebrack B, Robinson LL, et al. Behavioral and social outcomes in adolescent survivors of child-hood cancer: a report from the childhood cancer survivor study. *J. Clin. Oncol.* 2007; 25(24):3649-56.

[16] Ginsberg JP, Rai SN, Carlson CA, Meadows AT, Hinds PS, Spearing EM, et al. A comparative analysis of functional outcomes in adolescents and young adults with lower extremity bone sarcoma. *Pediatr. Blood Cancer.* 2007;49(7):964-9.

[17] Marulanda GA, Henderson ER, Johnson DA, Leston D, Cheong D. Orthopedic surgery options for treatment of primary osteosarcoma. *Cancer Control.* 2008; 15(1):13-9.

[18] Gerber LH, Hoffman K, Chaudhry U, Augustine E, Parks R, et al. Functional outcomes and life satisfaction in long-term survivors of pediatric sarcomas. *Arch. Phys. Rehabil.* 2006;87(12):1611-7.

[19] Oeffinger OC, Hudson MM. Long-term compli-cations following childhood and adolescent cancer: Foundation for providing Risk-based Health Care for Survivors. *CA Cancer J. Clin.* 2004;54:208-36.

[20] Biro K, Noszek L, Prekopp P, Nagyivanyi K, Geczi L, Gaudi I, Bodrogi I. Characteristics and risk factors of cisplatin-induced ototoxicity in testicular cancer patients detected by distortion product otoacoustic emission. *Oncology.* 2006;70(3):177-84.

[21] Bertolini P, Lassalle M, Mercier G, Raguin MA, Izzi G, Corradini N, et al. Platinum compound-related ototoxicity in children: long-term follow-up reveals continuous worsening of hearing loss. *J. Pediatr. Hematol. Oncol.* 2004;26(10):649-55.

[22] Lee SJ, Schover LR, Partridge AH, Patrizio P, Hamish Wallace W, et al. American Society of Clinical Oncology recommendations on fertility preservation. *J. Clin. Oncol.* 2006;24(18):2917-31.

Part IV. Endocrine, Nutritional and Metabolic Diseases

In: Adolescence and Chronic Illness
Editors: H. Omar et al.

ISBN: 978-1-60876-628-4
© 2010 Nova Science Publishers, Inc.

Chapter 3

ENDOCRINE ASPECTS OF CHRONIC DISEASE

Manmohan K. Kamboj[*]
Pediatric Endocrinology, Michigan State University,
Kalamazoo Center for Medical Studies, Kalamazoo,
Michigan, United States of America.

ABSTRACT

Endocrine problems are commonly seen in adolescents with chronic illness and disabilities. These problems may be due to the interference of normal endocrine function, either by the underlying pathology itself or because of the treatment modalities used. Therefore, it is of the utmost importance that a high index of suspicion for the development of these deficits be maintained in such patients. Growth and development should be very closely monitored for assuring early diagnosis and for the early initiation of adequate therapeutic measures to minimize further morbidity and mortality.

INTRODUCTION

Endocrine dysfunction commonly coexists in children and adolescents with severe illness. This co-existence has two perspectives. First, a primary non-endocrine chronic illness or disability can secondarily result in the compromise of a specific endocrine function, causing additional compromise or disability. On the contrary, a primary endocrine disorder may result in acute or chronic disability. Severe illnesses whether acute or chronic can cause abnormalities of endocrine function [1].

The new era of ever-advancing medical therapeutics has resulted in increasing cure rates for previously life-threatening medical conditions. In addition to increasing longevity, a higher incidence of side-effects including endocrine dysfunction is noted. Therefore, it is of the utmost importance that a high index of suspicion be maintained during long term medical

---

[*] *Correspondence:* Manmohan K. Kamboj, MD, Pediatric Endocrinology, Michigan State University, Kalamazoo Center for Medical Studies, 1000 Oakland Drive, Kalamazoo, MI 49008 United States of America. Tel: (269) 337-6450; Fax: (269) 337-6474; E-mail: kamboj@kcms.msu.edu

follow-up of these patients so that early diagnosis and treatment be initiated to minimize disability.

Endocrine dysfunction can be caused by one of many ways that can include the direct impediment of normal function caused by the underlying lesion, lack of adequate hormone production, overproduction of a particular hormone causing a hyper-functional state, effects of the treatment modalities used, or interference of multiple chemical compounds produced in the stress environment with the normal functioning of the complex hypothalamic-pituitary-peripheral endocrine gland axes [1]. The clinical presentation will vary depending on the underlying etiology. The common chronic illnesses in children and adolescents causing significant endocrine dysfunction are listed in table 1. Some of these conditions are discussed in this paper.

HEMATOLOGIC AND ONCOLOGIC DISORDERS

Cancer

Pediatric leukemias and central nervous system (CNS) tumors of the hypothalamo-pituitary-midbrain area are relatively common cancers in which endocrine dysfunction is frequently seen. Multiple pituitary hormone deficits result from the direct involvement of the hypothalamic-pituitary area by the primary lesion itself (e.g., craniopharyngioma) or resulting from radiation and/or chemotherapy. Newer treatment modalities for leukemias and cancers are resulting in increased survival and longevity of children and adolescents. These intensive regimens, on the other hand, result in significant secondary morbidity in the form of multiple medical problems. Two-thirds of all cancer survivors were found to have medical consequences of cancer therapy and the most common late effects were noted to be endocrine [2].

Growth and Growth Hormone (GH) Deficiency

Disorders of growth are the most common disorders of childhood cancer survivors [2]. Growth deficits may be evident in the early phase of the disease or treatment. These deficits, however, are usually not related to growth hormone deficiency. Early growth deficits are due to the acute catabolism of disease and poor nutrition. This phase is addressed by optimizing nutritional intake [3,4]. The growth deficits seen later in the course of illness or treatment, most commonly many years after completion of therapy, are due to GH deficiency.

The hypothalamo-pituitary-growth axis (HPGrowth) is the most sensitive of the hypothalamic-pituitary axes to the damaging effects of radiation therapy. The extent of damage depends on the dose and fractionation of radiation therapy used and the time elapsed since treatment [5-7]. The hypothalamus is more sensitive to damage by radiation (damaged by 1,200 to 1,800 centigray (CGy) than the pituitary gland (damaged by more than 5,000 CGy) [8]. A diagnosis of GH deficiency is common when radiation doses of more than 3,000 CGy are used. For doses between 1,800 and 2,400 CGy, however, the diagnosis is not as straightforward. These patients have subnormal growth velocities in the pre-pubertal period, which is followed by a poor pubertal growth spurt [9,10]. Spinal radiation induces growth deficits characterized by truncal shortening with normal limb growth by possibly inducing direct unresponsiveness in bone. Younger patients are affected more significantly by irradiation to the spine [11].

Total body irradiation (TBI) used as preparative therapy before hematopoetic stem cell transplantation (HSCT) is seen to cause growth deficits when single fraction doses of 1,000 CGy or fractionated doses of 1,200 CGy are used [12-15]. Chemo-preparative regimens for HSCT on the other hand are generally not associated with growth deficits [16,17]. The role of chemotherapy in causing growth deficits is debatable. There are mixed reports in various studies with results ranging from significant effect on growth to other reports showing no role of chemotherapy in causing growth deficits [18].

The key to early diagnosis is to maintain a high index of suspicion. Growth should be carefully measured and plotted on appropriately matched growth charts and compared with their mid-parental genetic target height. Super-added hypothyroidism may further enhance growth deficit, whereas disturbances of the hypothalamo-pituitary-gonadal axis causing precocious puberty may initially mask growth deficit, but finally result in a greater compromise of the final adult height.

Table 1. Chronic non-endocrine medical conditions associated with endocrine dysfunction. *Conditions discussed in this chapter

1)	Disorders of the Hematological/Oncological System	
	-Cancers*	
	-Hemoglobinopathies	
2)	Gastrointestinal Disorders*	
	-Celiac Disease	
	-Inflammatory Bowel Disease	
3)	Rheumatologic Disorders*	
	-Juvenile Rheumatoid Arthritis	
4)	Renal Disorders	
	-Chronic Renal Failure	
	-Nephrosis/Nephrotic Syndrome	
5)	Immunological Disorders	
	-HIV/AIDS	
6)	Disorders of the Respiratory System*	
	-Cystic Fibrosis	
	-Asthma	
7)	Nervous System Disorders	
	-Cerebral Palsy	
	-Congenital brain malformations	
8)	Eating Disorders	
	-Anorexia Nervosa*	
	-Obesity	
9)	Genetic Syndromes	
	-Turner Syndrome	
	-Klinefelter's Syndrome	
	-DiGeorge Syndrome	
	-Down Syndrome	
	-Beckwith Wiedemann Syndrome	
	-McCune Albright Syndrome	

Laboratory evaluations of patients treated with high dose radiation therapy usually reveal an obvious dysfunction of the hypothalamo-pituitary-growth axis with evidence of low insulin-like growth factor 1 (IGF-1), low IGFBP3 (insulin-like growth factor binding protein 3), and low GH levels on GH stimulation testing. On the other hand, lower radiation doses or TBI may result in poor growth that might not be easily demonstrated on laboratory testing [19,20]. Such patients may have normal IGF-1 and IGFBP3, as well as normal responses to GH stimulation. Twenty-four hour growth hormone profiles, however, reveal abnormal growth hormone secretion [21].

Growth hormone deficiency is treated by recombinant human growth hormone (rhGH). Children who have received craniospinal or TBI may not exhibit catch-up growth and may show poor growth even when on growth hormone [19,20]. It is recommended that treatment be initiated after the child/adolescent has been in remission for one year. Concern has been ongoing about possible tumor relapse or recurrence with GH therapy. Overall, presently there is no evidence that rhGH promotes leukemia or tumor relapse [22,23].

Thyroid Dysfunction

Thyroxine (T4) and triiodothyronine (T3) are the two major hormones produced by the thyroid gland. A wide range of thyroid dysfunction is seen following cancer therapy causing damage to the hypothalamo-pituitary-thyroid (HPT) axis including hypothyroidism (central or primary), hyperthyroidism, and thyroid nodules/ malignancies [1]. Central hypothyroidism may be caused by the underlying tumor in the area of the hypothalamus, pituitary or mid-brain; also, it may follow craniospinal irradiation (doses > 4,000 CGy) [24]. This condition is difficult to diagnose by routine free T4 (FT4) and thyroid stimulating hormone (TSH) testing. In patients with normal FT4 and TSH, central hypothyroidism has been documented by thyroid releasing hormone (TRH) stimulation testing [25]. It remains difficult to address the question of when to treat this latent hypothyroidism [26]. Primary hypothyroidism may result from irradiation to the neck directly or result from scattered radiation received from cranio-spinal radiation therapy [27].

Hyperthyroidism has also been reported in a group of radiation treated patients [28]. Thyroid nodules and malignancies are also reported with a higher incidence following irradiation. Thyroid cancer is seen in 0.4% of patients. A higher risk is seen in females, with higher dose of irradiation and younger age at time of radiation treatment [28].

A high index of suspicion, close watch for signs and symptoms albeit non-specific, and close monitoring of growth and growth velocity are key to early diagnosis. Careful thyroid examination should be performed for size and nodularity. Thyroid function tests should be evaluated carefully at least once a year. The possibility of latent central hypothyroidism in the face of normal FT4 and TSH needs to be considered.

Hypothyroidism is treated by replacement with thyroid hormone. The FT4 levels have to be titrated to mid-normal range in central hypothyroidism, where TSH is not useful for evaluation. Hyperthyroidism may be treated by antithyroid medication, radioactive iodine treatment, or surgery. Thyroid nodules and malignancies will have to be addressed as indicated.

Adrenal Dysfunction

Adrenal dysfunction is uncommon because the hypothalamo-pituitary-adrenal (HPA) axis is relatively resistant to the effects of cancer therapy. Central adrenal insufficiency may occur due to the presence of a tumor in the hypothalamus, pituitary, midbrain region or may follow surgical resection of the same. Radiation doses of over 3,500 CGy can result in central adrenal insufficiency as well. [8,29,30]. Adrenal insufficiency requires long term followup. Signs and symptoms may include lethargy, hypoglycemia, anorexia, failure to thrive, or acute decompensation with hypotension, shock, and seizures in face of a "stress" situation.

A high index of suspicion and laboratory evaluation with 8 a.m. cortisol and ACTH levels, metyrapone test, and/or ACTH stimulation testing may provide help with diagnosis [31-33]. Hydrocortisone replacement is required with maintenance doses of 8 to 12 mg/m2/day. Guidelines for increasing the dose to 3 to 5 times the normal dose during acute illness, injury, or surgery (30 to 50 mg/m2/day) are essential. Parenteral glucocorticoid administration for emergency use should be available and taught to caretakers.

Gonadal Dysfunction

Normal function of the hypothalamo-pituitary-gonadal (HPG) axis is two-fold. First, it provides sex steroids, which are essential for pubertal development, as well as maintenance of sexual function. Secondly, the HPG axis is essential for the development and maintenance of gametes for reproduction.

Gonadal Dysfunction in Females

Ovarian hormone production and oocyte development are closely related. Toxicity from cancer chemotherapy or radiotherapy to any one of these components is highly likely to be associated with toxicity to the other. A wide spectrum of pathology affecting the HPG axis is seen, varying from complete hypogonadism to precocious puberty. Damage at the level of the pituitary gland and/or the hypothalamus causes central or secondary hypogonadotropic hypogonadism, whereas direct damage to the ovaries causes primary or hypergonadotropic hypogonadism [1]. A varying extent of hypogonadism is seen depending on the extent of damage (partial or complete) at both these levels. On the other hand, disruption of the normal CNS inhibitory influences on pubertal onset caused by irradiation lead to precocious puberty [1].

Precocious Puberty

Precocious puberty in these patients, together with GH deficiency, leads to severe compromise of final adult height. Unless a high index of suspicion along with close clinical followup is maintained, these children/young adolescents may be given a false reassurance of growing normally. Such girls should be clinically followed every 6 months, and pubertal staging and growth velocity should be closely monitored. Laboratory assessment and imaging with measurement of gonadotropins, estrogen levels, bone age assessment, and pelvic ultrasound may be performed as needed. Gonadotropin releasing hormone (GnRh) agonists are used for purposes of suppressing puberty in such girls, in addition to an adequate replacement of the other pituitary hormone deficits.

Central/Hypogonadotropic Hypogonadism

The HPG axis may be damaged by cranial irradiation of more than 4000 CGy. The young girls present with delayed pubertal onset (> 13 years), slow tempo of pubertal progression, or even signs and symptoms of premature menopause after pubertal process has completed [26].

Close clinical followup of growth and pubertal progression along with a high index of suspicion help alert the clinician for possible hypogonadotropic hypogonadism. Gonadotropin and estrogen levels, bone-age assessment, and pelvic ultrasonography are helpful in further assessment. Estrogen-replacement therapy, starting with small doses and gradually increasing doses over about two years to mimic the normal pubertal process, is recommended. Progesterone is then added for menstrual cycling. Combined estrogen and progesterone preparations may be used in pubertal/post pubertal girls. Excessive doses cause accelerated skeletal maturation and must be avoided.

Hypergonadotropic Ovarian Hypogonadism

Ovarian damage can occur with radiation and/or chemotherapy [34,35]. Because ovarian hormone production is closely linked to oocyte development, it is difficult to differentiate between the effects of a specific treatment on each of these two components. Chemotherapy-induced ovarian toxicity is more of a risk in the pubertal versus the prepubertal ovary. Alkylating agents (cyclophosphamide) and busulfan can cause permanent ovarian damage [36].

Direct radiation to the ovaries (more than 700 CGy) is noted to cause partial ovarian dysfunction, whereas higher doses (2,000 CGy) lead to permanent ovarian damage [34]. Radiation exposure from spinal radiation can also lead to functional ovarian impairment [35]. Girls receiving preparative treatments for HSCT are reported to have compromised ovarian function with manifestations of delayed pubertal development or permanent gonadal failure [36-38]. Close follow-up of growth and development; lab assessment of gonadotropin and estrogen levels; bone-age assessment, and pelvic imaging are key to a timely diagnosis. Gonadotropin levels are high in primary gonadal failure and low in central hypogonadism. Treatment is with adequate hormonal replacement as in hypogonadotropic hypogonadism.

Gonadal Dysfunction in Males

Leydig Cells (responsible for testosterone production) and Sertoli cells (responsible for mature sperm production) have different sensitivities to cancer treatment. Sertoli cells are much more sensitive to chemotherapy as well as radiation treatment than Leydig cells [39].

Central/Hypogonadotropic Hypogonadism

Boys presenting with no signs of pubertal onset by 14 years of age with history of cranial irradiation of more than 4,000 CGy are at high risk for developing central hypogonadism [12]. Gonadotropin and testosterone levels will be helpful in establishing a baseline status. Boys can be treated with testosterone replacement therapy. The treatment is started with low doses and gradually increased to adult doses over 2 to 3 years. Post pubertal hypogonadism is treated with testosterone replacement in the form of intramuscular injections, patches, or gels.

Hypergonadotopic Hypogonadism

Sertoli cells are damaged by TBI; radiation exposure (300 to 1,000 CGy in abdominal or low spinal radiation); and by chemotherapy regimens (including alkylating agents, procarbazine, vinblastine cytarabine, and cisplatin) [40]. Leydig cells are generally more tolerant to chemotherapy but may be damaged by radiation (doses of over 2,000 CGy) or TBI [38]. Boys should be closely examined every 6 months to detect pubertal onset and then subsequently to follow the tempo of pubertal progression, and then annually after completion of puberty for early detection of hypogonadism or early andropause. High FSH levels indicate Sertoli cell damage; normal inhibin levels confirm the presence of Sertoli cell; high LH levels and low testosterone levels are indicative of leydig cell dysfunction. Treatment options include adequate testosterone replacement as in hypogonadotropic hypogonadism.

Concerns with Fertility

Concerns about fertility are significant for both males and females years after exposure to the initial gonadotoxic insult [41,42]. The options available to aid with fertility concerns in females include moving the ovaries out of the field of irradiation to protect from ovarian toxicity or cryopreservation of ovarian tissue for future use [42,43]. Sperm analysis is required to assess the potential for fertility in males and for evaluation for invitro fertilization [41,42]. Pretreatment sperm banking may be useful in older adolescents and young adults.

Central Diabetes Inspidus (DI)

Deficiency of antidiuretic hormone (ADH or AVP-Arginine Vasopressin) causes central DI. ADH is normally produced in the supraoptic, paraventricular, and suprachiasmatic hypothalamic nuclei and then transported via the pituitary stalk to be stored in the posterior pituitary. ADH deficiency is seen in children/adolescents before the initiation of any treatment because of tumors compressing the hypothalamus, pituitary gland, or stalk area causing central DI. Alternatively, damage caused in these areas after surgical procedures can cause DI as well. The typical triphasic response may be seen post-operatively characterized by DI-SIADH-DI (SIADH - syndrome of inappropriate antidiuretic hormone). Cranial irradiation is not accompanied by posterior pituitary dysfunction or DI.

A high index of suspicion for DI along with details of fluid intake and output may lead toward the diagnosis. Polyuria, polydipsia, nocturia, or secondary enuresis are usually present but may be subtle and missed. The quantification of fluid intake and urine output is very helpful in the diagnostic process. A water deprivation test may be required to uncover DI, especially if the thirst mechanism is intact and the patient has unrestricted access to fluids. Clinical expression of DI may be masked by the concomitant presence of thyroid and/or adrenal insufficiency. DI is clinically manifested once glucocorticoid and thyroid hormone replacement therapy is instituted. Laboratory evaluation reveals hypernatremia, plasma hypersomolality, and urine hypoosmolality.

Central DI can be treated by replacement with arginine vasopressin in the form of DDAVP (desmopressin acetate) in the form of oral, intranasal, or subcutaneous formulations.

Gastrointestinal (GI) Disorders

Celiac Disease

Celiac disease is an immune mediated enteropathy characterized by intolerance to dietary gluten. Celiac disease tends to coexist with other autoimmune conditions because of shared HLA (human leukocyte antigens), with a predisposition to autoimmune conditions [26]. The prevalence of celiac disease in the western population is about 1% (44). A 2% to 5% incidence of celiac disease has been reported in patients with type I diabetes mellitus and in patients with autoimmune thyroid dysfunction as well [45]. Hypocalcemia and vitamin D deficiency have also been reported in celiac disease, predisposing to a higher risk of fractures [46]. Menstrual disturbances, fertility issues, and hyperprolactinemia reported in celiac disease patients are due possibly to a deficiency of micro and macro nutrients secondary to malabsorption [47].

Children and adolescents with celiac disease may present in one of several ways [48]:

- with GI signs and symptoms, such as abdominal pain, bloating, distension, nausea, flatulence, bulky stools, weight loss, or history of intolerance to certain food stuffs
- with short stature and failure to thrive
- with other autoimmune conditions, as mentioned above and may be diagnosed with celiac disease as a part of routine screening or testing.

The institution of a gluten-free diet improves GI symptomatology, weight gain and linear growth, bone density, and reproductive function [49,50].

Crohn's Disease

Children and adolescents with Crohn's disease may present with poor linear growth, delayed puberty, and short stature [51]. Growth hormone testing reveals a picture consistent with mild GH resistance characterized by normal GH secretion and slightly low IGF-1 levels. The role of GH in adolescents with Crohn's disease remains unclear, with some reports suggesting benefit and other reports showing no/incomplete benefit of treatment. Thus far, Crohn's disease is not a United States Food and Drug Administration (FDA)-approved indication for GH treatment.

Rheumatologic Disorders

Chronic juvenile rheumatoid arthritis (JRA) will mainly be considered for discussion in this group. JRA in adolescents may present with varying degrees of growth retardation, depending on the severity of the chronic underlying disease process itself and/or the treatment modalities used including chronic/high dose glucocorticoid therapy. As an example, one can see an 8-year-old female child with severe JRA whose height is at −5 SD below the mean for her age. Such children/ adolescents can also exhibit osteopenia, osteoporosis, or low bone mineral density.

Growth hormone studies reveal a state of mild GH resistance with normal GH secretion and mildly low IGF-1 levels. Growth hormone treatment is not approved by the FDA for JRA but has been used in a clinical trial in which an increase in the rate of linear growth was shown [52,53].

RESPIRATORY DISORDERS

Asthma

Endocrine consequences secondary to asthma may be due to the effects of the chronic underlying illness itself, or more so, secondary to chronic glucocorticoid therapy.

Cystic Fibrosis (CF)

Cystic fibrosis is a genetic disorder caused by mutations in the cystic fibrosis transmembrane conductance regulator (CFTR) gene on chromosome 7; CF has an incidence of 1:2,500. A primary defect in the epithelial transport of electrolytes causes thick mucous secretions that lead to progressive organ damage to the lungs, pancreas, and reproductive organs [1]. The main endocrine concerns related to CF are due to the chronic illness itself, as well as to the progressive organ damage and include short stature, delayed puberty, cystic fibrosis related diabetes (CFRD), and male infertility. Short stature and constitutional delay of growth and development with poor linear growth, poor weight gain, and delayed puberty are seen secondary to poor nutritional status. Poor appetite, poor nutritional intake, and poor nutrient absorption along with increased energy expenditure result in a net poor nutritional state [1].

Such children are noted to have a mild GH resistance state with normal GH levels and low IFG-1 and IGFBP3 levels [54,55]. GH therapy is not FDA approved for use in patients with CF. Nutrition support is the mainstay treatment. Initial studies suggest some improvement in growth with GH, but trials are ongoing to see long term effect of GH on CF patients in terms of improved growth, increased weight gain, and possibly improved pulmonary function [56-59].

Cystic Fibrosis Related Diabetes (CFRD)

CFRD results from progressive fibrosis and fatty infiltration of the pancreas causing ß-cell destruction, leading to a partial insulin deficiency. Glucagon deficiency is also believed to be present, although relative sparing of non ß-cells may be seen. The incidence of CFRD is gradually increasing as the life expectancy of CF patients continues to improve [1]. CFRD develops gradually, with progression from normal to impaired glucose tolerance to frank diabetes mellitus, according to the diagnostic criteria defined by the American Diabetes

Association [60]. CFRD is associated with failure to thrive, poor weight gain, and deterioration of pulmonary function [26].

Treatment for CFRD has been shown to improve growth as well as lung function [61,62]. Treatment for CFRD should be individualized, and insulin therapy remains the mainstay of therapy as for type I diabetes mellitus. The role of oral agents is under current research. The insulin requirement is seen to increase significantly during acute pulmonary infections/ exacerbations, with or without associated increased steroid doses. The insulin dosing must be increased during these exacerbations to compensate for a higher insulin requirement.

ANOREXIA NERVOSA (AN)

Anorexia nervosa is a chronic disorder present in about 1% of adolescents, more common in females [63]. The diagnosis of AN is extremely challenging. Indeed, some of the secondary manifestations may be apparent before the diagnosis of AN itself is made. A number of endocrine disturbances can be seen in association with AN, including short stature, delayed puberty, abnormal thyroid function tests, secondary amenorrhea, and osteoporosis [1].

Adolescents presenting with short stature reveal a picture consistent with GH resistance with high GH levels and low IGF-1, IGFBP3, and growth hormone binding protein levels. These parameters are seen to normalize after nutrition rehabilitation [64,65]. Thyroid function in AN manifests a sick-euthyroid like picture with low total and free T4 and T3 levels, low normal TSH, and high rT3 (reverse T3) levels. The TRH stimulation test reveals a TSH response consistent with a hypothalamic hypothyroidism response [66].

The hypothalamo-pituitary-adrenal axis shows multiple changes resulting in hypercortisolemia, which is believed to be primarily hypothalamic in origin, as reflected in high corticotropin-releasing hormone (CRH) secretion. Serum cortisol levels are high but the circadian rhythm is preserved [63]. The disturbances of the hypothalamo-pituitary-gonadal axis present with a clinical picture consistent with hypothalamic hypogonadism reflected in low estrogen levels, low gonadotropin levels, and a normal response to GnRh stimulation. Adolescent girls may present with delayed puberty and hypothalamic amenorrhea [67,68].

Osteoporosis with decreased bone mineral density results from the interruption of multiple hormonal axes, including estrogen deficiency secondary to hypothalamic hypogonadism, suppression of hypothalamo-pituitary-GH-IGF-1 axis, inadequate intake of vitamin D as well as calcium, and low dehydroepiandrosterone (DHEA) [69,70]. The significance of these multiple deficiencies is very important in AN, as the peak incidence of AN overlaps the period of acquisition of peak bone mass. There may be long term implications of compromise in bone density unless anorexia is resolved early.

The biochemical laboratory evaluation is consistent with a picture of transient endocrine dysfunction, which seems to be an adaptive, physiologic response of the body to ensure minimum energy expenditure [63]. Nutrition rehabilitation remains the key mode of treatment for AN. The endocrine manifestations seen in AN normalize when adequate nutritional intake is instituted. Mixed results have been reported with use of different types of hormone replacement therapies, including estrogen replacement and combined estrogen-progesterone oral contraceptives [71]. Other modalities being investigated include rIGF-1 and DHEA [71].

Trials with alendronate bisphosphonate treatment show promising results for improvement in bone density [72].

CONCLUSIONS

Adolescents with chronic illness and disabilities should be closely monitored for growth and development. The key to reducing morbidity and mortality is to maintain a high index of suspicion for underlying endocrine deficits, their early diagnosis, and timely initiation of replacement hormonal therapy. Such comprehensive care, especially in the setting of multi-specialty clinic settings, help improve medical care to these groups of adolescents with special needs.

REFERENCES

[1] Zeitler PS, Meacham R, Allen DB, Pinhas-Hamiel O. Endocrine consequences of chronic illness. In: Kappy MS, Allen DB, Geffner ME, eds. Principles and practice of pediatric endocrinology. Spring-field, IL: Charles Thomas, 2005:857-909.

[2] Sklar CA. Overview of the effects of cancer therapies: the nature, scale and breadth of the problem. *Acta Pediatr.* 1999;88(Suppl 433):1-4.

[3] van Eys J. Nutrition in the treatment of cancer in children. *J. Am. Coll. Nutr.* 1984; 3(2):159-68.

[4] Reilly JJ, Weir J, McColl JH, Gibson BE. Preva-lence of protein-energy malnutrition at diagnosis in children with acute lymphoblastic leukemia. *J. Pediatr. Gastroenterol. Nutr.* 1999;29(2):194-7.

[5] Rappaport R, Brauner R. Growth and endocrine disorders secondary to cranial irradiation. *Pediatr. Res.* 1989;25(6):561-7.

[6] Shalet SM, Beardwell CG, Pearson D, Jones PH. The effect of varying doses of cerebral irradiation on growth hormone production in childhood. *Clin. Endocrinol. (Oxf)* 1976;5(3):287-90.

[7] Clayton PE, Shalet SM. Dose dependency of time of onset of radiation-induced growth hormone deficiency. *J. Pediatr.* 1991;118(2):226-8.

[8] Oberfield SE, Sklar CA. Endocrine sequelae in survivors of childhood cancer. *Adolesc. Med.* 2002;13(1):161-9.

[9] Katz JA, Pollock BH, Jacaruso D, Morad A. Final attained height in patients successfully treated for childhood acute lymphoblastic leukemia. *J. Pediatr.* 1993;123(4):546.52.

[10] Brauner R, Rappaport R, Prevot C, Czernichow P, Zucker JM, Bataini P, et al. A prospective study of the development of growth hormone deficiency in children given cranial irradiation, and its relation to statural growth. *J. Clin. Endocrinol. Metab.* 1989;68(2):346-51.

[11] Ogilvy-Stuart AL, Shalet SM. Growth and puberty after growth hormone treatment after irradiation for brain tumors. *Arch. Dis. Child.* 1995; 73(2):141-6.

[12] Sklar CA, Constine LS. Chronic neuroendocrino-logical sequelae of radiation therapy. *Int. J. Radiat. Oncol. Biol. Phys.* 1995;31(5):1113-21.

[13] Ogilvy-Stuart AL, Clark DJ, Wallace WH, Gibson BE, Stevens RF, Shalet SM, et al. Endocrine deficit after fractionated total body irradiation. *Arch. Dis. Child.* 1992;67(9):1107-10.

[14] Brauner R, Fontoura M, Zucker JM, Devergie A, Souberbielle JC, Prevot-Saucet C, et al. Growth and growth hormone secretion after bone marrow transplantation. *Arch. Dis. Child.* 1993;68 (4):458-63.

[15] Bakker B, Oostdijk W, Geskus Rb, Stokvis-Brantsma WH, Vossen JM, Wit JM. Patterns of growth and body proportions after total-body irradiation and hematopoietic stem cell trans-plantation during childhood. *Pediatr. Res.* 2006; 59(2):259-64.

[16] Adan L, de Lanversin ML, Thalassinos C, Souberbielle JC, Fischer A, Brauner R. Growth after bone marrow transplantation in young children conditioned with chemotherapy alone. *Bone Marrow Transplant.* 1997;19(3):253-6.

[17] Afify Z, Shaw PJ, Clavano-Harding A, Cowell CT. Growth and endocrine function in children with acute myeloid leukaemia after bone marrow transplantation using busulfan/cyclophosphamide. *Bone Marrow Transplant.* 2000;25(10):1087-92.

[18] Ogilvy-Stuart AL, Shalet SM. Effect of chemo-therapy on growth. *Acta Paediatr.* 1995;411:52-6.

[19] Sulmont V, Brauner R, Fontoura M, Rappaport R. Response to growth hormone treatment and final height after cranial or craniospinal irradiation. *Acta Pediatr. Scand.* 1990;79(5):542-9.

[20] Clayton PE, Shalet SM, Price DA. Growth response to growth hormone therapy following craniospinal irradiation. *Eur. J. Pediatr.* 1988;147 (6):597-601.

[21] Mo?ll C, Garwicz S, Westgren U, Wiebe T, Albertsson-Wikland K. Suppressed spontaneous secretion of growth hormone in girls after treatment for acute lymphoblastic leukaemia. *Arch. Dis. Child.* 1989;64(2):252-8.

[22] Ogilvy-Stuart AL, Ryder WD, Gattamaneni HR, Clayton PE, Shalet SM. Growth hormone and tumour recurrence. *BMJ.* 1992;304(6842):1601-5.

[23] Sklar CA, Mertens AC, Mitby P, Occhiogrosso G, Qin J, Heller G, et al. Risk of disease recurrence and second neoplasms in survivors of childhood cancer treated with growth hormone: a report from the Childhood Cancer Survivor Study. *J. Clin. Endocrinol. Metab.* 2002;87(7):3136-41.

[24] Sklar CA, Constine LS. Chronic neuroendocrino-logical sequelae of radiation therapy. *Int. J. Radiat. Oncol. Biol. Phys.* 1995;31:1113-21.

[25] Rose SR, Lustig RH, Pitukcheewanont P, Broome DC, Burghen GA, Li H et al. Diagnosis of hidden central hypothyroidism in survivors of childhood cancer. *J. Clin. Endocrinol. Metab.* 1999;84(12): 4472-9.

[26] Rappaport R, Thibaud E. Endocrine disorders after cancer therapy. In: Lifshitz F, ed. *Pediatric endocrinology.* vol 1, 5th ed. New York: Informa Healthcare, 2007.

[27] Schmiegelow M, Feldt-Rasmussen U, Rasmussen AK, Poulsen HS, Møller J. A population-based study of thyroid function after radiotherapy and chemotherapy for a childhood brain tumor. *J. Clin. Endocrinol. Metab.* 2003;88(1):136-40.

[28] Sklar C, Whitton J, Mertens A, Stovall M, Green D, Marina N et al. Abnormalities of the thyroid in survivors of Hodgkin's disease: data from the Childhood Cancer Survivor Study. *J. Clin. Endocrinol. Metab.* 2000;85(9):3227-32.

[29] Oberfield SE, Chin D, Uli N, David R, Sklar C. Endocrine late effects of childhood cancers. *J. Pediatr.* 1997;131:S37-41.

[30] Oberfield SE, Nirenberg A, Allen JC, Cohen H, Donahue B, Prasad V, et al. Hypothalamic-pituitary-adrenal function following cranial irradiation. *Horm. Res.* 1997;47(1):9-16.

[31] Constine LS, Woolf PD, Cann D, Mick G, McCormick K, Raubertas RF, et al. Hypothalamic-pituitary dysfunction after radiation for brain tumors. *N. Engl. J. Med.* 1993;328(2):87-94.

[32] Leong KS, Walker AB, Martin I, Wile D, Wilding J, MacFarlane IA. An audit of 500 subcutaneous glucagon stimulation tests to assess growth hormone and ACTH secretion in patients with hypothalamic-pituitary disease. *Clin. Endocrinol.* (Oxf) 2001;54(4):463-8.

[33] Schmiegelow M, Feldt-Rasmussen U, Rasmussen AK, Lange M, Poulsen HS, Møller J. Assessment of the hypothalamo-pituitary-adrenal axis in patients treated with radiotherapy and chemo-therapy for childhood brain tumor. *J. Clin. Endocrinol. Metab.* 2003;88(7):3149-54.

[34] Wallace WH, Shalet SM, Hendry JH, Morris-Jones PH, Gattamaneni HR. Ovarian failure following abdominal irradiation in childhood: the radiosensitivity of the human oocyte. *Br. J. Radiol.* 1989;62(743):995-8.

[35] Livesey EA, Brook CG. Gonadal dysfunction after treatment of intracranial tumours. *Arch. Dis. Child.* 1988;63(5):495-500.

[36] Thibaud E, Rodriguez-Macias K, Trivin C, Espérou H, Michon J, Brauner R. Ovarian function after bone marrow transplantation during childhood. *Bone Marrow Transplant.* 1998;21(3):287-90.

[37] Couto-Silva AC, Trivin C, Thibaud E, Esperou H, Michon J, Brauner R. Factors affecting gonadal function after bone marrow transplantation during childhood. *Bone Marrow Transplant.* 2001;28(1): 67-75.

[38] Sarafoglou K, Boulad F, Gillio A, Sklar C. Gonadal function after bone marrow transplantation for acute leukemia during childhood. *J. Pediatr.* 1997;130(2):210-6.

[39] Schmiegelow M, Lassen S, Poulsen HS, Schmiegelow K, Hertz H, Andersson AM, et al. Gonadal status in male survivors following child-hood brain tumors. *J. Clin. Endocrinol. Metab.* 2001; 86(6):2446-52.

[40] Goldman S, Johnson FL. Effects of chemotherapy and irradiation on the gonads. *Endocrinol. Metab. Clin. North Am.* 1993;22(3):617-29.

[41] Wallace WH, Shalet SM, Lendon M, Morris-Jones PH. Male fertility in long-term survivors of childhood acute lymphoblastic leukaemia. *Int. J. Androl.* 1991;14(5):312-9.

[42] Wallace WH, Anderson RA, Irvine DS. Fertility preservation for young patients with cancer: who is at risk and what can be offered? *Lancet Oncol.* 2005;6(4):209-18.

[43] Thibaud E, Ramirez M, Brauner R, Flamant F, Zucker JM, Fékété C, Rappaport R. Preservation of ovarian function by ovarian transposition performed before pelvic irradiation during childhood. *J. Pediatr.* 1992;121(6):880-4.

[44] Ch'ng CL, Jones MK, Kingham JG. Celiac disease and autoimmune thyroid disease. *Clin. Med. Res.* 2007;5(3):184-92.

[45] Collin P, Kaukinen K, Välimäki M, Salmi J. Endocrinological disorders and celiac disease. *Endocr. Rev.* 2002;23(4):464-83.

[46] Vasquez H, Mazure R, Gonzalez D, Flores D, Pedreira S, Niveloni S, et al. Risk of fractures in celiac disease patients: a cross-sectional, case-control study. *Am. J. Gastroenterol.* 2000;95(1):183-9.

[47] Rostami K, Steegers EA, Wong WY, Braat DD, Steegers-Theunissen RP. Coeliac disease and reproductive disorders: a neglected association. *Eur. J. Obstet. Gynecol. Reprod. Biol.* 2001;96(2):146-9.

[48] Iughetti L, Bulgarelli S, Forese S, Lorini R, Balli F, Bernasconi S. Endocrine aspects of coeliac disease. *J. Pediatr. Endocrinol. Metab.* 2003;16(6): 805-18.

[49] De Luca F, Astori M, Pandullo E, Sferlazzas C, Arrigo T, Sindoni A, et al. Effects of a gluten-free diet on catch-up growth and height prognosis in coeliac children with growth retardation recognized after the age of 5 years. *Eur. J. Pediatr.* 1988;147(2):188-91.

[50] Bradley RJ, Rosen MP. Subfertility and gastro-intestinal disease: 'unexplained' is often undiag-nosed. *Obstet. Gynecol. Surv.* 2004;59(2):108-17.

[51] Savage MO, Beattie RM, Camacho-H?bner C, Walker-Smith JA, Sanderson IR. Growth in Crohn's disease. *Acta Paediatr.* 1999;88 (Suppl 428):89-92.

[52] Simon D, Prieur A, Czernichow P. Treatment of juvenile rheumatoid arthritis with growth hormone. *Horm. Res.* 2000;53(Suppl 1):82-6.

[53] Bechtold S, Ripperger P, Muhlbayer D, Trucken-brodt H, Hafner R, Butenandt O, et al. GH therapy in juvenile chronic arthritis: results of a two-year controlled study on growth and bone. *J. Clin. Endocrinol. Metab.* 2001;86(12):5737-44.

[54] Laursen EM, Juul A, Lanng S, Høiby N, Koch C, Møller J, Skakkebaek NE. Diminished concen-trations of insulin-like growth factor I in cystic fibrosis. *Arch. Dis. Child.* 1995;72(6):494-7.

[55] Taylor AM, Bush A, Thomson A, Oades PJ, Marchant JL, Bruce-Morgan C, et al. Relation between insulin-like growth factor-I, body mass index, and clinical status in cystic fibrosis. *Arch. Dis. Child.* 1997;76(4):304-9.

[56] Hardin DS, Sy JP. Effects of growth hormone treatment in children with cystic fibrosis: the National Cooperative Growth Study experience. *J. Pediatr.* 1997;131(1 Pt 2):S65-9.

[57] Hardin DS. GH improves growth and clinical status in children with cystic fibrosis—a review of published studies. *Eur. J. Endocrinol.* 2004;151 (Suppl 1):S81-5.

[58] Hardin DS, Ellis KJ, Dyson M, Rice J, McConnell R, Seilheimer DK. Growth hormone decreases protein catabolism in children with cystic fibrosis. *J. Clin. Endocrinol. Metab.* 2001;86(9):4424-8.

[59] Hardin DS, Stratton R, Kramer JC, Reyes de la Rocha S, Govaerts K, Wilson DP. Growth hormone improves weight velocity and height velocity in prepubertal children with cystic fibrosis. *Horm. Metab. Res.* 1998;30(10):636-41.

[60] Moran A. Cystic fibrosis-related diabetes: an approach to diagnosis and management. *Pediatr. Diabetes.* 2000;1(1):41-8.

[61] Lanng S, Thorsteinsson B, Nerup J, Koch C. Diabetes mellitus in cystic fibrosis: Effect of insulin therapy on lung function and infections. *Acta Paediatr.* 1994;83(8):849-53.

[62] Ripa P, Robertson I, Cowley D, Harris M, Masters IB, Cotterill AM. The relationship between insulin secretion, the insulin-like growth factor axis and growth in children with cystic fibrosis. *Clin. Endocrinol.* (Oxf) 2002;56(3):383-9.

[63] Gungor N, Arsalanian S. Nutritional disorders – integration of energy metabolism and its disorders in childhood. In: Sperling M, ed. *Pediatric endocrinology*. 2nd ed. Philadelphia, PA: Saunders, 2002:689-724.

[64] Argente J, Caballo N, Barrios V, Muñoz MT, Pozo J, Chowen JA, et al. Multiple endocrine abnormalities of the growth hormone and insulin-like growth factor axis in patients with anorexia nervosa: effect of short- and long-term weight recuperation. *J. Clin. Endocrinol. Metab.* 1997;82 (7):2084-92.

[65] Counts DR, Gwirtsman H, Carlsson LM, Lesem M, Cutler GB Jr. The effect of anorexia nervosa and refeeding on growth hormone-binding protein, the insulin-like growth factors (IGFs), and the IGF-binding proteins. *J. Clin. Endocrinol. Metab.* 1992;75(3):762-7.

[66] Tamai H, Mori K, Matsubayashi S, Kiyohara K, Nakagawa T, Okimura MC, et al. Hypothalamic-pituitary-thyroidal dysfunctions in anorexia nervosa. *Psychother. Psychosom.* 1986;46(3):127-31.

[67] Poyastro Pinheiro A, Thornton LM, Plotonicov KH, Tozzi F, Klump L, Berrettini WH, et al. Patterns of menstrual disturbance in eating disorders. *Int. J. Eat. Disord.* 2007;40(5):424-34.

[68] Mitan LA. Menstrual dysfunction in anorexia nervosa. *J. Pediatr. Adolesc. Gynecol.* 2004;17(2): 81-5.

[69] Muñoz-Calvo MT. Anorexia nervosa: an endo-crine focus and procedure guidelines. *J. Pediatr. Endocrinol. Metab.* 2005;18(Suppl 1):1181-5.

[70] Miller KK, Lee EE, Lawson EA, Misra M, Minihan J, Grinspoon SK, et al. Determinants of skeletal loss and recovery in anorexia nervosa. *J. Clin. Endocrinol. Metab* 2006;91(8):2931-7.

[71] Grinspoon S, Thomas L, Miller K, Herzog D, Klibanski A. Effects of recombinant human IGF-1 and oral contraceptive administration on bone density in anorexia nervosa. *J. Clin. Endocrinol. Metab.* 2002;87;2883-91.

[72] Golden NH, Iglesias EA, Jacobson MS, Carey D, Meyer W, Schebendach J, et al. Alendronate for the treatment of osteopenia in anorexia nervosa: a randomized, double-blind placebo-controlled trial. *J. Clin. Endocrinol. Metab.* 2005;90(6):3179-85.

In: Adolescence and Chronic Illness
Editors: H. Omar et al.

ISBN: 978-1-60876-628-4
© 2010 Nova Science Publishers, Inc.

Chapter 4

ENDOCRINOLOGICAL ASPECTS OF INTELLECTUAL DISABILITY

Mohammed Morad[*,1,2,3], *Efrat Merrick-Kenig*[3] *and Joav Merrick*[2,3,4]

[1] Department of Family Medicine, Faculty of Health Sciences,
Ben Gurion University of the Negev, Beer-Sheva, Israel.
[2] Clalit Health Services, Beer-Sheva, Israel.
[3] National Institute of Child Health and Human Development,
Office of the Medical Director, Division for Mental Retardation,
Ministry of Social Affairs, Jerusalem, Israel.
[4] Kentucky Children's Hospital, University of Kentucky
College of Medicine, Lexington, U.S.A.

ABSTRACT

Persons with intellectual disability (ID) often have associated endocrine problems and sometimes the endocrine disease can be the cause of the intellectual disability. Several studies have shown that endocrine problems are common in the population of persons with intelletual disability both due to the same reasons as in the general population, but also specific and as part of several syndromes and conditions seen in this population. Since persons with intellectual disability today live longer and enter adolescence and adulthood they should therefore have a comprehensive evaluation of their endocrine function, which should also be followed up over time at regular intervals and being part of screening procedures as in the general population.

---

[*] Correspondence: Senior lecturer Mohammed Morad, MD, Medical director, Clalit Health Services Shatal Clinic, Rehov Similanski 79, IL-84223 Beer Sheva, Israel. E-mail: morad62@013.net.il

INTRODUCTION

Endocrinology actually began in China, when sex and pituitary hormones were isolated from human urine and used it for medicinal purposes already by the year 200 BCE. Persons with intellectual disability (ID) often have associated endocrine problems [1,2] and sometimes the endocrine disease can be the cause of the intellectual disability. Persons with intellectual disability may have [2]:

- their disability caused by endocrinopathies
- endocrine conditions associated with chromosomal and non-chromosomal syndromes
- other abnormalities of growth and development
- endocrine manifestations caused by medications taken
- endocrine disease as in the general population.

SCREENING AND THE MAGNITUDE

Primary congenital hypothyroidism occurs in approximately one of every 3,000-4,000 newborns in the United States [3]. Neonatal screening, which originated from Quebec in 1971 and implemented together with PKU (phenylketonuria) screening at birth will result in early diagnosis and treatment in order to prevent neurological, motor and growth deficits, including irreversible ID. With the implementation of tandem mass spectrometry and other techniques to screen large populations of children for various disorders and detect cases, very little is know about the long-term outsomes of these neonatal screening programs [4]. Of the CDC (Centers for Disease Control and Prevention) studies in Atlanta from the 1981-1995 birth cohorts 216 children tested positive for metabolic and endocrine disorders at their neonatal screening [4] and only nine children showed developmental disability less severe than intellectual disability.

Several large studies [5-7] of adults with ID aged 40 years and older in New York State (1,371 persons), Israel (2,282 persons) and Taiwan (1,128 persons) showed that the Israeli cohort had increased odds of dermatologic, endocrine, gastro-intestinal, and infectious diseases/conditions compared with the New York State cohort. Of these, endocrine and infectious diseases, as well as musculoskeletal and respiratory diseases, were two to three times more likely in males than females in the Israeli cohort when compared to the New York cohort, but in the Israeli cohort diabetes was at a lower frequency than the general Israeli population. Endocrine disorders were found with increased aging, in persons with Down syndrome and in the total cohort of all three studies 32% showed endocrine problems.

In smaller studies of patients referred for genetic evaluation a 9% prevalence of metabolic and endocrine disorders were found [8].

DISABILITY CAUSE BY ENDOCRINE DISEASE

The main two entities here are congenital hypothyroidism and neonatal hypoglycemia, which should be diagnosed in the early neonatal period and treated in order to prevent later intellectual disability.

Congenital hypothyroidism was not an easy diagnosis to make in the early period of life due to general symptoms, but the screening implemented in the 1970s has been able to detect more accurately the cases [3]. Congenital hypothyroidism seems to be a sporadic and not hereditary disease [9].

Glucose is the major energy source for the fetus and neonate, since the newborn brain depends upon glucose, but at birth glucose regulatory mechanisms are not always functioning well. The child is therefore susceptible to hypoglycemia, when glucose demands are increased. Severe or prolonged hypoglycemia may result in long term neurologic damage and intellectual disability. Symptoms are non specific and monitoring important to prevent hypoglycemia in the neonatal period and especially in children who are premature, small for gestional age or other neonatal risk factors in order to prevent long term consequences [2].

SYNDROMES

There are several syndromes with an endocrine component that the clinician should be aware of and anticipate, but due to space considerations only a few will be mentioned here.

Down syndrome is the classic example of a syndrome with several endocrinological and autoimmune manifestations, the most prominent hypothyroidism, but also diabetes mellitus, chronic lymphocytic thyrioditis, Graves disease and short stature [2]. Regular thyroid function tests should therefore be performed in persons with Down syndrome all through their life.

Turner syndrome, Klinefelter syndrome, Prader-Willi syndrome, Noonan syndrome and Williams syndrome [10] all have endocrine and other related disorders that the physician in charge of their health should be aware of and screen for.

GROWTH AND DEVELOPMENT

Intrauterine growth retardation can have long-term complications for development and health with increased prevalence of essential hypertension, impaired glucose tolerance, type 2 diabetes, polycysticovary syndrome, ischemic heart disease, hypertriglyceridemia and low-high density lipoprotein on top of the increased risk for seizures and developmental disability [2, 11].

Precocious puberty has also been described in association with intellectual disability [2,11,12] and it can be found together with any central nervous system abnormalities that also cause intellectual disability. Each case of development of secondary sexual characteristics before age 8-9 years should include a careful anamnesis, clinical and laboratory investigation. A recent study [13] has found that children with autism and autism spectrum disorder had significantly elevated level of growth-related hormones.

MEDICATIONS

Persons with intellectual disability have often associated medical problems that sometimes require medications, like for example epilepsia or mental health problems. In the last national survey of over 6,000 persons with ID living in residential care centers in Israel [14] it was found that nearly 80% received medication every day, 30% received anti-epileptic drugs and 51% received psychotropic medications. Many of the drugs used have thyroid-stimulating hormone suppression, thyroid suppression, effects on thyroid binding proteins, inactivation of vitamin D, osteoporosis, diabetes, obesity, galactorrhea and growth retardation [2].

OBESITY

Obesity is a problem in this population, basically due to the fact that there is habitual overeating and descrease daily activities resulting in obesity, but also several syndromes is complicated with obesity, like Down syndrome [15] and Prader-Will syndrome [10]. Prevention programs and physical activity should therefore be part of the interventions for these people.

DIABETES

As obesity and sedentary lifestyle is common in this population, so it would be expected to find a higher prevalence of diabetes. In the large cohort study of adults with ID in Israel diabetes was found with increasing age, decreased as ID became severe, but with a lower prevalence than the general Israeli population [6]. Regular screening should be conducted.

OSTEOPOROSIS

In an Australian study over a five year period of 337 persons (aged 19-83 years) with ID in a residential care center it was found that 57% were vitamin deficient [16]. The reasons being the reduced mobility, anti-epileptic medications and lack of sunlight. This situation results in increaased risks for fall and for fractures, which is higher in this population than the general population [16].

CONCLUSIONS

Several studies have shown that endocrine problems are common in the population of persons with intelletual disability both due to the same reasons as in the general population, but also specific and as part of several syndromes and conditions seen in this population.

Persons with intellectual disability should therefore have a comprehensive evaluation of their endocrine function, which should also be followed up over time at regular intervals and being part of screening procedures as in the general population.

REFERENCES

[1] McElduff A. Endocrinological issues. In: Prasher VP, Janicki MP, eds. *Physical health of adults with intellectual disabilities*. Oxford: Blackwell, 2002:160-80.

[2] Botero D, Fleischman A. Endocrinology. In: Rubin IL, Crocker AC, eds. *Medical care for children and adults with developmental disabilities*. Baltimore: Paul Brookes, 2006:387-98.

[3] US Preventive Services Task Force. Screening for congenital hypothyroidism (CH): U.S. Preventive Services Task Force reaffirmation recommendation statement. Ann Fam Med 2008;6(2):166. Available online at http://www.annfammed.org/cgi/content/full/6/2/166-a/DC1

[4] Braun KVN, Yeargin-Allscop M, Schendel D, Fernhoff P. Long-term developmental outcomes of children identified through a newborn screening program with a metabolic and endocrine disorder: A polulation-based approach. *J. Pediatrics*. 2003;143:236-42.

[5] Janicki MP, Davidson PW, Henderson CM, McCallion P, Taets JD, Force LT, Sulkes SB, Frangenberg E, Ladrigan PM. Health characteristics and health services utilization in older adults with intellectual disability living in community residences. *J. Intellect. Disabilit. Res.* 2002;47(4):287-98.

[6] Merrick J, Davidson PW, Morad M, Janicki MP, Wexler O, Henderson CM. Older adults with intellectual disability in residential care centers in Israel: Health status and service utilization. *Am. J. Ment. Retard.* 2004;109(5): 413-20.

[7] Wang KY, Hsieh K, Heller T, Davidson PW, Janicki MP. Carer reports of health status among adults with intellectual/developmental disabilities in Taiwan living at home and in institutions. *J. Intellect. Disabil. Res.* 2007;51(3):173-83.

[8] Maves SN, Williams MS, Willians JL, Lovonian PJ, Josephson KD. Analysis of 88 adult patients referred for genetic evaluation. *Am. J. Med. Genetics Part C.* 2007;145C:232-40.

[9] Gruters A, Biebermann H, Krude H. Neonatal thyriod disorders. *Horm. Res.* 2003;59(Suppl 1):24-9.

[10] Höybye C. Endocrine and metabolic aspects of adult Prader-Willi syndrome with special emphasis on the effect of growth hormone treatment. *Growth Horm. IGF Res.* 2004;5:1-15.

[11] Vining EP. You've come a long way, Baby: Or have you? *Epilepsy Curr.* 2008;8(5):118-9.

[12] Raphaelson MI, Stevens JC, Elders J, Comite F, Theodore WH. Familial spastic paraplegia, mental retardation, and precocious puberty. *Arch. Neurol.* 1983;40(13):809-10.

[13] Mills JL, Hediger ML, Molloy CA, Chrousos GP, Manning-Courtney P, Yu KF, Brasington M, England LJ. Eleveated levels of growth-related hormones in autism and autism spectrum disorder. *Clin. Endocrinol.* 2007;67:230-7.

[14] Morad M, Kandel I, Merrick J. National survey 2001 on medical services for persons with intellectual disability in residential care in Israel. *Int. J. Disabil. Hum. Dev.* 2007;6(3):317-22.

[15] Merrick J, Kandel I. Down syndrome and obesity. *Int. J. Child Health Hum. Dev.* 2008;1(4):xx-xx.

[16] Vanlint S. Vitamin D and people with intellectual disability. *Aust. Fam. Physician.* 2008;37(5):348-50.

In: Adolescence and Chronic Illness
Editors: H. Omar et al.

ISBN: 978-1-60876-628-4
© 2010 Nova Science Publishers, Inc.

Chapter 5

METABOLISM AND DISEASE

Efrat Merrick-Kenig[*1], *Mohammed Morad*[1,2,3] *and Joav Merrick*[1,4]

[1] National Institute of Child Health and Human Development,
Office of the Medical Director, Division for Mental Retardation,
Ministry of Social Affairs, Jerusalem, Israel.
[2] Department of Family Medicine, Faculty of Health Sciences,
Ben Gurion University of the Negev, Beer-Sheva, Israel.
[3] Clalit Health Services, Beer-Sheva, Israel.
[4] Kentucky Children's Hospital, University of Kentucky
College of Medicine, Lexington, U.S.A.

ABSTRACT

Metabolism refers to all biochemical processes and pathways in the body, where food eaten is processed and used for energy amd building blocks in the body. The major metabolic pathways for proteins, carbohydrates and lipids are closely integrated with key molecules and a genetic defect in any part of the major metabolic pathways can result in an inborn or congenital error of metabolism. Over the past nearly 100 years the scientific community has slowly discovered metabolic diseases, their reasons and pathways and their effects upon the human being and human development. It has been a battle to find the reasons and aome of the parts of the puzzle to the cure for intellectual disability. For a few diseases science has found solutions around early screening and detection, while for other we are still far away for a screening tool. With the increased knowledge we have also been able to find solutions in order to treat and prevent intellectual disability.

INTRODUCTION

There are today more than 1,400 inherited metabolic diseases described today. Metabolism refers to all biochemical processes and pathways in the body, where food eaten is

---

[*] *Correspondence:* Efrat Merrick-Kenig, MD, National Institute of Child Health and Human Development, Office of the Medical Director, Division for Mental Retardation, Ministry of Social Affairs, Box 1260, IL-91012 Jerusalem, Israel. E-mail: efratmerrick@gmail.com

processed and used for energy amd building blocks in the body. The major metabolic pathways for proteins, carbohydrates and lipids are closely integrated with key molecules and a genetic defect in any part of the major metabolic pathways can result in an inborn or congenital error of metabolism. The term inborn error of metabolism was coined by a British physician, Archibald Garrod (1857-1936), in the early 20th century. Metabolism is carried out by chemical substances called enzymes, which are made by the body. If a genetic abnormality affects the function of an enzyme or causes it to be deficient or missing altogether, various disorders can occur. Inborn errors of metabolism can be divided into three pathophysiological diagnostic groups:

- Disorders that disrupt the synthesis or catabolism of complex molecules with symptoms that are permanent, progressive, independent of intercurrent events and not related to food intake. These include lysosomal disorders, peroxisomal disorders and disorders of intracellular transport and processing.
- Disorders that lead to an acute or progressive accumulation of toxic compounds as a result of metabolic block. These include disorders of amino acid metabolism (phenylketonuria, homocystinuria, maple syrup urine disease), organic acidurias, congenital urea cycle defects and sugar intolerances (galactosaemia).
- Disorders with symptoms due to a deficiency of energy production or utilisation within the liver, myocardium, muscle or brain. These include congenital lactic acidemias, fatty acid oxidation defects, gluconeogenesis defects and mitochondrial respiratory chain disorders.

The mechanisms for brain damage resulting in intellectual disability are not understood well and relatively few metabolic conditions cause intellectual disability in isolation (Kahler & Fahey, 2003).

SCREENING

Metabolic disorders are a heterogeneous group of genetic conditions mostly occurring in childhood and individually rare, but collectively numerous resulting in substantial morbidity and mortality.

One study from the United Kingdon [1] looked at the 1999-2003 period and found the overall birth prevalence at 1 in 784 live births (95% confidence interval (CI) 619 to 970), based on a total of 396 new cases with the most frequent diagnoses mitochondrial disorders (1 in 4929; 95% CI 2776 to 8953), lysosomal storage disorders (1 in 5175; 95% CI 2874 to 9551), amino acid disorders excluding phenylketonuria (1 in 5354; 95% CI 2943 to 9990) and organic acid disorders (1 in 7962; 95% CI 3837 to 17 301). Most of the diagnoses (72%) were made by the age of 15 years and one-third by the age of 1 year. Another study from Luxembourg looked at all school children with intellectual disability in special school and residential care centers for person with intellectual disability and found that 1% showed metabolic abnormality (2Kutter & Metz, 1968).

As a classic example of how neonatal screening has progressed, let us take the example of phenylketonuria (PKU). PKU was discovered in 1934, when a Norwegian mother brought her intellectually disabled son and daughter to professor Ivar Asbjørn Følling (1888-1973) at the University of Oslo School of Medicine for a consultation [3]. In 1947, Jervis [4] showed that the administration of phenylalanine to normal humans led to a promt rise in blood tyrosine, whereas no increase in blood tyrosine could be detected in patients with PKU, indicating both the normal pathway of phenylalanine metabolism and the metabolic error in PKU. Several years later this inborn error of the amino acid metabolism, caused by the deficiency of the liver enzyme phenylalanine hydroxylase (PAH), changed to become a preventable form of intellectual disability, when Bickel et al [5] published the results of dietary treatment. The work of Jervis [4] and Bickel et al [5] was the incentive that led to the large field of investigations into the inborn errors of metabolism that became the basis for the understanding of a range of causes of mental retardation, developmental disability or intellectual disability, the possibility for treatment and prevention.

Several further studies stressed the importance of diet for these patients and a drive started to develop a diagnostic method to measure phenylalanine in the blood. Guthrie & Susi [6] developed a bacterial "inhibition assay" that facilitated a sensitive, specific, inexpensive and fast method for the determination of blood phenylalanine in large number of samples. Robert Guthrie (1916-1995), an American microbiologist, fought and won the battle for a screening tool motived by the fact that his son had intellectual disability.

From 1964-73 [3] different types of PKU were found and worldwide neonatal screening started resulting in early treatment and prevention of intellectual disability and since then more disease screening has been added. In Israel neonatal screening started in 1963. Whereas everyone can agree that treatment with phenylalanine (PHE) restricted diet must start as soon as possible (first two weeks of life), there is not universal agreement on when to stop, but in recent years we have come to understand the need for a "diet for life" [7].

Tandem mass spectrometry is now more and more being used as an analytical method implemented for neonatal screening. The method can determine the content of amino acids and acylcarnitines in neonatal screening samples in one integrated analysis. This allows detection of more than 20 inherited disorders of amino acid, fatty acid and organic acid metabolism.

METABOLIC DISEASE

Inborn errors of metabolism are inherited defects in human metabolism. To improve the prognosis for metabolic diseases, early recognition is necessary. Many infants with metabolic diseases can be diagnosed with routine biochemical tests and metabolic screening of urine. For some metabolic diseases, an early diagnosis will lead to specific treatment and improved prognosis, for others to genetic counseling and prenatal diagnosis.

Metabolic disorders can present with a great assortment of signs and symptoms that mimic non-genetic disorders. Common presenting symptoms are acute neonatal symptoms, failure to thrive, CNS symptoms such as developmental delay, movement or psychiatric disorder or cerebral palsy, sudden infant death syndrome (SIDS), episodic illness (anorexia, vomiting, lethargy, coma), cardiomyopathy, muscular (hypotonic, weakness, cramps), gastrointestinal (anorexia, vomiting, diarrhoea, malabsorption), liver disease, ophthalmic abnormalities, Reye's syndrome-like illness, dysmorphic features or metabolic manifestations (acidosis, hypoglycaemia).

Acute symptoms in the neonatal period can be very non-specific like respiratory distress, hypotonia, poor sucking reflex, vomiting, diarrhoea, dehydration, lethargy and seizures, which can be just the same symptoms as in infection. Children or babies with metabolic disorders of accumulation can show deterioration after a normal initial period that can last hours or weeks.

Another type of late onset symptoms are seem with metabolic disorders of toxic accumulation or energy production, where the child have a normal symptom free period for one year or more and even extend into late childhood, adolescence or even adulthood. Symptoms may be triggered by a viral infection, fever or diarrhoea, which result in the body reverting to the breakdown of stored protein within the cells and tissue. The child can improve without intervention and diagnosis missed or prolonged. General or chronic gastrointestinal, neurological and muscular complaints may also eventually lead to diagnosis.

In this short chapter we will not be able to list all the metabolic disease, but will describe each group mentioned above.

Lysosomal Storage Disorders

The lysosomal storage diseases are a heterogeneous group of disorders (over 40 known today) with a progressive accumulation of undegraded catabolites [8]. Due to the deficiency catabolites will be stored in the reticuloendothelial and nervous system with central nervous system damage and resulting intellectual disability. The lysosomal storage diseases are classified by the nature of the primary stored material involved into lipid storage disorders, mainly sphingolipidoses (including Gaucher's and Niemann-Pick diseases), gangliosidosis (like Tay-Sachs disease), leukodystrophies, mucopolysaccharidoses, glycoprotein storage disorders and mucolipidoses.

A cure has not been found for this group of metabolic diseases and treatment is therefore symptomatic. Bone marrow transplantation and enzyme replacement therapy have been tried with some success, but it is hoped that gene therapy (introduce the gene for a missing enzyme product in to blood, liver or other cells) may offer cures in the future [8].

Phenylketonuria

As mentioned above phenylketonuria (PKU) is a classic example of how a metabolic disease causing intellectual disability was discovered, diagnosed and universal screening and early detection implemented, which resulted in prevention of the consequences and early diet treatment. It also showed that when medicine solves one problem another arise. Due to the idea that the diet should only be implemented, while the brain was developing it resulted in children growing up with PKU and when the girls became pregnant (without having the diet before and during pregnancy) their offspring became affected [8] and "diet for life" [7] is therefore recommended for every child diagnosed with PKU.

Mitochondrial Disorders

Research in mitochondrial and metabolic medical conditions (called mitochondrial cytopathies) has taken a rapid development since the first case was diagnosed in 1959 [9]. A mitochondrion (singular of mitochondria) is part of every cell in the body that contains genetic material and responsible for processing oxygen and converting substances into energy for essential cell functions. Mitochondria produce energy in the form of adenosine triphosphate (ATP), which is then transported to the cytoplasm of a cell for use in numerous cell functions. Mitochondrial disorders now include more than 40 different identified diseases that have different genetic features (more than several hundred phenotypes). The common factor among these diseases is that the mitochondria are unable to completely burn food and oxygen in order to generate energy and the incompletely burned food accumulate inside the body.

Mitochondrial diseases might affect the cells of the brain, nerves (including the nerves to the stomach and intestines), muscles, kidneys, heart, liver, eyes, ears, or pancreas. In some patients, only one organ is affected, while in other patients all the organs are involved. Depending on how severe the mitochondrial disorder is, the illness can range in severity from mild to fatal.

Again symptoms are not specific, like poor growth, loss of muscle coordination and muscle weakness, visual and/or hearing problems, developmental delays, learning disabilities and intellectual disability, heart, liver or kidney disease, gastrointestinal disorders, respiratory disorders, diabetes, seizures and dementia. Diagnosis is technically and timewise a difficult task, but involving many disciplines. In adults, many diseases of aging have been found to have defects of mitochondrial function, like type 2 diabetes, Parkinson's disease, atherosclerotic heart disease, stroke, Alzheimer's disease and cancer.

There are no cures for mitochondrial diseases, but treatment can help reduce symptoms, or delay or prevent the progression of the disease, but must be individualized by specialists. There is no way today to predict the prognosis.

CONCLUSIONS

It this short chapter it has been impossible to review all the different metabolic diseases, where intellectual disability is part of the spectrum. Over the past nearly 100 years the scientific community has slowly discovered metabolic diseases, their reasons and pathways and their effects upon the human being and human development. It has been a battle to find the reasons and aome of the parts of the puzzle to the cure for intellectual disability [10].

For a few diseases science has found solutions around early screening and detection [10], while for other we are still far away for a screening tool. With the increased knowledge we have also been able to find solutions in order to treat and prevent intellectual disability.

Again there is a lot of unknown territory and much more to learn and investigate and it is hoped that the human genome project will help us part of the way and eventually provide a gene therapy for many of these diseases that today have severe consequences for the child, family and society.

REFERENCES

[1] Sanderson S, Green A, Preece MA Burton H. The incidence of inherited metabolic disorders in the West Midlands, UK. *Arch. Dis. Child.* 2006;91(11):896-9.
[2] Kutter D, Metz H. The frequency of some oligophrenias due to metabolic disease in the grand-duchy of Luxembourg. [Schweizer Archiv für Neurologie, Neurochirurgie und Psychiatrie]. *Schweiz. Arch. Neurol. Neurochir. Psychiatr.* 1968;101:369-82.
[3] Guttler F. Phenylketonuria: 50 years since Folling's discovery and still expanding our clinical and biochemical knowledge. Acta Paediatr Scand 1984;73:705-16.
[4] Jervis GA. Studies on phenylpyruvic oligophrenia. The position of the metabolic error. *J. Biol. Chemistry.* 1947;169:651-6.
[5] Bickel H, Gerrard J, Hickmans EM. The influence of phenylalanine intake on the chemestry and behavior of a phenylketonuria child. *Acta Paediatr. Scand.* 1954;43:64-77.
[6] Guthrie R, Susi A. A simple phenylalanine method for detecting phenylketonuria in populations of newborn infants. *Pediatrics.* 1963; 32:338-43.
[7] Merrick J, Aspler S, Schwarz G. Should adults with phenylketonuria have treatment? *Ment. Retard.* 2001;39(3):216-7.
[8] Kahler SG, Fahey MC. Metabolic disorders and mental retardation. *Am. J. Med. Genetics Part C.* (Semin Med Genet) 2003;117C:31-41.
[9] Shoffner JM. Metochondrial disorders. In: Rubin IL, Crocker AC, eds. *Medical care for children and adults with developmental disabilities.* Baltimore: Paul Brookes, 2006:130-37.
[10] Koch JH. Robert Guthrie. The PKU story. *A crusade against mental retardation.* Pasadena, CA: Hope Publ House, 1997.

Part V. Diseases of the Blood

In: Adolescence and Chronic Illness
Editors: H. Omar et al.

ISBN: 978-1-60876-628-4
© 2010 Nova Science Publishers, Inc.

Chapter 6

CHRONIC HEMATOLOGICAL DISORDERS

Elna N. Saah[*], *Renuka Gera, Ajovi B. Scott-Emuakpor and Roshni Kulkarni*

Division of Pediatric and Adolescent Hematology/Oncology,
Pediatric and Adolescent Sickle Cell Program,
MSU Center for Bleeding and Clotting Disorders,
Department of Pediatrics/Human Development,
Michigan State University, East Lansing,
Michigan, United States of America.

ABSTRACT

Disorders of hemostasis (coagulopathies) and those of hemoglobin (hemoglobinopathies) account for the majority of chronic hematological diseases seen in adolescents. Advances in clinical medicine have led to the effective management of children with these chronic hematological conditions. As a result, almost all of them survive beyond adolescence to adulthood. Both the coagulopathies and the hemoglobinopathies can lead to permanent disabilities in the adolescent, the full impact of which has not been fully researched. This review seeks to elucidate the range and kinds of disabilities experienced by children and adolescents with chronic hematological diseases. These disabilities are considered under the following headings: Intellectual and cognitive disability, psychosocial and emotional disability, physical mobility disability and major organ dysfunction.

---

[*] *Correspondence:* Elna N Saah, MD, Div. of Pediatric & Adolescent Hematology/Oncology, Pediatrics & Human Development, Michigan State University College of Human Medicine, B225 Clinical Center, 138 Service Rd, East Lansing, MI 48824-1313 United States. Tel:517-355-8998; Fax: 517-355-8312; E-mail: Elna.Saah@hc.msu.edu

INTRODUCTION

Disorders of hemostasis and those of hemoglobin, account for the majority of chronic hematological diseases seen in adolescents. Hemorrhagic and thrombotic diseases essentially deal with the ability of the body to prevent excessive bleeding or to prevent excessive clotting. The flow of blood through our veins is a delicate balance between the tendency to bleed and that to clot. The mechanisms that promote each of these two phenomena must exert opposite but equal influences on the body. Abnormalities do occur from time to time in these mechanisms, and when they occur are referred to as coagulopathies.

The function of hemoglobin is to carry oxygen and to distribute it throughout the body. The hemoglobin molecule is precisely structured and must maintain this structure to perform its function efficiently. Hemoglobin also must be present in sufficient quantities in the body for the optimum performance of its function. The structural derangement of hemoglobin will distort its functional quality, and insufficient production of any component of it will reduce its quantity. Together, these abnormalities are referred to as hemoglobinopathies.

Advances in clinical medicine have led to the effective management of children with these chronic hematological conditions. As a result, almost all these children survive beyond adolescence to adulthood. Both the coagulopathies and the hemoglobinopathies can lead to permanent disabilities in the adolescent, the full impact of which has not been fully realized. This review will therefore attempt to elucidate the range and kinds of disabilities experienced by children and adolescents with chronic hematological diseases.

Disability is defined, in the context of this discussion, as the "inability to carry out age-appropriate daily activities as a result of health condition or impairment" [1].

COAGULOPATHIES

Two main types of coagulopathies exist: diseases of excessive bleeding (hemophilia), and diseases of excessive clotting (thrombophilia). Among the several disorders of excessive bleeding, the most common are hemophilia A and hemophilia B. Both hemophilia A and hemophilia B are inherited as X-linked recessive bleeding disorders that respectively lead to a decreased synthesis of the normally functioning coagulation factors VIII and IX. The incidence is estimated at about 1 in 5000 live males births [2], and factor VIII deficiency accounts for 85% of these cases. Factor IX deficiency constitutes about 14%, and the 1% left is made up of very rare factor deficiencies, such as Factors V, VII, X, and XI.

Another bleeding disorder that may rarely cause some disabilities in adolescents is Von Willebrand disease. Von Willebrand disease (vWD) is the most common hereditary coagulation abnormality in humans, affecting 1% to 3% of the population. The disorder results from a qualitative or quantitative deficiency of von Willebrand factor (vWF), a multimeric protein that is required for platelet adhesion. Von Willebrand Factor is a protein critical to the initial stages of blood clotting. This glue-like protein, produced by the cells that line the blood vessel walls, interacts with platelets to form a plug that prevents the blood from flowing at the site of injury. People with von Willebrand Disease are unable to make this plug because they do not have enough vWF or, if they do have vWF, then it is abnormal. This disease is known to affect humans and in, veterinary medicine, dogs. Three types of hereditary vWD exist, which have been extensively described elsewhere [3].

In humans, the incidence of vWD is roughly between 1% and 2 %. Because most forms are rather mild, they are detected more often in women, whose bleeding tendency shows up in adolescence during menstruation. The disease may be more severe or apparent in people with blood group O. About two-thirds of adolescents with bleeding disorders have severe clinical disease with factor levels of < 1%; these individuals are the ones that experience spontaneous bleeding. This spontaneous bleeding or trauma-related bleeding is clinically associated with varying degrees of impaired function in the individual, depending on the site of the bleed.

The disorders of thrombosis can also be divided into two groups—the inherited thrombotic diseases and the acquired thrombotic diseases. Individuals in the first group have inherited a deficiency in one of the proteins responsible for anti-coagulation mechanism, such as antithrombin III (ATIII), protein C, or protein S.

More common than these three are two inherited disorders of anti-coagulation defect. One is an inherited syndrome of resistance to the anti-coagulation properties of protein C, referred to as factor V Leiden. In this disorder, the Leiden variant of factor V cannot be inactivated by activated protein C. Factor V Leiden, the most common hereditary hypercoagulability disorder found in humans, is present in 5% of the Caucasian population versus 1.2% of the African-American population. This factor increases the risk of venous thrombosis by 3- to 8-fold for heterozygous and substantially more, 30- to 140-fold, for homozygous individuals.

The other disorder is a prothrombin mutation that is the second most commonly inherited clotting abnormality, which is found in the heterozygous state in about 2% of the general population. This mutation is only a mild risk factor for blood clots, but together with other risk factors (such as oral contraceptives, surgery, trauma, high blood pressure, obesity, and smoking) or combined with other clotting disorders (such as factor V Leiden), the risk of clotting increases dramatically in these adolescents.

In the second group of thrombotic diseases belong individuals with an apparent high risk for developing thrombosis. For the most part, the mechanism for this increased risk for hypercoagulability is poorly under-stood. The underlying mechanism is an inherited abnormality in about one-third to one-half of children or adolescents with thrombosis. The hypercoagulable state leads to increased risks for blood clots, the location of which can be unpredictable. The kind of impairment, therefore, will depend, as in hemorrhagic diseases, on the location of the clot and the behavior of the clot.

To understand these disabilities, one must appreciate the manifestations of the coagulopathies. For excessive bleeding, these manifestations include easy bruising, spontaneous hemorrhage into tissues and joints, post-operative bleeding if not well managed pre-and intra-operatively, and a wide array of sociopsychological problems, such as occupational and economic issues. For excessive clotting, the manifestations also include a wide array of sociopsychological problems. In addition, there are manifestations caused by obstruction to blood flow, such as pain, swelling, and ischemia, as well as those caused by inflammation of the vessel wall or by embolization of the blood clot. Indeed, reports have shown that as many as 50% of all patients with deep vein thrombosis (DVT) of the legs will have embolization to the lungs [4], some of which are subclinical.

For the purpose of this chapter, impairments and disabilities will be divided into four broad categories:

1. Intellectual and cognitive disability
2. Psychosocial and emotional disability
3. Physical mobility disability
4. Major organ dysfunction

Intellectual and Cognitive Disability

Patients with hemostatic disorders are at risk for intellectual and cognitive disability, usually resulting from direct injury to the brain caused by an intracranial bleed or thrombotic event. The incidence of spontaneous intracranial hemorrhage (ICH) in hemophiliacs ranges between 2.6% to 13.8% [5]. In children, the incidence may be as high as 10% [6] and is nearly always preceded by trauma. In young adults, only about 50% of ICH cases are related to trauma [5,7]. Approximately one-third of ICH events will result in death, whereas 50% of the survivors will develop long-term neurologic sequelae [5]. Survivors without clinically recognizable neurologic deficits develop varying degrees of intellectual and cognitive impairments.

Data from the Hemophilia Treatment Center of Central Pennsylvania showed a disproportionately high incidence of attention deficit hyperactivity disorder (ADHD) (28.3%) and learning disability (15.8%) among their 66 hemophiliacs [8]. A higher incidence of ADHD in boys with hemophilia, ages 5-14 years, was reported in another study, which also showed that 38% of the boys were in special education programs [9].

The work of Shapiro and co-workers [10], a multicenter data collection, found a significant correlation between academic achievement and the number of bleeds in a cohort of school age boys with hemophilia. In the same study, the mathematics score of boys having less than 11 bleeds/year was significantly better than the score for boys with more than 11 bleeds/year. These are clearly troublesome problems for such adolescents. In the Universal Data Collection (UDC) of the Centers for Disease Control and Prevention (CDC), the average numbers of school/work days missed due to joint problems ranged from 6.7-11.4 days.

Thrombosis and thromboembolic events are believed to be responsible for focal ischemia of the brain [11]. Such events are very rare in children, but when they do occur, they leave serious physical and intellectual impairment. For instance, in adolescent girls with inherited thrombophilia, use of oral contraceptives is associated with increased risk for thrombosis, including cerebral venous sinus thrombosis that can result in neurological and cognitive deficits.

Psychosocial and Emotional Disability

Mental health issues in adolescents have been studied extensively. Even without the presence of a chronic disease, adolescence is the age of complex mental health issues [12]. It is important to understand that mental health and physical health have bi-directional relationships. The American Psychiatric Association states, "A compelling literature documents that there is much physical in mental disorders and much mental in physical disorders" [13]. Against this background, we have to remember that medical advances now allow children with these chronic hematological conditions to lead more productive and longer lives. Consequently, the psychological aspects of such living with a 'bad' disease must be understood, particularly as their emotional development is affected.

As these hematological conditions are primarily congenital, the child begins to feel the impact of the disease before learning any skills. Early childhood is the time when motor, speech, and cognitive skills develop rapidly and these serious diseases render the acquisition of such skills very vulnerable [14]. Any impairment in the acquisition of these skills will manifest itself as a disability in adolescence. This situation is not related to hematological diseases only but is also true for any chronic illness. Crucial developmental issues in adolescence include the following:

1   a need to navigate an independent existence;
2   identity formation, such as self and body image;
3   socialization; and
4   future orientation [15].

Achieving these normal tasks is severely compromised and complicated by any chronic illness of childhood, leading to psychological impairments.

Besides school absences due to bleeds that may reflect on academic achievement, the fear of bleeding in joints and pain in the joints secondary to bleeding may lead to passivity or in some cases, to risky behaviors. Added to this stress is the expense of treatment, the guilt of passing the disease to an offspring, as well as the fear of exposure to unknown pathogens from treatment. Anger, resentment, and social stigmatization may lead to considerable psychosocial maladjustment.

Physical Mobility Impairment

Spontaneous bleeding into a joint (hemarthrosis) and spontaneous muscle hematomas are characteristic of severe hemophilia A and hemophilia B. The knees are the most common sites of bleeding followed by, in descending order of frequency, elbows, ankles, shoulders, hips, and wrists [16]. This phenomenon can also be seen in moderate and severe deficiencies of fibrinogen, prothrombin, and factors V, VII, and X [17]. Such bleeding may also occur, though rarely, in severe Von Willebrand disease with associated factor VIII levels of < 5%. Although it is believed that such bleeds are spontaneous, they usually do not occur until the child begins to walk, and the bleeding may become worse with increased activity in adolescence.

Once bleeding occurs, inflammatory and proliferative changes take place in the joint, leading to synovial hyperplasia that is more friable and more prone to further bleeding. This vicious cycle of rebleeding becomes established, leading to hemophilic arthropathy [18]. Home-based care combined with prophylactic factor replacement therapy has reduced the incidence of hemophilic arthropathy and impaired joint function in the adolescent. However, the patient with hemophilia who has developed an 'inhibitor' to the factor will continue to remain at risk for spontaneous bleeding and arthropathy.

Intramuscular hemorrhages are second to hem-arthrosis as the most prevalent type of bleeding in hemophilia, accounting for about 40% of all bleeding events [19]. In large muscles, aside from the severe pain and morbidity, this bleeding may not constitute a serious problem. In smaller muscles, bleeding may occur in closed fascial compartment and may cause serious compression of vital structures, such as arteries and nerves, leading to gangrene and neuropathies (compartment syndrome) [20]. Bleeding into the ileopsoas muscle and retroperitoneal space can be very disabling and life threatening because of the large amount of blood that can be lost in the soft tissues of the retroperitoneal space [21]. Once again, because of extensive prophylactic use of factor replacement, these clinical presentations have significantly decreased in frequency.

Thrombosis can also lead to significant disabilities in movement. For instance, one chronic complication of DVT is called post-thrombotic syndrome (PTS). This condition is a consequence of damage to the venous valves leading to outflow obstructions and eventual venous insufficiency [22]. The symptoms are pain, which can be very severe, heaviness due to swelling, paresthesias, and cramping [23]. This is a significant disabling condition when it occurs in children and adolescents, leading to reduced activity and exercise intolerance. The incidence in adolescents and young adults with DVT is not known, but in older adults, PTS may be as high as 65-80% of all DVTs.

Major Organ Dysfunction

Any time that bleeding occurs in an organ, the chances of the event causing permanent damage to the organ are real. This probability is clearly illustrated by the report that persons with hemophilia who had chronic renal disease were more likely to be those who had been hospitalized with a kidney bleed [24]. Massive bleeding produces immediate symptoms and attracts immediate therapeutic interventions to stop the bleeding and save the organ. It is the slow and insidious bleed that, over time, exerts a damaging effect on organ function. Whereas the damage to an organ is slow in small bleeds, except in central nervous system (CNS) bleeds, thrombosis, on the other hand, has an immediate and dramatic effect on organ function. For instance, renal vein thrombosis presents with severe flank pain, hematuria, and sudden impairment of renal function [25]. Vague complaints from a child with a known bleeding disorder must be evaluated thoroughly to ascertain that no small bleeds into organs have occurred.

Very serious impairment occurs whenever there is bleeding into the CNS. The neurologic presentation is immediate and can be very serious, leaving long-term neurologic deficits in the child and adolescent. Aside from major bleeding into the joints and muscles, as previously discussed, small intramuscular hematomas are commonly seen and cause transient but significant pain. These hematomas usually resolve spontaneously. Rarely, intraosseous hemorrhages may occur, leading to a rare skeletal complication of hemophilia called hemophilic pseudotumor [26]. It is pertinent to mention here that the use of prophylactic factor replacement has rendered the occurrence of these dangerous bleeding events rare.

In thrombosis, the dysfunction of an affected organ can be immediate and dramatic. One of the notable features of thrombophilia is venous thrombosis in unusual places, such as those of the CNS and abdominal cavity. Symptoms of thrombosis outside the extremities are very vague, making diagnosis delayed.

Cerebral vein thrombosis is a well-recognized event that occurs in thrombophiliacs [27,28]. When cerebral vein thrombosis occurs, the venous pressure is markedly increased, which leads to cerebral edema and its physical consequences. Sometimes multiple cerebral infarctions can arise, leading to secondary hemorrhages. The neurologic deficits from such an event may be mild to severe, leaving permanent disabilities, such as learning, behavioral, and mobility disabilities. Central retinal vein thrombosis, leading to significant visual impairment has been reported in individuals with inherited thrombo-philia, such as prothrombin mutation [28] and activated protein C resistance mutation [29].

Abdominal thrombosis can be very challenging because the symptoms of mesenteric or portal vein thrombosis are very vague. The process can evolve over several days, sometimes leading to a surgical abdomen, before the thrombosis is recognized [30,31]. By contrast, hepatic vein thrombosis may have a fulminant presentation with sudden abdominal pain, enlarging painful liver, and massive ascites [32]. Mortality for this condition is as high as 67%, and survivors often suffer from chronic ascites and varying degrees of hepatic insufficiency. Renal vein thrombosis, when it occurs, is associated with severe dehydration in the neonate but, more commonly, is associated with the nephrotic syndrome. Renal vein thrombosis has a rapid effect on renal function, causing pain and hematuria immediately [25,33].

Thrombosis in the upper extremities used to be quite rare but now is a very common finding because of the widespread use of central venous catheters for chemotherapy and other treatment modalities requiring prolonged and frequent venous access. These thromboses are usually associated with long-term chronic pain and swelling of the arms and shoulders [34]. A complication of thrombosis that deserves mention is pulmonary embolism (PE), which is believed to occur in about 7% to 8% of adolescents and is marked by dyspnea and tachypnea and always associated with symptoms of deep vein thrombosis [35]. Permanent damage to the lungs and mortality from PE is very low in children, reflecting their better physiologic state [36,37].

HEMOGLOBINOPATHIES

The hemoglobinopathies, which include sickle cell disease (SCD) and thalassemia, are among the most common inherited human blood disorders. The thalassemias are quantitative defects in globin chain synthesis, whereas SCD is a qualitative defect that results in the synthesis of structurally abnormal globin chains. Chronic anemia is the hallmark of both disorders. Additionally, these disorders cause a wide spectrum of organ dysfunction, resulting in significant physical, emotional, and social impairments and disabilities. Since the 1970's, research has made significant progress in our understanding of the disease pathophysiology and management, which has led to remarkable improve-ment in the life expectancy of such patients, especially in developed parts of the world [38,39]. With inter-ventions that have decreased mortality, affected patients are living longer and are facing different challenges. These diseases and their interventions, over time, cause significant impairment in growth and development of adolescents and place them at risk for disruptions, difficulties, and poor quality of life.

It is imperative that all health care providers of this cohort of patients adequately and frequently assess the impact of these chronic disorders on growth, develop-ment, and quality of life. Their goal is to develop and institute programs to ensure normal growth and improve health related quality of life (HRQOL) (http://www.cdc.gov/hrqol/). Health related quality of life is an individual's self reported physical and emotional well-being. In children and adolescents, or more severely impaired adults, a parent or caregiver assessment is usually incorporated [40].

SICKLE CELL DISEASE (SCD)

Sickle cell disease is most prevalent in persons of African descent or Hispanic ethnicity, but affects people of all racial and ethnic backgrounds. The disease is seen in persons of African descent (sub-Saharan), the Medi-terranean, Arabian Peninsula, and the Indian subcon-tinent. Due to migration and shifts in population demographics, however, the disease is seen in many parts of the world, including Central and South America.

Sickle cell disease represents a group of hemo-globinopathies that are inherited as autosomal recessive conditions. Each of these diseases has one abnormal sickle hemoglobin (S) gene with another hemoglobin S gene in a homozygous state or with another abnormal non-S hemoglobin gene in a compound heterozygous state. The other abnormal hemoglobins include, but are not limited to, C, E, ß0, ß+, OArab, giving the hemoglobin genotypes of SS, SC, SE, Sß0, S ß+, SOArab, and many less frequent combinations, resulting in a wide spectrum of genotypes and phenotypes. The most severe of the SCDs are the homozygous SS and the compound heterozygous Sß0 forms.

The presence of the sickle hemoglobin leads to decreased red blood cell survival and, consequently, to anemia of varying degrees of severity. Even among the same genotype, phenotypic variation occurs, which is believed to be the result of other disease modulators playing a significant role in suppressing the expressivity. To date, many such modulators are known, the most frequently encountered being the persistence of fetal hemoglobin (HbF), the white blood cell count, baseline hemoglobin, and the inversely related reticulocyte count. Due to recent advances in the management of SCD, such as penicillin prophylaxis, pneumococcal vaccines, and prompt antibacterial therapy for febrile episodes, childhood mortality has decreased significantly. Newborn screening, the early identification of children at risk for stroke through the use of transcranial Doppler and the use of drugs like hydroxyurea to prevent painful episodes have contributed to reduced morbidity. Currently, bone-marrow or stem-cell transplantation affords the only cure for the disease. Despite these major advances, health care disparities remain an issue, and many adolescents with SCD continue to incur disabilities.

THALASSEMIAS

The thalassemias refer to a group of hemoglobinopathies characterized by imbalance in the synthesis of one or more globin chains (alpha or beta). These diseases, although encountered worldwide because of gene migration, predominantly affect people of Mediterranean, Indian, Asian, and African descent. Significant advances have also been made in the management of these disorders, and patients are now living longer [38]. Some of the strategies for the effective management of such patients include life-long transfusion to maintain the target hemoglobin concentration of 9-10g/dl to suppress erythropoiesis adequately, iron chelation therapy, the prevention of infection, and bone marrow transplantation. These modalities of treatment have significantly improved the growth and development and HRQOL of adolescents with these diseases.

For the purpose of this discussion, emphasis will be placed on ß-thalassemia and its variants. It is important to mention, however, that alpha thalassemia usually results in pregnancy loss from hydrops fetalis, unless in utero transfusions are commenced. For this reason, only a few patients are surviving worldwide.

In discussing the impact of SCD and thalassemia on the mental, social, and physical development in the adolescent, we have to point out that a great overlap exists between systems in the overall cause of disability. Hence, the major areas can best be analyzed under four broad categories:

1. Intellectual and cognitive impairment
2. Psychosocial and emotional impairment
3. Physical impairment
4. Major organ dysfunction

Intellectual and Cognitive Impairment

Both overt and silent cerebrovascular events are the most common causes of intellectual and cognitive impairment in patients with SCD [41]. School absenteeism for pain, hospitalization, or transfusions further increases the likelihood of poor academic performance and the risk of being held back in school. Neuroimaging studies have been performed in adults with thalassemia to evaluate the role of silent infarcts and their impact on neurocognitive function; however, this topic has not been evaluated in children and adolescents.

Psychosocial and Emotional Impairment

Some patients with SCD have been observed to have varying neuropsychological impairments, even in the absence of overt stroke [41]. In addition to the complex interplay of physical pain and psychological distress, children with SCD have delayed growth and develop-ment. Of utmost importance to the developing teen is stature and puberty. Impotence secondary to priapism in patients with SCD can further contribute to low self-image and interfere with personal relationships [42]. Poor self esteem and behavior issues, due to the factors stated above, may herald the onset of adjustment disorder. Parents report coping difficulties in up to 64% of patients [43]; maladjustment and other psychological problems appear to be more prevalent in boys than girls [44]. However, despite the growing body of evidence for increased psychosocial problems, most patients and families cope well. Being aware of positive coping mechanisms is important, as well as screening to identify patients at high risk. As a result, psychological evaluation should be part of the routine care of such children.

The source of psychological distress for children with thalassemia is multifactorial and complex, involving the interplay of burden of care, disease burden, and physical appearance.

The lifelong transfusion require-ment necessitates monthly visits to a hospital or a transfusion center and iron chelation therapy. Because of delayed growth and development, such children may have aberrant body perception. Probably in defiance to nightly subcutaneous injections for chelation, patients with thalassemia major were noted in one study to have an increased incidence of oppositional defiance disorder (ODD) [45].

Physical Impairment

Chronic anemia causes fatigue, reduced exercise tolerance, and exertional dyspnea; this deficiency can result in an inability to participate in age-appropriate athletic activities. Although most children by the time they enter adolescence are already aware of their limitations and have adjusted to their limitations, some may develop emotional problems. Additional physical disabilities result from organ damage caused by the disease or its interventions. Leg ulcers are a frequent cause of physical disability in both SCD and thalassemia.

Pain: Acute and Chronic

Pain is the hallmark of the clinical spectrum of SCD and is characterized by recurrent painful vaso-occlusive episodes that start early in life. By the time that such patients reach adolescence, some may develop the chronic pain syndrome. A recent prospective study of pain in adults with SCD found that daily pain, mostly managed at home, was far more prevalent and severe than prior large studies have indicated. The authors conclude that the prevalence of pain is probably underestimated by health care providers, resulting in misclassification, distorted communication, and under-treatment [46]. Recurrent pain crisis, hospitalizations, and the use of narcotic analgesic have a negative impact on the functional status and quality of life of an adolescent.

Acute Pain

As noted, the acute painful vaso-occlusive episode is the insignia of sickle cell disease. Although the frequency may decrease with age, this condition is still the most common cause for hos-pitalizations and is often underestimated, underreported, and under-treated [46,47]. Children and adolescents can experience on average five to seven episodes per year [48], but more important, sickle-related pain can occur as often as once in 14 days when monitored in a prospective fashion by keeping pain diaries [49]. The more common forms of painful episodes in adolescents include bony infarcts, priapism (in males), acute chest syndrome, and avascular necrosis. Such episodes are unpredictable in nature, usually spontaneous, and can be triggered by a variety of factors including, but not limited to, fatigue, temperature extremes, dehydration, and stress of any kind.

A great variability is seen in the degree and severity of the acute painful crisis between patients. Even within the same patient, there may be variability in painful experiences from crisis to crisis. Biological modulators of disease, intrinsic and extrinsic to the red blood cell, are an integral component in the phenotypic variation mentioned above. Psychological, social, cultural, and spiritual factors interplay to form a more complex pattern of inter-patient pain variability, coping, and health utilization [50,51]. Sickle-related pain results in increased missed school days, in addition to being highly disruptive of recreational and social activities [49].

Chronic Pain

Some chronic pain may be explained by obvious pathological sequelae of vasoocclusion, such as avascular necrosis, leg ulcers or chronic osteo-myelitis. Avascular necrosis affects the hips (femoral head) more commonly and is a major debilitating component of the disease. Avascular necrosis is seen more frequently and at an earlier age in patients with the SC and Sß+ genotypes. The relatively higher hematocrit in these variants of sickle cell disease is believed to be a predictor of this complication, with an onset as early as 9 years of age [52] and in addition to acute pain, may lead to chronic pain in its more advanced stages (grades III-IV) [53]. Children also have more frequently reported headaches and migraines [54].

Although seen more commonly in adults, the transition from acute to intractable chronic pain syndromes, in the absence of any physical signs, can begin in adolescence. This transition can occur following the inadequate management of recurrent acute painful episodes. What makes this phenomenon all the more debilitating is that once it has set in, the condition is still punctuated by recurrent acute painful episodes.

A small number of patients develop narcotic addiction or dependence. Such patients have very frequent contact with health professionals. The treatment of patients with drug addiction and a sickle cell syndrome poses a number of very difficult manage-ment problems because their pain episodes are less responsive to treatment. Additionally, drug withdrawal can precipitate severe acute pain episodes and other more life-threatening complications

The impact of chronic pain may have far reaching consequences in the developing teenager's HRQOL. Missed school days, poor coping, poor sense of overall well being, and poor peer relationships are some of the consequences. The management of chronic pain usually necessitates a multidisciplinary approach with ortho-pedics, physical therapy, and psychologists (for non pharmacologic modalities of pain management).

Although pain crisis is not a part of thalassemic syndromes, patients with thalassemia may suffer from leg ulcers and may develop physical disability. In parts of the world where adequate transfusions cannot be implemented sufficiently to suppress erythropoiesis, one encounters physical evidence of extramedullary hemato-poiesis with typical frontal bossing and maxillary hyperplasia (gnathopathy). The effects of the hemo-globinopathies on bone disease are only recently being appreciated. Evidence of decreased bone density in adolescents with ß-thalassemia major and intermedia is noted in patients with both normal and induced puberty [40]. Bone mineral density measurements are very important screening tools in patients with this disease because such abnormalities herald the more severe osteoporosis and pathological fractures seen later in life.

Major Organ Dysfunction

As patients with hemoglobinopathies grow older, they may develop end organ damage due to repeated vaso-occlusive crisis or sickling. Signs of end organ damage such as recurrent acute chest syndromes, retinopathy, and cardiac dysfunction may manifest in adolescence. Pulmonary hypertension and renal dysfunction may become apparent in adolescence. Iron overload is the main reason for organ dysfunction and mortality in patients with thalassemia. Iron deposition in liver, heart, pancreas, thyroid, and pituitary causes significant organ dysfunction. The patients require hormone replacement therapy for diabetes, hypogonadism, and hypothyroidism [55]. Although mortality from cardiac disease is rarely seen in adolescence, the early adult mortality stems from non-compliance with iron chelation therapy during the adolescent period [56].

Cerebrovascular accidents or strokes are the most catastrophic sequelae of SCD and occur in 11% of patients with hemoglobin SS and Sß0-thalassemia by 20 years of age. The strokes have an immense impact on the physical functioning of the child, in addition to contributing to more intellectual and cognitive deficits in affected children [57]. The landmark stroke pre-vention in children (STOP) study identified children at increased risk of stroke using transcranial Doppler screening. Chronic blood transfusion aimed at main-taining the relative proportion of hemoglobin S at < 30% has shown a significant risk reduction [58]. For this reason, the present recommendation is to perform transcranial Doppler screening on all patients aged 2-16 years.

Thrombotic events do occur in thalassemia albeit less frequently than SCD (2% versus 11%) and tend to occur after adolescence. Such events are more commonly seen in thalassemia intermedia than in thalassemia major. The multifactorial pathophysiological events induced by red cell hemolysis, inflammatory cytokines, and elevated platelet count increase the incidence of thrombotic events. Thrombotic events were found in a large prospective study to occur in about 4% of patients with intermedia (especially post splenectomy) and 1% of thalassemia major patients; this appears to be the case in sub-optimally transfused patients [59].

CONCLUSIONS

This discussion provides a general overview of the range of disabilities caused by chronic hematological disorders in adolescents. As morbidity and mortality continue to decline for the coagulopathies and hemo-globinopathies, health related quality of life in affected patients should be used as an endpoint to assess effective delivery of care. Comprehensive, multidisciplinary approaches to health care delivery with psychologists and therapists hold promise for the most holistic approach to these patients. The available instruments for assessing HRQOL should be part of evaluation of all adolescents with any chronic disease.

Several areas of importance are not discussed extensively because of a paucity of evidence-based information. For instance, adolescents with disabilities seem to be at greater risk of being obese than those without disabilities. Similarly, there appears to be a positive correlation between disabilities and adolescent smoking. There appears to be racial disparities in the care of adolescents with disabilities, which has not been adequately addressed by the health care system.

REFERENCES

[1] Perrin JM. Health services research for children with disabilities. *Milbank Q.* 2002;80(2):303-24.
[2] Soucie JM, Evatt B, Jackson D, and the Hemophilia Surveillance System Project Investigators. Occur-rence of hemophilia in the United States. *Am. J. Hematol.* 1998;59:288-94.
[3] Shankar M, Lee CA, Sabin CA, Eonomides DL, Kadir RA. von Willebrand disease in women with menorrhagia: a systematic review. *BJOG.* 2004; 111:734-40.
[4] Doyle DJ, Turpie AG, Hirsh J, Best C, Kinch D, Levine MN, et al. Adjusted subcutaneous heparin or continuous intravenous heparin in patients with acute deep vein thrombosis: a randomized trial. *Ann. Intern. Med.* 1989; 107(4):441-5.
[5] Eyster ME, Gill FM, Blott PM, Hilgartner MW, Ballard JO, Kinney TR. Central nervous system bleeding in hemophiliacs. *Blood.* 1978;51:1179-88.
[6] Klinge J, Auberger K, Auerswald G, Brackmann HH, Mauz-Körholz C, Kreuz W. Prevalence and outcomes of inttracranial haemorrhage in haemo-philiacs—a survey of the paediatric group of the German Society of Thrombosis and Haemostasis (GTH). *Eur. J. Pediatr.* 1999;158:S162-5.
[7] Bray GL, Luban NLC. Hemophilia presenting with intracranial hemorrhage: an approach to the infant with intracranial bleeding and coagulopathy. *Am. J. Dis. Child.* 1987;141:1215-7.
[8] Mayes SD, Handford HA, Schaefer JH, Scogno CA, Neagley SR, Michael-Good L, et al. The relationship of HIV status, type of coagulation disorder, and school absenteeism to cognition, educational performance, mood, and behavior of boys with hemophilia. *J. Genet. Psychol.* 1996; 157(2):137-51.
[9] Wodrich DL, Recht M, Gradowski M, Wagner L. Is attention deficit hyperactivity disorder over-represented among HIV-seronegative boys with haemophilia? Preliminary results from our centre. *Haemophilia.* 2003;9(5):593-4.
[10] Shapiro AD, Donfield SM, Lynn HS, Cool VA, Stehbens JA, Hunsberger SL, et al; Academic Achievement in Children with Hemophilia Study Group. Defining the impact of hemophilia: The Academic Achievement in Children with Hemo-philia Study. *Pediatrics.* 2001;108(6):E105.
[11] Denny-Brown D. Recurrent cerebrovascular episodes. *Arch. Neurol.* 1960;2:194-210
[12] Sigel EJ. Adolescent growth and development. In: Greydanus DE, Patel DR. Pratt HD, eds. *Essentials of adolescent medicine.* New York, McGraw Hill, 2006:3-27.
[13] American Psychiatric Association (APA). *Diag-nostic and statistical manual of mental disorders.* DSM-IV, 4th ed. Washington, DC: APA, 1994.
[14] Brunnquell D, Hall M. Issues in the psychological care of pediatric oncology patients. *Am. J. Ortho-psychiatry.* 1982;52:32-44.
[15] Sourkes B. Armfuls of time: *The psychological experience of the child with a life-threatening illness.* Pittsburgh, PA: Univ Pittsburgh Press, 1995.

[16] Handelsman JE. The knee joint in hemophilia. Orthop Clin North Am 1979;10:139-73.
[17] Peyvandi F, Duga S, Atchavan S, Mannucci PM. Rare coagulation deficiencies. *Hemophilia.* 2002; 8:308-21.
[18] Hilgartner MW. Recent advances in hemophilia. Part V. Discussion paper: Degenerative joint disease. *Ann. N.Y. Acad. Sci.* 1975;240:340-1.
[19] Handelsman JE, Glasser RA. Pathogenesis and treatment of hemophilia arthropathy and deep muscle hemorrhages. *Prog. Clin. Biol. Res.* 1990; 324:199-206.
[20] Gilbert MS. Musculoskeletal manifestations of hemophilia. *Mt. Sinai J. Med.* (N.Y.) 44:339-358, 1977.
[21] Goodfellow J, Fearn CB, Matthew JM. Iliacus haematoma: a common complication of hemophilia. *J. Bone Joint Surg. Br.* 1967; 49:748-56.
[22] Prandoni P, Frulla M, Sartor D, Concolato A, Girolami A. Vein abnormalities and the post-thrombotic syndrome. *J. Throm. Haemost.* 2005;3: 401-2.
[23] Kahn SR, Frinsberg JS. The post-thrombotic syndrome: current knowledge, controversies and directions for future research. *Blood Rev.* 2002; 16:155-65.
[24] Kulkarni, R, Soucie, MJ, Evatt, B. Renal disease among males with hemophilia. *Haemophilia.* 2003;9:703-10.
[25] Mahmoud, EI. Acute renal vein thrombosis in adults. *Int. Urol. Nephrol.* 1985;18:243.
[26] Ahlberg A. On the natural history of hemophilia pseudotumor. *J. Bone Joint Surg.* 1975;57A:1133.
[27] Ameri A., Bousser MG, Cerebral venous throm-bosis. *Neurol. Clin.* 1992;10:87-111.
[28] Incorvaia C, Lamberti G, Parmeggiani F, Ferraresi P, Calzolari E, Bernardi F, et al. Idiopathic central retinal vein occlusion in a thrombotic patient with heterozygous 20210 G/A prothrombin genotype. *Am. J. Ophthalmol.* 1999;128(2):247-8.
[29] Larson J, Olafsdottir E, Bauer B. Activated protein C resistance in young adults with retinal vein occlusion. *Br. J. Ophthalmol.* 1996;80: 200-2.
[30] Harward TR, Green D, Bergan JJ, Rizzo RJ, Yao JS. Mesenteric venous thrombosis. *J. Vasc. Surg.* 1989;9(2):328-33.
[31] Clavien PA, Durig M, Harder F. Venous mesen-teric infarction: a particular entity. *Br. J. Surg.* 1988; 75:252-5.
[32] Maddrey WC. Hepatic Vein thrombosis (Bud-Chiari Syndrome). *Hepatology.* 1984;4:44S-6.
[33] Keating MA, Althausen AF. The clinical spectrum of renal vein thrombosis. *J. Urol.* 1985;133:938-45.
[34] Joffe HV, Goldhaber SZ. Upper extremity deep vein thrombosis. *Circulation.* 2002;106:1874-80.
[35] Bernstein D, Coupey S, Schonberg S. Pulmonary embolism in adolescents. *Am. J. Dis. Child.* 1986; 140:665-6.
[36] Carson JL, Kelley MA, Duff A, Weg JG, Fulk-erson WJ, Palevsky HI, et al. The clinical course of pulmonary embolism. *N. Engl. J. Med.* 1992; 326:1240-5.
[37] Green RM, Meyer TJ, Dunn M, Glassroth J. Pulmonary embolism in younger adults. *Chest.* 1992;101:1507-11.
[38] Nathan DG, Thalassemia; The continued challenge. *Ann. N.Y. Acad. Sci.* 2005;1054:1-10.
[39] Powers DR, Chan LS, Hiti A. Outcome of sickle cell anemia: a 4-decade observational study of 1056 patients. *Medicine.* 2005;84(6): 363-76.

[40] Vogiatzi MG, Autio KA, Mait JE, Schneider R, Lesser M, Giardina PJ. Low bone mineral density in adolescents with beta-thalassemia. *Ann. N.Y. Acad. Sci.* 2005;1054:462-6.

[41] Noll RB, Stith L, Gartstein MA, Ris MD, Grueneich R, Vannatta K, et al. Neuropsycho-logical functioning of youths with sickle cell disease: Comparison with non-chronically ill peers. *J. Pediatr. Psychol.* 2001;26(2):69-78.

[42] Johnson C. Sickle cell disease. In: Stolov WC, Clovers MR, ed. Handbook of severe disability. *A text for rehabilitation counselors, other vocational practitioners and allied health professionals.* Washington, DC: US Dept Educ, 1981:349-62.

[43] Thompson RJ, Gil KM, Burbach DJ, Keith BR, Kinney TR. Role of child and maternal processes in the psychological adjustment of children with sickle cell disease. *J. Consult. Clin. Psychol.* 1993; 61:468-74.

[44] Midence K, Fuggle P, Davies SC. Psychosocial aspects of sickle cell disease (SCD) in childhood and adolescence: a review. *Br. J. Clin. Psychol.* 1993; 32(3):271-80.

[45] Aydin B, Yaprak I, Akarsu D, Okten N, Ulgen M. Psychosocial aspects and psychiatric disorders in children with thalassemia major. *Acta Paediatr. Jpn.* 1997;39(3):354-7.

[46] Smith WR, Penberthy LT, Bovbjerg VE, McClish DK, Roberts JD, Dahman B, et al. Daily assessment of pain in adults with sickle cell disease. *Ann. Intern. Med.* 2008;148(2):94-101.

[47] Ballas SK, Lusardi M. Hospital readmission for adult acute sickle cell painful episodes: frequency etiology and prognostic significance. *Am. J. Hematol.* 2005;79:17-25.

[48] Shapiro B. Management of painful episodes in sickle cell disease. In: Schechter NL, ed. *Pain in infants, children and adolescents.* Baltimore, MD: Williams Wilkins, 1993:385-410.

[49] Fuggle P, Shand PA, Gill, LJ, Davies SC. Pain, quality of life, and coping in sickle cell disease. *Arch. Dis. Child.* 1996;75(3):199-203.

[50] Patterson CC, Palermo TM. Parental reinforcement of recurrent pain: The moderating impact of child depression and anxiety on functional disability. *J. Pediatr. Psychol.* 2004;29(5):331-41.

[51] Hoff AL, Paleamo TM, Schuchter M, Zebracki K, Drotar D. Longitudinal relationships of depressive symptoms to pain intensity and functional disability among children with disease-related pain. *J. Pediatr. Psychol.* 2006;31(10):1046-56.

[52] Lee RE, Golding JS, Serjeant GR. The radiolog-ical features of avascular necrosis of the femoral head in homozygous sickle cell disease. *Clin. Radiol.* 1981;32(2):205-14.

[53] Sadat AM. Avascular necrosis of the femoral head in sickle cell disease. An integrated classification. *Clin. Orthop. Related Res.* 1993; 290:200-5.

[54] Palermo TM. Headache symptoms in pediatric sickle cell patients. *Pediatr. Hematol. Oncol.* 2005; 27(8):420-4.

[55] Borgna-Pignatti C. Survival and complications in thalassemia. *Ann. N.Y. Acad. Sci.* 2005;1054:40-7.

[56] Modell B, Khan M, Darlison M. Survival in beta-thalassemia major in the UK: Data from the UK Thalassemia Register. *Lancet.* 2000;360:516-20.

[57] Hariman LM, Griffith ER, Hurtig AL, Keehn MT. Functional outcomes of children with sickle cell disease affected by stroke. *Arch. Phys. Med. Rehabil.* 1991;72(7): 498-502.

[58] Adams RJ, McKie VC, Hsu L, Files B, Vichinsky E, Pegelow C, et al. Prevention of a first stroke by transfusions in children with sickle cell anemia and abnormal results on transcranial Doppler ultrasonography. *N. Engl. J. Med.* 1998;339(1):5-11.

[59] Cappellini MD, Grespi E, Cassinerio E, Bignamini D, Fiorelli G. Coagulation and splenectomy: an overview. *Ann. N.Y. Acad. Sci.* 2005;1054:317-24.

In: Adolescence and Chronic Illness
Editors: H. Omar et al.

ISBN: 978-1-60876-628-4
© 2010 Nova Science Publishers, Inc.

Chapter 7

SEVERE PAIN IN CHILDREN WITH SICKLE CELL DISEASE

Eufemia Jacob[*,1], *Marilyn Hockenberry*[2,3], *Brigitta U. Mueller*[4,5], *Thomas D. Coates*[6] *and Lonnie Zeltzer*[7,8,9]

[1] UCLA School of Nursing, Los Angeles, California.
[2] Departtment of Hematology/Oncology, Baylor College of Medicine.
[3] Center for Research and Evidence-Based Practice,
Texas Children's Hospital, Houston, Texas.
[4] Division of Clinical Services, Texas Children's Cancer Center
and Hematology Service, Baylor College of Medicine, Houston, Texas.
[5] Texas Children's Sickle Cell Center, Houston, Texas.
[6] Sickle Cell/Hemoglobinopathy Program, Childrens Center for
Cancer and Blood Diseases, Los Angeles, California.
[7] David Geffen School of Medicine at UCLA.
[8] Pediatric Pain Program, UCLA Mattel Children's Hospital and Patients.
[9] Survivors Program, UCLA Jonsson Cancer Center,
Los Angeles, California, United States of America.

ABSTRACT

Morphine given by Patient Controlled Analgesia (PCA) is widely used in hospital settings to manage severe pain during acute painful episodes. Wide variations in prescription patterns occur and some patients are often self-administering sub- or low-therapeutic doses. In this chapter, a descriptive design with repeated measures was used to examine the effects of different PCA morphine regimens on the intensity, location and quality of pain as well as on the perceived amount of relief and side effects in patients with sickle cell disease (N=13; mean age 13.7 years; eight males; five females). The preliminary data showed that a regimen with a high background infusion rate and low intermittent push dose (Regimen B) may provide better response to PCA morphine. The

---

[*] *Correspondence:* Assistant professor Eufemia Jacob, PhD, RN, UCLA School of Nursing, Factor Building 5-942, 700 Tiverton Avenue, Los Angeles, CA 90095-6919, United States. Tel: (310) 267-1823; Fax: (310) 206-3241; E-mail: ejacob@sonnet.ucla.edu

difference in trends between the worst and least pain intensity ratings were narrower in this regimen, suggesting that pain peaks and troughs were not occurring as in a regimen with an around the clock nurse administered dosing schedule (Regimen C). The amount of morphine that was administered per day was not significantly different ($p > 0.05$) among the three morphine regimens. The combination of a high background infusion rate and low intermittent push dose (as in Regimen B) within the first 24 hours of admission, may provide improved response and possibly shorter recovery from the painful episode than the regimen that would routinely be prescribed with lower background infusion rate and high intermittent push dose (as in regimen A).

INTRODUCTION

Sickle cell disease is an inherited disorder that affects one in 500 African Americans [1,2]. The acute painful episode is the most common problem in children with sickle cell disease. It may be a manifestation of vaso-occlusion or may be a symptom of another process, such as infection. The painful episode due to vaso-occlusion is the most frequent cause for emergency department visits and hospital admissions [3,4].

Painful episodes that are severe enough to require hospitalization typically last 3 to 7 days, but pain may persist for as long as several weeks [5]. Children may experience persistent pain of mild to moderate intensity on a daily basis, or may have intermittent acute exacerbations of more severe pain. In most cases during the acute painful episode, pain intensity increases rapidly, plateaus, and then falls, but the pattern may be unpredictable [6,7]. Morphine given by PCA is widely used in hospital settings to manage severe pain during acute painful episodes [8-10]. However, there were wide variations in prescription patterns, and patients were often self-administering sub- or low-therapeutic doses, commonly 35% on the average of what were prescribed. The most common PCA morphine regimen consisted of high intermittent push dose and low background infusion rate [8-10]. With this PCA morphine regimen, children were most likely falling asleep in between the intermittent push doses and waking up with pain, and leading to a "prn" dosing schedule and thus, not providing optimal relief. Therefore, pain intensity ratings remained at moderate to high levels through the course of hospitalization [8,9] and some patients with sickle cell disease had prolonged hospitalizations associated with persistent pain [10]. It is not known if other combinations of PCA settings, such as increasing the background infusion, or having larger amounts administered around the clock (ATC) may provide better response to morphine. Such regimens could achieve a more steady concentration of the drug associated with the "ATC" dosing schedule, rather than a "PRN" dosing schedule with peaks and troughs [11,12]. Therefore, the purpose of this preliminary study was to examine the effects of the different PCA regimens on the intensity, location and quality of pain as well as on the perceived amount of relief and side effects.

OUR STUDY

A descriptive design with repeated measures was used to examine the effects of the different PCA regimens during hospitalization for acute painful episodes. Patients with sickle cell disease were recruited from the hematology unit of a large children's hospital in the central southern United States. The Sickle Cell Program in this facility follows about 900 patients per year and provides comprehensive services for patients with sickle cell disease.

All hospitalized patients with sickle cell disease, eight years and older, were eligible. The age of eight years was chosen as the cut-off point because the outcome measures for pain were validated for patients eight years and older. In addition, patients younger than 8 years old were less likely prescribed patient controlled analgesia for pain management during acute painful episodes. Patients were included in the study if: 1) they were English-speaking (data collection instruments available only in English); 2) the primary reason for admission was for management of acute pain as documented by the attending physician in the admission records, and 3) the pain was severe enough to require the administration of intravenous morphine.

Patients with sickle cell disease were excluded if pain was not related to an acute painful episode (infection, surgery, burns, trauma). Patients were also excluded if they had cognitive and neurological impairments that precluded them from completing the pain tool. They were excluded if they were already receiving morphine at doses above the study entry dose (either an intermittent push dose setting greater than 0.07 mg/dose, a background infusion rate setting greater than 0.03 mg/kg/hr, or a four hour limit setting greater than 0.6 mg/kg (equivalent to 0.15 mg/kg one hour limit setting) . The decision to exclude patients was made by the PI in consultation with the hematology team. The study was approved by the Institutional Review Board of the medical center.

Patients were randomly assigned to one of three morphine regimens (Regimen A, B, or C). The differences among the regimens were in the combination of settings programmed in the PCA device. The settings differed in: 1) the amount given by background infusion, 2) the amount given by the intermittent push button, and 3) the lockout interval settings programmed in the PCA device (see table 1). The 4 hour maximum [converted to hourly equivalent] setting prescribed for each regimen was controlled to minimize the confounding effect of dose on the variation in response. The hourly limit setting was standardized in mg/kg/hour based on the amount that is recommended in the Pediatric Drug Dosage Handbook [13], a medication reference book which is widely used in children's hospitals as part of the formulary across the United States.

Patients in Regimen A were prescribed the regimen of higher intermittent push (HIP) dose (0.07 mg/kg/dose; proportionally two times the intermittent push dose prescribed for regimen B) and lower background infusion (LBI) rate (0.015 mg/kg/hr; proportionately half the amount prescribed for regimen B). The maximum 4-hour limit setting for this regimen was 0.6 mg/kg, equivalent to 0.15 mg/kg/hr x 4 hours [9,10]. The recommended therapeutic dose range from the Pediatric Drug Dosage Handbook commonly used by children's hospitals across the country is 0.1 to 0.2 mg/kg/hr [13]; thus the hourly dose selected for this study is in the midpoint of the therapeutic dose range.

Patients in regimen B were prescribed the opposite regimen of lower intermittent push (LIP) dose (0.03 mg/kg/dose; proportionally half from Regimen A) and higher background infusion (HBI) rate regimen (0.03 mg/kg/hr; proportionately two times the background rate in Regimen A). The 4-hour maximum limit setting for this regimen was also 0.6 mg/kg [0.15 mg/kg/hr x 4 hours], which was the same as the maximum 4-hour limiting setting for regimen A [13]. Thus, the hourly limit setting was standardized for the morphine PCA regimens in the study.

Table 1. Morphine patient controlled analgesia regimens

	Patient Controlled Analgesia Morphine Regimens		
	A (N=5)	B (N=5)	C (N=3)
Intermittent Push	0.07 mg/kg/dose	0.035 mg/kg/dose	0.15 mg/kg/dose
Background Rate	0.015 mg/kg/hr	0.03 mg/kg/hr	0.00 mg/kg/hr
Lock-out Interval	10 minutes	10 minutes	180 minutes [q 3 hrs]
4 hour Maximum [Hourly Maximum]	0.6 mg/kg [0.15 mg/kg/hr]	0.6 mg/kg [0.15 mg/kg/hr]	0.6 mg/kg
Example PCA Settings for a 40 kg patient for the different regimens:			
	Patient Controlled Analgesia Morphine Regimens		
	A	B	C
Intermittent Push	2.8 mg	1.4 mg	6 mg
Background Rate	0.6 mg/kg/hr	1.2 mg	0.0 mg/kg/hr
Lock-out Interval	10 minutes	10 minutes	180 minutes [q 3 hrs]
4 hour Maximum [Hourly Maximum]	24 mg [6 mg/kg/hr]	24 mg [6 mg/kg/hr]	

Patients in regimen C [Nurse Controlled Analgesia] were prescribed an around the clock (ATC) dose of 0.15 mg/kg/dose, based on the recommended parameters of 0.1 to 0.2 mg/kg/dose every 3 hours; maximum 15 mg/dose [13]. This dose was higher than the dose that could be delivered by PCA in a background infusion rate or in an intermittent push dose, but equivalent to the dose that would be prescribed if PCA was not available. However, for this study, regimen C was delivered using the PCA device with the intermittent push dose rate setting at 0.15 mg/kg/dose and background infusion rate set at 0.0; lockout interval was set at 180 minutes (three hours) to allow the nurse to push the dose every three hours, and simulate a "q 3 hour ATC" regimen, that was typically prescribed for patients without using the PCA device. Thus, no intermittent dose for patient to push and no background infusion rate were prescribed for Regimen C. In general, medications administered ATC achieve stead state levels after 4 to 5 half-lifes (half-life of morphine is two hours) [14]. Therefore, even though this regimen was administered intermittently every three hours ATC, the level of mophine in the blood is expected to reach steady state after two to three doses, a level that would be achieved if patient had a background infusion rate.

All patients were enrolled within 48 hours of initiation of PCA and they were prescribed the study dose for 24 hours. In the event that the patient required additional doses beyond the assigned study settings, a PRN dose was prescribed for all regimens at 0.05 mg/kg/dose (33% of the one hour limit study setting, i.e. 0.05 mg/kg/hr). This amount was based on the rescue dose recommended by the American Pain Society Guideline for the Management of Acute and Chronic Sickle Cell Disease, which is recommended at 25% to 50% of the hourly opioid dose [15]. If the patient required three additional doses in any one hour period beyond the study PCA settings before hour 24, the physician could change the PCA settings and the patient would be off study.

Outcome Measures

Children were asked to rate pain using 0 to 10 numerical rating scales (0=no pain to 10=a lot of pain) for 1) worst pain, 2) least pain, and 3) amount of pain relief during treatment (0=no relief to 10=complete relief). The 0 to 10 numeric rating scale is a well-established valid and reliable tool [16], and was previously used by children with sickle cell disease [8-10]. A checklist that consisted of common side effects of morphine (hypotension, bradycardia, respiratory depression, drowsiness, dizziness, tremors, sedation, pruritus, nausea, vomiting, constipation, urinary retention) was used to record side effects.

The patient was also asked to complete the Adolescent Pediatric Pain Tool (APPT) to measure the intensity, location, and quality of pain. Reliability and validity of the APPT is well established [17-20]. Previous APPT data from children with sickle cell disease showed that pain location and spatial distribution of pain changed during acute painful episodes even when pain intensity remained the same [8].

The patient's Medication Administration Record was reviewed for the dose, route, and time of all medications that were administered for pain (e.g. nonsteroidal anti-inflammatory drugs [NSAIDs] such as ibuprofen and ketorolac) and for side effects (e.g., diphenhydramine for itching, hydroxyzine and odansetron for emesis). In addition, the following information were also collected from the medical records: 1) demographic information such as age, gender, weight, height, hemoglobin genotype; and 2) health related information such as CBC, pain ratings in the ED, presence of fever, oxygen saturation, other signs and symptoms at time of admission, history of past complications and sickle cell related treatments.

Scatter plots were used to describe worst and least pain patterns across the five days. Descriptive statistics (frequencies, means, standard deviations) were used to describe worst and least pain, location of pain, and quality of pain, type and amount of medications, and amount of relief.

OUR FINDINGS

During the two year study period between August, 2005 and July, 2007, 326 sickle cell related admissions were screened in the hematology unit, with an average of 18.1 ± 5.6 admissions each month. These admissions represented 160 patients; 30% had three or more repeat admissions. Among the 160 patients, 68 (42.8%) patients were admitted for reasons other than acute painful episodes, 28 (17.6%) patients had acute painful episode, but did not have PCA morphine at time of screening and recruitment, 14 (8.8%) were excluded for various reasons (such as, developmental delay, communication disorder, behavioral problems, disruptive behavior, cognitive dysfunction, neurological impairments, patient not appropriate for randomization, parent noncompliant or not appropriate for consenting procedures, patient on legal custody and parent/legal guardian not known), 8 (5.0%) were weaned from pain medications and were planned to be discharged within 24 hours, 4 (2.5%) were eligible, but enrolled in a concurrent study, 2 (1.3%) did not have parents available for consent, 16 (10.1%) refused. A total of 15 patients were randomized in the PCA morphine regimens; two of them (1 from regimen C; the other from regimen A) had withdrawn early. The 13 patients who completed the study were randomly assigned to Regimen A (n=5), B (n=5), and C (n=5).

Baseline characteristics of patients in regimen A (n=5), B (n=5), and C (n=3) were not significantly different (N=13; mean age 13.7 years; eight males; five females; table 2). The Hemoglobin phenotype was predominantly HgbSS (n=9). Onset of pain was 1.7 to 3.4 days prior to admission. Lowest mean pain intensity ratings in the Emergency Department (ED) prior to admission ranged from 5.0 to 7.7, with the highest pain intensity ratings from 7.3 to 9.5 on 0 to 10 numerical ratings scales (NRS). Patients received 0.08 to 0.10 mg/kg/dose, which were lower or within the lower range of the recommended morphine dose of 0.1 to 0.2 mg/kg/dose [12]. Patients in regimen B had an overall mean shorter length of stay (see table 1); however this was not statistically significant ($p > 0.05$).

Table 2. Demographics

	A (N=5)	B (N=5)	C (N=3)
Age (years)	13.6 ± 2.1 (11 – 17)	13.0 ± 2.0 (10 – 16)	14.7 ± 4.2 (range 10 – 18)
Weight (kg)	49.5 ± 18.3 (31.0 to 76.0)	70.5 ± 18.6 (42.0 to 93.6)	48.1 ± 24.0 (26.5.0 to 74.0)
Height (cm)	158.5 ± 11.9 (145.5 to 169.0)	153.7 ± 20.7 (127.0 to 174.0)	151.1 ± 13.0 (141.0 to 166.0)
Gender			
Male	4	3	1
Female	1	2	2
Hemoglobin			
SS	4	2	3
SC	1	1	--
S Beta	--	1	--
Pain Onset (Number Days PTA)	1.8 ± 1.5 (1 to 4)	1.7 ± 0.6 (1 to 2)	3.4 ± 4.6 (1 to 9)
Lowest Pain in ER (0 to 10 NRS)	7.7 ± 2.1 (6 to 10)	7.0 ± 3.3 (0 to 7)	5.0 ± 1.4 (4 to 6)
Highest Pain in ER (0 to 10 NRS)	9.5 ± 1.0 (8 to 10)	7.3 ± 1.2 (6 to 8)	9.0 ± 1.4 (8 to10)
Morphine in ER (mg/kg/dose)	0.08	0.09	0.10
Length of Hospital Stay (days)	6.0 2.2 3 to 9	5.6 2.4 3 to 9	7.0 2.6 7 to 10

PTA: Prior to Admission; ER: Emergency Room.

Pain Intensity

The worst pain intensity ratings in Regimen B decreased significantly during the course of hospitalization (see figure 1). The worst pain intensity rating was 9.5 on day 1 and 5.5 on day 5, p=0.01 for Regimen B. The worst pain intensity ratings for patients on regimen A (9.8 to 9.0, $p > 0.05$) and regimen C (9.6 to 7.5, p>0.05) did not change significantly during hospitalization (see figure 1). The least pain intensity ratings of patients in regimen C were lower than patients in either regimen A or B (see figure 2). The difference in trends between the worst and least pain intensity ratings across the hospital days was widest in regimen C when compared to either Regimen A or B (see figure 2).

Pain Location

The most frequent areas marked for pain by patients in regimen A were the right upper arm (75%), right abdomen (50%), left thigh and knees (50%), right back chest (50%), and lower back (50%). The most frequent areas marked by patients in Regimen B were chest (83%), right knee (50%), and left thigh and knees (50%). Patients in regimen C marked the chest (66.7%), right upper arm (66.7%), right abdomen (66.7%), and lower back (66.7%).

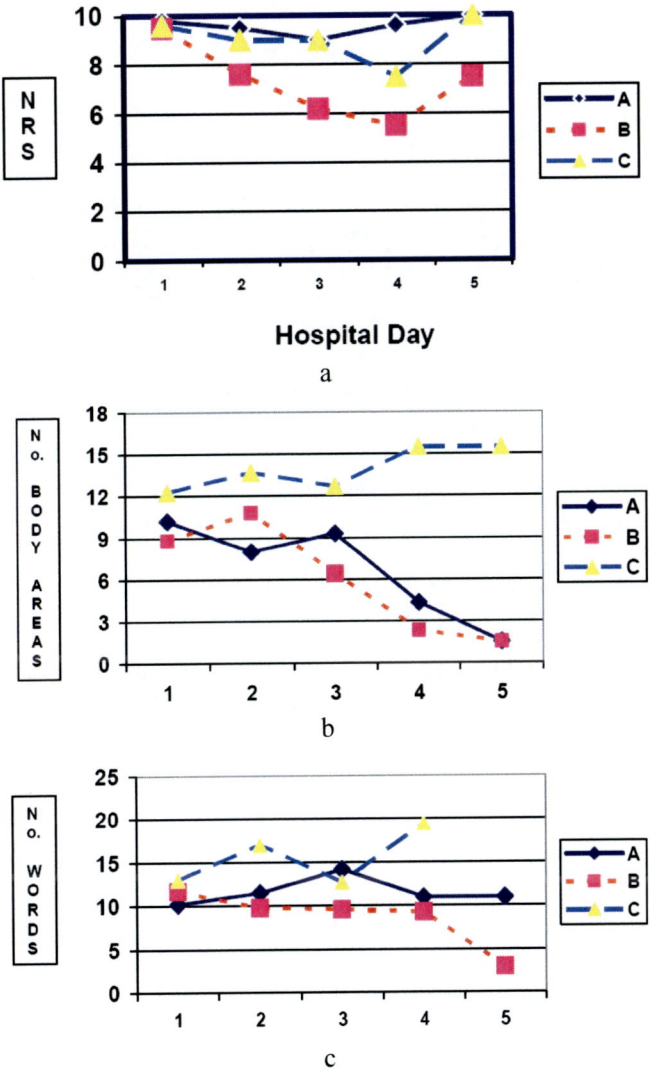

Figure 1. Pain intensity ratings (A), Number of body areas (B) and number of quality word descriptors (C) Day 1 to Day 5 of hospitalization.

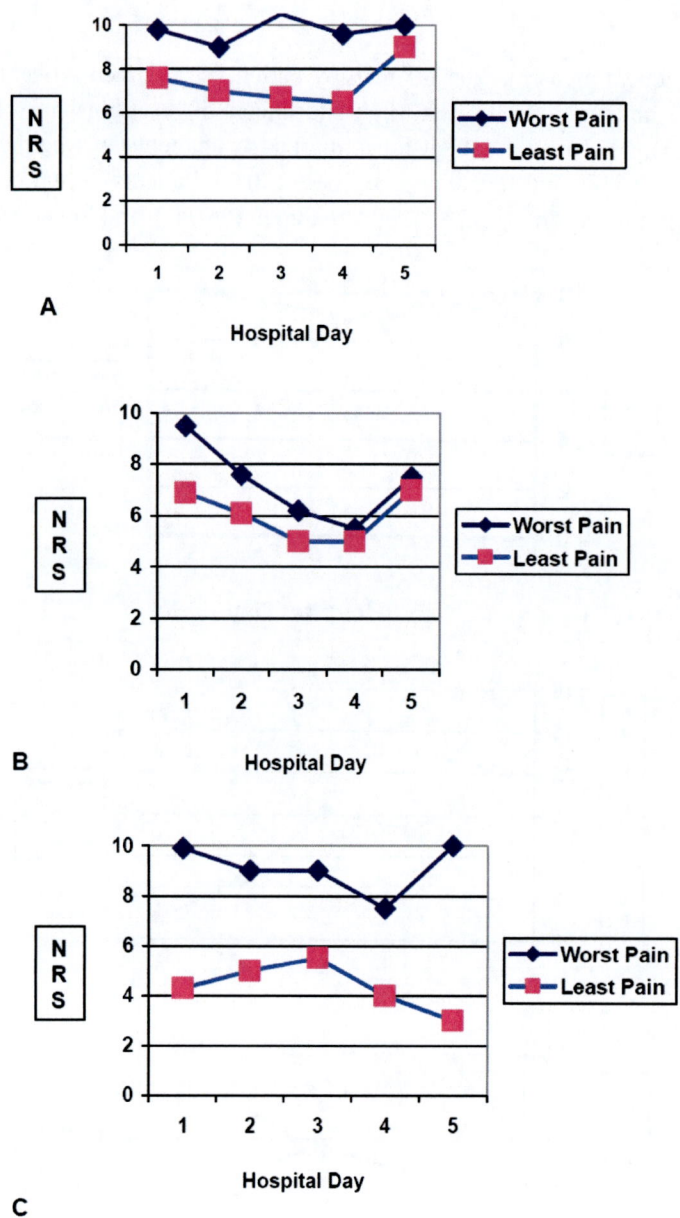

Figure 2. Comparison of worst and least pain ratings for regimen A, B, C.

The number of areas marked on the body outline diagram remained constant throughout hospitalization for regimen C (12.3 to 15.5 areas). The number of areas marked decreased for patients in regimen A (10.2 to 1.5) and B (8.8 to 1.5). Worst pain intensity ratings remained at moderate levels (see figure 1A) throughout hospitalization; however, the number of body areas marked with pain decreased for regimen A and B, but not for regimen C (see figure 1B).

Pain Quality

The number of words to describe the quality of pain remained similar throughout hospitalization from 10.2 on day 1 to 11.0 on day 5 ($p > 0.05$) for patients on regimen A (see figure 1C). The most frequent words were sensory quality (3.7 to 7.5), and fewer affective (1.75 to 2.5), evaluative (2.2 to 2.7), or temporal words (1.7 to 2.5). The number of words to describe the quality of pain decreased from 11.7 to 3.0 for patients on regimen B (see figure 1C). The most frequent words were also sensory quality (3.6 to 6.0) and fewer affective (0.8 to 1.3), evaluative (1.7 to 2.2), or temporal words (1.8 to 2.6). For patients in regimen C, the number of words remained similar throughout hospitalization, and slightly increased from 13.0 on day 1 to 19.2 on day 5 ($p>0.05$). The number of sensory (6.3 to 10.0), affective (2.3 to 3.0), evaluative (2.3 to 4.0), and temporal quality words (2.0 to 3.0) were slightly higher, but not significantly different ($p>0.05$) from the patients in regimen A and B.

The words that were selected by 75% of patients in regimen A to describe the quality of pain were hurting, sharp, pressure, awful, annoying and continuous. The majority of patients (66.7%) in regimen B selected aching, hurting, like a sharp knife, shooting, dizzy, annoying, and uncomfortable. The majority of patients in regimen C (66.7%) selected similar words. In addition, the majority of patients (66.7%) in regimen C also selected other words such as throbbing, tight, sore, like a pinch, stinging, shocking, and pounding from the sensory words; crying and sickening from the affective words; and never goes away, steady, and always from the temporal words.

Daily Morphine Consumption

The amount of morphine that was administered per day was not significantly different ($p>0.05$) among the three regimens (see figure 3A). Patients in regimen A were administered on the average from 59.4 mg on day 1 to 33.8 mg on day 5. This amount was equivalent to 1.2 mg/kg/day on day 1 to 1.1 mg/kg/day on day 5. The largest amount was administered on day 3 (77.3 mg/day or 1.4 mg/kg/day). Patients in regimen B had consistently decreased in the amount of morphine that was administered during hospitalization from 73.5 mg/day on day 1 to 23.5 mg/day on day 5 (equivalent to 1.1 on day 1 to 0.3 mg/kg/day on day 5). Patients in regimen C were administered on the average 55.7 mg (or 1.1 mg/kg/day) on day 1 and continued to have a slightly higher amount administered on day 4 (117.9 mg/day or 2.4 mg/kg/day) and day 5 (77.3 mg/day or 1.6 mg/kg/day).

Other Medications

Ketorolac (administered 15 to 30 mg every 6 hours) was the only other medication that all patients received for pain. A few patients had diphenhydramine for itching, and odansetron (8 mg prn) or promethazine (12 mg prn) for nausea/vomiting.

Pain Relief

The amount of pain relief did not change significantly (p > 0.05) during hospitalization (figure 3). The mean amount of pain relief (from 0 = no relief to 10 = complete relief) for each day of hospitalization was higher for regimen C (6.0 ± 2.0 to 6.5 ± 2.1), when compared with Regimen A (4.6 ± 2.5 to 5.7 ± 2.1) or B (4.6 ± 2.7 to 6.6 ± 1.9).

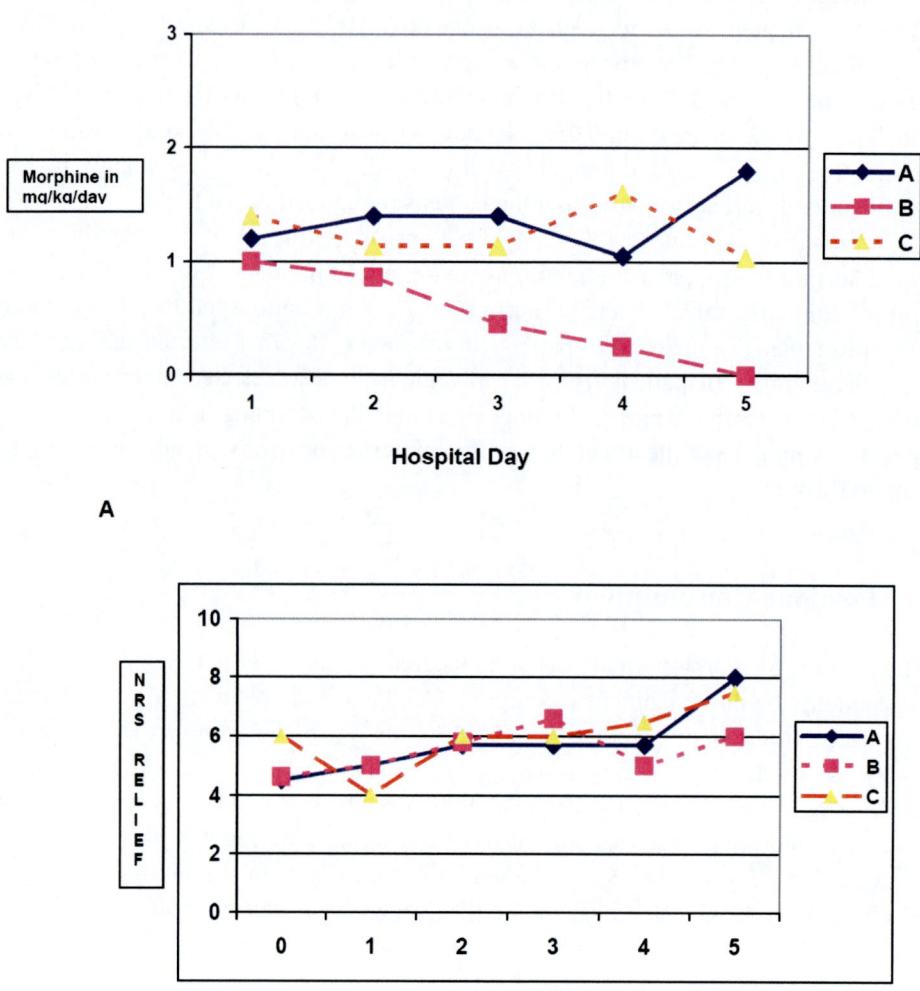

Figure 3. Amount of morphine in mg/kg/day (A) and perceived amount of relief [0 to 10 NRS] from medications (B).

Side Effects

Few patients were reporting side effects, mostly drowsiness, dizziness, itching, nausea, and vomiting. Two of five patients from regimen A and three of five patients from regimen B reported drowsiness prior to enrollment. Three patients on regimen A and two patients on regimen B also reported itching on day of enrollment. Two patients had nausea from regimen A and one each from regimen B and C had both nausea and vomiting. No one had low blood pressure, heart rate, or respiratory rate. One patient in regimen B had difficulty stooling, reported prior to enrollment.

DISCUSSION

This preliminary study evaluated the analgesic response to three different morphine regimens delivered by patient controlled analgesia (PCA). The worst pain intensity ratings in regimen B decreased during the course of hospitalization, while the worst pain intensity ratings in the other two regimens (A and C) did not change. This finding suggests that the regimen with higher background infusion rate (B) may provide a better response to PCA morphine. The difference in trends between the worst and least pain intensity ratings were also narrower in regimen B, suggesting that pain peaks and troughs were not occurring in regimen B, as they were most likely occurring in regimen C, with wide differences in highest pain and lowest pain ratings reported each day.

It is interesting to note that the trend in least pain intensity ratings reported by patients in regimen C was lower across hospitalization days than reported by patients in either regimen A or B (see figure 2). The difference in trends between the worst and least pain intensity ratings across the hospital days was widest in regimen C. This finding suggests that the higher intermittent doses were providing better relief than the amount that were delivered in either regimen A or B; however the every 3 hour interval was most likely not adequate to sustain the low intensity ratings, and may explain the high pain intensity ratings.

Patients in regimen A were reporting the highest worst and least pain intensity ratings and both remained consistently high throughout hospitalization. This finding is similar to previous reports [9,10], which also reported regimens similar to regimen A and worst and least pain intensity ratings that remained high to moderate throughout hospitalization. This implies that the routinely prescribed PCA regimen with lower background infusion and high intermittent push doses (similar to the doses prescribed in regimen A for this study) was not providing optimal pain control.

The chest, abdomen, and extremities were the most frequently marked areas for pain in all regimens, which are similar to the pain location marked by patients in previous reports [9,10]. The number of areas marked decreased for patients in regimens A and B. It is important to note that pain intensity ratings remained at high to moderate levels throughout hospitalization (figure 1A), but the number of body areas marked with pain decreased (figure 1B) for regimen A and B. This finding emphasizes the importance of assessing not only pain intensity dimension as routinely done in practice, but also assessing the location and spatial distribution of pain throughout hospitalization [8], which could be more informative in evaluating response to treatments. This data suggest that regimens A and B were providing better analgesia when compared to regimen C (figure 1B) when the dimension of pain location is used as the outcome criteria.

The most frequently used words selected to describe the quality of pain were predominantly sensory, and less frequently affective, evaluative, or temporal. Patients did not select words that suggest pain with neuropathic component (e.g. shooting, burning, or shock-like). This finding is similar to previous reports of patients with sickle cell disease [8,21].

The amount of morphine prescribed was standardized for all three regimens, which was selected so that the hourly maximum setting is midpoint of the therapeutic dose range [13]. We were anticipating that patients in regimen B would consume more morphine since the background infusion rate was higher. However, patients in regimen B showed a consistent decrease in their daily morphine consumption throughout hospitalization (figure 3A). Although not statistically significant, possibly due to small sample size, the length of stay for regimen B is shorter (table 1). This finding is suggesting that a higher background infusion rate (regimen B) than would routinely be prescribed (regimen A) within the first 24 hours of admission for acute painful episode may provide improved response and shorter recovery from the painful episode in patients with sickle cell disease.

An important finding in this study is that on the average, patients in the ED received 0.08 to 0.10 mg/kg/dose, which were lower or within the lower end of the recommended therapeutic dose range of 0.1 to 0.2 mg/kg/dose [13]. This finding is similar to previous studies which reported that in children and adolescents with sickle cell disease, the prescribed morphine doses were frequently prescribed and administered in the lower end of the therapeutic dose range [9,10]. It would be interesting to determine in future studies whether standardizing the ED protocol to increase the amount prescribed to at least the midpoint of the therapeutic dose range would lead to improved analgesia in the ED and thereby minimize the number of admissions related to acute painful episodes [4,22,23].

The patients in regimen C were reporting a higher relief than patients in regimens A and B. It is possible that the higher intermittent doses administered by the nurse around the clock were providing good relief. These pain relief data are consistent with their reports of least pain intensity ratings.

We did not examine the regimen with high background infusion rate and high intermittent push dose that would be within the therapeutic dose range, a regimen that may be optimal. Future studies need to examine this regimen using larger sample size. There were no differences in side effects reported by patients. The side effects (mostly drowsiness, dizziness, itching, nausea, and vomiting) were present prior to initiation of the doses prescribed in the regimens.

A major limitation in this study is the small sample size. We recommend larger samples in future studies. We screened and recruited patients from the hematology program serving a large population of patients with sickle cell disease. During the two year screening and recruitment period, we were only able to enroll 15 patients (including two early withdrawal patients). We recommend that in future studies, screening and recruitment be done in several sites as the pool of patients with sickle cell disease requiring patient controlled analgesia is relatively low compared to the overall number of all patients with sickle cell disease in a hospital setting.

Several studies including the current study, have documented that the most routinely prescribed regimen (similar to the doses prescribed in Regimen A with high intermittent push with low background infusion rates) was not optimal in providing analgesia. Our current study also showed that patients prescribed a nurse administered around the clock q 3 hour regimen (as prescribed in regimen C) were most likely experiencing pain peaks and troughs, and therefore such regimens should be avoided. We recommend future studies to examine a high background infusion rate with low intermittent push dose (as was prescribed for regimen

B) and alternative morphine regimens such as high background infusion with high intermittent push dose, while keeping within the recommended dose range [13]. Previous reports have documented that patients with sickle cell disease required higher dosing schedules due to the more intense pain [24], prolonged hospitalizations [10], and altered pharmacokinetics [25]. And finally, future studies are warranted that examine alternative PCA opioids such as hydromorphone [26], fentanyl [27], tramadol [28] or a combination of morphine and an adjuvant medication such as ketamine [29] in patients with sickle cell disease who experience severe pain that may be refractory to morphine PCA.

ACKNOWLEDGEMENTS

Funding from this study was provided by a Mentored Patient-Oriented Research Career Development Award (#5K23NR009192) from the National Institute of Nursing Research at the National Institute of Health.

REFERENCES

[1] Platt OS, Brambilla DJ, Rosse WF, Milner PF, Castro O, Steinberg MH et al. Mortality in sickle cell disease. Life expectancy and risk factors for early death. *N. Engl. J. Med.* 1994;330(23):1639-44.

[2] Platt OS, Thorington BD, Brambilla DJ, Milner PF, Rosse WF, Vichinsky E et al. Pain in sickle cell disease. Rates and risk factors. *N. Engl. J. Med.* 1991;325(1):11-16.

[3] Yang Y, Sha A, Watson M, Mankad V. Comparison of costs to the health sector of comprehensive and episodic health care for sickle cell disease patients. *Public Health Reports.* 1997;110:80-6.

[4] Blank FSJ, Li, H, Henneman, PL, Smithline, HA, Santoro, JS, Provost, D, Maynard, AM. A descriptive study of heavy emergency department users at an academic emergency department reveals heavy ED users have better access to care than average users. *J. Emerg. Nurs.* 2005;31(2):139-44.

[5] Beyer J, Simmons L, Woods GM, Woods PM. A chronology of pain/comfort in children with sickle cell disease. *Arch. Pediatr. Adolesc. Med.* 1999;153(9):913-20.

[6] Ballas S. The acute painful episode. In: *Sickle cell pain.* Seattle: IASP Press 1998;11:201-37.

[7] Conner-Warren RL. Pain intensity and home pain management of children with sickle cell disease. *Issues Compr. Pediatr. Nurs.* 1996;19(3):183-95.

[8] Jacob E, Miaskowski C, Savedra M, Beyer JE, Treadwell M, Styles L. Changes in intensity, location, and quality of vaso-occlusive pain. *Pain.* 2003;102(1-2):187-93.

[9] Jacob E, Miaskowski C, Savedra M, Beyer JE, Treadwell M, Styles L. Management of vaso-occlusive pain in hospitalized children with sickle cell disease. *J. Pediatr. Hematology/Oncology.* 2003;25(4):307-11.

[10] Jacob E, Mueller B. Pain and symptom experience in hospitalized children with sickle cell disease who had prolonged hospitalizations. *Pain Med.* 01 Feb 2007 [EPub ahead of print]

[11] Sutters KA, Miaskowski C, Holdridge-Zeuner D, Waite S, Paul SM, Savedra MC, Lanier B. A randomized clinical trial of the effectiveness of a scheduled oral analgesic dosing regimen for the management of postoperative pain in children following tonsillectomy. *Pain.* 2004l;110(1-2):49-55.

[12] Sutters KA, Miaskowski C, Holdridge-Zeuner D, Waite S, Paul SM, Savedra MC, Lanier B. Time-contingent dosing of an opioid analgesic after tonsillectomy does not increase moderate-to-severe side effects in children. *Pain Manag. Nurs.* 2005;6(2):49-57.

[13] Taketomo CK, Hodding JH, Kraus DM. *Pediatric dosage handbook*. Hudson, Ohio: Lexi-comp, 2007.

[14] Brunton L, Lazo J, Lazo, JS. *Goodman and Gilman's the Pharmacological basis of therapeutics,* 11th ed. New York: McGraw-Hill, 2005:569-20.

[15] Benjamin LJ, Dampier CD, Jacox AK, Odesina V, Phoenix D, Shapiro B et al. Guideline for the management of acute and chronic pain in sickle cell disease. Glenview, Ill: *Am. Pain Society.* 1999:42.

[16] Burns N, Groves S. *The practice of nursing research*. Philadelphia, PA: WB Saunders, 2003:292.

[17] Savedra M, Tesler M, Holzemer WL, Wilkie DJ, Ward JA. Testing a tool to assess postoperative pediatric and adolescent pain. In: Tyler DC, Krane EJ, eds. Advances in pain research and therapy: *Pediatric pain*. New York: Raven Press, 1990.

[18] Savedra MC, Holzemer WL, Tesler MD, Wilkie DJ. Assessment of postoperation pain in children and adolescents using the adolescent pediatric pain tool. *Nurs. Res.* 1993;42(1):5-9.

[19] Savedra MC, Tesler MD, Holzemer WL, Wilkie DJ, Ward JA. Pain location: Validity and reliability of body outline markings by hospitalized children and adolescents. *Res. Nurs. Health.* 1989;12: 307-14.

[20] Wilkie DJ, Holzemer WL, Tesler MD, Ward JA, Paul SM, Savedra MC. Measuring pain quality: Validity and reliability of children's and adolescents' pain language. *Pain.* 1990;41:151-9.

[21] Franck LS, Treadwell M, Jacob E, Vichinsky E. Assessment of sickle cell pain in children and young adults using the adolescent pediatric pain tool. *J. Pain Sympt. Manage* 2002;23:114-20.

[22] Givens M, Rutherford C, Joshi G, Delaney K. Impact of an emergency department pain management protocol on the pattern of visits by patients with sickle cell disease. *J. Emerg. Med.* 2006;32(3):239-43.

[23] Melzer-Lange MD, Walsh-Kelly CM, Lean G, Hillery CA, Scott JP. Patient-controlled analgesia for sickle cell pain crisis in a pediatric emergency department. *Pediatr. Emerg. Care.* 2004;20(1):2-4.

[24] Crawford MC, Galton S, Nascr B. Postoperative morphine consumption in children with sickle cell disease. *Pediatric Anesthesia.* 2006;16:152-7.

[25] Dampier CD, Setty BN, Logan J, Ioli JG, Dean R. Intravenous morphine pharmacokinetics in pediatric patients with sickle cell disease. *J. Pediatr.* 1995;126(3):461-7.

[26] Perlman KM, Myers-Phariss S, Rhodes JC. *A shift from meperidine to hydromorphone improves pain control and decreases admissions for patients in sickle cell crisis.* 2004;30(5):439-46.

[27] Ruggiero A, Barone G, Liotti L, Chiaretti A, Lazzareschi I, Riccardi R. Safety and efficacy of fentanyl administered by patient controlled analgesia in children with cancer pain. *Supportive Care Cancer*. 2007;15:569-73.

[28] Ozalevli M, Unlugenc H, Tuncer U, Gunes Y, Ozcengiz D. Comparison of morphine and tramadol by patient controlled analgesia for postoperative analgesia after tonsillectomy in children. *Pediatric Anesthesia*. 2005;15:979-84.

[29] Subramaniam K, Subramaniam B, Stenbrook RA. Ketamine as adjuvant analgesic to opioids: A quantitative and qualitative systematic review. *Anesthesia Analgesia*. 2004;99:482-95.

Part VI. Mental Disorders

In: Adolescence and Chronic Illness
Editors: H. Omar et al.

ISBN: 978-1-60876-628-4
© 2010 Nova Science Publishers, Inc.

Chapter 8

MENTAL HEALTH AND CHRONIC DISEASE

Marlene B. Huff, Kimberly K. McClanahan and Hatim A. Omar*

Department of Pediatrics, Division of Adolescent Medicine,
University of Kentucky, Lexington, Kentucky, United States of America.

ABSTRACT

By 2015, worldwide, 1.2 billion children aged 5-14 years will have some kind of significant chronic disease. Although scientific evidence indicates that children with chronic illness have more mental health issues than their healthy peers, many controversies and gaps in the literature exist. It is imperative that an understanding of the effects of chronic illness upon the mental health status of children and adolescents be undertaken. This chapter uses a biopsychosocial perspective to investigate the connection between chronic illness and mental health. The intent of the chapter is to suggest ways that medical and mental health professionals can provide services to chronically ill children and adolescents that foster positive mental health through the achievement of all developmental tasks with as little psychological stress as possible.

INTRODUCTION

The major tasks of childhood involve achieving healthy development and functioning in the physical, cognitive, emotional, and psychosocial domains. Past research indicates that childhood chronic illness can severely impair psychosocial functioning and impede further development in all domains of functioning [1,2]. Considering the biological, psychological, and social (herein referred to as 'biopsychosocial') concerns and effects in the management of chronic illness and simultaneously fostering positive mental health includes continuous assessment and management of the biopsychosocial factors which all influence one another and are integral to the healthy emotional functioning of children and adolescents.

---

* *Correspondence:* Marlene B. Huff, PhD, LCSW, Department of Pediatrics, Division of Adolescent Medicine, University of Kentucky, Lexington, KY, USA. E-mail: marlene.huff@uky.edu

This chapter uses a biopsychosocial perspective to investigate the connection between chronic illness and mental health. The intent of the chapter is to suggest ways that medical and mental health professionals can provide services to chronically ill children and adolescents that foster positive mental health through the achievement of all developmental tasks with as little psychological stress as possible. The medical management goal is to minimize the impact of the disease on the physical and emotional development and functioning of children and adolescents while the mental health goal is to achieve balance between disease management and positive mental health. These goals can only be met through the facilitation of interactions that occur in each of the four domains of adaptive functioning.

A focus on the developmental and biopsychosocial domains that all chronic childhood illnesses share will assist in drawing conclusions about mental health that apply regardless of the specific illness. It should be noted, however, that tremendous complexity exists among chronic illnesses including the type, severity, and progression of the illness, the resources of the family and community to support the child or adolescent, and the capacity of the health care provider team.

CHILDHOOD CHRONIC ILLNESS

The causes of chronic illness are discussed extensively in research involving the medical aspects of childhood chronic illness [3-5]. The causes typically include genetic or hereditary dispositions, birth traumas and other conditions present at birth, accidents and injuries, disease and illnesses, and conditions associated with the aging process. Detailed discussion of these causes is beyond the scope of this article. Despite the varied and complex causes of childhood and adolescent chronic illness, there are striking similarities among the effects that chronic illness has on the mental health status of this population.

Common Chronic Illnesses

The most common and disruptive chronic illnesses that have their onset in childhood or adolescence in the United States are respiratory allergies (9%), asthma (4%), eczema and skin allergies (3%), heart disease (2%), epilepsy (0.2%), and diabetes (0.1%) [2]. These chronic illnesses often co-occur with mental illness. For instance, depression and anxiety are associated with heart disease [6], type 2 diabetes [7,8], renal disease [9], obesity [10,11], and asthma [12-14].

Effects of Chronic Illness

By 2015, worldwide, 1.2 billion children aged 5-14 years will have some kind of significant chronic disease [15]. National population-based studies from western countries show that 20% to 30% of adolescents have a chronic illness, defined as one that lasts longer than six months, and 10% to 13% of those adolescents report having a chronic illness that substantially limits their daily life or requires extended periods of care and supervision. The increasing prevalence of chronic illness across the globe further indicates the need for research that fully explores the relation between mental health and chronic illness.

Children with chronic illnesses have an increased risk of emotional and behavioral problems [16]. This risk has been documented in epidemiological studies [1], as well as in studies of clinic samples [17]. The assessment and treatment of emotional and behavioral problems is recognized as an essential part of treating children and adolescents with chronic illness [17]. Even though children and adolescents with chronic illness may be in regular contact with general and specialty healthcare providers, the children may not have access to needed mental health support services, and many children and adolescents do not report mental health issues to medical providers [1]. Glazebrook and colleagues [17], for example, suggest that pediatricians detect only approximately 25% of psychosocial problems among their chronically ill patients.

Developmental Issues and Mental Health

Regardless of the specific developmental stage, children and adolescents must adapt to the nature and limitations of the chronic illness with its physical and emotional sequelae, as well as comply with recommended medical treatments to attain adult functionality. In addition, children and adolescents must fulfill normative tasks of individual growth and development. Incomplete adaptation to the chronic illness, non-adherence to medical advice, and/or failure to accomplish normative developmental tasks can result in significant emotional disorders, psychosocial impairment, and developmental delay [1]. Whereas adequate adaptive functioning in the psychosocial domain promotes mental health as well as effective management of the chronic illness, inadequate adaptive functioning within this domain can become a precursor to future mental health difficulties and/or play a significant role in assessing and managing current mental health concerns.

The response to living with a chronic illness depends on several factors, including but not limited to personality characteristics, the specific illness, and the family. Extremely important to the complex set of sequelae is the particular developmental stage in which the child or adolescent is operating that requires energy. Infants and toddlers, for example, are beginning to develop trust and an overall sense of security. They generally have very little understanding of their illness. Children in this stage of development experience pain, restricted emotion, and separation from parents as challenges to developing trust and security.

Preschool children are beginning to develop a sense of independence. They may understand what it means to get sick but they may not understand the cause and effect nature of illness. Being in the hospital or adjusting to a medication schedule, for example, can challenge the child's developing independence.

Early school-aged children are developing a sense of mastery over their environment. They can describe reasons for illness, but these reasons may not be entirely logical. Children this age often have "magical thinking." They may believe they caused the illness by thinking bad thoughts, by hitting their brother, or by not eating their vegetables. Children also begin to sense that they are different from their peers.

Older school-aged children are beginning to focus on peer relationships. They are now more capable of understanding their illness and its treatment but they should not be expected to respond as adults do. They may feel left out when they miss school or activities with their peers as developing and maintaining peer relationships is one of the most important psychosocial developmental tasks that will continue into adolescence.

Adolescents begin to develop their own identity separate from their families. Self-image becomes extremely important during the teenage years. The perception of the peer group is of paramount importance and is an issue when the adolescent's appearance is altered by illness or medication.

MENTAL HEALTH ISSUES

As stated previously, children and adolescents with chronic illness have the same developmental needs as other same age peers. In many ways, the accomplishment of developmental tasks is made more difficult by an extra set of demands and hardships associated with the chronic illness [18].

Typical developmental tasks may interact with issues related to chronic illness, producing increased demands and stress upon children and adolescents. If the additional stress is not managed effectively, then the risk for mental health problems increases. Although many chronically ill children and adolescents do not experience mental health problems secondary to development-related stress, several epidemiologic studies have found indications of approximately a two-fold increase in mental health problems among this group of children [1,19].

Although chronically ill children and adolescents can develop any type of mental health problem, the following discussion illustrates some of the areas in which the chronically ill may be most vulnerable.

Body Image Issues

One of the major developmental tasks of childhood and adolescence is the establishment of an individual identity while major changes are also occurring physically. Chronic illness may intensify concerns about personal and sexual identities with fears or distortions related to the illness. Research during the last two decades has demonstrated variability in body size preference and in body image dissatisfaction among children and adolescents based on age, pubertal status, presence or absence of a chronic illness or disability, gender, ethnicity, body mass index (BMI) or weight, and family relationships [20]. Specific body image concerns among chronically ill children or adolescents have not been investigated.

Adolescents report greater body image dissatisfaction than do younger children [21]. In addition, dissatisfaction with one's body image and the desire for thinness, with its perceived approval from others, increases as children approach puberty [22]. Girls report greater dissatisfaction than boys [23,24] and a greater desire for thinness [21]. Body mass index, at risk for overweight, or being overweight have positive associations with body image dissatisfaction among youth, according to some studies [25,26].

Children and adolescents with chronic illness may struggle with body image, especially if there is a visible difference or limitation in activity. This is especially apparent for adolescents who are concerned with membership in a particular peer group. For those adolescents who may take medication on a long-term basis to manage their illness, adherence with the drug regimen may be erratic. If the medication has undesirable side effects, such as weight gain or an increase in acne, adolescents may be acutely aware of body image issues.

Chronically ill children and adolescents may attempt to manage poor body images through the development of an eating disorder: a group of disorders that has a disturbance in eating behavior that endanger physical and mental health. Eating disorders include the following:

- Anorexia Nervosa—a condition in which a person purposely limits food intake and refuses to maintain a weight within a healthy range for height and age. People with Anorexia Nervosa may also binge and purge.
- Bulimia Nervosa—a condition that involves cycles of bingeing and behaviors that follow to prevent weight gain and can include such behaviors as vomiting, using laxatives, diuretics, or involvement in excessive exercise.
- Binge Eating Disorder—a condition in which a person binge eats but does not attempt to control weight through unhealthy purging behaviors. As many as one third of obese people may have this eating disorder but have gone undiagnosed.
- Eating Disorder NOS (not otherwise specified)—a term used with individuals who have disordered eating behaviors, dissatisfaction with body weight or shape, and harmful weight control behaviors that do not meet full criteria for one of the more severe eating disorders above.

Development of Independence

Chronic illness frequently interferes with the attainment of independence and autonomy. Parents may be less willing to grant autonomy to children and adolescents who have a chronic illness. While children and adolescents try to function autonomously, parents or caregivers may be reluctant for this to happen because they fear that the specific child or adolescent will not manage the chronic illness effectively. Because chronic illness may delay the onset of puberty with its immense increase in growth and development, parents may be even more likely to remain protective as children and adolescents may not appear to be capable of autonomous functioning. In addition, children and adolescents may become physically dependent upon the family for companionship, friendship, and social support if there is not a strong connection to the peer group.

Relationships with Peers

Chronic illness and the assessment, treatment, and management of that illness often interferes with time spent in the school setting, which is children's and adolescents' primary social environment. Self-esteem issues related to acceptance of self and concerns about acceptance by others are intensified in chronic illness. In addition, if they have limited access to the school setting or other social environments because they are ill, then their ability to establish and maintain peer relationships is impaired.

Given the central role that peer relationships play in the psychological development of children and adolescents, and because peer rejection and isolation have been associated with subsequent adjustment problems, chronically ill children and adolescents are at an increased risk for difficult psychological development. Meijer et al [27] and his colleagues report that the level of psychological adjustment among chronically ill children and adolescents is variable. This variability may be due, in part, to the presence of protective factors, such as the use of adequate coping strategies.

Promoting Positive Mental Health

Promoting positive mental health among children and adolescents with chronic illness means promoting adaptation and/or competence in living with that illness. Promoting competence requires the development and maintenance of sufficient capabilities to meet cumulative and persistent demands. It may also mean reducing demands or removing barriers to successful adaptation, such as minimizing hospital visits while encouraging family involvement, increasing opportunities for peer interaction, and maximizing independence in living.

There are four strategies to consider when promoting positive mental health: (1) encourage typical life experiences, (2) increase coping skills, (3) increase use of social support, and (4) empower families.

Encouragement of Typical Life Experiences

Children and adolescents with chronic illness have the same developmental needs as other same-age peers. Activities that challenge them to develop social skills, master new approaches to social situations, build self-esteem, and form separate and healthy identities away from caregivers while engaging with others (e.g., peers, family members, other adults) promote successful accomplishment of developmental tasks as well as positive mental health. As children and adolescents with chronic illness become fully integrated into family, school, and community activities, engaging in typical life experiences will become more routine and expected. Until then, however, it is often left up to the medical and mental health treatment teams to encourage parents and other caregivers to allow active participation in diverse life experiences by children with chronic illness.

Increase Coping Skills

Teaching children and adolescents with chronic illness and their family members how to cope with the demands of the illness is frequently a strategy used to promote mental health. Coping is behavior directed at restoring a balance between excess demands placed on children and adolescents secondary to achieving developmental tasks and managing the chronic illness with, often, inadequate resources.

If children or adolescents and their families manage to balance these needs, then the number and use of coping skills is adequate. There are times, however, when parents, caregivers, friends, or extended kinship networks are unable or unprepared to deal with the intense emotional response of chronically ill children and adolescents. Depending upon the type and severity of the chronic illness, just understanding and managing the illness can take so much time and emotional energy that the psychological aspects of the developing person are neglected [28]. The neglect of these psychological aspects may result in depression, anxiety, or other disorders requiring early treatment in order to prevent long-term negative sequelae.

Increase Use of Social Supports

Of all the resources for promoting positive mental health, none has received more attention than social support [29]. There have been many conceptualizations of social support, most of which incorporate the support that is given as well as the person who gives it. Three broad categories of support are listed below:

- emotional support that provides information that one is loved and valued, that children or adolescents matter to and are connected with others;
- informational support that helps chronically ill children and adolescents solve problems and find other tangible services and resources and can give feedback about how they are doing in managing the illness; and
- instrumental support or tangible support during times of extreme stress.

Social supports can be from formal or informal sources. Formal supports include assistance that can be accessed through the school system or the hospital setting. Informal support networks refer to family, friends, relatives, neighbors, churches, clubs, and organizations with whom a person voluntarily interacts. A combination of formal and informal supports is necessary for the optimal management of a chronic illness.

Empowerment of Families

The notion of empowerment of families of chronically ill children and adolescents is becoming associated with service delivery across many medical and mental health settings or professions [30]. Rather than parents or caregivers doing everything for chronically ill children or adolescents, thus maintaining dependency, a process is begun whereby the children or adolescents with a chronic illness discover and build on their own strengths, leading to a greater sense of mastery and control over their lives. They have confidence in their own ability to acquire and use resources to meet needs, to solve problems, and to make decisions. Empowered families of chronically ill children and adolescents are not helpless and dependent, nor are they totally independent. Rather, the goal of empowerment is interdependence among self, family, informal support, and formal service providers.

CONCLUSIONS

Growing up is a stressful developmental process even for physically healthy children and adolescents. Chronic illness further complicates the developmental process. The chronic illness, treatment requirements, hospitalization, and surgery, when necessary, all intensify concerns about physical appearance, interfere with the process of gaining independence, and disrupt changing relationships with parents and peers. In addition, developmental issues complicate the transition of children and adolescents toward taking responsibility for managing their illness and learning to comply with the medical and mental health treatment plans.

The prevalence of chronically ill children and adolescents with mental health issues, worldwide, is increasing as larger numbers of such children live until and beyond adolescence. In addition, the prevalence of certain chronic illnesses in adolescence, such as diabetes (types 1 and 2) and asthma, has increased, as have survival rates from cancer.

Although scientific evidence indicates that children with chronic illness have more mental health issues than their healthy peers, many controversies and gaps in the literature exist. A full understanding of the relation between chronic illness and mental health is yet to be available. Second, the specific types of mental health issues associated with specific chronic illnesses continue to be delineated. Third, there is inconsistency and a paucity of data regarding the connection between mental health and social issues among specific clinical groups of chronically ill children and adolescents. As research continues to illustrate the relation between chronic illness and mental health, appropriate services will be more available to meet the needs of children and adolescents.

REFERENCES

[1] Cadman D, Boyle M, Szatmari P, Offord DR. Chronic illness, disability and mental and social well-being: Findings of the Ontario child health study. *Pediatrics*. 1987;79:805-13.
[2] Rolland JS. Toward a psychosocial typology of chronic and life-threatening illness. *Fam. Syst. Med.* 1984;2:245-62.
[3] Bowe F. Physical, sensory, and health disabilities: *An introduction*. Upper Saddle River, NJ: Merrill, 2002.
[4] Eisenberg MG, Glueckauf RL, Zarensky HH, eds. Medical aspects of disability: *A handbook for the rehabilitation professional*. New York: Springer, 1999.
[5] Falvo D. Medical and psychosocial aspects of chronic illness and disability, 2nd ed. *Gaithersburg*, MD: Aspen, 1999.
[6] Muehrer P. Research on co-morbidity, contextual barriers, and stigma: A introduction to the special issue. *J. Psych. Res.* 2002; 53:843-5.
[7] Hippisley-Cox J, Fielding K, Pringle M. Depression as a risk factor for ischaemic heart disease in men: Population based case-control study. *BMJ*. 1998;316-1714-9.
[8] Strik JJ, Denollet J, Lousberg R, Honig A. Comparing symptoms of depression and anxiety as predictors of cardiac events and increased health care consumption after myocardial infarction. *J. Am. Coll. Cardiol.* 2003;42:1801-7.

[9] Guzman SJ, Nicassio PM. The contribution of negative and positive illness schemas to depression in patients with end-stage renal disease. *J. Behav. Med.* 2003;26:517-34.

[10] Linde JA, Jeffery RW, Levy RL, Sherwood NE, Utter J, Pronk NP, et al. Binge eating disorder, weight control self-efficacy, and depression in overweight men and women. *Int. J. Obes. Relat. Metab. Disord.* 2004;28:418-25.

[11] Yanovski SZ, Nelson JE, Dubbert BK, Spitzer RL. Association of binge eating disorder and psychiatric comorbidity in obese subjects. *Am. J. Psych.* 1993;150:1472-9.

[12] Ortega AN, Huertas SE, Canino G, Ramirez R, Rubio-Stippec M. Childhood asthma, chronic illness, and psychiatric disorders. *J. Nerv. Ment. Dis.* 2002;190:275-81.

[13] Goodwin RD, Jacobi F, Thefeld W. Mental disorders and asthma in the community. *Psychol. Med.* 2003;33:879-85.

[14] Goodwin RD, Fergusson DM, Horwood LJ. Asthma and depressive and anxiety disorders among young persons in the community. *Psychol. Med.* 2004;34:1465-74.

[15] Judson L. Global childhood chronic illness. *Nurs. Adm. Q.* 2004; 28:60-6.

[16] Lavigne JV, Faier-Routman J. Psychological adjustment to pediatric physical disorders: A meta-analytic review. *J. Pediatr. Psychol.* 1992; 17:133-57.

[17] Glazebrook C, Hollis C, Heussler H, Goodman R, Coates L. Detecting emotional and behavioral problems in pediatric clinics. *Child Care Health Dev.* 2003;29:141-9.

[18] Briggs-Gowan MJ, Horwitz SM, Schwab-Stone ME, Leventhal JM, Leaf PJ. Mental health in pediatric settings: Distribution of disorders and factors related to service use. *J. Am. Acad. Child Adolesc. Psychiatry*. 2000;39:841-9.

[19] Gortmaker SL, Walker DK, Weitzman M, Sobol AM. Chronic conditions socioeconomic risks, and behavioral problems in children and adolescents. *Pediatrics*. 1990;85:267-76.

[20] Doll HA, Petersen SE, Stewart-Brown SL. Obesity and physical and emotional well-being: Associations between BMI, chronic illness and the physical and mental components of the SF-36 questionnaire. *Obes. Res.* 2000;8:160-70.

[21] Cohn, LD, Adler NE. Female and male per-ceptions of ideal body shapes: Distorted views among Caucasian college students. *Psych. Women Q.* 1992;16:69-79.

[22] Gardner RM, Friedman BN, Jackson NA. Hispanic and white children's judgments of perceived and ideal body size in self and others. *Psychol. Record.* 1999;49.

[23] Hausenblas HA, Symons-Downs D, Fleming DS, Connaughton DP. Body image in middle school children. *Eat. Weight Disord.* 2002;7(3):244-8.

[24] Siegel J, Yancey A, Aneshensel C, Schuler R. Body image, perceived pubertal timing and adolescent mental health. *J. Adolesc. Health*. 1999; 25:155-65.

[25] Garner DM, Rosen LW, Barry D Eating disorders among athletes: Research and recommendations. *Child Adolesc. Psychiatr. N. Am.* 1998;7:839.

[26] Presnell K, Stice E. An experimental test of the effectiveness of dieting on bulimic pathology: Tipping the scales in a different direction. *J. Abnorm. Psychol.* 2003;112:166-70.

[27] Meijer SA, Sinnema G, Bijstra J, Mellenbergh GJ, Wolters WH. Coping styles and locus of control as predictors for psychological adjustment of adolescents with a chronic illness. *Soc. Sci. Med.* 2002;54:1453-61.

[28] Newacheck PW, Taylor WR. Childhood chronic illness: Prevalence, severity, and impact. *Am. J. Pub. Health*. 1992;82:364-71.

[29] McClellan C, Cohen L. Family functioning children with chronic illness compared with healthy controls: A critical review. *J. Pediatrics.* 2007;150(3):221-3.
[30] Bauman LJ, Drotar D, Leventhal JM, Perrin EC, Pless IB. A review of psychosocial interventions for children with chronic health conditions. *Pediatrics.* 1997;100(2):244-51.

In: Adolescence and Chronic Illness
Editors: H. Omar et al.

ISBN: 978-1-60876-628-4
© 2010 Nova Science Publishers, Inc.

Chapter 9

PSYCHIATRIC ISSUES IN CHRONICALLY ILL CHILDREN, ADOLESCENTS AND YOUNG ADULTS

Joseph L. Calles, Jr.

Associate Professor of Psychiatry, College of Human Medicine, Michigan State University, East Lansing, Michigan, U.S.A. Director, Child and Adolescent Psychiatry, Psychiatry Residency Training Program, Michigan State University/Kalamazoo Center for Medical Studies, Kalamazoo, Michigan, U.S.A.

INTRODUCTION

For those of us who provide medical care to younger patients, our quest to eradicate illness in that population has been a proverbial "double-edged sword." As noted by the World Health Organization [1], there has been a decline in acute medical conditions in children and adolescents, cured or prevented by improved nutrition, hygiene and antimicrobial agents. Conversely, there has been an emergence of chronic, often disabling, and sometimes fatal medical conditions in adolescence and early adulthood. This trend is already affecting developed countries, financially straining healthcare and social service systems. In the United States, one indicator of having a disabling condition is the receipt of monthly Supplemental Security Income (SSI) payments, which have been available to qualified, under-18 years of age individuals since 1974. Reviewing the data from that first year until 2005 (the last year reported) shows an increase in SSI payments to under-18 year-olds from 1.8% of the total number of recipients in 1974 to 14.6% of the total in 2005 [2].

The increased numbers of chronically ill children and adolescents presents another challenge: their maturation into adulthood, which will require the seamless transition of care from pediatric specialists to adult medical specialists in order to produce the best possible outcomes [3]. That follow-up care should also include psychiatric treatment, as many young adults with chronic illnesses will also suffer from emotional and behavioral problems that had their origins in earlier life. Following is a brief discussion of chronic medical conditions and their associated psychiatric symptoms and disorders in children, adolescents and young adults.

Specific Disorders

Asthma

The prevalence rates of asthma symptoms are quite variable around the world, although the differences are getting smaller. In the 13-14 year age group, rates of lifetime diagnoses of asthma range from 5.9% in Northern and Eastern Europe to 32.4% in Oceania [4]. The diagnosis and management of asthma in adolescents poses many challenges, including denial of symptoms, smoking, and treatment noncompliance [5].

Psychological issues may have negative effects on asthma management. A study of 11-17 year-olds with asthma found that, in the 5% who identified themselves as smokers, 37.8% met criteria for a depressive or anxiety disorder versus 14.5% of nonsmokers [6]. The smoking group was also less compliant with routine medication use (but used more "rescue" medications), more symptomatic, and less functional than those in the nonsmoking group.

In another study [7] groups of asthmatic adolescents (12-18 years of age), with/without a history of life-threatening asthma attacks, were compared to healthy controls. In those who had required intensive medical treatment of the asthma, or had experienced serious medical consequences (e.g. intubation), 20% met criteria for post-traumatic stress disorder (PTSD), versus 11% in the asthma controls and 8% in the healthy controls. What is relevant to this discussion is that PTSD symptoms accounted for 5% of the variance in functional asthma morbidity, and beside severity of illness (20% of the variance) was the only significant predictor of functional morbidity.

The exact causal relationship between asthma and depression is unclear [8]; nevertheless, it is important for clinicians to screen for depressive symptoms in their asthmatic patients, keeping in mind the effect that depression can have on compliance and symptomatology. It is equally important to screen for anxiety disorders [9], especially for PTSD in high-risk patients.

Sickle Cell Disease

Originating in parts of the world where malaria is endemic (especially in Africa), the gene mutation for sickle cell (SC) disease has been carried to other parts of the globe via immigration. For example, about 60,000 people in the United States and about 10,000 in the United Kingdom suffer from the disease [10]. As in many other chronic illnesses, especially those associated with pain and disability, rates of psychiatric comorbidity are high in SC disease.

When compared to healthy matched controls (from the same classrooms), children and adolescents (8-14 years-old) treated for SC disease at a comprehensive center showed significantly higher rates of total psychological problems as well as internalizing problems (i.e. depression and anxiety), and lower levels of competence per caregiver reports [11].

In a study involving a small number of children and adolescents (ages 7.5 to 15.5 years) who had been hospitalized at least once for a painful crisis [12], 27% met criteria for PTSD, a rate that is similar to that seen in patients who have had severe asthma attacks (as previously described). It appears that the PTSD symptoms were less related to severity of pain than to the perception that it could have been life-threatening, i.e. the development of PTSD was more reliant on psychological state than actual physical status.

Lastly, patients with SC disease (5-17 years of age) had rates of nocturnal enuresis that were significantly higher than those found in the general population [13]. The importance of this finding is that parents often restrict fluids to try and prevent bedwetting episodes; however, this contradicts the strategy of keeping SC patients well-hydrated in order to try and prevent sickling crises.

Although the connection between anxiety/depression and SC disease has been questioned [14], clinicians should still screen for those treatable psychiatric disorders, both for their own sake and for the sake of overall disease management.

Diabetes Mellitus

The incidence of diabetes mellitus, type 1 (DM-1) varies widely around the world. In most populations studied the incidence increases with age [15], placing adolescents at greater risk for developing the disease. Diabetes mellitus, type 2 (DM-2), once an uncommon cause of new-onset diabetes in children and adolescents, has become much more common worldwide, representing 45% of new cases in the United States and 80% in Japan [16]. Management of the illness becomes more difficult during adolescence, when patients not uncommonly stop following dietary, glucose monitoring and medication regimens.

Adolescents with either type of DM are at risk for developing depression, which contributes to the poor self-care that leads to hyperglycemia [17]. Depression is also a risk factor for the development of DM-2, which could set up patients for the bidirectional exacerbation of both disorders. Young people who endorse depressive symptoms at the time of DM-1 diagnosis also endorse high rates (almost one-third of patients) of suicidal ideation [18]. When followed over time patients with suicidal ideation tended not to progress to suicidal attempts, but did tend to have poor compliance with their medical regimens. An important note, however, is that in the few who did attempt suicide almost one-half induced hypoglycemia, either with insulin overdose or by refusing to eat.

Even in the absence of suicidal ideation, eating problems are common in both types of DM. Adolescent females with DM-1 are likely to engage in dieting, withholding of insulin and/or binge eating [19], while many patients of either sex with DM-2 will meet criteria for Binge eating disorder (BED) [20]. Many of the disordered eating behaviors may be related to dissatisfaction with body image and low self-esteem.

Proper evaluation, identification, and treatment of psychiatric issues in diabetic adolescents increase the likelihood that glycemic control will be achieved and maintained.

Epilepsy

Every year about 40% of newly recognized seizures occur in those under the age of 18 years, and most active cases of epilepsy- even in adults- have their onset in childhood [21]. Improvements in diagnosis and treatment have produced favorable medical outcomes (about 70% will achieve remission); however, early-onset epilepsy is associated with long-term psychological, cognitive and behavioral dysfunction.

A review of studies that explored the presence of psychological issues in epileptic youth [22] found that the risk for depression and suicidal ideation and behaviors was much greater than in non-epileptic controls, especially in females. An even more disconcerting finding was that in a significant number of patients the depression was not identified or treated.

Along with affective disorders, anxiety disorders are also common in patients (ages 5-16 years) with either complex partial or absence epilepsy, and in combination with a disruptive behavior disorder (Attention-deficit/hyperactivity disorder [ADHD], Oppositional defiant disorder [ODD], or Conduct disorder [CD]) are associated with higher rates of suicidal ideation [23].

Academic difficulties are common in young people with epilepsy, and are likely due to a combination of factors, including the seizure activity itself and side-effects of anti-epileptic drugs. There are two neuropsychiatric conditions that also contribute to school problems: ADHD and learning disorders. Although the rates of disruptive behavior disorders in young epileptic patients are highly variable, depending on the informant (e.g. parent vs. teacher), attentional problems- including formal ADHD- are seen at higher rates (30%-40%) than in healthy controls [24]. The ADHD is more likely to be of the inattentive type, rather than the hyperactive-impulsive or combined types, which could delay its recognition.

The school-age person with epilepsy is also at risk for having a learning disorder (LD). Even when excluding children and adolescents who have combined mental retardation and seizure disorders, about 25% of those with epilepsy alone will have a LD, the most common of which involves reading [25].

Arthritis

Juvenile idiopathic arthritis (JIA), with its various subtypes, is the most common arthritis encountered in younger people around the globe [26]. The prevalence of JIA is highly variable, with estimated worldwide rates of 7-401 per 100,000 and U.S. rates of 9.2-220 per 100,000 [27]. Youth with chronic arthritis are at risk of developing psychiatric problems; the risk derives not only from illness-related factors (e.g. reduced mobility) but also non-illness-related factors such as environmental stress.

In a study of 75 patients (ages 8-18 years) with chronic arthritis (three-fourths with some form of rheumatoid arthritis), the majority did not endorse significant symptoms of depression or anxiety. However, in those that did report clinically significant symptoms, depression and anxiety were related to older age, increased stressors, and negative attitudes about illness [28]. The level of depression in JIA can also be related to the level of physical pain experienced, which in turn can exacerbate the patient's depression [29]. In addition to pain, level of physical disability is moderately correlated to depression, anxiety, and behavioral disturbances in youth with JIA [30]. As adolescents with JIA transition into early adulthood the rate of depression declines, but the rate of anxiety remains quite high (present in almost one-third of patients) [31]. Anxiety and depression, in young adults, are perpetuated by patients' negative perceptions of body image, social support, and self-management [32].

Cancer

Although cancer is rare before the age of 20 years, for those 1-19 years of age cancer is the fourth leading cause of death and the most common cause of illness-related mortality [33]. What is often under-appreciated is that long-term (≥ 5 years) survivors of childhood cancer are at risk for developing late-occurring treatment sequelae. For example, psychosocial and cognitive disturbances are 2½ to 3-times more likely to occur by young adulthood in those who, as children, received radiotherapy of the head/neck region [34].

It would be reasonable to assume that youth diagnosed with- and treated for- cancer would have high rates of depression. Even though studies to date have been marred by methodological concerns, it appears that young cancer patients actually report less depression than do controls [35]. One possible explanation for this finding is that youth with cancer may have a repressive personality style, i.e. they counter-intuitively manifest desirable qualities during undesirable situations (e.g. acting happy while dealing with serious medical illness) [36]. Denial is an unconscious strategy used to avoid unpleasant thoughts and feelings. All young people with cancer should therefore be screened for the presence of depression.

Psychological disturbances, such as PTSD [37], can derive from the intensive medical interventions that cancer patients are subjected to. In those that develop post-traumatic symptoms, short-term adaptations to stressful life events are impaired [38], and longer-term effects are evidenced by early adulthood, wherein one-fifth of early cancer survivors have developed PTSD, with its associated high levels of anxiety and adverse effects on development [39,40].

Another manifestation of cancer-related stress is the number of adolescent survivors who smoke cigarettes and drink alcohol; they report that the negative behaviors are associated with fears of developing adverse late-effects of treatment and of recurrence of cancer [41]. That smoking and drinking behaviors place those young people at greater risk of developing cancer (as well as addictions) speaks to the high level of anxiety and worry that they experience, as well as to the need for healthier coping strategies.

Cerebral Palsy

World-wide estimates of the prevalence of cerebral palsy (CP) derive from population-based registries and from population-based, cross-sectional surveys; prevalence is in the range of 1.5-2.5 per 1000 live births [42]. In addition to the muscular spasticity seen in the majority of CP patients, there is a fairly high incidence of other physical problems, including visual and hearing impairments, epilepsy, speech abnormalities, and reduced linear growth [43].

Young patients with CP are also at risk for developing emotional and behavioral problems. When compared to controls (ages 4-17 years), patients with CP were 3.5 times more likely to be anxious and 5 times more likely to be hyperactive [44]. The perceptions of self-worth and competence (minus athletic competence) do not seem to vary between youth with CP and those from a normative sample. However, the presence of anxiety and/or depression tends to diminish the perceptions of both self-worth and competence in CP patients [45], which could limit or even suspend their involvement in social activities. The transition into young adulthood for those with CP can be especially challenging. In one study [46], concurrent with declining physical functioning, rates of anxiety increased to 63% and depression emerged in 10% of the sample.

Cystic Fibrosis

The prevalence of cystic fibrosis (CF) has been estimated in different regions around the world, although the illness most commonly affects Caucasians. In the European Union the mean prevalence was found to be 0.737 per 10,000 people [47]; in the United States, based on an estimated 2006 population of 299,398,484 [48] and 24,487 CF patients registered that same year with the Cystic Fibrosis Foundation [49], prevalence can be calculated at 0.818 per 10,000 people.

The literature on psychopathology in CF is contradictory [50], with some studies showing rates of anxiety and depression equal to those in normal controls, whereas others report higher rates. Pearson, et al [51], evaluated CF patients divided by age into two groups: 8-15 years and 16-40 years. The older group reported higher rates of anxiety (22.2% vs. 6.9%) and depression (42.4% vs. 14.8%) when compared to the younger group; symptoms were not related to severity or duration of illness. More recently, Bregnballe and colleagues [52] found that boys and girls 7-10 years of age and boys 7-14 years of age with CF had higher levels of anxiety than did healthy children. In the 11-14 years-old group there was an inverse correlation between anxiety and FEV_1 (forced expiratory volume at 1 second).

In the Pearson study [51], younger patients were more likely to develop symptoms of anorexia nervosa than were older patients (16.4% vs. 2.8%, respectively). Other studies are inconsistent, reporting both high rates [53] and low rates [54] of eating disorders in CF patients. Screening for eating disorders in CF patients should be considered in those who are making inadequate weight gains or who are losing weight.

Inflammatory Bowel Disease

The incidence of inflammatory bowel disease (IBD) is extremely rare before puberty; rates may be increasing, although differing definitions and methodologies limit the accuracy of reporting [55]. No matter what the actual incidence is, it has been known for some time that the illness starts in childhood in up to one-quarter of IBD cases [56]. Along with physical morbidities, IBD patients have higher rates of psychiatric morbidities.

Burke, et al [57], compared the lifetime prevalence rates of depression in three groups of chronically-ill children and adolescents: those with Crohn's disease (CD), those with ulcerative colitis (UC), and those with CF. That study found significantly higher rates of: depression in CD vs. CF; dysthymia (chronic depression) in UC vs. both CD and CF; and, "atypical depression" in both CD and UC vs. CF. No significant differences were found between groups regarding anxiety disorders.

Similar to that noted previously about CF, there are discrepant reports in the literature about rates of psychopathology in IBD patients. One possible confounder is that younger patients with IBD may minimize or even deny psychological symptoms, possibly related to the socially embarrassing nature of their physical symptoms [58]. It is incumbent upon the treating physician to gently question the patient with IBD about emotional issues, especially anxiety and worry.

Traumatic Brain Injury

The reality of traumatic brain injury (TBI) is very frustrating, given that much of it should be prevented; it is equally frightening, given the profound effects it can have on a person's functioning. Younger people are at high risk for sustaining cerebral injuries. As reported by the U.S. Centers for Disease Control and Prevention for the year 2002 [59], for 12 U.S. states, the age group 15-24 years had the second-highest rate of hospitalization for TBI (about 1 per 1,000 population), and was far and away the group with the highest rate of TBI related to motor vehicle accidents.

It is interesting to note that there is a high rate of psychiatric disorders in younger TBI patients that pre-date the head injuries [60,61], with ADHD being the most common premorbid condition. After brain trauma ADHD is also the most common psychiatric disorder, with more than one-third of survivors developing new problems with attention and impulse control [61]. Post-traumatic depression is also common (about one-fourth of new diagnoses), with the majority of cases resolving over time [61].

Other types of psychopathology following TBI include PTSD [62], other anxiety disorders [63], personality changes [64], and possibly psychosis [65]. Given the wide range and high rates of cognitive, emotional, and behavioral problems seen after head injury, the evaluation and management of TBI patients is best accomplished in a specialized, multidisciplinary setting. The primary pediatrician should have a working knowledge of local TBI-related resources.

Congenital Heart Disease

Since the beginning of the antibiotic era, congenital heart disease (CHD) has replaced rheumatic heart disease as the most common form of heart disease in children. The CHD prevalence of around 4 per 1,000 live births is surprisingly similar from countries half a world apart: India [66] and Brazil [67]. Having a CHD impacts not only healthcare resources and interpersonal functioning, but also intrapersonal factors such as mood and self-esteem, which are inversely correlated with severity of illness [68].

A group of adolescents with severe CHD was compared to an adolescent group with surgically repaired atrial septal defect (ASD) that was otherwise healthy [69]. A parent-completed checklist did not identify significant differences in psychopathology between groups. However, when results of semi-structured clinical interviews were compared, the rates of psychiatric problems (especially anxiety and depression) in the CHD group were significantly greater than those found in the ASD group. A Canadian study similarly found high rates of anxiety, depression and behavioral problems in children (average age 10 years) with CHD vs. healthy controls [70]. The levels of fear and anxiety were significantly greater in the children who had cyanotic CHD vs. the non-cyanotic group.

The findings from these two studies are consistent with meta-analytic findings that show that older children and adolescents (average age > 10 years) with CHD are more likely to experience internalizing symptoms than are CHD patients who are younger (average age < 6 years) [71]. Another vulnerable group is children who have cardiac surgery for CHD, in that there is a risk (> 10%) of developing PTSD, especially if the post-operative ICU stay is prolonged [72]. Externalizing problems, e.g. inattention and aggression, are also more common in CHD patients who have had cardiac surgery [73].

HIV Infection

One of the most unsettling aspects of HIV infection in children is that the vast majority who are infected, i.e. those living in sub-Saharan Africa, are the least likely to obtain adequate treatment [74]. Even in industrialized countries, such as the United States, greatly reduced mortality from HIV infection does not guarantee absence of morbidity; in fact, HIV-infected youth are at risk for developing neurocognitive and psychiatric disorders [75].

Children and adolescents with HIV infection are at high risk of developing depression [76,77], ADHD [77,78], other behavioral disorders [76,78], and anxiety disorders [78]. Although large, controlled studies have yet to be carried out, the average prevalence of ADHD, depression, and anxiety disorders in pediatric HIV/AIDS has been calculated as 28.6%, 25%, and 24.3%, respectively [79]; all of these are much greater than rates seen in the general population. Rates of psychiatric hospitalization are also higher in young people with HIV infection vs. those without infection [76].

The effective management of pediatric patients with HIV infection requires attention to multiple factors. Along with the disease process itself, the clinician should monitor for neuropsychiatric side effects of the anti-retroviral medications, family strain and dysfunction, reactions to the social stigma attached to HIV infection, and the patient's fear of separation from loved ones (e.g. through hospitalization or death) [80], in addition to the psychiatric issues noted above.

Hearing Impairment

Sensorineural hearing loss (SNHL) is caused by environmental factors (e.g. prenatal viral infections) in half of the cases and by genetic factors in the other half [81]. In developed countries there has been a dramatic decline in the numbers of cases of acquired SNHL, with an associated relative increase in inherited forms. In poorer developing countries both forms of SNHL remain high. No matter the cause or setting, growing up deaf is incredibly challenging and has consequences in terms of mental health [82]. Sadly, appropriate assessment and treatment services for the hearing impaired with psychiatric issues are not always available [83].

When compared to the general adolescent population using a standardized written questionnaire, severely and profoundly deaf Australian adolescents scored similarly in terms of psychopathology [84]. However, when the same instrument was converted into an interactive form, using sign language, the deaf adolescents endorsed much higher rates of withdrawal/depression, somatic symptoms, social problems and thought problems. In a study of mild-to-moderately hearing impaired Swedish adolescents [85], those who were hard-of-hearing (HH) had more mental symptoms (anxiety, depression, irritability) and school problems (truancy, poor grades) than did those without any disability. The presence of any other disability along with being HH also increased the risk of substance abuse. Finally, in a Dutch sample of deaf adolescents, the most accurate evaluation for psychopathology used reports from parents and teachers, as well as a semi-structured interview using sign-language interpretation [86]. Using this approach, 27% of the subjects were identified with an emotional disorder, 11% with a behavioral disorder.

SUMMARY

This chapter briefly discusses common, chronic illnesses that affect younger people worldwide. They all share the increased risk of comorbidity with psychiatric disorders, especially depression and anxiety. They also share the need for a comprehensive, multidisciplinary treatment approach, which includes input from mental health professionals. It is hoped that this information will be the impetus for asking chronically ill child, adolescent, and young adult patients about their moods, thoughts, and behaviors, and that the information elicited will lead to better medical management and clinical outcomes.

REFERENCES

[1] Michaud P-A, Suris JC, Viner R. The adolescent with a chronic condition. *Epidemiology, developmental issues and health care provision.* WHO discussion papers on adolescence, Department of Child and Adolescent Health and Development, World Health Organization, Geneva, Switzerland, 2007.

[2] Children Receiving SSI, 2005. SSA Publication No. 13-11830, Social Security Administration, Washington, DC, 2006. Available at: http://www.ssa.gov/policy/docs/statcomps/ ssi_children/2005/ssi_children.pdf Accessed December 30, 2007.

[3] Turkel S, Pao M. Late consequences of chronic pediatric illness. *Psychiatr. Clin. North Am.* 2007;30(4):819-835.

[4] Pearce N, Ait-Khaled N, Beasley R, et al. Worldwide trends in the prevalence of asthma symptoms: phase III of the International Study of Asthma and Allergies in Childhood (ISAAC). *Thorax.* 2007;62(9):758-766. Epub 2007 May 15.

[5] de Benedictis D, Bush A. The challenge of asthma in adolescence. *Pediatr. Pulmonol.* 2007;42(8):683-692.

[6] Bush T, Richardson L, Katon W, et al. Anxiety and depressive disorders are associated with smoking in adolescents with asthma. *J. Adolesc. Health.* 2007;40(5):425-432. Epub 2007 Feb 15.

[7] Kean EM, Kelsay K, Wamboldt F, Wamboldt MZ. Posttraumatic stress in adolescents with asthma and their parents. *J. Am. Acad. Child Adolesc. Psychiatry.* 2006;45(1):78-86.

[8] Opolski M, Wilson I. Asthma and depression: a pragmatic review of the literature and recommendations for future research. *Clin. Pract. Epidemol. Ment. Health.* 2005;1:18.

[9] Ross CJ, Davis TM, Hogg DY. Screening and assessing adolescent asthmatics for anxiety disorders. *Clin. Nurs. Res.* 2007;16(1):5-24; discussion 25-28.

[10] Meremikwu MM. Sickle cell disease. *BMJ Clin. Evid.* 2007;08:2402.

[11] Trzepacz AM, Vannatta K, Gerhardt CA, Ramey C, Noll RB. Emotional, social, and behavioral functioning of children with sickle cell disease and comparison peers. *J. Pediatr. Hematol. Oncol.* 2004;26(10):642-648.

[12] Hofmann M, de Montalembert M, Beauquier-Maccotta B, de Villartay P, Golse B. Posttraumatic stress disorder in children affected by sickle-cell disease and their parents. *Am. J. Hematol.* 2007;82(2):171-172.

[13] Jordan SS, Hilker KA, Stoppelbein L, Elkin TD, Applegate H, Iyer R. Nocturnal enuresis and psychosocial problems in pediatric sickle cell disease and sibling controls. *J. Dev. Behav. Pediatr.* 2005;26(6):404-411.

[14] Benton TD, Ifeagwu JA, Smith-Whitley K. Anxiety and depression in children and adolescents with sickle cell disease. *Curr. Psychiatry Rep.* 2007;9(2):114-121.

[15] Karvonen M, Viik-Kajander M, Moltchanova E, Libman I, LaPorte R, Tuomilehto J. Incidence of childhood type 1 diabetes worldwide: Diabetes Mondiale (DiaMond) Project Group. *Diabetes Care.* 2000;23:1516-1526.

[16] Pinhas-Hamiel O, Zeitler P. The global spread of type 2 diabetes mellitus in children and adolescents. *J. Pediatrics.* 2005;146(5):693-700.

[17] Stewart SM, Rao U, White P. Depression and diabetes in children and adolescents. *Curr. Opin. Pediatr.* 2005;17(5):626-631.

[18] Goldston DB, Kovacs M, Ho VY, Parrone PL, Stiffler L. Suicidal ideation and suicide attempts among youth with insulin-dependent diabetes mellitus. *J. Am. Acad. Child Adolesc. Psychiatry.* 1994;33(2):240-246.

[19] Jones JM, Lawson ML, Daneman D, Olmsted MP, Rodin G. Eating disorders in adolescent females with and without type 1 diabetes: cross sectional study. *BMJ.* 2000;320(7249):1563-1566.

[20] Crow S, Kendall D, Praus B, Thuras P. Binge eating and other psychopathology in patients with type II diabetes mellitus. *Int. J. Eat. Disord.* 2001;30(2):222-226.

[21] Shinnar S, Pellock JM. Update on the epidemiology and prognosis of pediatric epilepsy. *J. Child Neurology.* 2002;17(Suppl 1):S4-S17.

[22] Baker GA. Depression and suicide in adolescents with epilepsy. *Neurology.* 2006;66(6 Suppl 3):S5-12.

[23] Caplan R, Siddarth P, Gurbani S, Hanson R, Sankar R, Shields WD. Depression and anxiety disorders in pediatric epilepsy. *Epilepsia.* 2005;46(5):720-730.

[24] Dunn DW, Kronenberger WG. Childhood epilepsy, attention problems, and ADHD: review and practical considerations. *Semin. Pediatr. Neurol.* 2005;12(4):222-228.

[25] Beghi M, Cornaggia CM, Frigeni B, Beghi E. Learning disorders in epilepsy. *Epilepsia.* 2006;47 Suppl 2:14-18.

[26] Sawhney S, Magalhaes CS. Paediatric rheumatology- a global perspective. *Best Pract. Res. Clin. Rheumatol.* 2006;20(2):201-221.

[27] Sacks J, Helmick C, Yao-Hua L, Ilowite N, Bowyer S. Prevalence of and annual ambulatory health care visits for pediatric arthritis and other rheumatologic conditions in the US in 2001-2004. *Arthritis Rheum.* 2007;57(8):1439-1445.

[28] LeBovidge JS, Lavigne JV, Miller ML. Adjustment to chronic arthritis of childhood: the roles of illness-related stress and attitude toward illness. *J. Ped. Psychol.* 2005;30(3):273-286.

[29] Margetic B, Aukst-Margetic B, Bilic E, Jelusic M, Bukovac LT. Depression, anxiety and pain in children with juvenile idiopathic arthritis (JIA). *Eur. Psychiatry.* 2005;20(3):274-276.

[30] Ding T, Hall A, Jacobs K, David J. Psychological functioning of children and adolescents with juvenile idiopathic arthritis is related to physical disability but not to disease status. *Rheumatology.* 2008;47:660-664.

[31] Packham JC, Hall MA, Pimm TJ. Long-term follow-up of 246 adults with juvenile idiopathic arthritis: predictive factors for mood and pain. *Rheumatology.* 2002;41:1444-1449.

[32] Packham JC. Overview of the psychosocial concerns of young adults with juvenile arthritis. *Musculoskeletal Care.* 2004;2(1):6-16.

[33] Ries LAG, Smith MA, Gurney JG, Linet M, Tamra T, Young JL, Bunin GR (eds). *Cancer Incidence and Survival among Children and Adolescents:* United States SEER Program 1975-1995, National Cancer Institute, SEER Program. NIH Pub. No. 99-4649. Bethesda, MD, 1999.

[34] Geenen MM, Cardous-Ubbink MC, Kremer LCM, et al. Medical assessment of adverse health outcomes in long-term survivors of childhood cancer. *JAMA.* 2007;297:2705-2715.

[35] de Jong M, Fombonne E. Depression in paediatric cancer: an overview. *Psychooncology.* 2006;15:553-566.

[36] Phipps S, Srivastava DK. Repressive adaptation in children with cancer. *Health Psychol.* 1997;16(6):521-528.

[37] Taieb O, Moro MR, Baubet T, Revah-Levy A, Flament MF. Posttraumatic stress symptoms after childhood cancer. *Eur. Child Adolesc. Psychiatry.* 2003;12(6):255-264.

[38] Barakat LP, Kazak AE, Gallagher PR, Meeske K, Stuber M. Posttraumatic stress symptoms and stressful life events predict the long-term adjustment of survivors of childhood cancer and their mothers. *J. Clin. Psychol. Med. Settings.* 2000;7(4):189-196.

[39] Hobbie WL, Stuber M, Meeske K, et al. Symptoms of posttraumatic stress in young adult survivors of childhood cancer. *J. Clin. Oncol.* 2000;18:4060-4066.

[40] Schwartz L, Drotar D. Posttraumatic stress and related impairment in survivors of childhood cancer in early adulthood compared to healthy peers. *J. Ped. Psychol.* 2006;31(4):356-366.

[41] Cox CL, McLaughlin RA, Steen BD, Hudson MM. Predicting and modifying substance use in childhood cancer survivors: application of a conceptual model. *Oncol. Nurs. Forum.* 2006;33(1):51-60.

[42] Paneth N, Hong T, Korzeniewski S. The descriptive epidemiology of cerebral palsy. *Clin. Perinatol.* 2006;33(2):251-67.

[43] Odding E, Roebroeck ME, Stam HJ. The epidemiology of cerebral palsy: incidence, impairments and risk factors. *Disabil. Rehabil.* 2006;28(4):183-91.

[44] McDermott S, Coker AL, Mani S, et al. A population-based analysis of behavior problems in children with cerebral palsy. *J. Pediatr. Psychol.* 1996;21:447-463.

[45] Schuengel C, Voorman J, Stolk J, Dallmeijer A, Vermeer A, Becher J. Self-worth, perceived competence, and behaviour problems in children with cerebral palsy. *Disabil. Rehab.* 2006;28(20):1251-1258.

[46] Krakovsky G, Huth MM, Lin L, Levin RS. Functional changes in children, adolescents, and young adults with cerebral palsy. *Res. Dev. Disabil.* 2007;28:331-340.

[47] Farrell PM. The prevalence of cystic fibrosis in the European Union. *J. Cyst. Fibros.* 2008. Article in press.

[48] U.S. Census Bureau. Annual Estimates of the Population for the United States, Regions, States, and for Puerto Rico: April 1, 2000 to July 1, 2006 (NST-EST2006-01). Available at: http://www.census.gov/popest/states/tables/NST-EST2006-01.xls. Accessed May 21, 2008.

[49] Cystic Fibrosis Foundation, Patient Registry 2006 *Annual Report,* Bethesda, Maryland.

[50] Pfeffer PE, Pfeffer JM, Hodson ME. The psychosocial and psychiatric side of cystic fibrosis in adolescents and adults. *J. Cyst. Fibros.* 2003;2:61-68.

[51] Pearson DA, Pumariega AJ, Seilheimer DK. The development of psychiatric symptomatology in patients with cystic fibrosis. *J. Am. Acad. Child Adolesc. Psychiatry.* 1991;30(2):290-297.

[52] Bregnballe V, Thastum M, Schiotz PO. Psychosocial problems in children with cystic fibrosis. *Acta Paediatrica.* 2007;96(1):58-61.

[53] Pumariega AJ, Pursell J, Spock A, Jones JD. Eating disorders in adolescents with cystic fibrosis. *J. Am. Acad. Child Psychiatry.* 1986;25(2):269-275.

[54] Raymond NC, Chang PN, Crow SJ, et al. Eating disorders in patients with cystic fibrosis. *J. Adolesc.* 2000;23(3):359-63.

[55] Lakatos PL. Recent trends in the epidemiology of inflammatory bowel diseases: Up or down? *World J. Gastroenterol.* 2006;12(38):6102-6108.

[56] Kim SC, Ferry GD. Inflammatory bowel diseases in pediatric and adolescent patients: Clinical, therapeutic, and psychosocial considerations. *Gastroenterology.* 2004;126(6):1550-1560.

[57] Burke P, Meyer V, Kocoshis S, et al. Depression and anxiety in pediatric inflammatory bowel disease and cystic fibrosis. *J. Am. Acad. Child Adolesc. Psychiatry.* 1989;28(6):948-951.

[58] Engstrom I. Mental health and psychological functioning in children and adolescents with inflammatory bowel disease: a comparison with children having other chronic illnesses and with healthy children. *J. Child Psychol. Psychiatry.* 1992;33(3):563-82.

[59] Centers for Disease Control and Prevention. Incidence rates of hospitalization related to traumatic brain injury- 12 states, 2002. *MMWR.* 2006;55:201-204.

[60] Gerring JP, Brady KD, Chen A, et al. Premorbid prevalence of ADHD and development of secondary ADHD after closed head injury. *J. Am. Acad. Child Adolesc. Psychiatry.* 1998;37(6):647-654.

[61] Bloom DR, Levin HS, Ewing-Cobbs L, et al. Lifetime and novel psychiatric disorders after pediatric traumatic brain injury. *J. Am. Acad. Child Adolesc. Psychiatry.* 2001;40(5):572-579.

[62] Gerring JP, Slomine B, Vasa RA, et al. Clinical predictors of posttraumatic stress disorder after closed head injury in children. *J. Am. Acad. Child Adolesc. Psychiatry.* 2002;41(2):157-165.

[63] Vasa RA, Gerring JP, Grados M, et al. Anxiety after severe pediatric closed head injury. *J. Am. Acad. Child Adolesc. Psychiatry.* 2002;41(2):148-156.

[64] Max JE, Koele SL, Castillo CC, et al. Personality change disorder in children and adolescents following traumatic brain injury. *J. Int. Neuropsychol. Soc.* 2000;6:279-289.

[65] AbdelMalik P, Husted J, Chow EWC, Bassett AS. Childhood head injury and expression of schizophrenia in multiply affected families. *Arch. Gen. Psychiatry.* 2003;60:231-236.

[66] Chadha SL, Singh N, Shukla DK. Epidemiological study of congenital heart disease. *Indian J. Ped.* 2001;68(6):507-510.

[67] Miyague NI, Cardoso SM, Meyer F, et al. Epidemiological study of congenital heart defects in children and adolescents. Analysis of 4,538 cases. *Arq. Bras. Cardiol.* 2003;80(3):274-278.

[68] Birkeland AL, Rydberg A, Hagglof B. The complexity of the psychosocial situation in children and adolescents with heart disease. *Acta Pædiatr.* 2005;94:1495-1501.

[69] Spurkland I, Bjornstad PG, Lindberg H, Seem E. Mental health and psychosocial functioning in adolescents with congenital heart disease. A comparison between adolescents born with severe heart defect and atrial septal defect. *Acta Paediatr.* 1993;82(1):71-6.

[70] Gupta S, Giuffre RM, Crawford S, Waters J. Covert fears, anxiety and depression in congenital heart disease. *Cardiol. Young.* 1998;8(4):491-9.

[71] Karsdorp PA, Everaerd W, Kindt M, Mulder BJ. Psychological and cognitive functioning in children and adolescents with congenital heart disease: a meta-analysis. *J. Pediatr. Psychol.* 2007;32(5):527-41.

[72] Connolly D, McClowry S, Hayman L, Mahony L, Artman M. Posttraumatic stress disorder in children after cardiac surgery. *J. Pediatr.* 2004;144(4):480-484.

[73] Miatton M, De Wolf D, François K, Thiery E, Vingerhoets G. Behavior and self-perception in children with a surgically corrected congenital heart disease. *J. Dev. Behav. Pediatr.* 2007;28(4):294-301.

[74] Prendergast A, Tudor-Williams G, Jeena P, Burchett S, Goulder P. International perspectives, progress, and future challenges of paediatric HIV infection. *Lancet.* 2007;370(9581):68-80.

[75] Donenberg GR, Pao M. Youths and HIV/AIDS: Psychiatry's role in a changing epidemic. *J. Am. Acad. Child Adolesc. Psychiatry.* 2005;44(8):728-747.

[76] Gaughan DM, Hughes MD, Oleske JM, et al. Psychiatric hospitalizations among children and youths with human immunodeficiency virus infection. *Pediatrics.* 2004 Jun;113(6):e544-51.

[77] Misdrahi D, Vila G, Funk-Brentano I, Tardieu M, Blanche S, Mouren-Simeoni MC. DSM-IV mental disorders and neurological complications in children and adolescents with human immunodeficiency virus type 1 infection (HIV-1). *Eur. Psychiatry.* 2004 May;19(3):182-4.

[78] Mellins CA, Brackis-Cott E, Dolezal C, Abrams EJ. Psychiatric disorders in youth with perinatally acquired human immunodeficiency virus infection. *Pediatr. Infect. Dis. J.* 2006 May;25(5):432-7.

[79] Scharko AM. DSM psychiatric disorders in the context of pediatric HIV/AIDS. *AIDS Care.* 2006 Jul;18(5):441-5.

[80] Rao R, Sagar R, Kabra SK, Lodha R. Psychiatric morbidity in HIV-infected children. *AIDS Care.* 2007;19(6):828-33.

[81] Smith RJH, Bale JF, White KR. Sensorineural hearing loss in children. *Lancet.* 2005;365:879-90.

[82] du Feu M, Fergusson K. Sensory impairment and mental health. *Advances in Psychiatric Treatment.* 2003;9:95-103.

[83] Briffa D. Deaf and mentally ill: are their needs being met? *Australas Psychiatry.* 1999;7(1):7-10.

[84] Cornes A, Rohan MJ, Napier J, Rey JM. Reading the signs: impact of signed versus written questionnaires on the prevalence of psychopathology among deaf adolescents. *Aust. N. Z. J. Psychiatry.* 2006;40(8):665-73.

[85] Brunnberg E, Bostrom ML, Berglund M. Self-rated mental health, school adjustment, and substance use in hard-of-hearing adolescents. *J. Deaf. Stud. Deaf. Educ. Advance Access* published on December 13, 2007.

[86] van Gent T, Goedhart AW, Hindley PA, Treffers PD. Prevalence and correlates of psychopathology in a sample of deaf adolescents. *J. Child Psychol. Psychiatry.* 2007;48(9):950-8.

In: Adolescence and Chronic Illness
Editors: H. Omar et al.

ISBN: 978-1-60876-628-4
© 2010 Nova Science Publishers, Inc.

Chapter 10

EATING DISORDERS AND THERAPEUTIC HEALTH OUTCOME

Bruce Kirkcaldy[*1], *Marlies Pinnow*[2] *and Georg R. Siefen*

[1] International Centre for the Study of Occupational and Mental Health, Düsseldorf.
[2] Faculty of Psychology, Ruhr-University of Bochum.
[3] Department of Pediatrics, Ruhr-University Bochum,
St Josef Hospital, Bochum, Germany.

ABSTRACT

In a German child and adolescent psychiatric clinic, female adolescents were much more likely than males to exhibit eating disorders, affective disorders and personality disturbances. Suicidal behaviour was least common among the clinical groups of eating disorder (8.3%) and hyperkinetic /social disorder (2.9%). Moreover, significantly more of the adolescents with eating disorders revealed higher intelligence quotients (22.2% in excess of 115 IQ points) compared to other clinical groups e.g. neurotics and stress related disorders (7.2%) and emotional/social disorders (4.3%). Personality profiles of neurotic/stress and eating disordered groups revealed differences on the individual difference variables, physical ailments, schizoid-compulsive, social inhibition and delinquency. Overall, eating disordered adolescents were inclined to be low in externalisation (and somewhat higher on internalisation). Significant differences were also observed on the scales insecurity, depression, compulsiveness and aggression – individuals with eating problems scoring higher on all scales with the exception of aggression, which was substantially lower. Eating disordered individuals were less likely than other clinical groups to originate from families with abnormal inner family relationships, inadequate and/or maladaptive family communication, parental overprotectiveness and/or acute stressful life events. Medical and psychological expert ratings of health outcome revealed that almost two-thirds of the eating disordered group had shown "full recovery" or "significant improvement" in contrast to the clinical group "neurotic/stress" (42.6%) and the emotional and social disturbed (31.5%). The

---

* *Correspondence:* Bruce David Kirkcaldy, MA, PhD, FBPsS, International Centre for the Study of Occupational and Mental Health, Haydnstrasse 61, D-40593 Düsseldorf, Germany. E-mail: brucedavidkirkcaldy@yahoo.de

implications of these findings are discussed in terms of psychotherapeutic treatment plans for adolescents in clinical care.

INTRODUCTION

Eating disorders is a psychological disorder with diverse forms of manifestations [1] and the Diagnostic and Statistical Manual of Mental Disorders (DSM-IV) of the American Psychiatric Association and the World Health Organisation's International Classifications of Diseases (ICD-10) distinguish between anorexia nervosa, bulimia nervosa and eating disorders not otherwise specified, the latter presenting a group of less differentiated eating disorders. Despite the heterogeneity in the phenomenology of eating disorders, they all have their origins in dietary and regimented eating behaviour. In the subsequent development of the disorder, the changes in life-important nutritional intake lead to enormous psychosomatic problems with somatic, psychological and social implications. There is evidence that the psychological similarities between eating disorders e.g. anorexia nervosa and bulimia nervosa are more pronounced than the differences [2].

In addition to the enormous personal costs for eating disorders the financial burden for the community health services has to be taken into account. For 2001 the direct cost of a patient receiving 12 week's specialist in-patient British NHS treatment was estimated as approximately 25,000 pounds, with private patient costs for the same period ranging between 24,500-45,500 pounds [3]. In a German adolescent clinic an average 10-11 week hospitalisation would cost approximately 22,500 euro (the majority of these patients were either still at school or doing apprenticeships, hence there are scarce additional financial costs incurred through loss of working time).

Incidence of the Eating Disorder and Gender Differences

The Royal College of Physicians found three times as many women as men who displayed a body mass index (BMI) of less than 20 (8.1 and 2.4% respectively). At the same time there has been an almost obsessive preoccupation in Western culture concerning the idealisation of a thin female or muscular male physique, suggesting that the concern over body image is not restricted to women. Furthermore consequences of self-perceived attractiveness are important. There is evidence that young adolescents, who were being teased about their weight are likely to be more dissatisfied with their bodies and were more likely to contemplate or attempt suicide compared to those who had not been teased [4].

Cash [5] found in a large scale survey, that 34 percent of men and 38 percent of women expressed dissatisfaction with their overall physical appearance. There had been a marked increase in body image satisfaction in the period from 1972 to 1986. A substantial proportion of men and women report dissatisfaction with their body weight even when they are within the healthy weight region. Sixty percent of women and 25 percent of men who had normal weight perceived themselves as being too fat and/or exhibited self-disparaging thoughts and feelings about their appearance. Moreover, there is a wealth of research suggesting that a prevalence of clinical symptoms such as social anxiety, depression and sexual dysfunction are frequently found in association with negative body image, and this is particularly evident in eating disorders such as anorexia and bulimia [6].

It has generally been asserted that only a minority of the population [7-9] will display eating disorders (both anorexia and bulimia nervosa) though estimates inevitably differ [10]. For young females, van Hoeken, Lucas and Hoek [11] provide typical rates of anorexia from between 2 and 8 per 1,000 (0.2-0.8%). In a review of the literature, Palmer [12] suggested that the incidence rates of anorexia nervosa in health service, including primary care, amount to around 4-10 cases per 100,000 inhabitants per year. More recently, Teachman, Schwartz, Gordic and Coyle [13] reported that the incidence rate of anorexia nervosa among young women (late adolescence and early adulthood) in America is between 0.4-1.0 percent. The rate of bulimia nervosa among college students is significantly higher, about 3-4% [14]. As mentioned, it is a mistaken assumption that males are never prone to anorexia [15].

The US National Institute for Mental Health [16] cites estimates of between 0.5 and 3.7% of females suffering from anorexia nervosa and an estimated 1.1 - 4.2% have bulimia during their lifetimes. In contrast, 2-5 percent of Americans experience binge-eating in a six-month period [17]. There is some evidence that a higher prevalence of homosexuality among men with bulimia nervosa exists which may be attributable to greater dysfunction in psychosexual development than among females [18].

In a South Australian Survey of eating disorder behaviour, Hay [19] reported figures of 3.2% of respondents who had regular episodes of binge eating, 1.6% having professed to fasting regularly or using a strict diet, 0.8% purging, 0.3% had bulimia nervosa and 1.0% binge eating disorder. Strict dieting was less common for those persons who were married or cohabiting, may be because living with someone can inhibit extreme dieting behaviour or mediates behaviour, or it had been suggested that the behaviour is mediated through things such as emotional support and/or improved self-esteem.

Contemporary research studies have not be able to clearly identify the main causes of anorexia nervosa so that currently a multidimensional aetiological model of the disorder prevails, incorporating biological. Individual, familial and socio-cultural factors [20,21]. As a result of the complex aetiology and a more favourable prognosis for those individuals with a shorter history of the disorder (time between onset of illness and the onset of therapy), there has been increased effort by researchers to focus their attention on the identification of those pathogenic mechanisms which lead to a maintenance of the disorder and a subsequent deterioration of health.

The multidimensional model of eating disorders is clearly due to eating being controlled by diverse factors including appetite, availability of nutritional resources, family and cultural practices, peer pressures and attempts at voluntary control [16].

Co-Morbidity and Individual Differences

Overall, it is asserted that eating disorders such as anorexia nervosa show considerable heterogeneity in symptomatology and co-morbid psychopathology, including substance abuse, mood disorders, anxiety disorders and personality disorders.

Eating disorders are frequently associated with other psychological disorders such as substance abuse, anxiety and depression disorders [22]. The most prevalent disorders are anxiety and affective disorders as well as anxious-fearful-obsessive personality disorders

[23]. There are suggestions that anorexia is a manifestation of obsessive-compulsive disorder. Anorexics for example display "stereotypically rigid, ritualistic, perfectionist and meticulous" attributes with an "obsessional concern with food and focus on control" personality traits. Less specific features of OCD are negativism, rebelliousness and intense dedication to physical activity [24]. Some studies [25] reported that approximately 10 percent of female patients with OCD had displayed a history of anorexia.

Teachman et al [13] reported individual factors that exerted a role in children and adolescents with anorexic disorders, which included high expectations and perfectionism, extreme desire to conform, high degree of restraint and inhibition, avoidance of risk taking and dependence on outward rewards and compliments. In addition to high expectations, bulimics are characterised by interpersonal sensitivity, an outgoing personality coupled with impulsivity, emotional lability and low self-esteem.

There is some evidence that personality factors associated with anorexia nervosa include social isolation, low self-esteem and perfectionism. High rates of avoidant personality disorders were reported among eating disordered individuals, but anorexics showed greater compulsivity ("serious and rule conscious") than did bulimics [26]. Wonderlich et al [27] found a common phenotype in the restricting-type of anorexia nervosa characterised by high restraint, obsessionality and perfectionism. They found evidence that variability in the anorexic diagnostic type could be related to personality traits. Milos et al [28] examined comorbidity and eating disorder inventory profiles in eating disordered patients. It has been suggested that some EDI subscales are influenced by other psychiatric disorders such as depression, obsessive-compulsive disorders or personality disorders. The psychological subscales of the EDI seem to be associated with problems in intrapersonal and interpersonal relationships that can result particularly from anxious and affective disorders [27].

Marano [29] refers to two-thirds of people suffering from eating disorders that exhibit some source of clinical anxiety such as obsessive-compulsive disorder or social phobia. For those eating disordered individuals who did not show a clearly diagnosable anxiety disorder, they had anxiety-related traits such as generalised anxiety, anxiety-avoidance and perfectionism.

Some researchers e.g. Schmidt et al [30] argued that maladaptive eating behaviour represents a way of coping with stress, particularly negative emotions. Individuals with eating disorders are assumed to have difficulties expressing their feelings (alexthymia). Anorexia is frequently associated with the trait of "autistic" or "lacking empathy" [31]. Crisp [32] claimed the single-minded rejection of food characterizing anorexia nervosa is a biologically based avoidance behaviour propelled by a phobia of normal bodily weight.

Some researchers [33] argue that despite the co-occurrence of eating disorder and depression, there would seem little empirical support that either anorexia or bulimia nervosa represents an underlying depressive disorder. Therapeutic outcome studies have shown that bulimic patients who have improved during their treatment generally exhibit a disappearance of this co-occurring psychiatric disorder indicating that the depression was a secondary consequence of the eating disorder.

Developmental and Intellectual Factors

Eating disorders generally begin between early adolescence, 13-18 years and early adulthood. In instances of early onset (7-12 years) features of depression and/or obsessional behaviour can be apparent. Selvini-Palazolli and co-workers [34] reported the average age of outbreak of anorexia among their patients was 16 years, with symptoms initially appearing between 12 and 18 years, most frequently at 14 years of age. Anorexia nervosa has an age-adjusted incidence of 14.6 per 100,000 for females in the age group 15-24 years [35].

Walitza et al [36] found that among 140 adolescents in a German university clinic suffering from eating disorders, the anorectic patients were higher than average on IQ, as well as their revealing more enmeshment and over-protectiveness in family relations, greater separation anxiety and inferior communication skills. The bulimic patients showed inferior scholastic performance and more disciplinary difficulties at school. Other researchers have shown that anorexics are more intelligent and also high-achievers.

Many descriptive cross-sectional studies have tended to neglect contemporary theories of neurobiological developmental psychology which have been shown useful in "addictive" research. It has, for instance, been observed that youths and adolescents are inclined to display dependency disorders in this period of their development, suggesting that adolescence represents a critical phase of vulnerability [37]. Moreover, the disorder anorexia nervosa typically emerges during early and middle stages of puberty and adolescence [38]. Cortical developmental processes have been shown to undergo changes during this period which are associated with motivation, impulsivity and dependency [37], which in turn appear related to intentional behaviour and executive functions [39]. Patients exhibiting eating disorders during this phase develop a potent functional cycle coupled with dysfunctional eating behaviour in which both psychological as well as physiological reinforcing mechanisms are established and maintained [40].

Among the psychological factors, self-assuredness and self-efficacy seem to play a major role, and among individuals suffering from anorexia nervosa, they are likely to implement diverse methods of newly acquired behaviours including nutritional habits and manipulating body weight as methods of influencing their self-concept.

Family, Socio-Cultural Functioning and Birth Order

Jacobi et al [41] in a review of the literature focused on the extremely dominant position of the mother or another female member of the family, and this in turn results in difficulties in the necessary identification the daughter has with her mother. Further, the communication structures within such families are frequently "enmeshed" and frequently characterised by rigid systems. The individual's development towards autonomy and self-sufficiency is inhibited by the family's reluctance to yield strivings towards independence which are perceived as threatening. The authors underline that although these findings are common among eating disordered individuals, they are not specific for such young clinical groups. Indeed any observed pathological family relationship may be a reaction to the illness itself.

Palmer [12] asserts that the theories underlining (dysfunctional) family influences on eating disorders are not supported by empirical systematic research, and have frequently been counterproductive, imposing an additional burden on the current family suffering. There is an indication, however, that recollections of childhood are inclined to feature diverse negative characteristics, common to other psychiatric disorders. Some specific recollections include low contact and higher expectations of parents. On the other hand, there is also evidence [41,42] that sufferers of anorexia nervosa report less overt difficulties in their childhood.

Men who display eating disorders are more inclined to display dependent, avoidant and passive aggressive personality styles. They have often experienced unfavourable reactions to their bodies from their peers during their development and did not conform to the cultural expectations for masculinity. They also more frequently reported feeling closer to their mothers than fathers. Overall their passive-dependency and tendency towards non-athleticism may result in increased feelings of social isolation and ridicule concerning their body [43].

In a retrospective study of some 250 anorexic patients, Gower et al [44] focused on family structure and birth order. There was little evidence of a relationship to birth order, nor was there evidence of a preponderance of female siblings within the families of anorexic patients. Selvini-Palazzoli et al [34] found that there was a tendency for eating disorder patients with no siblings to display inferior general health feelings than those with sisters/brothers. On the other hand, having only sisters among their siblings did not affect subjective reports of well-being. They found that 54% of patients reported a favourable attitude towards their family and 32% were "mixed" with only 14% expressing negative feelings.

Twin studies suggest that biological factors do exert a significant role in eating disorders. For example, Schepank [45] and Kendler et al [46] have shown a higher concordance for mono- and indeed dizygotic twins. Kendler et al [47] found that for the disorder bulimia nervosa a significant effect emerged for familial environmental factors as a predictor of the ailment. Kassett et al [48] found higher rates of substance abuse and depression in first-degree relatives of patients with anorexia and bulimia.

Self-Injury and Suicidal Behavior

Dancyger and Fornani [49] examined eating disorders and suicide. Age of onset of eating disorder, co-morbid psychopathology, age of individuals at onset of study, duration of follow-up are all factors which influence the relationship between suicidal behaviour and eating disorder. They provided a meta-analysis of studies of suicide and eating disorders in adolescence and young adulthood. Overall suicide rates varied between 2.2% to a high of 15%. For bulimia nervosa rates were between 0.45 to 2.2%. Rates of mortality and suicide are significantly higher than for the general population but how do these figures compare to other clinical populations?

Moreover, gender has also been shown to exert a major effect on suicidal behaviour, for instance, males with eating disorders had more than double the number of attempted suicides than females - as indeed were the number of completed suicides among males. Furthermore, bulimic and anorectic individuals both display elevated scores on depression and anxiety. Malnutrition and emaciation may elicit symptoms which are difficult to distinguish from depression. There are problem of causality here because depression may be pre-morbid to the eating problem. The authors suggest that because eating disorders are related to higher incidences of co-morbid psychopathology (e.g. mood disorders, substance abuse, anxiety disorders and personality disorders) it may be the coexisting clinical disorders which are associated with increase in suicidal behavior and suicidal ideation [49,50].

Health Outcome and Therapy Success Rate

For the area of specialisation of child and adolescent psychiatry, anorexia nervosa (AN) occupies a conspicuous position, in that it emerges predominantly during early adolescence and is mainly witnessed among females with a chronic progressive deterioration in physical and psychological well-being. The mean mortality rate "hovering" around 6 percent, raises anorexia nervosa to the heights of one of the psychological disorders with a high mortality rate [51]. Despite a particularly extensive and prolonged therapeutic treatment programme, some would argue that anorexia nervosa has a low positive prognosis rate [52]. Some current follow-up studies have asserted that only one-third of patients suffering from symptoms of eating disorders are symptom-free two years after completion of treatment [53].

Personality factors have been shown to have an important impact on the success rate of therapy treatment, so that female patients who are less likely to comply with therapy are more anxious, and have lower scores on those factors associated with self-responsibility such as self-acceptance and tolerance [54]. Earlier onset of anorexia nervosa has been associated with higher recovery rates and a lower mortality. Herpertz-Dahlman [23] found that adolescent anorexic patients who overcame their eating problem did not differ from normal controls with regard to psychosocial functioning (partnership, family relationships and occupational status).

Fichter and coworkers [55] examined the long-term development of anorexia nervosa over a period of 12 years among just over 100 patients. They observed substantial improvement during the therapy, followed by a moderate decline during the 2 years after treatment, and further improvement between 3 to 12 years after treatment completion. The evaluation statistics over 12 years revealed 27.5% had a good outcome, 25.3% intermediate outcome, almost 40% had poor outcome and 7.7% had deceased. The major predictors of treatment outcome after 12 years were impulsivity, sexual difficulties, (long) duration of inpatient treatment and duration of eating disorder.

Selvini Palazzoli et al [34] reported that of 143 patients in their follow-up study, 89% were symptom free (anorexic symptoms), 4.3% showed restrictive anorexia, 5.3% bulimia and 1.4% had died. As regards global feeling of well-being, 56% were rated "good", a further 25% satisfactory, and 12% still had problems with 6% seriously incapacitated. In a previous study, Santonasto et al (56) found just over two-thirds (68%) of their patients had recovered after a follow-up study 6.8 years later.

The National Institute for Mental Health [16] cites a mortality rate for anorexics of 0.56% per year or 5.6 percent over a decade, which would seem to correspond closely to the figures for Germany [55]. These fatalities are due to complications caused by the disorder including cardiac arrest, electrolyte imbalance and suicide [57]. Teachman et al [13] report studies suggesting that 80 percent of individuals suffering from bulimia nervosa and 73% of those with anorexia nervosa show full or partial recovery.

Cognitive behavioural therapies have demonstrated good maintenance of therapeutic change at 6 and 12 month follow-up. Fairburn et al [58,59] have conducted rigorous post-treatment assessment studies and found binge eating and purging had declined over 90% after one year, and over one-third (36%) of patients had ceased all binge-eating and purging.

In a review of the course and outcome of the eating disorders, Palmer [12] reports that at about five years after treatment, the majority of individuals are recovered or nearly so, with some 25% still highly symptomatic (chronic course over many years). Outcome studies of anorexia show that recovery rates after ten years range between 18-76% with death rates ranging from 0-6%. In this chapter we will look at the following hypotheses

- Within a clinical population, male and female adolescents will differ in their clinical diagnoses. More specifically, females will be overrepresented in the eating disordered group
- What percentage of clinical population exhibit eating disorders?
- Is suicidal and self-injurious behaviour higher among eating disordered compared to other clinical groups?
- Anorexics will display higher intelligence quotient compared to other groups.
- Anorexics will be more inclined to display negative affect, reflected in elevated anxiety and depression scores and social inhibition.
- Eating disorders will be associated with compulsive and impulsive tendencies and inhibited overt aggression.
- Eating disorders will originate from dysfunctional families characterised by maladaptive intra-family communication.
- The likelihood of therapy success will be low among the eating disorder group compared to other clinical diagnoses.

OUR STUDY

The sample comprises approximately 2,500 children and adolescents in hospitalised care with a recognised medical/psychiatric diagnosis. Data were collected from the clinic in the Marl area of West Germany, Westfalia Clinic for Child and Adolescent Psychiatry and Psychotherapy, one of the two largest specialised medical centres of its kind in Germany. It has over 129 beds in 12 wards, with diverse specialised treatment units and 48 day clinic placements. The clinic is required to cater for the needs of 2.2 million inhabitants of an area from Southern Münster to the Northern districts of the Ruhr. This geographical region in the middle of the Rhein-Ruhr area represents a typical semi-rural area in the northern, Protestant part of Germany. The patients would all have reported a psychological problem which was so distressing that clinical attention had been recommended. Admission was to the clinic for child and adolescent psychiatry and psychosomatics during the period from July 2001 until the end of 2003. The sample includes all admissions with the exception of those crisis interventions that lasted shorter than two weeks. Therapists were required to complete a socio-medical and psychological status evaluation programme involving expert ratings on a standardised medical-psychological documentation scheme ("Ba-Do"). This structured interview inventory covered comprehensive areas of family lifestyle, educational status, family history of mental and physical illnesses, and socio-demographic data. In addition, a self-report questionnaire including items relating to self-injurious behaviour, suicidal intent and socially disruptive and threatening behaviour (FAPS) and the symptom checklist (SCL-90) were administered to a representative sample of the clinic population, consisting of the patients between 12 and 19 years of age being treated on four of the twelve wards. Treatment generally is eclectic combining elements of CBT with psychoanalytical and systemic diagnostical and therapeutical approaches. Individual and group-oriented therapy is conducted together with parental counselling within each ward, as well as more general somatic and creativity-related therapy programmes.

Overall there are more males than females in the child and adolescent clinic. The average age was 13.4 years, and although the range is from 3-24, the majority (almost 80%) – and the focus of this study - were between 12 and 18 years of age. The mother's age at birth of the "target" child was approximately 26 years. Just over 70 percent had average IQs (defined as within the range of 85-114), with 8.1% displaying an intelligence quotient in excess of 114 points. At the other end of the distribution, 20.3% yielded IQs below 85. Focussing on the 12-18 year old group, about a 38% of the students were attending either a technical or a grammar school, and the remainder a secondary or comprehensive school. There was an average of 2.3 other siblings in the family. The four most frequent psychiatric diagnoses were emotional and social disturbances in childhood, neurotic, stress and somatoform disorders, hyperactivity and social disorders, and eating disorders (bulimia and anorexia nervosa). The mean duration of hospitalisation was around 50 days (maximal stay around 40 weeks).

The questionnaires written in the German language explored socio-demographic variables (gender, age, nationality, number of siblings, and educational status); family variables (e.g. parental child-rearing style, intra-family communication), and mental well-being (problems of introversion and anxiety/depression). These psychometric questionnaires had been recommended by a group of clinical psychologists whose central interests were the identification and treatment schedules for self-injurious and/or mutilating behaviour. For this purpose, only a select sample of adolescents for a specific period (few months) and for several wards were given the entire sequence of questionnaires. The documentation basic health screening (Ba-Do) on the other hand was used for practically all admissions with the exception of short-term crisis interventions. The basic medical documentation programme is in accord with the original interview construction by the Frankfurt Medical College. More recently, attempts have been made to develop a revised, short computerised form of the Ba-Do which is expected to be the standard benchmarking procedure for screenng in adolescent psychiatric clinics.

For the more detailed psychometric analyses, a fixed time frame was chosen. Over a specific time frame of 10-12 weeks, a select intake of adolescents was made filtering out the affective disorders, schizophrenia, chemical abuse (the hyperactive group being significantly younger). During this period 80% of the sample were diagnosed as falling in this broad category of "neurotic and related disorders" (37.7% neurotic, 20.1% eating disordered, and 22.1% emotional disordered). Of the 152 eating disordered group, all but 3 were diagnosed with F50.0 and F50.01, therefore labelled "anorexic".

Symptom Check List (Health)

The Symptom Checklist (SCL-90-R) [60, 61] comprises 90 items of physical and psychological ailments which are rated on a 1-5 Likert scale (never, slightly, somewhat, strongly and very strongly). The inventory includes items from the area of general well-being, vegetative complaints, bodily pains, emotionality and common complaints. Previous factor analysis has revealed a 9-factor solution of "ailments" containing several items (ranging from 6 items for the aggression/anger and paranoia scales to -13 items for the depression scale) in the following areas; somaticisation (e.g. "headaches", "breathing difficulties", "nausea"), obsessive-compulsive (e.g. "concentration difficulties", "compulsion to repeatedly check actions"), interpersonal sensitivity (e.g. "hypercritical of others", "feelings of inferiority"), depression (e.g. "feeling of isolation", "hopelessness regarding future"), anxiety (e.g. "tense or agitated", "nervous or inner shakiness"), anger-hostility (e.g. "need to shout or throw objects around", "feeling of being easily aroused or angered"), phobic anxiety (e.g. "fear of open places or streets", "places, things, tasks to avoid"), paranoid ideation (e.g. "feeling of being observed", "ideas and views that others don't have") and psychoticism (e.g. "feeling of isolation even in the company of others", "hearing voices that others cannot hear"). We chose to rate the answers of a scale from 0-4 and then aggregate scores for overall scale scales.

As Hessel et al [62] demonstrated in a representative national sample, despite some psychometric insufficiencies regarding factorial structure and a high interrelationship between subscales of the SCL-90-R, there is strong evidence of the reliability and validity of the total scale score as a measure of global mental distress of health symptoms. The total scale score displays high internal reliability (alpha=0.97). The consistency coefficients of the subscales range from 0.77 to 0.88 which are assumed to be attributable to item-subsets of the homogeneous total scale.

Psychological and Physical Health

The German version of the Child Behaviour Checklist [63] was used in the study to assess the areas of social problem behaviour (behavioural inhibition) and (anxiety)-depression. For this purpose, the eight original YSR [63] scales were implemented involving ratings on a 3-point scale ("0" not applicable, "1" occasionally, and "2" frequently), "social inhibition" (9 items), "physical complaints" (9 items), "anxious-depressive" and 16 items relating to introversion, perfectionism, guilt-proneness, anxiety, emotionality, etc) "social problems" (8 items), "schizoid-compulsive" (7 items), "attentional problems" (10 items), "asocial behaviour" (11 items) and aggression (19 items). Alpha reliability coefficients have been shown to range from 0.69 and 0.85 (anxiety-depression).

German Inventory for Subjective Reports of Self-Injurious Behavior (FAPS)

In addition to the expert interview ratings of self-injurious, para-suicide, death ideation and suicidal behaviour, several items were included in the self-report questionnaire.

Socio-Psychological, Medical and Educational Attitudes ("Ba-Do" Documentation)

The psychological health screening inventory includes details of whether attempts have been made for self-injury including mutilating behaviour, suicidal attempts prior to admission, physically assaulting behaviour (against animals, objects and/or persons), details of family and socio-economic status (number of siblings, age of parents, birth order, disabilities of other family members, educational status) and school behaviour (aggression, concentration problems, interpersonal disturbances, hypermotoric behaviour, school anxiety) and results of intelligence testing (IQ).

Further items are encompassed, constituting the area related to family issues and social competencies on a 3 point scale (no, yes, unknown). One of the domains is related to "abnormal psychosocial circumstances" including "abnormal intrafamilial relationships" e.g. sexual abuse, disharmony between the adults within a family unit, parental rejection; "mental illness or handicaps within the family" (e.g. disability of a sibling, social deviant behaviour or mental ailment of a parent), "inadequate, distorted intrafamilial communication", "abnormal child-rearing practices" (overprotective parents, inadequate supervision by parents, inferior educational practises), "acute life events" (loss of a significant other, events that impose threat to self-worth), "chronic educational pressures" (abnormal conflicts with pupils, scapegoat for teacher) and "stressful circumstances" (institutional care, events that threaten self-esteem).

OUR FINDINGS

Figure 1 shows the prevalence of different diagnostic clinical groups among children and adolescents observed for the psychiatric and psychosomatic clinic.

The most frequent diagnoses were the neurotic and stress disorders, emotional and social disturbances, hyperkinetic disorders and eating disorders. Males were more likely to exhibit emotional and social disorders as well as hyperkinetic ailments, and chemical abuse, in contrast to females who were more likely than males to display eating disorders, neurotic stress disorders and personality disorders.

The gender distribution (see table 1) for each psychiatric category revealed that female adolescents were much more likely to exhibit eating disorders (96.6:3.4) approx. 30 times more likely than males, and higher rates of affective disorders (c. 2:1) and personality disorders (2:1), but males were overly represented in some other ailments such as hyperkinetic and social disorders (9:1), chemical abuse and dependency (2:1) and emotional and social disturbances in childhood development (2:1). These findings are consistent with other clinical reports.

Of the entire clinical sample involved in the survey, 6% percent displayed eating disorders, predominantly anorexia nervosa. The largest clinical diagnoses were emotional and social disorders (35.2%), neurotic/stress disorders (32.6%) and hyperkinetic disorders (15.3%).

Table 2 shows the history of "suicidal behavior prior to admission" was most common among affective disorders, followed by personality disorders and then neurotic and stress disorders.

It was least likely to be manifested by the group of eating disorders and hyperkinetic/social disturbances. If we focus on the 3 main clinical groups, the suicidal attempts prior to admission were lowest for the eating disorder group (1:12) in contrast to the children with emotional problems who displayed 19.7% suicidal, that is, approx. 1 in 5.

Finally, the neurotic and stress disordered individuals showed the highest incidence of suicidal behaviour (1:3). This may reflect the population of adolescents who are hospitalised due to psychological disorders. It does suggest that patients who exhibit eating disorders do not appear substantially more likely to attempt suicide, although the physiological and somatic ailments associated with such illnesses as anorexia nervosa do appear to be one of the precipitating reasons for being sent into psychiatric care. There would not appear to be a clear relationship to past suicidal attempt and eating disorders per se.

Looking at table 3 we see that for the neurotic and emotional disordered groups, they display suicidal histories between 20-39%, in contrast, the eating disordered group displayed "only" 8-9% histories of suicidal attempt. Self-mutilation incidence was roughly equivalent for both the eating disordered and the emotional disordered group (c. 27%) with neurotic stress groups revealing rates of 35%. With regard to overt aggression, 60% was reported for emotional disorders and 43% for neurotic stress disorders, in contrast to eating disorders with almost 8 % (overt aggression).

Age and Intelligence Factors

The mean age of the eating disordered group corresponds closely to other studies. They are on average older than the other two clinical groups (M eating 16.45 SD 1.56, n=138, M neurotic M15.23 SD 1.62, n=655, and M emotional 14.49 SD 1.67 years, n=635; $F(2,1425)=91.41, p<0.001$).

A between group comparison of eating and general neurotic and stress disordered adolescents revealed that the eating disorders were generally around 1.5 years older, were likely to stay in the clinic for a significantly longer period (75 compared to 47 days). The intelligence quotient was higher among the eating disordered individuals, but there was no major difference in terms of the age of their mother at birth or the number of brothers and sisters.

As expected a significantly greater proportion of adolescents with eating disorders displayed higher intelligence (see table 4), 22.2% high or very high IQ, defined as IQ in excess of 115. In contrast, the figures for neurotic/stress disorders were 7.2% and emotional disorders 4.3%). The difference in IQ between groups was statistically significant ($t(924) =6.66, p<0.001$). A greater proportion of children with emotional and social disturbances were an only child, 1 in 5 compared to c. 1 in 8 for other diagnoses. There was a greater tendency for those with eating disorders to be the youngest member of a family (see table 5).

Sibship size (number of siblings within family) tended to differ between those with eating disorders (M 1.68) and neurotic/stress disorders (M 1.90) ($t(\text{df } 668) = 1.68, p>0.10$).

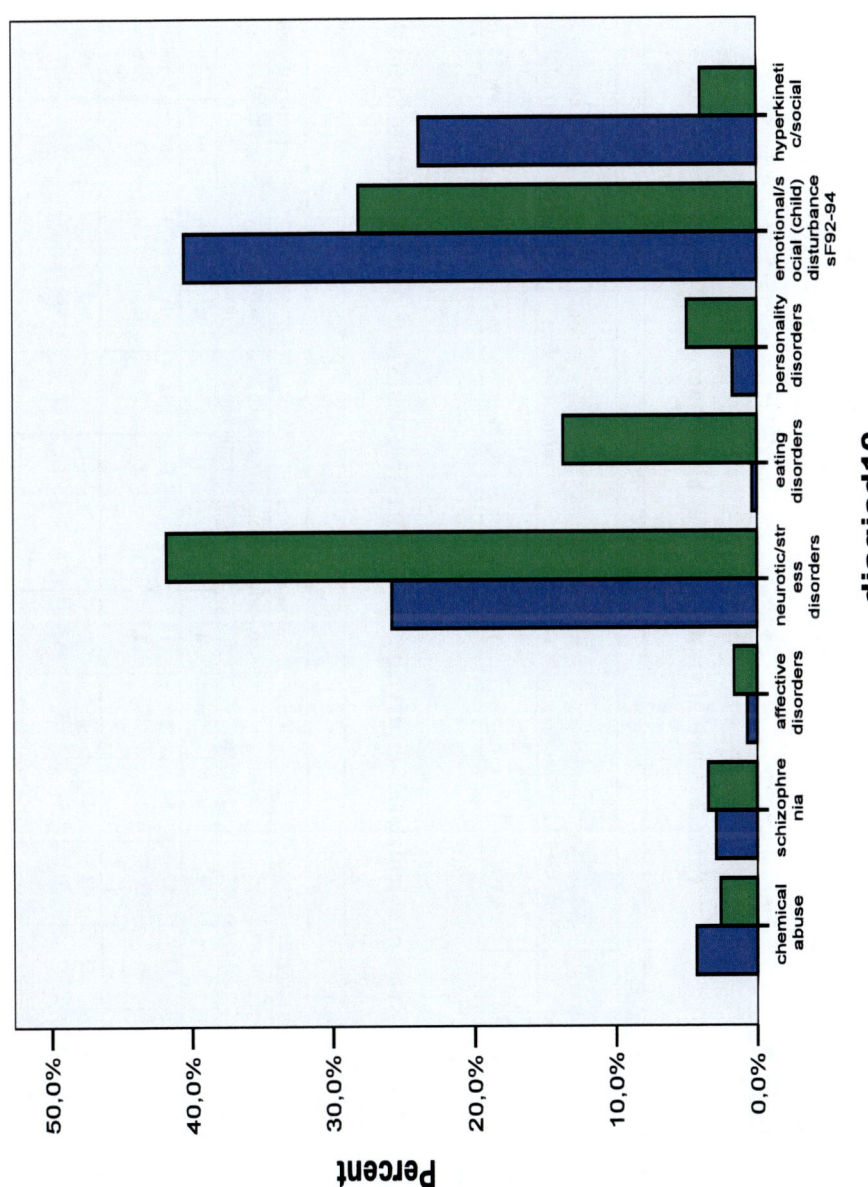

Figure 1. Distribution of the incidence of clinical diagnoses for males and females.

Table 1. Gender differences in the incidence of clinical disorders for hospitalised patients

Gender	Diagnosis							
	chemical abuse	schizo-phrenia	affective disorders	neurotic/ stress disorders	eating disorders	personality disorders	emotional/ social (child) disturbances	hyper-kinetic/ social
male	69,0%	53,2%	37,0%	45,4%	3,4%	32,0%	66,0%	89,1%
female	31,0%	46,8%	63,0%	54,6%	96,6%	68,0%	34,0%	10,9%

Table 2. Suicidal vs. non-suicidal history across all clinical diagnoses

	Diagnosis							
	chemical abuse	Schizo-phrenia	affective disorders	neurotic/stress disorders	eating disorders	personality disorders	emotional/social (child) disturbances[+]	Hyper-kinetic/ social
non-suicidal	88,0%	74,7%	38,5%	66,0%	91,7%	61,1%	80,3%	97,1%
suicidal	12,0%	25,3%	61,5%	34,0%	8,3%	38,9%	19,7%	2,9%

Note+: ICD10 F92-94.

Table 3. Rates of suicidal, self-injury and overt aggressive behaviour prior to admission for 3 clinical groups

	Diagnosis												
	neurotic/stress disorders						eating disorders						
	suicidal		overt aggression		self-mutilate		suicidal		overt-aggression		self-mutilate		
	n	%	n	%	n	%	n	%	n	%	n	%	
absent	521	66.0	449	57.3	503	64.7	132	91.7	132	92.3	106	73.1	
present	268	34.0	334	42.7	275	35.3	12	8.3	11	7.7	39	26.9	

	emotional/social (child) disturbances					
	suicidal		overt aggression		self-mutilate	
	n	%	n	%	n	%
absent	679	80.3	343	40.9	626	75.3
present	167	19.7	495	59.1	205	24.7

Table 4. Intelligence quotients across the three main clinical groups

	Diagnosis					
	neurotic/stress disorders		eating disorders		emotional/social (child) disturbances	
	n	%	n	%	n	%
IQ over 129	1	0.2%	3	2.2%	2	0.3%
115 - 129	45	7.0%	27	20.0%	25	4.0%
85 - 114	480	74.9%	99	73.3%	427	67.8%
70 – 84	84	13.1%	6	4.4%	140	22.2%
50 - 69	25	3.9%	0	0.0%	32	5.1%
35 - 49	6	0.9%	0	0.0%	4	0.6%

Table 5. Sibling and birth order across clinical diagnoses

	Diagnosis					
	neurotic/stress disorders		eating disorders		emotional/social (child) disturbances F92-94	
	n	%	n	%	n	%
Only child	70	12,3%	18	13,6%	102	19,2%
Youngest	147	25,9%	41	31,1%	130	24,5%
middle	148	26,1%	23	17,4%	123	23,2%
Oldest	202	35,6%	50	37,9%	175	33,0%

Duration in Clinic

The period of hospitalisation is shown below for each of the psychiatric groups. The stay is shortest for the chemical abuse group (15.93 SD 9.67 days) and longest for the eating disorders (c. 74.54 SD 49.99). The neurotic/stress disordered group stayed an average of 47.18 days (SD 32.51), and the emotional/social disturbances for 46.31 (SD 29.61) days. On average children and adolescents are hospitalised for around 49.69 days (SD 34.22). The main effect for "duration of hospitalisation" F-test comparison showed statistically significant between clinical-group differences $(F/7, 2442)=36.12, p<0.001)$.

Personality Differences

Using the secondary scales, internalisation and externalisation, the clinical groups differed significantly on both scales (see table 6).
Of the three clinical diagnostic groups, eating disorders emerged as significantly higher on internalisation (M anorex 26.31 SD 10.03, M emotion 17.73 SD 11.55, M neurot 20.42 SD 12.04; $F(2,226)= 8.48, p<0.001$) and lowest on externalisation (M anorex 14.58 SD 6.99, M emotion 22.58 SD 10.90, M neurot 17.70 SD 9.71; $F(2,281)= 13.60, p<0.001$). On the other hand, because the eating disorder group is almost entirely made up of females and the other clinical groups were substantially larger than the eating disordered group, a decision was made to "screen out" the males of the other two clinical groups and repeat the statistical

analysis (removing any artefact due to gender differences). Univariate statistical comparisons between the three clinical groups (neurotic/stress, eating disorders and emotional/social disturbances) revealed that although consistent with table 8 (significant differences on scales such as delinquency, aggressivity attention disorder and social inhibition), the main effect for anxiety-depression and physical ailments failed to reach statistical significance (for scales of behaviour checklist).

Table 6. A comparison of internalisation and externalisation scores between three main clinical groups

Secondary scales		n	M	SD
internalisation	neurotic/stress disorders	107	20.42	12.04
	eating disorders	51	26.31	10.03
	emotional/social (child) disturbances	71	17.73	11.55
externalisation	neurotic/stress disorders	133	17.70	9.71
	eating disorders	60	14.58	6.99
	emotional/social (child) disturbances	91	22.58	10.90

We now see a difference persists only for externalisation which is much lower for the eating disordered group (M eating 14.71 SD 6.98, M neurotic M 17.25 SD 9.67, and M emotional 25.34 SD 10.88 years; $F(2,186)= 17.01$, $p<0.001$). The eating disorders continue to display higher internalisation scores but the difference does not merge as statistically significant (M eating 26.68 SD 9.78, M neurotic M 23.66 SD 12.45, and M emotional 22.93 SD 12.25 years; $F= 1.34$, $p>0.05$).

A sample of individuals were provided with the SCL-90-R from each group and a between group comparison made. The linear discriminant function analysis revealed that 45% of the variance between groups could be explained by the differences exhibited in SCL profiles (Rc 0.45, eigenvalue 0.25, Wilk's lambda =0.798, chi-squared (9)= 22.01, $p<0.01$).

The three clinical groups, emotional disorders, eating disorders and neurotic groups (see table 7) differed with respect to the scales, insecurity/uncertainty and depressive (but not anxiety cf. Checklist Scales. Adolescents with eating disorders displayed higher scores on both these scales suggesting uncertainty and depression may be the scales which distinguish eating disorders from other psychiatric groups. It could be argued that these reference groups, e.g. other children attending a clinic, are better control groups than comparing eating disorders with healthy population norms, because these differences could be attributable to psychological illness per se, rather than specific factors related to eating disorders.

The magnitude of the standardised canonical coefficients reveal that those potent discriminants of the clinical diagnostic groups were obsessive-compulsive (+0.86), depression (+0.81), interpersonal sensitivity (+0.73) and (reduced) anger-hostility (-0.90) and anxiety (-0.68).

Table 7. Personality profiles (Symptom Checklist) between neurotic/stress and eating disordered patients (bold print represents those scales which emerged as significant determinants in the canonical coefficient)

	Neurotic stress disorder	Eating disorders	Emotional disorder		
	Mean	Mean	Mean	F(2,192)	p
Somaticisation	10.24	12.53	8.40	2.64	0.10
Obsessive-compulsive	9.02	12.33	9.68	2.59	0.10
Interpersonal sensitivity	10.32	14.40	8.65	5.36	0.01**
Depression	15.33	21.59	14.61	4.50	0.02*
Anxiety	9.58	10.24	10.17	<1	n.s.
Anger-hostility	6.09	5.53	6.96	<1	n.s.
Phobic anxiety	4.61	5.25	4.51	<1	n.s.
Paranoid ideation	5.90	6.50	6.67	<1	n.s.
Psychoticism	7.62	7.62	8.81	<1	n.s.

The second questionnaire (Achenbach (64)) was also administered and the following differences were found. On the scales physical ailments, anxiety-depression, schizoid-compulsive, social inhibition, delinquency and aggressivity were differences, with eating disorder group and neurotic somatoform ailments. The eating disordered group were more inclined to show more physical ailments, higher anxiety-depression and compulsive scores, physical ailments, higher social inhibition and lowered delinquency/ aggressivity scores. The clinical groups showed significantly different profiles (Rc=0.49, eigenwert =0.32, Wilk's lambda =0.760, chi-squared (8)=29.63, p<0.001). The standardised coefficients revealed that the scales which were influenced mostly were social problems (+0.95), delinquency (+0.86), social inhibition (-0.65) and schizoid-compulsive (-0,42) (see table 8).

Table 8. An univariate analysis of personality scales between eating disorders and neurotic/stress disorders

	Mean			F(1,319)	p
	neurotic/stress disorders	eating disorders	Emotional disordered		
anxiety-depression	12.16	15.44	11.05	7.28	0.001***
physical ailments	3.88	5.47	3.64	5.53	0.01**
social problems	2.81	2.77	3.17	0.84	n.s.
schizoid-compulsive	2.13	3.54	1.80	8.43	0.001***
social inhibition	5.54	6.86	4.58	10.66	0.001***
attention disorder	6.61	6.25	7.27	1.86	n.s.
delinquency	7.28	5.22	8.29	10.02	0.001***
aggressivity	10.55	9.16	14.00	15.16	0.001***

Health Outcome

Overall, "no change" or a "deterioration" of symptoms was observed in 24% of those cases with emotional and social disorders, 17.4% eating disorders, and 15.8% of neurotic and stress disorders (see table 9). Almost two-thirds of the patients with eating disorders (61.6%) had reported both a marked or full improvement after their stay in the clinic compared to only one-third of emotional and socially disturbed (31.5%) and the neurotic/stress disorders (42.6%).

Table 9. Health outcome as a function of clinical diagnosis

Evaluation of health outcome	Diagnosis					
	neurotic/stress disorders		eating disorders		emotional/social (child) disturbancesF92-94	
	n	%	n	%	n	%
Full improvement	21	3,3%	11	8,0%	4	0,6%
Marked improvement	251	39,3%	74	53,6%	193	30,9%
Partial improvement	265	41,5%	29	21,0%	278	44,5%
Unchanged	99	15,5%	20	14,5%	148	23,7%
worsening	2	0,3%	4	2,9%	2	0,3%

In order to explore the relationship between personality scales and health outcome, correlational analyses were conducted between the secondary scales, externalisation and internalisation and therapeutic success (symptom reduction). Therapy success was significantly correlated ($r=+0.12$, $p<0.02$) with low externalisation. A subsequent stepwise linear regression analysis was computed incorporating the subscales of the Aschenbach Questionnaire as predictor variables and symptom improvement health outcome variable. Two subscales emerged (see table 10) as significant predictors of health outcome, (low) aggressivity and social problems.

Table 10. Two subscales: Predictors of health outcome

	$R=0.21$	Adj. $R^2=0.04$	$F(2,221)=4.99**$	
		beta	t	p
Aggressivity		+0.19	2.76	0.01**
Social problems		-0.16	-2.28	0.05*

Family Structure and Developmental History

A discriminant analysis was performed using the overall item scores for each domain as revealed in table 11. The means ranged from 1 (not true) to 2 (true) and hence higher average scores indicate that the scale was more likely to be endorsed by that particular group.

On all scales the eating disorders scored lower than the neurotic group in terms of such elements as inadequate inner familial communication, institutional education, overprotective parents, acute stressful situation, etc. (Rc=0.25, eigenwert 0.068, Wilk's lambda = 0.936, chi-squared (9)= 61.78, $p<0.001$) (see table 11).

Table 11. Family- and school-related differences between clinical groups

Risk factor	Diagnosis	N	Mean	SD	F	p
Abnormal inner family relationships	neurotic/stress disorders	393	1.62	.49		
	eating disorders	137	1.50	.50		
	emotional/social (child) disturbancesF92-94	230	1.63	.49		
					3.77	.03*
Psychological disorder. deviant behaviour or disability within the family	neurotic/stress disorders	394	1.44	.50		
	eating disorders	137	1.26	.44		
	emotional/social (child) disturbancesF92-94	232	1.37	.48		
					6.80	.001***
Inadequate / maladaptive family communication	neurotic/stress disorders	395	1.65	.48		
	eating disorders	137	1.49	.50		
	emotional/social (child) disturbancesF92-94	232	1.70	.46		
					8.42	.001***
Parental overprotectiveness	neurotic/stress disorders	393	1.64	.48		
	eating disorders	137	1.47	.50		
	emotional/social (child) disturbancesF92-94	229	1.71	.46		
					10.41	.001***
Abnormal immediate surroundings	neurotic/stress disorders	393	1.51	.50		
	eating disorders	136	1.32	.47		
	emotional/social (child) disturbancesF92-94	231	1.45	.50		
					7.32	.001***
Acute. stressful life events	neurotic/stress disorders	394	1.44	.50		
	eating disorders	137	1.24	.43		
	emotional/social (child)					

Table 11. (Continued).

Risk factor	Diagnosis	N	Mean	SD	F	p
	disturbancesF92-94	230	1.29	.46		
					12.99	.001***
Societal stressors	neurotic/stress disorders	395	1.09	.29		
	eating disorders	136	1.07	.26		
	emotional/social (child)					
	disturbancesF92-94	232	1.07	.26		
					.30	n.s.
Chronic pressures in relationship with school or work	neurotic/stress disorders					
		395	1.19	.39		
	eating disorders	137	1.10	.30		
	emotional/social (child)					
	disturbancesF92-94	232	1.19	.39		
					2.93	0.06(*)
Stressful life event as a consequence of a behavioural disorder or handicap of a child	neurotic/stress disorders					
		395	1.12	.32		
	eating disorders	137	1.04	.19		
	emotional/social (child)					
	disturbancesF92-94	232	1.15	.35		
					5.45	.01**

DISCUSSION

Gender Differences

The first hypothesis was substantiated, that is, gender differences were observed across a variety of clinical diagnoses. Females were significantly more likely than males to exhibit eating disorders, as well as affective and personality disorders. Males were more commonly found among the acting out disorders such as hyperkinetic disorders, chemical abuse and emotional and social disturbances (ICD classifications). The statistics for eating disorders are consistent with many research findings [15] with substantially less than 10% of males showing such disorders.

The eating disorders are among the most common (6.0% rate) of the clinical groups (H2), but the incidence rate in clinical care is lower than other groups such as neurotic and stress disorders and emotional and social disturbances. Previous research suggests figures between 0.2 and 3.7% [16] for the incidence of eating disorders among normal populations.

Suicide, Self-Injury and Overt Aggression

Moving onto the third hypothesis, that suicidal behaviour will be high among eating disordered individuals, we found that the rate of suicidal behaviour prior to admission to the clinic was high (8.3%) in relation to a normal population of adolescents. On the other hand, compared to the other clinical groups e.g. affective and personality disorders, the incidence of suicidal behaviour was low. Clearly, although self-injurious and suicidal behaviour are found among individuals with eating problems, such behaviour is not specific to the disorder itself. There are certainly other clinical disorders with a much higher rate of suicidal behaviour (and self-inflicting injury rates). Our finding of a pre-suicidal rate of about 8% was in alignment with other reports [49,50] suggesting figures ranging from 2.2-15%. Furthermore, the covert aggressive behaviour was much less frequent among adolescents with eating disorders.

It is likely that the statistic if anything is an inflation of the rate of self-inflicted injuries because of the bias towards females which are over-represented in the eating disordered patients. Other studies have found that females are much more likely to report suicidal attempts than males both in clinical and non-clinical samples [64].

Intellectual Competence and Age

The fourth hypothesis addresses the issue of intellectual capacity. The eating disordered group displayed significantly higher intelligence quotients than any of the other clinical categories. One in five displayed an intelligence quotient in excess of 115 points. This cognitive "superiority" may be responsible for the high expectations (scholastic and otherwise) and desire for perfectionism frequently reported among anorexics [25]. It may serve as a propelling factor towards educational and personal striving, whilst counterproductive for normal daily functioning and social relationships. Whatever the reason, there does appear support for the claim that female adolescents with eating disorders exhibit higher scores on diverse tests of intelligence.

Personality Factors

The fifth and sixth hypotheses are directed at specific personality characteristics that may distinguish those adolescents with eating disorders. Adolescents displaying eating disorders are likely to display personality profiles that will distinguish them from other clinical groups, that is, in terms of physical ailments, schizoid-compulsivity, social inhibition and low overt aggression (delinquency). Moreover, they were more inclined to score higher on factors of insecurity, depression and compulsiveness in agreement with others [25,26]. These findings were substantiated together with low externalisation (and high internalisation). The higher scores on the physical ailments scale (to some extent due to the disproportionate number of females in the eating disorder group) and the high compulsive scores seem consistent with the concept of their being preoccupied with their body image.

The problems frequently reported to be associated with adolescents displaying eating disorders e.g. interpersonal relationships, may be explained by social anxieties manifested in elevated insecurity and social inhibition. There was little evidence that they were more anxious compared to other clinical groups, but they did exhibit elevated depression scores and were socially more restrained. On the other hand, one of the questionnaires used a scale which was a fusion of anxiety and depression and thus may have confounded differences more clearly attributable to either the facet of anxiety or of depression.

Family Functioning

The seventh hypothesis postulates that eating disordered individuals are more likely to originate from dysfunctional families in which overprotectiveness is frequently observed and intra-familial communications are maladaptive. The findings showed no indication that female adolescents with eating problems came from dysfunctional families, nor indeed were their parents/mothers seen as overprotective or was there evidence of problems in family communications [21]. Palmer [12] had found little empirical support showing a clear association between eating disorders and high dysfunctionality within their families. Jacobi et al [15] had suggested previous findings, which had reported a significant relationship between family communication and functioning and eating disturbances, were likely to be non-specific, that is, not associated with eating disorders per se.

Moreover, exploring the sibling status, there was scarce support that status or birth order played a role in the development of an eating disorder [65]. There was a tendency for adolescents with eating disorders to be the youngest member of the family. No attempt had been made to document the specific gender of other siblings, hence more detailed analyses were not possible. Selvini et al [34] have reported a tendency for eating disordered individuals to originate from families with several sisters among their siblings.

Health Outcome

The final hypothesis focuses on the treatment outcome rates. In contrast to Agras [52] we found relatively favorable (high) rates of therapeutic outcome. About two-thirds (66%) of the clinical sample revealed a significant or full improvement after their hospitalisation. Albeit some 1 in 6 showed no improvement or the condition deteriorated. Our results would seem consistent with Teachman [13] and Fichter and co-workers [55] being intermediate to their results of 73% and 53% for both studies respectively. Fichter's study [55] was based on a follow-up study stretching over 3-12 years after treatment. Overall, these findings would appear to offer good chances of significant improvement in the condition of eating disordered subjects, rates of recovery that compare favourably with other clinical diagnoses. The treatment success rates may be attributable to a longer stay in the clinic; or more severe, chronic cases may avoid institutionalised care (or be self-selectively screened out of treatment, which in turn may account for inflated mortality rates among eating disordered), or the early treatment onset. Studies have revealed that there is a better prognosis for those individuals attending therapy early.

Overall there was an indication that therapy success was significantly correlated with (low) externalisation, for specifically the scales social problems and aggressivity. This may suggest that negative emotions such as anger and aggressivity may cause patients to be less compliant to therapy programmes. These scales may be associated in non-conformity [66]. Adolescents expressing more social problems on the other hand, were more likely to display improvements in their symptoms during the course of therapy.

Due to the complexity of factors involved in the manifestation of eating disorders, the inclusion of cognitive-behavioural therapy as well as family-oriented therapeutic concepts coupled with medical treatment would appear to offer an intervention inventory which would be most effective in offering adolescents optimal treatment programmes [67,68].

Future studies may benefit from making clear distinctions between distinct groups of eating disordered patients. For example, using the model of personality postulated by Cloninger, German researchers [69] had reported distinct differences between adult patient samples with anorexia and those with bulimia nervosa as well as a healthy control population. In a second study with adolescent young females (12-18 years) with eating disorders, they were able to confirm that there are differential temperamental dimensions affording credence to the assumption that personality factors exert a significant role between eating disorders types. They used the German version of the Junior Temperament and Character Inventory (JTCI). Significant differences had been displayed between anorexia nervosa restricting types and bulimia nervosa patients, the latter group scoring higher on novelty seeking but lower on persistence, whereas binge eating/purging types revealed intermediate profile scores. In contrast to the restricting type of anorexia, both binge-eating/purging type and bulimia nervosa exhibited low scores on self-directedness.

REFERENCES

[1] Lindau F. Zur Subklassifikation von Essstörungen: Eine Untersuchung von Patienten in einer Spezialambulanz für Essstörungen in Hinblick auf Unterschiede in allgemeiner und spezifischer Psychopathologie. Freiburg: Dept. Psychosomatic. *Med. Ther.* Albert Ludwig University, 2005. [German].

[2] Assmann B, Dähne A, Hinz A, Ettrich C. Eating disorder specific diagnostics in anorexia nervosa and bulimia nervosa. *Suchtmed Forschung Praxis.* 2001;5(3):185-91. [German].

[3] EDA. Eating Disorder Association. Norwich, 2003. www.edauk.com

[4] Eisenberg ME, Neumark-Sztainer D, Story M. Associations of weight-based teasing and emotional well-being among adolescents. *Arch. Pediatr. Adolesc. Med.* 2003;157(8):733-8.

[5] Cash, T.F. (1997) The Body Image Workbook. *MJF Books,* New York.

[6] Garner DM. The 1997 body image survey results. *Psychol. Today.* 1997;30:30-41.

[7] Fairburn CG, Wilson GT, eds. *Binge eating; Nature, assessment and treatment.* New York: Guilford, 1993.

[8] Hsu LKG. Epidemiology of the eating disorders. *Psychiatr. Clin. North Am.* 1996;19:681-700.
[9] Szmukler GI, Patton G. Sociocultural models of eating disorders. In: Szmukler G, Dare C, Treasure J, eds. *Handbook of eating disorders: Theory, treatment and research.* New York: Wiley, 1994:177-92.
[10] Willi J, Grossman S. Epidemiology of anorexia nervosa in a defined region of Switzerland. *Am. J. Psychiatry.* 1983;140:564-7.
[11] van Hoeken D, Lucas AR, Hoek HW. Epidemiology. In: Hoek HW, Treasure JL, Katzman MA, eds. *Neurobiology in the treatment of eating disorders.* Chichester, UK: John Wiley, 1988:97-126.
[12] Palmer B. Helping people with eating disorders. *A clinical guide to assessment and treatment.* Chichester, UK: Wiley, 2000.
[13] Teachman BA, Schwartz MB, Gordic BS, Coyle BS. Helping your child overcome an eating disorder. *What you can do at home?* Oakland, Calif: New Harbinger, 2003.
[14] Drewnowski A, Yee DK, Krahn DD. Bulimia in college women: Incidence and recovery rate. *Am. J. Psychiatry.* 1988;145:753-5.
[15] Jacobi C, Thiel A, Paul T. Kognitive Verhaltenstherapie bei Anorexia und Bulimia nervosa. Beltz, pvu, Weinheim, 2000. [German]
[16] NIMH. Eating disorders: Facts about eating disorders and the search for solutions. Bethesda, MD: *Nat. Inst. Ment. Health, Dept. Health Hum. Serv.,* 2006.
[17] Spitzer RL, Yanovski S, Wadden T, Wing R, Marcus MD, Stunkard, A, Devlin M, Mitchell J, Hasin D, Horne RL. Binge eating disorder: Its further validation in a multisite study. *Int. J. Eating Disord.* 1993;13(2):137-53.
[18] Fichter MM, Hofman R. Bulimia (nervosa) in the male. In: Fichter MM, ed. Bulimia nervosa: *Basic research, diagnosis and therapy.* Chichester, UK: Wiley, 1990:99-111.
[19] Hay P. The epidemiology of eating disorder behaviour: An Australian community based survey. *Int. J. Eating Disord.* 1998;23:371-82.
[20] Gerlinghoff M, Backmund H. Essstörungen im Kindes- und Jugendalter. *Bundesgesundheitsblatt Gesundheitsforschung Gesundheitsschutz.* 2004;3:246-50. [German].
[21] Herpertz-Dahlmann B, Hagenah U, Vloet T, Holtkamp K. Jugendliche Essstörungen. *Zeitsch Kinderpsychol Kinderpsychiatr.* 2005;54(4):248-67. [German].
[22] American Psychiatric Association Work Group on Eating Disorders. *Am. J. Psychiatry.* 2000;157(Suppl):1-39.
[23] Herpertz-Dahlmann B. Outcome in adolescent anorexia nervosa. *Acta Neuropsychiatr.* 2002;14:90-2.
[24] Shah A. The relationship between anorexia nervosa and obsessive compulsive disorder. *Health Psychology Homepage.* Vanderbilt Univ, 2002.
[25] Fahy TA, Osacar A, Marks I. History of eating disorders in female patients with obsessive compulsive disorder. *Int. J. Eating Disord.* 1993;14:439-43.
[26] Pryor R, Wiederman MW. Personality factors and expressed concerns of adolescents with eating disorders. *Adolescence.* 1998;33(130):291-300.
[27] Wonderlich SA, Lilenfeld LR, Riso LP, Engel S, Mitchell JE. Personality and anorexia nervosa. *Int. J. Eating Disord.* 2005;37:68-71.

[28] Milos G, Spindler A, Schnyder U. Psychiatric comorbidity and eating disorder inventory (EDI) profiles in eating disorder patients. *Can. J. Psychiatry.* 2004;49:179-84.
[29] Marano HE. Body image: Before the obsession. *Psychol. Today.* 10 Dec 2004.
[30] Schmidt U, Jiwany A, Treasure J. A controlled study of alexithymia in eating disorders. *Compr. Psychiatry.* 1993;34(1):54-8.
[31] Gillberg IC, Rastam M, Gillberg C. Anorexia nervosa 6 years after onset: Part I, Personality disorders. *Compr. Psychiatry.* 1995;36:61-9.
[32] Crisp A. Treatment for anorexia nervosa appears to have improved outcome. *Alert Public release.* Wiley Publishers, 23rd May 2006.
[33] Wilson GT, Pike KM. Eating disorders. In: Barlow DH, ed. Clinical handbook of psychological disorders. *A step-by-step treatment manual.* New York: Guilford, 1993:278-317.
[34] Selvini-Palazzoli M, Cirillo S, Sellini M, Sorrentino AM. Anorexie und Bulimie. *Neue familientherapeutische Perspektiven.* Stuttgart: Klett-Cotta, 1999. [German]
[35] Lucas AR, Beard CM, O'Fallon WM. 50-year trends in the incidence of anorexia nervosa in Rochester, Minn. A population-based study. *Am. J. Psychiatry.* 1991;148:917-29.
[36] Walitza S, Schulze U, Warnke A. Unterschiede zwischen jugendlichen Patientinnen mit Anorexia and Bulimia nervosa im Hinblick auf psychologische und psychosoziale Merkmale. *Zeitsch. Kinder Jugendpsychiatr.* 2001;29(2):117-25. [German]
[37] Chambers RA, Taylor JR, Potenza MN. Developmental neuro-circuitry of motivation in adolescence: A critical period of addiction vulnerability. *Am. J. Psychiatry.* 2003;160(6):1041-52.
[38] Davison GC, Neale JM. *Klinische Psychologie: ein Lehrbuch.* Weinheim: Beltz, PVU, 2002. [German]
[39] Gogtay N, Giedd JN, Lusk L, Hayashi KM, Greenstein D, Vaituzis AC, Nugent TF, Herman DH, Clasen LS, Toga AW, Rapoport JL, Thompson PM. Dynamic mapping of human cortical development during childhood through early adulthood. *Proc. Nat. Acad. Sci. U.S.A.* 2004;101(21), 8174-9.
[40] Halmi KA. The multimodal treatment of eating disorders. *World Psychiatry.* 2005;4(2):69-73.
[41] Jacobi C. Zur Spezifität und Veränderbarkeit von Beeinträchtigungen des Selbstkontrollkonzepts bei Essstörungen. Regensburg. S. Roderer, 1999 [German].
[42] Webster J, Palmer RL. The childhood and family background of women with clinical eating disorders. A comparison with women with major depression and women without psychiatric disorder. *Psychol. Med.* 2000;30:57-60.
[43] Kearney-Cooke A, Steichen-Asch P. Men, body image and eating disorders. In: Andersen A, ed. *Males with eating disorders.* New York: Brunner/Mazel, 1990:47.
[44] Gowers S, Kadambari SR, Crisp AH. Family structure and birth order of patients with anorexia nervosa. *J. Psychiatr. Rev.* 1985;19(2-3):247-51.
[45] Schepank H. Genetic determinants in anorexia nervosa: Results of studies with twins. In: Herzog W, Deter DC, Vandereycken W, eds. *The course of eating disorders.* Berlin: Springer, 1992.
[46] Kendler KS, MacClean C, Neale M, Kessler R, Heath A, Eaves L. The genetic epidemiology of bulimia nervosa. *Am. J. Psychiatry.* 1991;148:1627-37.

[47] Kendler KS, Walters EE, Neale M, Kessler R, Heath AC, Eaves L. The structure of the genetic and environmental risk factors for six major psychiatric disorders in women. *Arch. Gen. Psychiatry.* 1995;52:372-83.
[48] Kassett JA, Gershorn ES, Maxwell ME, Guroff JJ, Kazuba DM, Smith AL, Brandt HA, Jimerson DC. Psychiatric disorders in the first degree relatives of probands with bulimia nervosa. *Am. J. Psychiatr.* 1989;146:1468-71.
[49] Dancyger IF, Fornari VM. A review of eating disorders and suicide risk in adolescence. *Scientific World Journal.* 2005;5:803-11.
[50] Latzer Y, Hochdorf Z. Dying to be thin: attachment to death in anorexia nervosa. *Scientific World Journal.* 2005;5:820-7.
[51] Keel PK, Dorer DJ, Eddy KT, Franko D, Charatan DL, Herzog DB. Predictors of mortality in eating disorders. *Arch. Gen. Psychiatry.* 2003;60(2):179-83.
[52] Agras WS. The consequences and costs of the eating disorders. *Psychiatr. Clinics North. Am.* 2001;24(2):371-9.
[53] von Wietersheim C, von Uexküll T. Lehrbuch *Psychosomatische Medizin.* München und Jena: Urban Fischer, 2003. [German]
[54] Fassino S, Abbare Daga G, Piero A, Rovera GG. Dropout from brief psychotherapy in anorexia nervosa. *Psychother Psychosom.* 2002;71:200-6.
[55] Fichter MM, Quadflieg N, Hedlund S. Twelve-year course and outcome predictors of anorexia nervosa. *Int. J. Eating Disord.* 2005;39(2):87-100.
[56] Santonasto P, Favaretto G, Canton G. Anorexia nervosa in Italy: Clinical features and outcome in a long-term follow-up. *Psychopathol.* 1987;20:8-17.
[57] Sullivan PF. Mortality in anorexia nervosa. *Am. J. Psychiatry.* 1995;152(7):1073-4.
[58] Fairburn CG, Peveler RC, Jones R, Hope RA, Doll H. Predictors of 12-month outcome in bulimia nervosa and the influence of attitudes to shape and weight. *J. Consult. Clin. Psychol.* 1993;61:696-8.
[59] Fairburn CG, Jones R, Peveler RC, Hope RA, O'Connor M. Psychotherapy and bulimia nervosa. Longer-term effects of interpersonal psychotherapy, behavior therapy, and cognitive behavior therapy. *Arch. Gen. Psychiatry.* 1993;50(6):419-28.
[60] Derogatis LR. SCL-90. Administration, scoring and procedure manual – I for the R(revised) version. Baltimore: John Hopkins Univ. School Med,1983.
[61] Franke GH. SCL-90-R. Die Symptom-Checkliste von Derogatis - Deutsche Version. Göttingen: Beltz Test, 1995. [German].
[62] Hessel A, Schumacher J, Geyer M, Brähler E. Symptom-Checkliste SCL-90-R: Testtheoretische Überprüfung und Normierung an einer bevölkerungsrepräsentativen Stichprobe. *Diagnostica.* 2001;47:27-39. [German].
[63] Achenbach TM. Deutsche Child Behaviour Checklist. KJFD (Arbeitsgruppe Kinder-, Jugendlichen- und Familiendiagnostik): Cologne, 1991. [German].
[64] Kirkcaldy BD, Siefen RG, Urkin J, Merrick J. Risk factors for suicidal behavior in adolescence. *Minerva Pediatrica.* 2006;58:443-50.
[65] Gowers S, Kadambari SR, Crisp AH. Family structure and birth order of patients with anorexia nervosa. *J. Psychiatr. Rev.* 1985;19(2-3):247-51.
[66] Kirkcaldy BD. Self-Image and personality. *Pers. Individ. Dif.* 1990;11(4):321-6.
[67] Herzog DB, Nussbaum KM, Marmor AK. Comorbidity an outcome in eating disorders. *Psychiatr. Clin. North Am.* 1996;19(4):843-59.

[68] Ratsunariya RH, Eisler I, Szmukler GI, Russell GFM. Anorexia nervosa: Outcome and prognostic factors after 20 Years. *Br. J. Psychiatry.* 1991;158:495-502.

[69] Hueg A, Resch F, Haffner J, Poustka L, Parzer P, Brunner R. Temperaments- und Charaktermerkmale jugendlicher Patientinnen mit Anorexia und Bulimia Nervosa. *Zeitschrift Kinder Jugendpsychiatr. Psychother.* 2006;34(2):127-37. [German]

In: Adolescence and Chronic Illness
Editors: H. Omar et al.

ISBN: 978-1-60876-628-4
© 2010 Nova Science Publishers, Inc.

Chapter 11

PSYCHOLOGICAL ISSUES IN CHRONICALLY ILL ADOLESCENTS

Helen D. Pratt[*]

Pediatrics and Human Development, College of Human Medicine,
Michigan State University, East Lansing Michigan, Kalamazoo Campus,
Kalamazoo, Michigan, United States of America.

ABSTRACT

Adolescence is a period of tremendous growth and represents a time of transition from childhood to adulthood. Youth who do not experience typical development as a result of chronic illness may experience psychological problems. Adolescents with chronic illness versus typically developing adolescents may need a greater degree of support, resources and guidance to ensure that they grow into psychologically healthy adults. Those youth who receive such help have a greater chance of developing the ability to live relatively healthy and productive lives. Youth who do not experience typical development as a result of chronic illness may experience psychological problems.

INTRODUCTION

Adolescence is a period of tremendous growth and represents a time of transition from childhood to adulthood [1-8]. Youth who do not experience typical development as a result of chronic illness (see table 1) may experience psychological problems [3,5,9-13]. They may also need a greater degree of support, resources and guidance to ensure that they grow into psychologically healthy adults as compared to "typically" developing adolescents [10-15]. Those youth who receive such help have a greater chance of developing the ability to live relatively healthy and productive lives.

---

[*] *Correspondence:* Professor Helen D Pratt, PhD, Behavioral Developmental Pediatrics, Pediatrics Program, Michigan State University/Kalamazoo Center for Medical Studies, 1000 Oakland Dr, Kalamazoo, Michigan 49008 United States. Tel: (269) 337-6450; Fax: (269) 337-6474; E-mail: pratt@kcms.msu.edu

Psychological Development

Psychological development deals more specifically with the progressive organization of cognitive, emotional, and social aspects of function (see table 2). The synthesis of physical, biological, hormonal factors in the individual with the functional domains produces predictable types of behavioral and personality characteristics in each individual, the expression of which is unique [2-4,7,15-17]. Research by noted personality theorist provides us with models of how these general expressions can be categorized [17-20].

Individuals manifest emotional reactions and coping skills that are goverened by their a) cognitive capacity, b) intelligence, c) mental flexibility, d) temperament, e) attachment to family, peers, community, f) sense of autonomy, g) social competence, h) problem solving skills, i) coping skills and j) exposure to violence, substance, and poverty (see table 3) [8,15]. Psychological development continues well into adulthood. During middle and late adolescence cognitive capacity expands to include abstract thinking, and more complex thinking skills. Youth who had chronic illnesses during childhood, may not have mastered age appropriate psychological skills (cognitive, emotional, social, integrative adaptive) (see table 4) [13,19,22]. This means that these youth must expend their engery in skill acquisition versus refinement of their psychological development. Cognitive and emotional responses to their environment may appear "childish" and parents may complain that their adolescent is not being responsible.

Table 1. Sample Of Chronic Illnesses And Disorders That May Have A Psychological Impact On Adolescent Development [9-13]

Medical		Mental /Behavioral
AIDS	Muscular Dystrophies	Anxiety Disorders
Asthma	Neurological Disorders	Attention Deficit/Hyperactivity Disorder
Chronic pain	Non Migraine Headaches	Body Dysmorphic Disorder
Cancer	Neurocutaneious Syndromes	Chronic Depression
Crohn's Disease	Obesity	Disruptive Behavior Disorders
Congenital Heart Disease	Osteoid Osteoma	Eating Disorders
Cystic Fibrosis	Psoriasis	Elimination Disorders
Diabetes Melitus	Scoliosis	Communication Disorders
Epilepsy	Seizures	Learning Disorders
Guillain-Barr'e Syndrome	Sickle Cell Disease	Mental Retardation
Hemophilia	Sleep Disorders	Motor Skills Disorders
Hepatitis	Spina bifida	Other Psychotic Disorders
Hypertension	Syncope	Personality Disorders
Juvenile Rheumatoid Arthritis	Thyroid Disorders	Pervasive Developmental Disorders
Leukemia		Reactive Attachment Disorders
Lupus		Schizophrenia
Migraine Headaches		Sexual And Gender Identity Disorders
Multiple Sclerosis		Tic Disorders

Table 2. Stages of Adolescent Development [1, 2,3 4, 5, 8, 13, 16]

Early Adolescence 10 – 14 year of Age
Onset of puberty
Neurobiological changes in the brain impact: speech, language
Psychological Components
Cognitive Growth results in major changes in mental abilities and thought processes:
- Preoccupation with rapidly changing events of puberty
- Increased abilities to perform more complex mental tasks (thinking skills and problem solving skills)
- Improved mental processing speed and alertness
- Longer attention span
- Better judgment
- Better ability to adopt another person's spatial perspective
- A clear sense of their own body image
- Clear sense of social standing with peer
- Comparison with peers and worry over perceived abnormalities

Development of initial abstract thought
The process of emancipation begins
Establishment and maintenance of same-sex friendships
Exposure to bullying and teasing (perpetrator, victim, or both)

Middle Adolescence 14 – 18 year of Age
Somatic growth spurt.
Females, and males who engage in body image activities may find it difficult to maintain a personally desired weight or body size; this may result in dieting, excessive exercise, purging or other pathogenic weight control measures or body image problems.

Psychological Components
- Significant symbolic movement away from the home environment
- Considerable need for independence
- Strong reliance on peers setting personal rules
- Heterosexual experimentation predominates
- Altruistic nature emerges
- Identification with non-parental adult role models
- Expermentation with sex, substance use or abuse
- Major changes in cognitive abilities and fantasy life
- Can engage in fantasy
- May become preoccupied with comparing their physical characteristics with peers
- Is developing theories about life
- Able to independently weigh consequences of decisions before taking action
- Ability to engage in inductive and deductive reasoning is expanding
- Can think about what they would like to do when they become adults
- May know and understand the consequences of risk taking behaviors, but their caution may be overridden by their stronger need for popularity and peer recognition
- May experience sexual fantasies
- These fantasies may occupy much of their time
- Some youth will fantasize about same sex peers and become very disturbed over these events
- Beginning to development of a positive self-image and increased confidence occurs as he or she consistently experiences success
- Is highly sensitive to negative comments from others and peer rejection, bullying, and traumatic personal experiences

Table 2. (Continued).

> Late Adolescence 18 – 21
> Final pubertal changes physiologic fine tuning) occur
> Psychological Components
> - Issue of emancipation from parents are essentially resolved
> - Finalization of secure, acceptable body image and gender role
> - Establishment of adult versus narcissistic sexual relationships
> - Acquisition of adult lifestyle
> - Considerable energy spent in establishment of vocational skills for training
> - Cognitive abilities are more complex.
>   - Abstract thought has been established
>   - Empathy skills are well developed
>   - Personal values clearer and well defined.
>   - Is future oriented
>   - Perceives and reacts upon long range options.
>   - Beginning to resolve conflicts between themselves and their parents.
>   - Contining to develop th ability to think and function independently
>   - Less influenced by peers
>   - Uses own judgement for setting personal rules.
>   - More actively participating is sexual experimentation
>   - Predominate altruistic nature emerges.
>   - Relationships with romantic partners are less narcissistic and more geared towards mutual respect and gratification.
>   - Prefers the association with groups and or couples and prefers intimacy versus isolation.
>   - Most adolescents at this stage of maturation have developed a strong sense of personal identity.
>   - Capable of establishing and maintaining stable, mutually caring and satisfying interpersonal (including sexual) relationships.

Impact of Puberty/Sexual Maturation

All youth matriculate through three major stages (early, middle and late) of adolescence which occur in a dynamic, sequential, orderly and time-dependent manner (see table 2) [1-5,8,13,18]. However, there is considerable individual variation in the onset, rate, and progression of an adolescents move through this process. That variation is significantly impacted by many factors: a) internal (including biological, neurological, physical growth, mental development) or external (changes in the adolescent's personal, family, peer, school, and neighborhood environment, exposure to violence, trauma, chemicals, etc.) [1,3-7,13,15]. The effects can result in changes in any one of the essential components in the domains of function (see table 3) [8,15]. The presence of a chronic illness can cause many of the factors mentioned above to impact psychological development of the adolescent.

The hallmark of adolescence is the onset of puberty, which can begin as early as age 8 years or as late as age 15 years in females and as early as age 9.5 years and as late as age 15 years in males. Puberty ends when the adolescent reaches full physical and developmental maturity (which can be as late as age 21 years) (see table 2). Youth diagnosed with chronic illnesses such as intellectual disability, malnutrition, diabetes mellitus (when glycemic control is poor) cystic fribrosis, sickle cell disease, or anorexia nervosa may experience delayed sexual maturation [23]. This may mean that the adolescent becomes emotionally distressed over not experiencing physcial changes in their bodies similar to those of their typically developing peers. Adolescents who do not experience the hormonal changes of puberty may not experience co-occuring changes in brain function [23]. As adolescents work to adjust to physical and hormonal changes caused by puberty, the presence of a chronic illness may significantly alter their ability to master the tasks of adolescence: Individuation, emotional and behavioral regulation, ability to initiate and maintain reciprocal intimate relations and to develop skills that support independence [4,9,21,24,25]. Chronic illness may also result in over involvement of parents in to personal functioning (especially when bathing and toileting are involved) impeding the adolescent's ability to develop self confidence, feeling of independence, and opportunities for healthy sexuality development.

Table 3. Domains of Function [8, 15]

Psychological Components	
Cognitive	**Social/Emotional**
	Ability to regulate, modulate and control emotions
Attention	Ability to establish new friendships
The ability to focus selectively and generally on events, actions and or information in the environment	Ability to maintain peer relationships
	Ability to establish and maintain healthy family relationships
Mental Processing Speed (alertness)	Integration and coordination of all of these skills
The ability to respond in an effective manner to physical, mental, emotional and physiological events in self to process information in a manner that allows for the appropriate adaptation of behavior to maximize positive outcomes and minimize negative outcomes	
	Integrative/Adaptive
	Ability to adapt skills and functions to meet demands of specific situations or conditions
Memory	**Other Domains of Function**
The ability to acquire, store, and recall recent, remote, and long term events, actions, information in an organized an useful manner.	Auditory
	Language
Thinking	Motor
	Perceptual Motor
Knowledge of specifics, Comprehension, Application, Analysis, Synthesis, Evaluation, Decision Making, Problem Solving, Ability to monitor multiple events & people simultaneously	Visual

Impact on the Adolescents Relationships with Family

The impact of chronic illness on on family relationships is dependent the specific illness, its severity, how it affects the adolescent's body, how and if the functional limitations are preceived, what kinds of treatments are involved, and whether the symptoms of the illness or the result of treatment are manifested publically. For instance, spina bifida may impair an adolescent's ability to walk or siblings who see their "sick" sibling (preceived by siblings as sick/different) on crutches or in a wheel chair may be embarrased by the visual images, when they are around peers and the public. Those siblings may then treat the "sick" sibling differently; the adolescent with chronic illness may feel angry or saddened by this reaction. Youth who have loss their hair because of their chronic illness (alapegia) or chemotherapy also presents visuals for the individuals that can result in peer rejection, embarrassemnt and other emotions in sibling and thus cause reciprocal emotions in the chronically ill teen. Members of the family, especially parents may restrict/limit the ability of their teen to individuate and move towards emancipation. Parents may also become overprotective and limit their teen's access to activities that may give them opportunities to be with other youth of similar interests. The well intentioned family members may actually cause frustration for the teen and impede possibility of "typical" development.

Although the illnesses of asthma or diabetes may not be readily visible, if the teen has public displays of their illness in front of peers (i.e. a) an asthma attack, or b) the teen with diabetes begins to shake and get confused as the result of hypoglycemia) those illnesses also become visible or public. If the teen has to go to the office to take shots or use an inhaler before exercise or an outing, the illness becomes public. Other teens will "know." Most adolescents between ages 10 and 16 years will become very upset about these events (exhibiting symptoms of chronic illness), because being different or a public spectacle is something to be avoided at all costs. Younger adolescents may be too embarrassed to return to the setting of a psychologically traumatic event (public display of their illness). However, if these same events occur when the teen is 17 years of age, they might be less psychologically traumatic and result in the teen simply asking for help and explaining to peers what just happened (case example1).

Psychological development may also be impeded when there are visible signs of chronic illness - such as the loss of hair from chemotherapy, obesity due to medications (such as corticosteroids), or congenital conditions or injuries; these signs may result in the adolescent retreating from social situations. He or she may avoid contact even with former friends. Older adolescent may rationalize emotions about these visible signs of their illness and be prepared to address them with peers and others. Youth who appear younger than their chronilogical age may face various forms of discrimination or be treated like a younger child by adults who interact with them (case example 2).

Case Example 1

For instance the youth who develops type I or insulin dependent diabetes at age 9 years usually adjusts well at this age and dissplays very responsible eating and exercise habits (with supportive parental help). Then at age 15 years, Mark begins to eat extra unhealthy foods, does not tell his parents; he also does not adjust his fast acting insulin to compensate for the extra foods. He told his parents that he did not want to be differenct from his peers, he wanted to be like everyone else. He hated having diabetes. Mark is told he can adjust his insulin to allow some variation in his diet, yet he lies to his parents and physician about his diet and blood sugar levels. When his parents find out, they are livid, scared, and distressed. Many arguments result. Mark becomes very moody and resentful. Yet he repeatedly engages in this behavior and suffers the wrath of his parents and physician. When his parents present in the physician's office with Mark, they describe their son as a liar, a sneak, and an irresponsible teen who is killing himself.

The physician referred the family for counseling. A comprehensive psychologal evaluation that included developmental assessments was conducted. Results of testing and interviewing showed that Mark has above average intellectual function (verbal and non verbal), is mildly depressed but basically he is a very mentally healthy person who responds cognitively to emotional destress as a 9 or 10 year old. The psychologist tells Mark and his family that Mark's resistance to parental direction and non-compliance with his medical regime is the result of Mark's emotional development. Mark had not yet gotten past a concrete stage of intellectual development because when he was at that stage, he experienced the psychological trauma of being diagnosed with a chronic illness. When he acted out, Mark was not able to understand the long term consequences of not controlling his blood sugars. He could only focus on not wanting to be different from his peers.

Most of the literature on treatment responsibility (self effacicy) recommends that parents help their children be as independent with treatment regimes as possible. However, parents may need help to know when they have turned over too much care or have decreased their emotional involvement too much. Mark's parents were encouraged to make shot time and glucose testing times opportunties to spend "quality" time with their teen. They did not have to administer the procedures, but might sit with the teen and ask him about various events in his life or tell him about events in their lives. Mark was encouraged to help make these pleasant times also. The psychologist helped the parents understand that although the intervention was time intensive, the end goal of fading that level of involvement as their teen complied with treatment, was what they were all working toward..

Psychoeducation was used as a major technique to help Mark . This included the teaching of coping skills, nurturing abstract thinking and helping him understand the relationship between his everyday behavior/actions and his longterm health. Mark was also helped to understand the motives of his parents and their fears about his longterm health. The clinician pointed out that his parents were reacting out of fear for their son's life, not because they hated him. With education, Mark's parents were able to view their son's emotional needs, and understand his behavior as a part of normal adolescence development; they were given straegies to intervene with Mark that respected their teen's chronical age and met his emotional need of more concrete instructions, more parental attention to the medication regime

Case Example 2

Charles is a 15 year old male diagnosed with cystic fribrosis. Charles was short stature, had a high pitched voice, no facial hairs, and had not yet started to experience puberty. He was being seen by a clinician for help with anger management. Charles has a slight frame and facial features more like a nine or ten year old. At their first meeting the clinician greeted Charles as she does most "children" of his perceived age. She bent down to shake his hand, leaned in and said "Hello, young man. How are you today." When she escorted Charles and his mother to their respective seats, she told him he was welcome to sit any where he liked or could stay close to his mother if he felt safer. Charles began to get angry, he glared at the clinican. The clinician had not read his referral letter in a couple of weeks and went by her perceptions of his age and developmental stage. Next, she said "Now, I am going to ask you some hard questions (she was joking) that most kids your age might struggle with, but I bet you know the answers."

Charles had enough! He said, "Look, stop being condesending to me! I am not a child, I am 15 years old and would appreciate you respecting me as a young man and not treating me like a child!" The clinician, realized the error of her ways, quickly appoligized and told Charles she had read his referral letter a couple of weeks ago and was treating him inappropriately. She asked for his forgiveness and said, "Charles, would you allow me to start over?" Charles agreed and the rest of the meeting went well. He completed evaluation and therapy and at followup, he said he was able to effectively employ the anger management techniques he learned. His mother supported the claim. Charles completed therapy with the clinician and both he and his mother gave her a high satisfaction rating.

Developing Psychologically Healthy Adolescents with Chronic Illness

Youth who are born with chronic illnesses can grow up to be psychologically healthy if they have all of the characteristics and factors in their lives that researchers have found to be present in resilient youth. Those youth that develop a chronic illness a different stages in their lives may experience psychological problems, because of the loss of function, However some researchers have found that those youth who do not perceive a loss of function and who peer acceptance will be able lead socially and emotionally healthy lives.

Research on resilience in adolescents (with and without chronic illness) shows that resilient youth are better able to handle the complexities of growing up (see table 5) [26-29]. Youth with chronic illnesses who are also resilient show the same qualities. The ability to be resielient is a very important component of survival for all youth but especially those with chronic illness. Resilience is the capacity to successfully undertake the work of each successive developmental stage (see table 4) in the face of significant factors that predispose to vulnerability and adapt to those conditions in a manner that improves their trajectory [13,15,21, 22,25-27].

Table 4. Psychosocial Issues that may be experienced
by Chronically Ill Youth [13, 19, 28]

Personal	Parents	Siblings	Peers
Being disappointed in their bodies.	Feeling parents are angry at they because their chronic illness monopolizes parent's lives	Feeling stress of sibling because of their adjustment and stigmatizing guilt and fear of having a chronically ill sibling	Social Rejection
Dealing with complex medical procedures	Detecting parental stress because of adjustment to chronically ill teen and stigmatizing guilt and fear about having a chronically ill teen	Detecting their siblings' anger at them for monopolizing parental attention	Being made fun of because of their chronic illness

Table 4. (Continued).

Personal	Parents	Siblings	Peers
Feeling vulnerable	Realizing their parent's fatigue from having to deal with acute and chronic stressors of implimenting daily medical regimes	Realizing their siblings are embarrassed about their condition	Acceptance
Feeling illness is unfair	Recognizing their parent's financial distress	Being rejected by healthy sibling	Collegial relationships
Having to continuously adapt	Knowing their parents are unhappy because of their inability to meet needs of spouse or their other children	Acceptance	
Lack of esteem	Rejecting their parent's over-protectiveness	Collegial relationships	Lack of esteem
Lack of confidence	Feeling rejection from parents because they are not what their parents expected		
Loss of life freedoms that are associated with excellent health	Acceptance		
Periodic, and often unpredictable, crisis events.	Collegial relationships		
Permanent lifestyle changes	Loving parental relationship		
Problems with emancipation			
Slowed or altered physical development and appearance			
Social limitations			
Social stigma			
Unpredictable course of illness			
Self acceptance			
Joy of living			
Self confidence			
Success			

Intimate Relationships

Peer relationships provide the second most important influence on adolescent development [15]. Peer interactions afford the opportunity to interact in an equal status relationship and reinforce cultural norms. The support network of chronically ill youth usually includes parents, siblings, peers, counselors, caring health care professionals, and pets. A survey of these youth supported that chronically ill youth said their pets also played an important role in providing a listening ear and emotional comfort [11]. They further reported that they need direct communication from their doctors, teachers and other care givers; and benefited best from honesty, attention to their reports of physical and emotional pain. The researchers concluded that these teens understand both the value of the scientific and interpersonal aspect of care [12,28,31,32].

Impact on Experimentation and Risk Behavior

Adolescence is a time where youth begin to experiment with making personal decisions, challenging the religious beliefs of their parents, making a variety of friends, defying parental rules and beliefs, trying different styles of dressing, hair, makeup, and talking. Some youth will want to get tattoos or body piercings, experiment with their sexuality, engage in sexual acts, use substances (smoke or chew tobacco, marijuana, heroin, cocaine, drink alcohol) , and or other drugs [10,32]. Having a chronic illness does not prevent experimental behaviors during adolescence; these youth can be expected, as will their peers, to test their own limits. The opportunities to have access to peers, purchase items, go shopping without parental supervision, be alone with a sexual partners, or be alone with peers may be impeded by the severity of their illness and their physical limitations; however experimental behaviors are not rarer in adolescents with a chronic condition [31,32]. It is important that these youth be afforded privacy to experiment with age appropriate intimate relationships so that they do not get involved in experimenting sexually with age inappropriate youth or public masturbation.

CONCLUSIONS

Youth who do not experience typical development as a result of chronic illness may experience psychological or psychosocial problems (see table 1) [3,5,9-13]. As adolescents work to adjust to physical and hormonal changes caused by puberty the presence of a chronic illness may significantly alter their ability to master the tasks of adolescence: Individuation, emotional and behavioral regulation, ability to initiate and maintain reciprocal intimate relations, development of skills that support independence. External factors such as family support and resources, peer acceptance, and academic support and resources can have a major impact on the psychological development of these teens. When working with youth who have chronic illnesses, it is vital that clinicians remember that these youth are subject to the same statistical risk from experimentation with sex, drugs, and other risk taking behavior. They must also be aware of the impact of those chronic illnesses on the psychological development of each individual adolescent. Youth diagnosed with chronic illness can lead very psychologically healthy lives given a) individual strengths of cognitive flexibility, intelligence and hope (see table 5); b) a supportive family environment and resources; and c) peers who accept and value them; and d) teachers and classmates who provide a positive learning environment with resources to meet or adapt to the needs of these youth.

Table 5. Characteristics of Resilient Youth [25, 26, 29, 31]

Internal
Gender
Being male
Psychological
Sense of Autonomy
Positive sense of independence
Emerging feelings of efficacy
High self-esteem
Impulse Control
Planning and goal setting
Belief in future
Social Competence
Responsiveness to others
Conceptual and intellectual flexibility
Caring for others
Good communication skills
Sense of humor
Problem-Solving Skills
Ability to apply abstract thinking
Ability to engage in reflective thought
Critical reasoning skills
Ability to develop alternative solutions in frustrating situations
External
A. Family
A healthy family environmen
Parental aceptance of and ability to cope with their adolescents chronic illness (es) both emotionally and financially.
Strong family connectedness and cohesion
Socio-economic class (access to and possession of resources to meet family an chronically ill adolescent's needs)
B. Community/School
Acceptance by classmates and peers of the adolescents special needs.
Positive peer relationships
Lack of exposure to violence
Lack of exposure to substance
Mimimal exposure to trauma
Teachers who provide academic adaptations that meets adolescent's needs
A supportive social network
Peers who do not engage in maladaptive behavior

REFERENCES

[1] Acosta M, Gallo V, Batshaw ML. Brain development and the ontogency of developmental disabilities. *Adv. Pediatr.* 2002;49:1-57.

[2] Erickson EH. *Identity, youth and crisis,* New York: WW Norton, 1968.

[3] Gemelli R. Normal child and adolescent development. Washington, DC: *Am. Psychiatr.* Press, 1996.

[4] King A. Adolescence. In: Lewis M, ed. Child and adolescent psychiatry. *A comprehensive textbook,* 3rd ed. Philadelphia, PA: Lippincott Williams Wilkins, 2002:332-42.

[5] Kreipe RE. Normal somatic adolescent growth and development. In: McAnarney ER, Kreipe RE, Orr DP, Comerci GD, eds. *Textbook of adolescent medicine*. Philadelphia, PA: WB Saunders, 1994:4-67.
[6] Sarnat HB. Normal development of the nervous system. In: Coffey CE, Brumback RA, eds. Textbook of pediatric neuropsychiatry. Washington DC: *Am. Psychiatr. Press*, 1998:26-36.
[7] Werry JS, Zametkin A, Ernst M. Brain and behavior. In: Lewis M, ed. Child and adolescent psychiatry. *A comprehensive textbook,* 3rd ed. Philadelphia, PA: Lippincott Williams Wilkins, 2002:120-5.
[8] Pratt HD, Patel DR, Greydanus DE. Sports and the neurodevelopment of the child and adolescent. In: Delee JC, Drez DD, Miller MD, eds. *Orthopaedic sports medicine,* 2nd ed. Philadelphia, PA: WB Saunders, 2002:624-43.
[9] LeBlanc LA, Goldsmith T, Patel DR. Behavioral aspects of chronic illness in children and adolescents. *Pediatr. Clin. North Am.* 2003;50(4):859-78.
[10] Brener ND, Kann L, Garcia D, MacDonald G, Ramsey F, Honeycutt S, Hawkins J, Kinchen S, Harris WA. Youth Risk Behavior Surveillance. Selected steps communities, 2005. *Surveillance Summaries,* 2005;56/SS-2
[11] Kyngäs H. Support network of adolescents with chronic disease: Adolescents' perspective. *Nurs. Health Sci.* 2004;6:287-93.
[12] Britto MT, DeVellis RF, Hornung RW, DeFriese G, Atherton HD, Slap GB. Health care preferences and priorities of adolescents with chronic illnesses. *Pediatrics.* 2004;114(5):1272-80.
[13] Dixon SD. Gender and sexuality: normal development to problems and concerns. In: Behrman RE, Kliegman RM, Jenson HB, eds. *Nelson textbook of pediatrics,* 17th ed. Philadelphia, PA: WB Saunders, 2004:470-6.
[14] Miauton L, Narring F, Michaud PA. Chronic illness, life style and emotional health in adolescence: results of a cross-sectional survey on the health of 15-20-year-olds in Switzerland. *Eur. J. Pediatr.* 2003; 162(10):682-9.
[15] Pratt HD. Neurodevelopmental issues in the assessment and treatment of deficits in attention, cognition, and learning during adolescence. Adoles Med 2002;13(3):579-98.
[16] Piaget J. Intellectual evaluation from adolescence to adulthood. *Hum. Dev.* 1972;15:1-12.
[17] Greydanus DE, Pratt HD, Patel DR. The first three years of life and the early adolescent: Comparisons and differences. Lessons for child rearing. *Int. Pediatr.* 2004;19(2):68-80.
[18] Blos P. On adolescence. *Glencoe,* NY: Free Press, 1962.
[19] Boeree CG. Personality theories. 1997. Accessed on 2008 Jul 28. http://www.ship.edu/~cgboeree/perscontents.html
[20] Millon T, Davis RD. Disorders of personality: *DSM-IV and beyond,* 2nd ed. New York: Wiley, 1996
[21] Minuchin P. Families and individual development: provocations from the field of family therapy. *Child Dev.* 1985;56:289-302.
[22] Kaplan MS, McFarland BH, Huguet N, Newsom JT. Physical illness, functional limitations, and suicide risk: A population-based study. *Am. J. Orthopsychiatry.* 2007;77(1):56–60.

[23] Rosen DS. Pubertal growth and sexual maturation for adolescents with chronic illness or disability. *Pediatrician.* 1991;18:105-20.

[24] Bandura A. Influence of model's reinforcement contingencies on the acquisition of imitative processes. *J. Pers. Soc. Psychol.* 1965;1:589-95.

[25] Resnick MD. Protective factors, resiliency, and healthy youth development. *Adolesc. Med.* 2000;11:157-64.

[26] Blum RW, McNeely C, Nonnemaker J. Vulnerability, risk and protection. *J. Adolesc. Health.* 2002;31S(1):28-39.

[27] Masten AS, Hubbard JJ, Gest SD, Tellegen A, Garmezy N, Ramirez M. Competence in the context of adversity: pathways to resilience and maladaptation from childhood to late adolescence. *Dev. Psychopathol.* 1999;11(1):143-69.

[28] Mandleco BL, Peery JC. An organizational framework for conceptualizing resilience in children. *J. Child Adolesc. Psychiatr. Nurs.* 2000;13(3):99-111.

[29] Masten AS. Ordinary magic. Resilience processes in development. *Am. Psychol.* 2001;56(3):227-38.

[30] Luthar SS, Cicchetti D. The construct of resilience: implications for interventions and social policies. *Dev. Psychopathol.* 2000;12(4):857-85.

[31] Wirrell E, Cheung C, Spier S. How do teens view the physical and social impact of asthma compared to other chronic diseases? *J. Asthma.* 2006;43:155-60.

[32] Wyman PA, Cowen EL, Work WC, Hoyt-Meyers L, Magnus KB, Fagen DB. Caregiving and developmental factors differentiating young at-risk urban children showing resilient versus stress-affected outcomes: a replication and extension. *Child Dev.* 1999;70(3):645-59.

Part VII. Nervous System

In: Adolescence and Chronic Illness
Editors: H. Omar et al.

ISBN: 978-1-60876-628-4
© 2010 Nova Science Publishers, Inc.

Chapter 12

NEUROLOGICAL IMPAIRMENT AND DISABILITY

Dilip R. Patel and *Donald E. Greydanus*
Department of Pediatrics and Human Development,
Michigan State University College of Human Medicine,
Kalamazoo Center for Medical Studies, Kalamazoo,
Michigan, United States of America.

ABSTRACT

A number of neurological conditions can cause a wide range of functional impairments and disability in adolescents. Depending on the specific condition and neurological deficits, these can have significant implications for the normal progression of adolescent growth and development as well as social participation. Some of the major neurological conditions that can cause functional impairments and disability include epilepsy, traumatic brain injury, complications of infections, cerebrovascular accidents, brain neoplasms, neuromuscular diseases, neurodegenerative diseases, movement disorders, and various neurobehavioral disorders. The major functional domains affected include motor, sensory, cognitive, and psychosocial. Relevant aspects of epilepsy, Tourette syndrome, and cerebral palsy are reviewed briefly to highlight some these issues.

INTRODUCTION

Numerous neurological conditions that can lead to functional impairment and disability in adolescents are listed in table 1 [1-3]. The specific types of impairments will vary depending up on the neurological disorder and its severity. The broad categories of functional domains that are affected by various neurological conditions are listed in table 2. To highlight some of the impairments and disability associated with neurological conditions, we have briefly reviewed epilepsy, Tourette syndrome, and cerebral palsy [4-8].

---

* *Correspondence:* Professor Dilip R. Patel, MD, MSU/ KCMS/ Pediatrics, 1000, Oakland Drive, Kalamazoo, MI 49008 United States. E-mail: patel@kcms.msu.edu

Epilepsy

Epilepsy is characterized by the occurrence of recurrent seizures; its annual incidence in adolescents ranges from 18.6 to 24.7 per 100,000 (2). Epilepsy in adolescents provides an example of the wide ranging psychosocial implications that can be associated with a neurological disorder. Epilepsy can affect the daily activities of the teenager; for example, exposure to flickering lights of video games can increase the risk for seizures in some adolescents, and such photic stimulation may have to be avoided by this teenager [1,4,5]. Adolescents by their very nature are often sleep-deprived, which is another trigger for increased risk for seizure. The management of epilepsy is compounded by abuse of illicit drugs by some adolescents.

Sports participation is very important part of an adolescent's life. Adolescents with good seizure control can participate in most sports with no restrictions; however, certain sport scenarios pose increased risks for injury. In general, activities for which immediate help may not be available in case of a seizure can be potentially risky such as sky diving, hang gliding, rope climbing, and underwater swimming. Adolescents should be educated about the risks and should have a partner while participating in certain activities.

Driving is another area that is very critical in the life the adolescent. In most instances, the adolescent is eligible for a license to drive if he or she is seizure free for 1-2 years with or without medications. The time required to be seizure free varies from State to State (in the United States) and range from 3 months to 2 years. Any restriction on the ability of the adolescent to drive can have a significant emotional and social impact, including reduced self-esteem, limited socialization, limited job opportunities, and decreased adherence with the driving regulations [1,4,5].

Table 1. Neurological conditions that can be associated with various types of functional impairments and disabilities in adolescents (selected examples)

INBORN ERRORS OF METABOLISM (phenylketonuria, lysosomal storage diseases, mucopolysaccharidoses)
CONGENITAL BRAIN MALFORMATIONS (agenesis of corpus callosum, Dandy-Walker malformation, mild forms of holoprocencephaly)
GENETIC SYNDROMES (various mental retardation syndromes, Down syndrome, Fragile X syndrome)
NEUROCUTANEOUS DISORDERS (neurofibromatosis, Klippel-Trenaunay-Weber syndrome, Sturge-Weber syndrome)
EPILEPSY (generalized seizures, partial seizures, absence seizures)
WHITE MATTER DISEASES (adrenoleukodystrophies)
MOVEMENT AND BALANCE DISORDERS (Tourette syndrome, Frederick ataxia, ataxia-telengiectasia, Sydenham chorea, dystonia)
SLEEP DISORDERS (narcolepsy, restless legs syndrome)
NEUROMUSCULAR DISORDERS (peripheral neuropathies, myasthenia gravis, spinal muscular atrophy)
MUSCULAR DYSTROPHIES (Duchenne, Emery-Dreifuss, Limb-girdle, Fascioscapulohumeral)
NEUROBEHAVIORAL DISORDERS (attention deficit hyperactivity disorder, autism spectrum disorder, learning disabilities)
TRAUMA (traumatic brain injury, spinal cord injury)
INFECTIONS (complications of meningitis, encephalitis)
NEOPLASTIC DISEASES (benign and malignant brain and spinal cord neoplasms)
CEREBROVASCULAR DISEASES (stroke)

For adolescent females who are sexually active, epilepsy poses additional problems related to contraception and pregnancy risks. Pregnancy can increase the risks for seizures, and the use of antiseizure medications can have teratogenic effects on the fetus. Hormonal contraception should be offered to adolescent females who are sexually active, and the girls should be educated about the increased risks of seizures with pregnancy. The effectiveness of hormonal contraceptives should be carefully monitored because antiseizure medications can reduce the effectiveness of such contraceptives by the process of hepatic enzyme induction.

Epilepsy can be associated with subtle neurocognitive difficulties and learning disabilities [2,4,5] that will have implications for effective learning and academic functioning. Such difficulties can be compounded by the psychological impact of having epilepsy and the reaction of others toward the adolescent who has epilepsy. Schools should make appropriate accommodations for the adolescent with epilepsy to provide an optimal learning environment. Adolescents with epilepsy can also suffer from mental health problems, such as depression and anxiety, and these should be recognized and treated appropriately.

Table 2. Domains of function affected by neurological diseases (examples)

Motor functions (mobility, feeding, ambulation)
Sensory functions (hearing loss, blindness, loss of taste sensation, loss of peripheral sensation)
Cognitive abilities (mental retardation, learning disabilities)
Psychosocial development and functioning (ability to drive, ability to communicate, depression)

Tourette Syndrome

Tourette syndrome is the most severe form of tic disorder with an incidence of 5 in 10,000 with a 3-4:1 male to female ratio [1-3,7]. The prevalence of attention deficit hyperactivity disorder, obsessive compulsive disorder, learning disabilities, enuresis, aggressive and oppositional behaviors, and sleep disorders is high in adolescents with Tourette syndrome [7]. Tourette syndrome is characterized by a combination of multiple, simple or complex motor tics (involving the head, neck, trunk, and upper or lower extremities) and vocal tics (coughing, grunting, shouting, crying, barking, throat clearing, sniffing, and others). More complex vocal tics include echolalia, palilalia, and coprolalia. Some common motor tics include eye blinking, lip smacking, head tossing, and grimacing.

The behavioral symptoms of Tourette syndrome can be significantly distressing for the adolescent in the social context. This situation can lead to embarrassment, isolation, anxiety, and depression. The associated neuro-behavioral disorders can further complicate academic and psychosocial development. The management of adolescents with Tourette syndrome must include a comprehensive behavioral evaluation and treatment of the specific disorders identified. The tics can be controlled in most cases by use of medications like haloperidol, risperidone, clonidine, or pimozide [1,7].

Cerebral Palsy

A large number of children with cerebral palsy now survive into adulthood [8]. Adolescents with cerebral palsy present special management challenges. Depending upon the severity and type of neuromotor deficits, there can be a range of functional impairments affecting activities of daily living, academic participation, and social participation. Mild degrees of cerebral palsy may not be diagnosed until adolescence when the adolescent presents with subtle motor dysfunction. In broad terms, cerebral palsy encompasses a range of primarily motor deficits characteristically increased tone, spasticity, incoordination, abnormal reflexes, and gait disturbances. The associated problems further complicate the growth, development, and functional capacity of adolescents with cerebral palsy. Some of the associated problems include dysarthria, mental retardation, seizures, progressive joint contractures, neuromuscular scoliosis, hip dislocations, visual motor incoordination, bowel and bladder dysfunction, and feeding difficulties. Adolescents with cerebral palsy are best managed in a multidisciplinary team setting with comprehensive and coordinated care.

CONCLUSIONS

Various neurological disorders can induce functional impairments and disabilities in adolescents with considerable dysfunction in such parameters as growth and development, socialization, and mental health. Some of the major neurological conditions that can cause functional impairments and disability include epilepsy, traumatic brain injury, complications of infections, cerebrovascular accidents, brain neoplasms, neuromuscular diseases, neurodegenerative diseases, movement disorders, and various neurobehavioral disorders. The major functional domains affected include motor, sensory, cognitive, and psychosocial. Relevant aspects of epilepsy, Tourette syndrome, and cerebral palsy are reviewed briefly to highlight some these issues.

REFERENCES

[1] Swaiman KF, Ashwal S, Ferriero DM, eds. Pediatric neurology: Principles and practice, 4th ed. Philadelphia, PA: *Mosby Elsevier,* 2006.
[2] Greydanus DE, Van Dyke DH. Neurologic disorders. In: Greydanus DE, Patel DR, Pratt HD, eds. *Essential adolescent medicine.* New York: McGraw Hall, 2006:235-80.
[3] Greydanus DE, Pratt HD, Van Dyke HD, eds. Neurologic and neurodevelopmental dilemmas in the adolescent. In: Greydanus DE, Pratt HD, Van Dyke HD, eds. *Adolescent medicine.* Philadelphia, PA: Elsevier, 2002:413-686.
[4] Liebenson MH, Rosman NP. Seizures in adoles-cents. *Adolesc. Med.* 1991;2:629-48.
[5] Nordli DRJr. Special needs of the adolescent with epilepsy. *Epilepsia.* 2001;42(Suppl 8):10-7.
[6] Paolicchi JM. Epilepsy in adolescents: diagnosis and treatment. *Adolesc. Med.* 2002;13:443-59.
[7] Kuperman S. Tic disorders in the adolescent. *Adolesc. Med.* 2002;13:537-51.

[8] Bottos M, Feliciangeli A, Sciuto LS, et al. Functional status of adults with cerebral palsy and implications for treating children. *Dev. Med. Child Neurol.* 2001;431:516-28.

Chapter 13

YOUTH WITH CHRONIC PAIN

Paula Forgeron* and Patrick J. McGrath

Pediatric Complex Pain Management Team and IWK Health Centre,
Dalhousie University, Halifax, Nova Scotia, Canada.

ABSTRACT

This chapter describe a focus group interview to explore the self-identified needs of adolescents living with chronic pain. Nineteen youth, who receive care through the Chronic Pain Clinic at a tertiary care children's hospital were invited to participate. Six youth, age 13-17 years, consented to participate. The discussions were transcribed verbatim and thematic analysis was conducted. Two major themes emerged from the data; struggling to be normal, and dealing with the pain. Participants view themselves as different and unhealthy compared to their peers. Health is seen as "being normal"; "able to do whatever you want". Distraction was the primary strategy for coping with pain. Friends were seen as essential to well being but understanding was limited. Half of the participants felt that peers who had pain would provide a major source of support. Those not in favour of this support cited the idiosyncratic nature of pain. School was uniformly identified as the greatest source of stress. The thought of transition to adult care was overwhelming. They were unsure what skills they needed in order to transition, and asserted they were not ready to transition to adult service.

INTRODUCTION

Adolescents with chronic pain face many challenges; they suffer from a disease process that is not well understood, has an uncertain illness trajectory, and is not usually accompanied by obvious physical signs. Hence many teens face disbelief from friends, family, and health professionals [1,2]. In addition, although up to 25% of children and or adolescents may develop chronic pain at some point in their childhood [3,4], most adolescents with chronic

---

* *Correspondence:* Paula Forgeron, RN, MN, Clinical Nurse Specialist, Pediatric Complex Pain Management Team, IWK Health Centre, 5850/5980 University Avenue, POBox 9700, Halifax, Nova Scotia, B3K 6R8, Canada. Tel: (902) 470-6350; Fax (902) 470-7911; E-mail: pforgero@dal.ca

pain feel isolated as they do not have peers with a similar chronic pain experience [1,2]. As a result, youth with chronic pain must learn ways to cope with these many challenges. We could not find any studies that identified what youth believe their needs to be. Understanding the self-identified needs of youth with chronic pain will assist in designing ways to meet these needs.

Our qualitative study captured what youth identified as helpful in coping with chronic pain and which areas of their lives they needed help. Youth identified that they struggled with being the same as their peers. Despite finding ways to cope with pain, issues such as academic workload, talking to friends, dealing with peers who were not friends, and preparing to transition to adult services were challenging.

Chronic pain in children and adolescents results from "a dynamic integration of biological processes, psychological factors, and sociocultural context considered within a developmental trajectory" [5]. Coping is a process of changing behavioral and cognitive efforts to manage specific external and/or internal demands that an individual appraises as taxing or beyond their resources [6]. Hence coping is contextually based, and therefore an understanding of coping would be enhanced by examining the description of thoughts and actions that take place in stressful encounters [6]. Pain also changes over time and may depend on the context. Given the variable nature of coping and pain we believe understanding what is needed to improve pain coping is embedded in the experiences of those living with pain.

OUR STUDY

We used a fundamental qualitative approach [7] to provide a descriptive analysis of the data to discover and understanding the phenomena from the perspective of our specific population [8]. A focus group was used to elicit the experiences and needs of the adolescents with chronic pain. Interactions among participants can generate more in-depth information than one could obtain in a survey [9], and provides an opportunity to clarify agreement, or disagreement within the group, by observing body language, as well as, listening to the dialogue among participants as they respond to questions and comments [10].

The study took place at the only pediatric chronic pain clinic for the Maritime Provinces in Canada. A purposeful sample was obtained by inviting all current eligible adolescent patients from the pediatric chronic pain clinic to participate. The medical director of the clinic endorsed the study and mailed letters to the patients. This letter included a brief description of the study along with the contact information of the researchers; interested patients were instructed to contact the researchers directly.

Eligible patients between the ages of 12-18 years of age who spoke English fluently were invited to participate. Youth with cognitive impairments or cancer pain were excluded. The letter announcing the study was sent to 19 eligible youth. Eight called to receive consent packages. Two of these patients were unable to participate due to prior commitments on the day of the focus group. Six youth participated in the focus group. Travel expenses were reimbursed for participants.

Five of the six participants were female and ranged in age from 13 to 18 years. Participants were in grade 8 to 12, which was appropriate for their age. They were all from Caucasian middle-class socioeconomic families and lived at home with both parents.

A self-administered eleven-item demographic questionnaire was completed prior to the focus group discussion. A semi-structured interview guide was used to keep the discussion flowing. The discussion was audiotaped and transcribed verbatim. Refreshments were provided. The adolescents had never met prior to the focus group so the session started with introductions, followed by a review of the rationale for the focus group, and a discussion on respecting everyone's comments and experiences. Confidentiality was reviewed. Participants were reassured that their would be no names or identifying features attached to their comments and quotes in discussions, papers and presentations.

The youth were shy at first but opened up to sharing their experiences. Often the participants shared experiences with each other as opposed to answering the questions posed by the facilitator. All participants contributed to the discussion. No adolescents left or declined to answer any of the questions.

The focus group discussion was thematically analyzed. Open coding [11] was conducted on the transcripts by the first author by reading the entirety of the transcript several times to gain an impression of the overall experiences of the participants. A list of identified labels was developed from the data during this process and the categorizing scheme was continually refined during analysis. The data were then clustered under the established category headings and themes identified. Validity of the themes was determined through constant comparison, which has been described as the distribution of data into specific categories based on whether the contents "look-alike" or "feel-alike" until all data are accounted for [12].

OUR FINDINGS

The participants had been attending the pain clinic for over a year and had experienced pain from 13 months to 10 years. Pain location varied and included pelvic area, shoulders, neck, back, hands, feet, left knee, and stomach. Two participants had pain in only one location and one participant had short periods of no pain. All participants had pain on daily basis, ranging from 3-9/10 on a 0 to 10 scale, with exacerbations escalating between 6-10/10. Despite individual difference, they all experienced pain that interfered with daily life and prevented them from participating in their favorite activities and sports with school absences between 2 to 13 days/month. Five of the participants were on medication and the sixth had trials of various medications. All participants received instruction on psychological pain management techniques by the pediatric pain psychologist, and all but one received physiotherapy.

There were two over-riding themes that emerged from the focus group data: "struggling to be normal" and "dealing with the pain". These themes transcended the stories that the adolescents shared and shed light on the needs of these adolescents to enhance coping.

Struggling to Be Normal

All of the participants told stories of wanting to be like their peers, who they viewed as normal. Pain interrupted their ability to function to the extent that they felt abnormal. Their pain caused them to take medications, attend various appointments, miss out on activities, or be absent from school, which only served to remind them that their lives were deeply altered and different from their peers. Several sub themes emerged in their struggle to be normal.

Healthy Is Being Normal

Overall the participants did not see themselves as healthy at the time of the focus group. From their definitions, health was synonymous with being normal and is exemplified in this female participant's quote "The key word is normal. You have to be able to feel like you're normal and not outside of like everyone else." The salient characteristic of being healthy centered on activity. As the male in the group explained, " I think it [health] means that you can do whatever you want". Pain was not only seen as preventing engagement in activities but also restricting the amount of time they had for activities by attending to the demands of treatment. "Like, most 17 year olds don't go to physiotherapy 3, 4, 5 times a week, and you know, go to the pain clinic. Most normal teenagers don't do that. I am far from the norm—far, far from the norm" (female participant). These statements on health illustrate that the adolescents viewed health through the lens of normal adolescent behavior, not physiologic impairments. Even for the two adolescents who had other chronic illnesses, it was the restrictions caused by their pain that made them feel unhealthy.

Trying to Be Normal at School

Although they all wanted to be seen as normal, and did not want attention drawn to themselves in the classroom, each voiced a need to have modifications to their academic requirements and all were stressed and frustrated when modifications were not offered. One of the participants started the discussion about school by saying, "school is a killer". This comment was received with laughter, sighs of understanding, and agreement by nodding of heads from others. They struggled academically because of their pain and this struggle interfered dramatically with their desire to be normal. Trying to keep up marks was difficult due to the cognitive effects of pain, which was exacerbated by the amount of school absence. As one participants comment, "When I was trying to make the honor role last year it [pain] was bad, like before every test I was like I'm gonna puke." Another noted that "Grade eleven sucks, I can usually concentrate when I am there but when I miss like a week of chemistry [due to pain], I'm lost."

Despite not wanting to differ from their peers, they all acknowledged that this was impractical at times. Being absent from school, needing to leave class, getting up to stretch, or inability to participate in physical education class were impossible to hide. However, for a few this was made worse by teachers who were described as fussing over them, asking in class if they were OK, or not getting upset with their behavior when other pupils would have been disciplined for the same action. These situations increased their unease with standing out.

Not all the participants experienced the 'over caring' teachers. Most struggled with teachers not providing agreed upon accommodations for their pain. This was perceived as disbelief from their teachers. As one adolescent shared, "Like if I'm sick then too bad—oh well, they don't care. They say like that's your problem." This was very problematic for this young woman who was in her final year of high school and trying to attain the necessary grades to be accepted into university. She felt that her marks had dropped as a result of missed class time and that her teachers did not want to assist her in obtaining the missed content. Others voiced similar experiences resulting in an increase in stress related pain, a decrease in marks, and, for some, disengagement from academic pursuits. One of the youth said that he did not study for tests anymore as he would get "pissed off because half of the things [notes] I don't have", the result of not receiving information or help for missed content. Another participant empathized and stated that there is "no sense in studying if you don't have the stuff." Even when they try to find the material for themselves one said, "You have to write all these notes from your friends and that's going to take even longer and you're going to get less time to study". Another noted, "it's frustrating because you know you can, like, make a certain mark and usually you do really awesome and then with pain sometimes you can't finish this or you can't finish that. You are capable of so much more but you're kind of screwed."

Although all of the participants shared stories of struggles at school, two of the participants shared how things had improved once their teachers understood, or, at least, made agreed upon accommodations. Provision of notes, decreased workload, and flexible assignment and test dates were essential components of supportive academic accommodations. Even though other factors, such as absences from school and being excused from physical education, still made them stand out as different, these two adolescents now felt positive about their academic abilities.

Relating to Peers and Society Interferes with Being Normal

There was a unanimous agreement that relating to peers who were not friends and society in general reminded them that they were different and they struggled with how to relate. This occurred everywhere in their communities: at the grocery store, pharmacy, church, group activities, and school. They spoke of these interactions as different from those with their teachers and friends, as they were willing to share some of their health history with teachers and friends to gain their support and understanding. The participants shared stories of relative strangers asking them personal health questions. One participant explained, "people that you don't even talk to or even know, they just come up and ask you how you are doing." Some of these interactions occurred after discharge from hospital, but other interactions occurred for no apparent reason reason, as illustrated by the following quote:

> Some random girl walked up like, I was in the hospital three years ago and she was like are you still sick? I hadn't been in the hospital for like three years and she asks are you better yet? I never talk to her; I don't know how the hell she knew I was ever in the hospital. I was like I've been out of the hospital for like three years and she was like

oh, I didn't know that. She then asked me what's wrong with you? I just didn't want to talk to her and I just walked away and she was swearing at me and stuff. (male participant)

Another participant recounted her first outing after being in hospital for her pain. She went to the pharmacy with her mother and felt as though everyone in the pharmacy came up and asked her what was wrong with her. Although she believed most were trying to show concern the questioning was overwhelming and left her wanting to leave and remembered saying, "Mom, take me home because I don't want to be around anyone." The other participants revealed similar experiences and as one adolescent said, "Yeah, like they're always asking and I really hate it because I don't want to tell the whole world that I'm sick [in pain]. I just want to be back to normal, a normal teenager living my life without everyone having to know that I'm sick [in pain]".

These interactions reminded them that they were different than their peers, as virtual strangers did not ask other adolescents such personal questions. In addition, not only were these interactions an invasion of their privacy they resulted in other negative experiences. As noted in one of the exchanges the adolescent was subjected to cursing when he ignored a girl's questions. Another participant explained how people pitied her. "A lot of people give me pity and that's not something I want. I don't want to be pitied or treated any different than anyone else just because of what's going on." All of participants expressed that they did not want to have to explain their pain condition to everyone. They had already experienced disbelief from people they either knew or trusted, such as health care professionals, and desired privacy from strangers.

Dealing with the Pain

Dealing with the pain was a daily occurrence. Some felt that the pain had a life of its own, while others verbalized a more cavalier attitude towards their pain, stating that it was "not ruling their life". Regardless of their professed belief they shared stories that illustrated that their pain did dictate aspects of their lives. Yet, their stories were also filled with courage and a desire to move forward.

Management Strategies

The participants found strategies to deal with their pain but none had found these to be successful in all situations or all the time. All but one of the participants took analgesics to help manage their pain. Although generally helpful, these medications were not useful during exacerbations. As one participant explained, "When it [the pain] hits a certain level then its gonna go its own path" and the medications were no longer very effective.

Activity was a challenge for each of the group but in varying degrees. One of the female participants commented, "I am active to the degree that I can be without being in pain." Although the concept of pacing had been reviewed, they found it difficult to pace their activities incorporate pacing into their lives, and unconvinced of the benefit. One girl clarified the difficulties with pacing by saying "I can't really help [by pacing activity], because you don't know when it [the pain] is going to come, it comes from anything." However, another stated "I can't pack it in because I get really, really tired and tired just doesn't help the pain and then this whole spiral effect starts to happen." So, for all but one participant they had fun when they felt good. As one girl noted, she did activities even if it resulted in increased pain, "I went to the movies the other night and I said I know I'm going to hurt [as I was overdoing it] but I really wanted to go to the movies." Dealing with increased pain was seen as a necessary consequence of engaging in activities: "There is a level of pain that like goes up if I do certain things, but I know it is going to go back to normal pain, so like she was saying, I do like to get out and do stuff, like remain sane."

The one strategy that they all used and agreed was most effective after their medication was distraction. As one stated, "Distraction is my main thing. Anything to get my mind off of it." In most instances the participants had found unique ways to distract themselves. They shared their best distraction strategies, and these ranged from playing piano, listening to music, going for run, using the computer, going to a tanning bed, to having their friends tell them stories while they were in school. One girl described distraction while at school, "If I'm at school and get an episode [of pain] I'm like OK, talk and talk with my friend and I'm focusing on her and not what's going on with my pain."

Relating to Friends

Pain complicated the adolescents' relationships with their friends. Friends' disbelief and, or, inability to grasp the impact of pain was a common and distressing experience. As one participant revealed, "they don't really understand when you say I can't go because I'm going to end up getting sick." Although some said it was helpful to talk to their friends about the frustrations of living with pain this was not true all the time, or, for all participants. One shared that her friends are "useless from a pain point of view". None of the participants had a visible abnormality to account for their pain and believed that this contributed to the disbelief they encounter from friends and society. This was exemplified by this participant's account.

> They all [my friends] think that I'm full of it, they all think that I don't have any pain and uh, that I must be making it up because I don't take medication, because I refuse to. But they don't see the side effects. The side effects that hit me are like I sit on my kitchen floor because my room is spinning. Like it's horrible and they thinking I'm making it up.

Despite the struggles with friends the participants were quick to excuse their friends' lack of understanding. One participant explained that, "friends are helpful to a point but they can't fully understand because they haven't gone through it." Trying to explain everything to their friends became tiring and was reported at times to increase confusion amongst their friends. " Well like, the first year I had pain and at the hospital and stuff that was the only time we ever talked about where I was and what happened. But they did not really understand they just wanted to know how much it hurt and can you still play basketball? "(male participant).

Three participants in the group had a friend who also struggled with a health condition; one of these three had a friend with chronic pain. These friendships were described as being different from their other friends. "One best friend, she's like my sister she like lives at our house. She kind of gets what it's like to be different. She has diabetes and kidney disease so she knows what it's like to have to miss school for appointments and such".

The participant who had a chronic pain friend described the relationship as helpful in the following way. "Oh my gosh, she has made a world of difference in my life. I found talking with her helped. I could tell her anything. I didn't think it would be that awesome or great to have someone with pain to talk to, [but] that's what really helps me—not feeling so alone".

A few of the participants expressed that it would be "cool to meet someone who has close to the same thing" but others were skeptical of finding such a person, as they believed that their pain was unique and rare. Other reasons for not being keen on the idea of a pain buddy included not wanting to be reminded of their pain by talking about it or talking with strangers about their condition. It is unclear if some of these participants felt that meeting someone else with pain would once again make them feel abnormal, as healthy peers do not have this sort of 'special' friend.

Transitioning—Not Yet

When transitioning to adult care was introduced most of the participants expressed discomfort with the idea. All believed that one should be an adult before moving to adult care facilities and none of them felt that they were adults yet. There was an acknowledgement from the older participants that they felt too old for a pediatric hospital but too young for an adult hospital. As one noted "Not until I am 18 years old, 20 is technically an adult. Like I am not an adult when I am 16, I would be still a teenager in an adult hospital." Most others agreed with this statement and included criteria such as being out of high school and able to drive themselves to appointments as signs of adulthood. One suggested, "they should give you a choice of when you want to leave, but the limit would be like 20. So, if you're ready to leave when you're 16 then you can". The other participants agreed that they should have more say in when to transition.

The participants cited other discomforts with transitioning. They did not look forward to getting to know new health professionals and having to tell their story again. They voiced concerns over what the adult health care professionals would be like, in particular, would they be believed. This concern was exemplified by one participant who had been seen in an adult clinic for a second opinion, "Like the way they worded things, like they were almost trying to trick you to like thinking like their way, and I'm like no [I really have pain]."

None of the participants cited self-advocacy, or self-management skills as necessary to interact successfully in an adult system. Parents still attended appointments, called for the youth's prescription renewals, and were responsible to contact health professionals when questions arose. Only one had independently called to ask questions or discuss her needs with the members of the pain care team. When asked if these skills were required before transitioning they agreed but were surprised that their parents' involvement in their care might change when they were transitioned. The group felt that it would be important to start taking more ownership of their care but wanted this to evolve slowly, such as attending a portion of their appointments by themselves.

The adolescents were concerned about their futures; would pain still be present, would it decrease, would they be able to manage and pursue their dreams. Transitioning to adult care was yet another challenge that they had to mount in dealing with pain. They spoke of the impending event with great reservation and viewed the physical environment as void of caring. As one of the participants noted, "Yeah, but the bad thing about the adult care system is that there are so many colours here it makes you feel happier but in there [adult clinic] it is just white".

DISCUSSION

Our research identified several needs of this group of adolescents suffering with chronic pain. They view themselves as unhealthy and different compared to their peers. Although other studies [1,2] have identified that adolescents with chronic pain feel isolated from their peers at times, the participants in this study spoke of struggles that encompassed more than feelings of isolation. Their stories shed light on how deeply they viewed themselves as different. They felt alienated from the mainstream and did not see themselves as being normal members of society. They even described health as being normal. However, part of their definition of health, being able to engage in activities that they want, is similar to that found that in other studies with chronically ill children and adolescents [13,14].

Although viewing themselves as different they did not want to be seen as different, or sick, and tried to do what they could to appear similar to peers. This desire to not be seen as sick is not unique to adolescents with chronic pain [15]. Despite not wanting to appear sick there were constant reminders that they were different. Their pain complicated conversations with friends and resulted, at times, in self-imposed isolation to avoid personal questions. Lazrus [6] asserted, that when an individual believes little or nothing can be done the emphasis is apt to be placed on emotion-focused coping processes, whereas when the situation is believed to be changeable problem-focused approaches are apt to prevail. It is not known if these adolescents would have engage more fully with others if they thought differently about the situation or felt competent in their skill to discuss their pain with others.

Perceived disbelief among teachers and non-friend peers contributed to sources of stress at school. Trying to catch up on missed information and teach themselves concepts while dealing with the cognitive effects of pain, increased stress related pain. These adolescents cited accommodations as essential to achieve academic success and prevent them from falling behind their peers. Teachers' willingness to make accommodations were viewed as an acknowledgement that their pain was real, otherwise they felt punished for their condition. Despite being at different stages of adolescence and illness trajectory they all agreed that a problem-focused coping strategy including the provision of notes, flexible timelines, and a decreased workload were needed and that a more active involvement by health care professionals helped secure these accommodations. The individuality of this coping process was in the degree of accommodation required.

Greco, Freeman, and Dufton [16] found that children and adolescents with undiagnosed abdominal pain were subject to increases in overt and relational victimization, while Kashikar-Zuck et al [17] discovered that youth with fibromyalgia are not as likable compared to normative classmates. Comparatively, the adolescents in this study described being misunderstood by friends in relation to their pain versus feeling disliked. Overall, they remarked that non-friend peers and others in their communities asked questions and made comments that made them feel stigmatized for having pain.

Peer support has been conceptualized as providing informational, emotional, and appraisal functions and identified as improving health outcomes through numerous actions including reinforcing help-seeking behaviors, encouraging effective coping, promoting social comparisons, and aiding self esteem [18]. Half of the participants felt that peers who had pain would provide a major source of support. Those not in favour of this cited the idiosyncratic nature of pain. Lazarus [6] asserts that individuals tend not to seek social support if their self-esteem is at stake. Recent research suggests that chronic pain in adults has a negative impact on one's self and identity which is made worse in the public arena [19]. It would be important to know if adolescents not interested in peer support appraised the sharing of their pain as somehow shameful.

Regardless of the positive impact of peer support on various health conditions it remains unclear what form of peer support adolescents with chronic pain would benefit from. We know little about the actual peer relationships of adolescents with chronic pain and even less about what needs would be met through peer support, or, the best method for delivering peer support to these adolescents. There is evidence emerging within adolescent populations that suggests some negative effects of peer support exchanges [20-22]. More research is needed before peer support becomes a mainstay in adolescent chronic pain care.

The thought of transition to adult care was overwhelming. They were unsure what skills they needed, were skeptical about adult health care professionals, and asserted they were not ready to transition but felt strongly that they should be involved in the decision of when to transition. Similar to adolescents with other chronic illnesses, chronological age was not seen as the best determinant of readiness; as self-management and advocacy skills are essential for adolescents, regardless of their chronic illness, to navigating the adult care system [23,24]. It has also been suggested that some adolescents, by the very nature of their illness, may not receive the same level of expertise by adult health care professionals, such as those living with cystic fibrosis [23]. This is pertinent for adolescents with chronic pain as recognition of pain as a disease is fairly recent. Thus, health professionals working in adult chronic pain clinics have not had the opportunity to work with adolescent patients and be aware of their unique needs. Trusting a new adult health care team was concerning, as they had encountered disbelief from health professionals in the past.

Although living with pain present challenges, the adolescents in this study found positive management strategies. Evidence supports the effectiveness of various cognitive behavioral techniques such as guided imagery and relaxation [25,26] but distraction was the primary pain coping strategy and it was adaptable to most situations. Given that coping is an individual process, which changes over time and context, the usefulness of distraction is not surprising.

Even though pacing is regarded as an important strategy for managing chronic pain [27] only one participate found this to be true. The rest stated that they no longer paced activity, as it was not beneficial. These participants approached activity by "packing it in". Pacing may remind them of how they are different from their peers and thus rejected. Recent literature suggests that a formal approach to pacing may be used by some individuals to avoid activity by focusing on rest or shirking pain producing activities, while a functional approach to pacing, which focuses on pacing as a way to reduce pain's influence, may improve functioning [28]. How important pacing is remains a matter for discussion, as Nielson et al [29] found that pacing only contributed to 2-4% of the explained variance in functioning of a 110 adults with fibromyalgia after controlling for sex, gender, pain severity, and scores on the Chronic Pain Coping Inventory. It may be that 'packing it' is the adolescents' perception of functional pacing. The one participant who found pacing helpful described purposefully missing out on activities and thus may be using pacing as a reason to avoid activities. It remains unknown how, or to what degree, pacing improves functioning in adolescents with chronic pain.

Since we only gathered data during one session it may be that additionally needs would have been uncovered in subsequent discussions. The goal of qualitative research is not to reach generalizable conclusions; a quantitative study to determine if other adolescents with chronic pain have similar needs is warranted.

CONCLUSIONS

Youth attending a tertiary care pain clinic had multiple needs. They struggled to be normal while dealing with their pain. They identified needing help with school and communicating with friends and others about their pain. Friends were important but friendships were negatively impacted by the adolescents' chronic pain. Half the participants viewed support from another peer with chronic pain as positive. Distraction was the favored strategy for coping; pacing was least valued. Transition to adult care evoked several concerns including timing of transition and the needed skills to engage in adult health systems. It would be important for health care professionals to be aware of these self-identified needs in order improve outcomes for adolescents with chronic pain.

ACKNOWLEDGEMENTS

This research has been funded by a Rising Researcher Support Award from the Child Health Clinician Scientist Program to Paula Forgeron and her PhD studies are support by a Canadian Institutes of Health Research—Doctoral Research Fellowship.

REFERENCES

[1] Sällfors C, Fasth A, Hallberg LR. Oscillating between hope and despair—a qualitative study. *Child Care Health Dev.* 2002;28:495-505.

[2] Carter B, Lambrenos K, Thursfield J. A pain workshop: An approach to eliciting the views of young people with chronic pain. *J. Clin. Nurs.* 2002;11:753-62.

[3] Perquin CW, Hazebroek-Kampschreur AA, Hunfeld JA, Bohnen AM, van Suijlekom-Smit LW, Passchier J, van der Wouden JC. Pain in children and adolescents: A common experience. *Pain.* 2000;87: 51-8.

[4] Goodman JE, McGrath PJ. The epidemiology of pain in children and adolescents: A review. *Pain.* 1991;46:247-64.

[5] Bursch B. Pain in infants, children, and adolescents SIG: Policy statement on peditaric chronic pain. APS Bulletin,10, retrieved October 10, 2007 http://www.ampainsoc.org/pub/bulletin/may00/sig1.

[6] Lazarus RS. Coping with the stress of illness. In: Kaplun A, ed. *Health promotion and chronic illness*. Geneva: WHO, 1992.

[7] Sandelowski M. Whatever happened to qualitative description? *Res. Nurs. Health.* 2000;23:334-40.

[8] Merriam SB. *Qualitative research and case study application in education*. San Francisco: Jossey-Bass, 1998.

[9] Morgan DL. Focus groups. *Ann. Rev. Sociol.* 1996;22:129-52.

[10] Morgan DL. Focus groups. In: Hesse-Biber SN, Leavy P, eds. Approaches to qualitative research: *A reader on theory and practice*. New York: Oxford Univ Press, 2004:263-85.

[11] Holloway I, Wheeler S. *Qualitative research in nursing,* 2nd ed. Oxford: Blackwell, 2002.

[12] Lincoln Y, Guba E. *Naturalistic inquiry*. London: Sage, 1985.

[13] Christensen PH. Childhood and the cultural constitutions of vulnerable bodies. In: Prout A, ed. *The body, childhood and society*. Basingstoke, UK: MacMillan, 2000:38-59.

[14] James A. Embodied being(s): Understanding the self and the body in childhood. In: Prout A, ed. *The body, childhood and society*. Basingstoke, UK: MacMillan, 2000:19-37).

[15] Guell C. Painful childhood: children living with juvenile arthritis. *Qual. Health Res.* 2007;17:884-92.

[16] Greco LA, Kari E, Freeman MS, Dufton L. Overt and relational victimization among children with frequent abdominal pain: Links to social skills, academic functioning, and health service use. *J. Pediatr. Psychol.* 2007;32:319-29.

[17] Kashikar-Zuck S, Lynch A, Graham B, Swain N, Mullen SA. Social functioning and peer relationships of adolescents with juvenile fibromyalgia syndrome. *Arthritis Rheum.* 2007;57:474-80.

[18] Dennis C. Peer support within a health care context: a concept analysis. *Int. J. Nurs. Stud.* 2003;40:321-32.

[19] Smith J, Osborn M. Pain as an assault on the self: An interpretative phenomenological analysis of the psychological impact of chronic benign low back pain. *Psychol. Health.* 2007;22(5):517-34.

[20] Rose AJ, Carlson W, Waller EM. Prospective associations of co-rumination with friendship and emotional adjustment: Considering the socioemotional trade-offs of co-rumination. *Dev. Psychol.* 2007;43:1019-31.

[21] Rose AJ. Co-rumination in the friendships of girls and boys. *Child Dev.* 2002;73:1830-43.

[22] Gramic I, Dishion TJ. Deviant talk in adolescent friendships: A step toward measuring a pathogenic attractor process. *Soc. Dev.* 2003;12, 314-34.

[23] Reiss JG, Gibson RW, Walker L. Health care transition: Youth, family, and provider perspectives. *Pediatrics.* 2005;15:112-20.

[24] McDonagh JE. Transition of care from paediatric to adult rheumatology. *Arch. Dis. Child.* 2007;92:802-7.

[25] McGrath PJ, Humphreys P, Keene D, Goodman JT, Lascelles MA, Cunningham SJ. The efficacy and efficiency of a self-administered treatment for adolescent migraine. *Pain.* 1992;49;321-4.

[26] Hicks CL, von Baeyer C, McGrath PJ. Online psychological treatment for pediatric recurrent pain: A randomized evaluation. *J. Pediatr. Psychol.* 2006;31:724-36.

[27] Hanson RW, Gerber KE. *Coping with chronic pain: a guide to self-management.* New York: Guilford, 1990.

[28] McCracken LM, Samuel VM. The role of avoidance, pacing, and other activity patterns in chronic pain. *Pain.* 2007;130:119-25.

[29] Nielson WR, Jensen MP, Hill ML. An activity pacing scale for the chornic pain coping inventory: development in a sample of patients with fibromyalgia syndrome. *Pain.* 2001;89:111-5.

VIII. Circulatory System

In: Adolescence and Chronic Illness
Editors: H. Omar et al.

ISBN: 978-1-60876-628-4
© 2010 Nova Science Publishers, Inc.

Chapter 14

A Comprehensive Approach to Obesity, Hypertension, and Mental Health Evaluation

Stefan G. Kiessling[1], Kimberly K. McClanahan[2] and Hatim A. Omar[*2]

[1] Division of Nephrology
[2] Division of Adolescent Medicine, Department of Pediatrics,
Kentucky Children's Hospital, Lexington, Kentucky, United States.

Abstract

The global epidemic of childhood and adolescent obesity in developing and developed countries has become a major public health concern. Given the relationship between obesity and hypertension as documented in several landmark studies, it is no surprise that, as the prevalence of obesity has increased in the pediatric population, rates of hypertension have also increased substantially. Hypertension is one of the most important risk factors for cardiovascular diseases and stroke; therefore, evaluation and initiation of appropriate treatment are extremely important in the pediatric population. Evaluation for secondary causes of hypertension, including renovascular, renoparenchymal, and endocrine disease, is the approach most commonly utilized in health care settings with the goal to detect abnormalities that already have or might, if left unrecognized, affect the physical health of the child in the future. Children and adolescents are commonly evaluated for organic disease even in situations where secondary hypertension is unlikely and overweight or obesity is most likely the primary factor contributing to hypertension. Psychological and psychosocial factors, which may play an important role in the etiology of obesity and related blood pressure elevation, are often addressed inadequately or completely ignored, potentially reducing long-term therapy success and increasing the incidence of avoidable complications. It is proposed that a comprehensive evaluation by a behavioral health provider will improve outcomes

---

[*] *Correspondence:* Hatim Omar, MD, Professor, Pediatrics & Obsterics/Gynecology, Director of Adolescent Medicine and Young Parent Program, J422 Kentucky Clinic, University of Kentucky,Lexington, KY 40536-0284, United States. Tel: 859-323-5643; Fax: 859-257-7706; Email: haomar2@uky.edu

and potentially reduce long-term morbidity and hypertension-related end organ disease. A framework for mental health evaluation is provided.

INTRODUCTION

Obesity has become one of the most common diseases and disease-associated conditions in the United States (US) and other countries. It should be noted that overweight and obesity are usually defined as a body mass index (BMI) equal to or greater than the 95th percentile, compared to pediatric population reference data when plotted on the appropriate age and gender chart; children and adolescents with a BMI between the 85th and 95th percentile are considered to be at risk for obesity according to the Center for Disease Control (CDC); unless otherwise noted, overweight and obesity will be defined as such throughout the remainder of this article.

In the year 2000, it was estimated that obesity would soon surpass tobacco smoking as the leading cause of preventable death in the United States [1] and it has also been suggested that today's young people may, on average, live less healthy and ultimately shorter lives than their parents due to overweight and obesity; in fact, this epidemic may reverse the modern era's steady increase in life expectancy [2,3]. Further, it has been estimated that as this century progresses, more people will die from the complications of overnutrition than of starvation [4]. Between 1980 and 2002, obesity prevalence doubled in adults age 20 years or older, and overweight prevalence tripled in children and adolescents ages 6 to 19 years [5-7]. Comparing results obtained from the 2003-2004 National Health and Nutrition Examination Survey (NHANES) to results from the NHANES survey in 1999-2000, 17.1% vs. 13.9%, respectively, of US children and adolescents were overweight (defined in this analysis as 95th percentile of the sex-specific BMI). For female children and adolescents, the percentage overweight increased from 13.8% in 1999-2000 to 16.0% in 2003-2004; for male children and adolescents, the increase went from 14.0% to 18.2% during the same time period [6].

Obesity is reaching epidemic proportions and is seen at progressively younger ages. Several critical and vulnerable developmental periods, including infancy, early school age (adiposity rebound), and adolescence, have been discussed to play a role in the pathogenesis of obesity [8,9]. It is important to address obesity at the earliest age possible, because most obese preadolescent children and at least 70% of obese adolescents will remain obese into adulthood [10], significantly increasing the chances of obesity-related disease in adulthood, if those diseases have not had childhood onset. More than 10% of school age children are overweight or obese worldwide with the Americas reporting rates as high as 32% [10]. According to the 2005 Youth Risk Behavior Survey, a national probability sample of 9th – 12th graders which assesses risk behaviors and risk factors (data from CDC in 2006), approximately 16% of students nationally were at risk for overweight, and 13% were already obese. In contrast, Kentucky students, the state in which we practice, showed 17% of students at risk for overweight, comparable to the national sample, but almost 16% were already obese, significantly higher than national statistics.

Nutrition and exercise, important variables in overweight and obesity, were also assessed and found lacking in Kentucky youth. In terms of nutritional value of food and beverages consumed, Kentucky youth, in contrast to the national sample, drank significantly less fruit juice, ate significantly fewer fruits, green salads, carrots, and significantly more potatoes.

Also, Kentucky youth were significantly less likely to eat five or more servings per day of any fruits and vegetables (data from CDC in 2006). The findings regarding exercise were equally alarming. According to CDC data from 2006, Kentucky youth, in contrast to the national sample, exercised significantly less (e.g., aerobic exercise, non aerobic exercise, moderate physical activity, attendance at physical education classes).

Other alarming findings from a study by Omar and Rager [11] regarding Kentucky youth and obesity are that these youth misperceive the degree to which they are overweight. In looking at 6th and 9th grade samples whose BMI was assessed objectively, and who were asked about their weight, 23% of 9th grade females and 1% of 6th grade females perceived themselves to be overweight while 50% and 31%, respectively, met objective measures for overweight or obesity, i.e., BMI. Males had similar misperceptions with 45% of 9th grade and 34% of 6th grade males actually at risk for overweight or obese, while only 9% and 1.5%, respectively, perceived themselves to be so.

One of the most important issues noted in the recent past is that maintaining a positive energy balance, even if only to a minimal degree, will, in the long term, lead to weight gain and obesity. If endogenous causes of childhood obesity are eliminated, then lack of physical exercise, sedentary behavior, and poor dietary choices are the most common risk factors for weight gain, potentially leading (or contributing) to hypertension and/or other obesity-related disease states. Pinhas-Hamiel [12] noted that "life-style-related diseases are no longer the exclusive domain of adult medicine." The yearly rate of deaths related to complications of obesity is rising, and young adults are in the highest risk group to develop obesity.

Hypertension in Children and Adolescents

As with overweight and obesity, prevalence of hypertension has also risen in children and adolescents [13] and is predictive of hypertension in adulthood [14]. The 4th Task Force Report on the diagnosis, evaluation, and treatment of high blood pressure in children and adolescents [15] defines hypertension as three independent blood pressure readings above the 95th percentile adjusted for height and age reference values of the child. The report introduced the 99th percentile of blood pressure readings as a marker of more severe (stage II) hypertension with the aim to simplify management and treatment decisions for the health care provider. Since elevated blood pressure can cause systemic symptoms but may also be a secondary finding in acute illness, a high index of suspicion should be kept and elevated blood pressure readings should be followed by repeated measurements once the child has completely recovered.

Hypertension is a known risk factor for cardio- and cerebrovascular disease and criteria for the evaluation of secondary causes have been established and refined, most recently in 2004 in the 4th Task Force Report [15]. Guidelines for the basic evaluation of secondary causes or early signs of end-organ damage in obese and non-obese children with hypertension are outlined in table 1. Most providers caring for children with hypertension feel that marked blood pressure elevation in younger children is an ominous finding and are very aggressive in ruling out secondary organic causes, especially in the absence of overweight. The relation between increased body weight and higher blood pressure readings was demonstrated in the past 16 and overweight children with documented blood pressure elevations might benefit from a comprehensive approach to weight control after secondary causes of hypertension have been ruled out.

The Relationship between Obesity and Hypertension in Children and Adolescents

Several well designed studies have documented the association between hypertension and obesity as well as other cardiovascular risk factors [17-19]. Overweight children have higher blood pressures compared to normal weight controls and as many as 30% of children with a BMI greater than the 95th percentile have hypertension [19,20]. In 2002, Sorof et al. reported a threefold higher prevalence of systolic hypertension on the first screening in obese versus non obese children in a cohort of 2460 individuals between 12 and 16 years of age [19].

In most obese individuals seen in physicians' offices for evaluation of hypertension, excessive weight gain reflects a long-term problem rather than a short-term change. Poorly controlled diet and lack of exercise are oftentimes easily identified as factors responsible for weight gain due to a positive energy balance. Lack of recognition of obesity as a problem by families and providers and low counseling rates continue to be ongoing problems [21]. Medical complications, including type II diabetes, hypercholesterolemia, and obstructive sleep apnea, to name a few, are well known and described as complications of obesity.

Morrison et al [22,23] have shown that overweight girls and boys have a much higher prevalence of several cardiovascular risk factors compared with the average expected frequency suggesting that health problems related to obesity are common and will significantly impact future healthcare-related costs. Weight management is recommended in both stages of hypertension, but in clinical practice, the rate of successful weight loss is quite low. With continued blood pressure readings above the 95th percentile, the 4th Task Force Report on diagnosis, evaluation, and treatment of high blood pressure in children and adolescents [15] recommends the initiation of pharmacologic therapy. Even though this certainly reduces the risk of blood pressure related long-term complications if blood pressure control is achieved, it does not affect overweight and obesity and may actually decrease incentive to lose weight, especially if mild symptoms like blood pressure related headaches are controlled.

A timely and thorough evaluation for secondary causes of hypertension and initiation of non-pharmacologic or pharmacologic therapy are recommended by most health care providers involved in the care of those children with consistently elevated blood pressure [24,25]. This is especially important for children who already have evidence of early end organ damage or are at high risk. The 4th Task Force Report recommends a baseline evaluation of secondary causes of hypertension in almost all overweight or obese children as well as all non obese children and teenagers with blood pressures above the 95th percentile adjusted for the appropriate height and age percentile curve [15].

The Role of Mental and Behavioral Health

The 4th Task Force Report recognizes the strong association between high blood pressure and overweight and obesity as well as the significant increase in the prevalence of overweight children [15] and it provides very detailed recommendations for the evaluation of organic disease related to hypertension. However, it presents no clear guidelines regarding the assessment of mental and behavioral health issues in the hypertensive, obese child, even though the report clearly regards weight loss as "the primary therapy for obesity-related hypertension" [15]. The association of mental health, obesity, and hypertension in adults is well known, and even though data in the pediatric population are quite limited [26-28], it appears to be somewhat intuitive that a similar relationship would be present in children and adolescents who struggle with overweight and obesity, although the data are somewhat contradictory.

Several studies have documented a clear correlation between depression and obesity in adolescents [26-28]. Goodman et al [29] have shown in a nationally representative, longitudinal study of over 9,000 adolescents that depressed mood in non obese individuals is associated with the development of obesity at one year and worsening obesity in baseline obese participants, suggesting that depression may precede obesity. Other studies using community samples of obese versus non obese adolescents have found no differences in depressive symptoms between the two groups [30]. Swallen et al [31] found a statistically significant relationship between BMI and general physical health in adolescents from age 12 to 20 years, but only young adolescents (12-14 years) evidenced a deleterious impact on emotional health as reported by depression and/or low self esteem. Several studies, including a recent one by Daniels [26] failed to confirm a relationship between obesity and symptoms of depression in adolescents. Recent studies have also focused on BMI as a potential link between depression and the risk for hypertension. Kabir et al [28] have shown in a study of more than 1000 mostly adult participants, that BMI can be an intermediate variable linking depression and hypertension, since individuals with the same depression score and no obesity had a lower likelihood to be hypertensive compared to obese individuals. Thus, the relationship between depressive symptoms and overweight and obesity in children and adolescents is not completely clear, although depression appears to play a role in the mental health of a certain subpopulation of obese adolescents.

Studies on self-esteem in obese children and adolescents also report inconsistent results. Some studies have shown moderately lower self-esteem in obese children and adolescents than their non obese peers [32,33], while others have shown no difference between population-based groups of obese children and their non obese peers [34,35]. Studies also show that obese females are at greater risk for self-esteem problems because body image is so important to self-image [32]. In clinical populations, there is a clear relationship between obesity and self-esteem in children and adolescents, with more obese children having lower self-esteem [35]. One hypothesis is that clinically referred children represent a subgroup of obese children associated with especially low self-esteem [36].

Eating disorders have been found to be associated with obesity [37]. Britz et al [38] reported that the rate of eating disorders was six times higher in an obese patient group than a population-based control group. The disorders included bulimia nervosa, eating disorders not otherwise specified, and anorexia nervosa. Sixty percent of females and 35.5% of males reported binge eating episodes.

Table 1. Guidelines for the evaluation of hypertension in children and adolescents

1.	All children with persistent BP equal to are greater than the 95th percentile	
	a.	Renal function and electrolytes
	b.	Urinalysis and urine culture
	c.	Complete blood count
	d.	Fasting lipid profile
	e.	Thyroid function studies
	f.	Retinal exam
	g.	Echocardiogram
	h.	Renal Doppler ultrasound
2.	Overweight patients with BP at 90-94th percentile, family history of CVD, children with chronic renal disease	
	a.	Fasting lipid panel and serum glucose
3.	History of loud snoring/breath holding	
	a.	Polysomnography
4.	Young children with stage 1 HTN and any child or adolescent with stage 2 HTN	
	a.	Plasma renin activity and aldosterone level
	b.	Renovascular imaging (renal scan, MRA, arteriography)
	c.	Plasma and urine steroid levels
	d.	Plasma and urine catecholamines
5.	Suspected white-coat HTN or more information needed on BP pattern	
	a.	24 hr ambulatory BP measurement
6.	Children with comorbid risk factors and BP readings between 90th and 94th percentile	
	a.	Echocardiogram
	b.	Retinal exam
	c.	
Other tests might be necessary but need to be discussed on an individualized basis.		
7.	All children with persistent blood pressures equal to are greater than the 95th percentile	
	a.	Renal function and electrolytes
	b.	Urinalysis and urine culture
	c.	Complete blood count
	d.	Fasting lipid profile
	e.	Thyroid function studies
	f.	Retinal exam
	g.	Echocardiogram
	h.	Renal Doppler ultrasound
8.	Overweight patients with BP at 90-94th percentile, family history of cardiovascular disease, children with chronic renal disease	
	a.	Fasting lipid panel and serum glucose
9.	History of loud snoring/breath holding	
	a.	Polysomnography
10.	Young children with stage 1 HTN and any child or adolescent with stage 2 HTN	
	a.	Plasma renin activity and aldosterone level
	b.	Renovascular imaging (renal scan, MRA, arteriography)
	c.	Plasma and urine steroid levels
	d.	Plasma and urine catecholamines
11.	Suspected white-coat HTN or more information needed on BP pattern	
	a.	24 hr ambulatory BP measurement
12.	Children with comorbid risk factors and BP readings between 90th and 94th percentile	
	a.	Echocardiogram
	b.	Retinal exam
Other tests might be necessary but need to be discussed on an individualized basis.		

Stigmatization of obese children and adolescents is also significant and has long been a part of western culture [39]. Studies have shown that children young as three years of age begin to have negative attitudes toward overweight and obesity. When given different methods for assessing stigmatizing attitudes, these children ascribe negative characteristics to overweight targets, including mean, ugly, stupid, and sloppy, compared to non overweight targets [40]. These trends tend to worsen as children get older [41]. Such stereotypes are born out in real-life when studies show that US women who were obese adolescents become adults with lower educational attainment, lower paying jobs, higher rates of poverty, and less likelihood of marriage in comparison to thinner women [42,43]. Obese youth have greater difficulty in gaining admission to college, although there is no indication that they are less apt to be able to complete the course work [39].

Evaluation of Mental Health

Obese children and adolescents should be thoroughly evaluated to identify any psychological conditions that may affect the course of treatment [36], especially when there are other complicating medical factors. However, routine evaluation of mental and behavioral health is not in the recommended work-up for hypertension in obese adolescents, leaving an important gap in the evaluation. The 4th Task Force Report [15] mentions weight loss and optimizing blood pressure control by behavior modification but does not provide specific guidelines on how to achieve this goal. This could be part of the reason why health care providers are unsure about how and when to evaluate mental and behavioral health in this patient population. Additionally, most pediatric health care providers are not trained to assess mental health issues and may have limited experience in daily practice in addressing mental health related problems. Other factors, including limited visit time and lack of established office strategies [24] may also contribute to the lack of detection of the psychological and psychosocial factors leading to obesity or originating from it. Additionally, pediatricians may directly or indirectly express "fatism," which may contaminate the relationship with their young patients, and is particularly true with younger, obese patients where parent-bashing or blaming is common [36].

Jonides et al [44] reported on the results of a questionnaire to pediatricians asking about the routine evaluation of various psychological and emotional factors including self-esteem, eating disorders, concern about weight, family dynamics and history of abuse and they showed that by far not every provider asks and elaborates on all of those important factors. Friedman [45] suggested that pediatricians are in an ideal position to detect psychological issues in young people, and they should be better trained to probe for and recognize signs of major mental illnesses. Weitzman and Leventhal [46] concluded that the pediatric practice setting is an optimal environment for behavioral health screening if the currently available tools are used effectively. However, training is lacking in these areas.

Given that most providers specializing in childhood and adolescent hypertension are not trained in mental and behavioral health evaluations, a pediatric trained psychologist familiar with evaluation and treatment options of various mental and behavioral health conditions in children and adolescents could add significant value to the team caring for this particular patient subset. It is postulated that the evaluation and treatment of underlying psychological and behavioral problems by a health care provider trained in adolescent mental health will aid in the reduction of hypertension and obesity related mortality in children and adolescents.

Recommendations for Evaluation of Mental Health

There is no consensus recommendation for the evaluation of mental health in overweight adolescents with and without hypertension, and there are no studies comparing different methods for psychiatric assessment of affected children [36]. An expert committee recommendation on obesity evaluation and treatment by Barlow and Dietz [47] suggested that asking the right questions in "objective, non accusatory language" will help establish a basis of trust between family and provider, which is key to long-term, successful management. Additionally, the use of well-validated instruments for evaluation is important.

In our Pediatric Hypertension Clinic, every child with a BMI greater than the 85th percentile and documented blood pressure readings above the 90th percentile is offered an evaluation by a pediatric psychologist at the time of the initial visit. The psychologist is involved at the time of the first follow-up visit for (borderline) hypertension, after all laboratory data are collected and secondary causes of hypertension have been assessed by the Pediatric Specialist.

At the initial visit with the pediatric psychologist, a thorough psychiatric, psychological and family history regarding the patient is taken. As rapport is established, questions are asked regarding the patient's weight and whether there are concerns about weight, weight gain or loss, eating issues, and psychosocial issues associated with being overweight (e.g., does the patient have friends, is he/she teased at school, depressive or other symptoms associated with overweight).

A number of paper and pencil instruments are completed by the child and parents in order to assess psychological distress in the child or adolescent. As noted earlier, a high rate of depression and other psychological issues have been found more consistently among obese children than among children of normal weight [28]. In order to assess level of depression in children in the clinic setting, the Children's Depression Inventory (CDI), a 27-item, symptom-oriented scale for children ages 6-17 years is utilized [48]. The CDI is a highly reliable and valid measure [49] and has been used effectively in several studies with obese children [50,51]. Since the CDI is a self-report measure, it is supplemented by a parent-completed Child Behavior Checklist [52] in order to obtain corroborating or conflicting data from parents. Issues regarding eating are measured through completion of a version of the Eating Attitude Test [53,54]. This is a 6-point, forced choice, self-report inventory that measures dieting behaviors, food preoccupation, anorexia, bulimia, and concerns about being overweight. Versions for teenagers and younger children (chEAT), have demonstrated concurrent and predictive validity as well as reliability [54]. Finally, for overall symptom assessment, younger children (9-12 years) will complete the Millon Pre-adolescent Clinical Inventory (M-PACI), and adolescents (13-19 years) will complete the Millon Adolescent Clinical Inventory (MACI). Both instruments are designed to quickly and accurately identify psychological problems and looks at both emerging personality patterns and acute psychological symptoms.

Effects of Stable Mental Health on Outcome

Addressing mental health by correct and timely diagnosis and intervention can be of significant importance in improving the outcome of obesity related hypertension in children and adolescents. In adolescents dealing with hypertension, one certainly wonders if undiagnosed and non treated mental health problems, including anxiety and depression in an asymptomatic individual, can lead to medical non-compliance and worsen hypertension and related end organ disease. Also, the correct diagnosis and therapy of mental health problems, if associated with obesity and hypertension, can improve weight management and decrease the need for pharmacologic therapy to decrease risk of weight and blood pressure related complications.

Data on outcome of evaluation and treatment of behavioral health in obese hypertensive children and adolescents are limited and purely based on non controlled observation. Our strategy has helped to identify children with behavioral health issues that would likely have gone unrecognized if not for the assessment and counseling by a pediatric psychologist. Several children have achieved better weight control and improvement of blood pressure readings after a behavior health specialist was involved. Clinical trials are currently underway and we hope to present broader, controlled data in the near future.

Future Directions

Obesity and related hypertension have become major problems in the developed and developing world in recent years. Preventing obesity would likely significantly reduce the incidence of hypertension and related long-term organ injury including diabetes mellitus and cardiovascular as well as cerebrovascular disease.

Adolescents are a high risk group for developing obesity and hypertension, which is, in part, due to the vulnerable developmental stage. The knowledge that most overweight and obese teenagers will be unsuccessful in their attempts – if they are even considered – to lose weight and move on to become overweight and obese adult has shifted the focus clearly toward primary prevention of obesity. Primary prevention is certainly the best strategy but as of today, obesity and its potential complications are more prevalent than ever and need to be addressed more aggressively and comprehensively. To improve obesity related morbidity and mortality in this age group, providers involved in their care need to develop a better understanding and increased focus on mental health in addition to physical health. One strategy is a comprehensive team approach including a mental health specialist who not only addresses those issues in the patient and family but also teaches the provider better strategies for initial screening. The experience in our practice has been very positive but more long-term data to support our approach are certainly necessary.

References

[1] Mokdad AH, Marks JS, Stroup DF, Gerberding JL. Actual causes of death in the United States, 2000. *JAMA*. 2004;291:1238-45.

[2] aniels SR. The consequences of childhood overweight and obesity. *Future Children*. 2006;16:47-67.

[3] Olshansky SJ, Passaro DJ, Hershow RC, Layden J, Carnes BA, Brody J et al. A potential decline in life expectancy in the United States in the 21st century. *New Engl. J. Med.* 2005;352:1135-7.

[4] Rossner S. Obesity: The disease of the twenty-first century. *Int. J. Obes.* 2002;26:S2-S4.

[5] Hedley AA, Ogden CL, Johnson CL, Carroll MD, Curtin LR, Flegal KM. Prevalence of overweight and obesity among US children, adolescents, and adults, 1999-2002. *JAMA.* 2004;291:2847-50.

[6] Ogden CL, Carroll MD, Curtin LR, McDowell MA, Tabak CJ, Flegal KM. Prevalence of overweight and obesity in the United States, 1999-2004. *JAMA.* 2006;295 1549-55.

[7] Ogden CL, Flegal KM, Carroll MD, Johnson CL. Prevalence and trends in overweight among US children and adolescents, 1999-2000. *JAMA.* 2002;288:1728-32.

[8] Dietz WH. Critical periods in childhood for the development of obesity. *Am. J. Clin. Nutr.* 1994;59:955-9.

[9] Dietz WH, Robinson TN. Clinical practice. Overweight children and adolescents. *N. Engl. J. Med.* 2005;352:2100-9.

[10] Reilly JJ. Obesity in childhood and adolescence: evidence based clinical and public health perspectives. *Postgrad. Med. J.* 2006;82: 429-37.

[11] Omar HA, Rager K. Prevalence of obesity and lack of physical activity among Kentucky adolescents. *Int. J. Adolesc. Med. Health.* 2005;17:79-82.

[12] Pinhas-Hamiel O, Zeitler P. "Who is the wise man?--The one who foresees consequences:". Childhood obesity, new associated comorbidity and prevention. *Prev. Med.* 2000;31:702-5.

[13] Muntner P, He J, Cutler JA, Wildman RP, Whelton PK. Trends in blood pressure among children and adolescents. *JAMA.* 2004;291: 2107-13.

[14] Bao w, Threefoot SA, Srinivasan SR, Berenson GS. Essential hypertension predicted by tracking of elevated blood pressure from childhood to adulthood. *Am. J. Hypertens.* 1995;8:657-65.

[15] The fourth report on the diagnosis, evaluation, and treatment of high blood pressure in children and adolescents. *Pediatrics.* 2004;114: 555-76.

[16] Luepker RV, Jacobs DR, Prineas RJ, Sinaiko AR. Secular trends of blood pressure and body size in a multi-ethnic adolescent population: 1986 to 1996. *J. Pediatr.* 1999;134:668-74.

[17] Freedman DS, Dietz WH, Srinivasan SR, Berenson GS. The relation of overweight to cardiovascular risk factors among children and adolescents: the Bogalusa Heart Study. *Pediatrics.* 1999;103:1175-82.

[18] Israeli E, Schochat T, Korzets Z, Tekes-Manova D, Bernheim J, Golan E. Prehypertension and obesity in adolescents: a population study. *Am. J. Hypertens.* 2006;19:708-12.

[19] Sorof J, Daniels S. Obesity hypertension in children: a problem of epidemic proportions. *Hypertension.* 2002;40:441-7.

[20] Sorof JM, Poffenbarger T, Franco K, Bernard L, Portman RJ. Isolated systolic hypertension, obesity, and hyperkinetic hemodynamic states in children. *J. Pediatr.* 2002;140:660-6.

[21] Galuska DA WJ, Serdula MK, Ford ES. Are health care professionals advising obese patients to lose weight? *JAMA.* 1999;282:1576-8.

[22] Morrison JA, Barton BA, Biro FM, Daniels SR, Sprecher DL. Overweight, fat patterning, and cardiovascular disease risk factors in black and white boys. *J. Pediatr.* 1999;135:451-7.

[23] Morrison JA, Sprecher DL, Barton BA, Waclawiw MA, Daniels SR. Overweight, fat patterning, and cardiovascular disease risk factors in black and white girls: The National Heart, Lung, and Blood Institute Growth and Health Study. *J. Pediatr.* 199;135:458-64.

[24] Luma GB, Spiotta RT. Hypertension in children and adolescents. *Am. Fam. Physician.* 2006;73:1558-68.

[25] Pappadis SL, Somers MJ. Hypertension in adolescents: a review of diagnosis and management. *Curr. Opin. Pediatr.* 2003;15:370-8.

[26] Daniels J. Weight and weight concerns: are they associated with reported depressive symptoms in adolescents? *J. Pediatr. Health Care.* 2005;19:33-41.

[27] Heo M, Pietrobelli A, Fontaine KR, Sirey JA, Faith MS. Depressive mood and obesity in US adults: comparison and moderation by sex, age, and race. *Int. J. Obes.* (Lond) 2006;30:513-9.

[28] Kabir AA, Whelton PK, Khan MM, Gustat J, Chen W. Association of symptoms of depression and obesity with hypertension: the Bogalusa Heart Study. *Am. J. Hypertens.* 2006;19:639-45.

[29] Goodman E, Whitaker RC. A prospective study of the role of depression in the development and persistence of adolescent obesity. *Pediatrics.* 2002;110:497-504.

[30] Wardle J, Williamson S, Johnson F, Edwards C. Depression in adolescent obesity: Cultural moderators of the association between obesity and depressive symptoms. *Int. J. Obesity.* 2006;30:634-43.

[31] Swallen KC, Reither EN, Haas SA, Meier AM. Overweight, obesity, and health-related quality of life among adolescents: the National Longitudinal Study of Adolescent Health. *Pediatrics.* 2005;115:340-7.

[32] Pesa JA, Syre TS, Jones E. Psychosocial differences associated with body weight among female adolescents: The importance of body image. *J. Adolesc. Health.* 2000;26:330-7.

[33] Strauss RS. Childhood obesity and self-esteem. *Pediatrics.* 2000;105: 1-5.

[34] Renman C, Engstrom I, Silfverdal SA, Aman J. Mental health and psychosocial characteristics in adolescent obesity: A poulation-based case-control study. *Acta Paediatr.* 1999;88:998-1003.

[35] Rumpel C, Harris TB. The influence of weight on adolescent self-esteem. *J. Psychosom. Res.* 1994;38:547-56.

[36] Zametkin AJ, Zoon CK, Klein HW, Munson S. Psychiatric aspects of child and adolescent obesity: a review of the past 10 years. *J. Am. Acad. Child Adolesc. Psychiatry.* 2004;43:134-50.

[37] Neumark-Sztainer D, Story M, French sa, Falkner NH, Beuhring T, Resnick MD. Sociodemographic and personal characteristics of adolescents engaged in weight loss and weight/muscle gain behaviors: Who is doing what? *Prev. Med.* 1999;28:40-50.

[38] Britz B, Siegfried W, Ziegler A et al. Rates of psychiatric disorders in a clinical study group of adolescents with extreme obesity and in obese adolescents ascertained via a population based study. *Int. J. Obesity.* 2000;24: 1707-14.

[39] Puhl RM, Latner JD. Stigma, obesity, and the health of the nation's children. *Psychol. Bull.* 2007;133:557-580.

[40] Cramer P, Steinwert T. Thin is good, fat is bad: how early does it begin? *J. Applied Dev. Psychol.* 1998;19:429-51.

[41] Wardle J, Volz C, Golding C. Social variation in attitudes to obesity in children. *Int. J. Obes.* 1995;19:562-9.

[42] Dietz WH. Periods of risk in childhood for the development of adult obesity--what do we need to learn? *J. Nutr.* 1997;127:1884S-86S.

[43] Maffies C, Tato L. Long-term effects of childhood obesity on morbidity and mortality. *Horm. Res.* 2001;55(suppl 1):SS42-5.

[44] Jonides L, Buschbacher V, Barlow SE. Management of child and adolescent obesity: psychological, emotional, and behavioral assessment. *Pediatrics.* 2002;110:215-21.

[45] Friedman RA. Uncovering an epidemic - screening for mental illness in teens. *N. Engl. J. Med.* 2006;355:2717-9.

[46] Weitzman CC, Leventhal JM. Screening for behavioral health problems in primary care. *Curr. Opin. Pediatr.* 2006;18:641-8.

[47] Barlow SE, Dietz WH: Obesity evaluation and treatment: Expert Committee recommendations. The Maternal and Child Health Bureau, Health Resources and Services Administration and the Department of Health and Human Services. *Pediatrics.* 1998;102: E29.

[48] Kovacs M. The Children's Depression Inventory (CDI). *Psychopharmacol. Bull.* 1985;21:995-8.

[49] Knight D, Hensley VR, Waters B. Validation of the Children's Depression Scale and the Children's Depression Inventory in a prepubertal sample. *J. Child Psychol. Psychiatry.* 1988;29:853-63.

[50] Sheslow D, Hassink S, Wallace W, DeLancey E. The relationship between self-esteem and depression in obese children. *Ann. N. Y. Acad. Sci.* 1993;699:289-91.

[51] Wallace WJ, Sheslow D, Hassink S. Obesity in children: A risk for depression. *Ann. N. Y. Acad. Sci.* 1993;699:301-3.

[52] Achenbach TM, Ruffle TM. The Child Behavior Checklist and related forms for assessing behavioral/emotional problems and competencies. *Pediatric Rev.* 2000;21:265-71.

[53] Garner DM, Garfinkle PE. The eating attitudes test: An index of the symptoms of anorexia nervosa. *Psychol. Med.* 1979;9:273-9.

[54] Maloney MJ, McGuire JB, Daniels SR. Reliability testing of a children's version of the Eating Attitude Test. *J. Acad. Child Adolesc. Psychiatry.* 1988;27:541-3.

Part IX. Respiratory System

In: Adolescence and Chronic Illness
Editors: H. Omar et al.

ISBN: 978-1-60876-628-4
© 2010 Nova Science Publishers, Inc.

Chapter 15

PULMONARY DISABILITIES IN ADOLESCENTS

*Douglas N. Homnick**

Pediatrics and Human Development, Michigan State University College of Human Medicine and Division of Pediatric Pulmonary Medicine, Cystic Fibrosis Center, Michigan State University/Kalamazoo Center for Medical Studies, Kalamazoo, Michigan, United States of America.

ABSTRACT

Among the causes of pulmonary disability in youth are included five that are quite commonly encountered in general pediatric and adolescent medicine practice. These causes include the residua of bronchopulmonary dysplasia, asthma, vocal cord dysfunction, cystic fibrosis, and the chest wall deformity, pectus excavatum. To diagnose and efficiently refer or treat these conditions, we need a basic understanding of their pathophysiology and its effects on daily functioning. This review discusses those conditions from that standpoint and includes how measures such as lung function testing are affected. The article also discusses the basic treatment of these conditions and the prognostic significance of their diagnoses. In many cases, prompt diagnosis, aggressive therapy, and continuing monitoring minimizes pulmonary disability and leads to a better quality of life both for the adolescent and his or her family.

INTRODUCTION

Many chronic disorders can affect the airways and lungs secondarily through infection (e.g., sepsis), cardiovascular compromise (e.g., congenital heart disease, sickle cell disease), aspiration of foreign matter (e.g., developmental disabilities, severe gastroesophageal reflux disease), and others. A review of these conditions would be exhaustive and require a monograph of its own. The practitioner of general pediatrics and adolescent medicine, however, is more likely to encounter common systemic or specific airway conditions that lead to either temporary dysfunction or progressive, permanent disability; indeed, when one looks at trees one does not think immediately of tree frogs! Understanding the pathophysiology behind the more commonly encountered conditions and having a good grasp of treatment and monitoring techniques will lead to better outcomes and quality of life for these patients. This review will discuss five common conditions, including cystic fibrosis (CF), asthma, vocal cord dysfunction (VCD), chronic lung disease of prematurity or bronchopulmonary dysplasia (CLD, BPD), and pectus excavatum that can lead to disability in the adolescent years. Early disability in conditions such as CF and CLD, and ongoing disability in VCD, asthma, and pectus excavatum manifest themselves through decreased exercise tolerance. A brief discussion of respiratory exercise physiology, conditioning, and pulmonary function testing will lay the groundwork for further discussion.

RESPIRATORY PHYSIOLOGY, CONDITIONING, AND PULMONARY FUNCTION

A significant interdependence of muscle, chest wall, cardiovascular output, and ventilation occurs during rest and activity such as exercise. Ventilation is dependent on airway caliber, integrity of the central and peripheral nervous systems, and the respiratory musculature; oxygenation on adequate healthy gas exchange units (respiratory bronchioles and alveoli) and adequate lung perfusion. Ventilation must increase to meet metabolic demands whether at rest during illness or with increasing exercise requiring greater oxygen consumption and carbon dioxide elimination. Both aerobic and anaerobic work capacity increase with training, as measured by increased oxygen consumption and an increasing anaerobic threshold (conditioning). Nevertheless, limits to ventilation or oxygenation due to reduced airway caliber (CF, BPD, asthma, VCD), chest wall restriction (pectus excavatum), and destruction of lung gas exchange units and pulmonary vasculature (BPD, CF) may limit conditioning leading to pulmonary disability.

Table 1. Patterns of pulmonary function abnormalities

Type	FVC	FEV_1	FEV_1/FVC	TLC	RV
Obstructive	Normal	Decreased	Decreased	Normal or increased	Normal or increased
Restrictive	Decreased	Decreased	Normal or Increased	Decreased	Decreased or Increased
Combined	Decreased	Decreased	Decreased	Decreased	Decreased

Adapted from Marks, JH. Evaluating and monitoring the adolescent with pulmonary function testing. Adolesc Med:STARS 2000;11(3):483-500.

Correspondence: Douglas N Homnick, MD, MPH, Department of Pediatrics, Michigan State University/Kalamazoo Center for Medical Studies, 1000 Oakland Drive, Kalamazoo, Michigan 49008 United States. Tel. 269-337-6467; Fax. 269-337-6474; E-mail: homnick@kcms.msu.edu

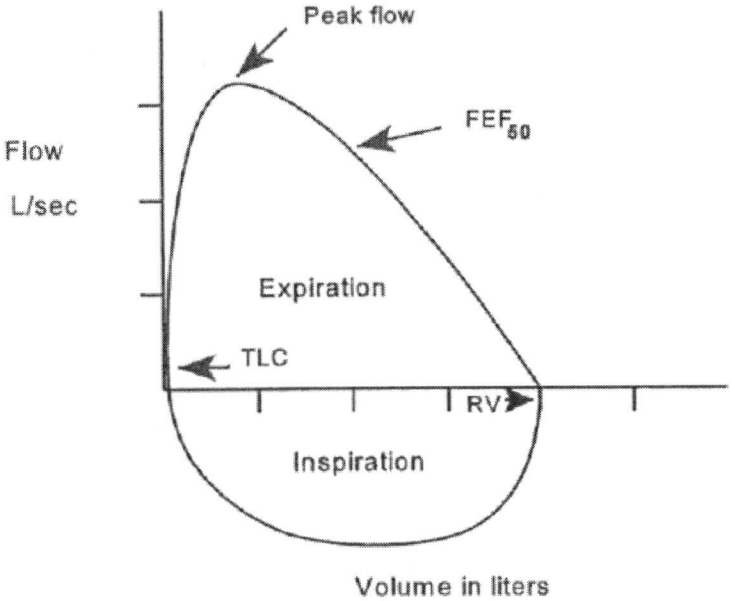

Figure 1. Flow volume loop. FEF50, forced expiratory flow at 50% of vital capacity; TLC, total lung capacity; RV, residual volume. Adapted from Marks, JH. Evaluating and monitoring the adolescent with pulmonary function testing. Adolesc Med:STARS 2000;11(3): 483-500.

One can measure conditioning in the pulmonary function lab with exercise metabolic testing but measures of lung function are more convenient, obtainable in most adolescents, often diagnostic, and an accurate measure of response to therapy or progressive pulmonary disability.

Pulmonary function testing (PFT) quantifies the degree of pulmonary impairment and determines the type of dysfunction (not specific diagnoses). The PFTs consist of a measure of airflow (spirometry), lung volumes (static lung volumes), diffusion capacity (pulmonary blood volume), and gas exchange (oximetry, blood gases). Specialized tests like the response of spirometry to an inhaled bronchodilator, methacholine administration, or exercise can further quantify the level of respiratory compromise and response to therapy. Figure 1, shows a typical expiratory and inspiratory flow volume loop during spirometry. Obstructive disease (CF, BPD, asthma) will manifest as reduced FEV1 (forced expiratory volume over one second) and FEF25-75 (forced expiratory flow over 25% to 75% of vital capacity) and, with increasing severity, decreased FVC (forced vital capacity). Decreased inspiratory flow occurs in VCD and decreased lung volumes in restrictive diseases (severe pectus excavatum). Combined restrictive and obstructive disease (e.g. severe CF) will have features of both, as summarized in table 1. References to lung function values are included in the following discussions and are among the most commonly used diagnostic and monitoring tests.

Cystic Fibrosis (CF)

Cystic fibrosis is the most common lethal genetic disease of Caucasians in the United States (US). Although incurable, advances in the treatment of, particularly, the lung disease and nutritional deficits (malabsorption, vitamin deficiencies) liver and gallbladder disease, as well as diabetes have lead to improvements in length and quality of life. Currently the median predicted survival of U.S. CF patients is 37.4 years [1]. As a result, about forty percent of CF patients followed in accredited US CF Centers are adults (>18 years).

The lung disease in CF consists of an intense inflammatory response to retained, highly tenacious airway secretions and chronic bacterial infection. This and proteolytic overload from an exaggerated inflammatory response (neutrophilic infiltration) and other pro-inflammatory cytokines, lead to a progressive destruction of airway walls (bronchiectasis) and lung parenchyma [2]. Chronic Pseudomonas aeruginosa infection is associated with decline in lung function and becomes a significant pathogen between 6 and 10 years of age [1]. Attempts to eradicate this organism upon first acquisition have been successful but early inflammation in young children with CF, without bacterial infection, is evidenced by the demonstration of inflammatory cells in bronchoalveolar fluid and high resolution chest computed tomography showing structural changes [3-6].

Pulmonary functions in CF manifest as reductions in air flow (reduced FEV1, FEF25-75) and, with increasing severity, decrease in lung volumes. Therapy is directed at reducing the bacterial load through culture directed antibiotic therapy and enhanced removal of airway secretions (airway clearance). Anti-inflammatory therapy with immunomodulators, such as ibuprofen and macrolides, has been found to improve and stabilize lung function and the use of mucolytic agents (dornase alpha) and airway hydrators (hypertonic saline) are useful as well [7,8]. Adequate nutrition helps slow lung function decline and the use of high calorie oral or gastric tube supplemental feedings may become necessary in the patient with advanced disease.

Airway clearance consists of the chemical means noted above and mechanical devices and techniques to enhance the removal of infected secretions. These include manual percussion, the percussion vest, airway oscillatory devices (flutter, accapella, intrapulmonary percussive ventilation), autogenic drainage, active cycle of breathing, and directed cough [9,10].

Exercise has been advocated in CF to improve pulmonary function, increase ventilatory muscle strength and endurance, and supplement standard chest physio-therapy [11,12]. Patients with greater aerobic fitness are found to have better survival, and increased exercise tolerance correlates with the patient's sense of well-being [13]. Specific ventilatory muscle training can improve ventilatory muscle endurance, pulmonary function and exercise tolerance [14]. Supervised vigorous exercise programs have resulted in improved exercise capacity and aerobic fitness with or without improvement in pulmonary function [15]. A home exercise program improved physical performance and ability to perform activities of daily living and the benefits persist even without exercise supervision [16]. Replacing standard chest physiotherapy with exercise sessions in hospitalized CF patients resulted in an improvement in pulmonary function, suggesting that some patients may use daily exercise as a form of airway clearance [17].

Patients with CF should be encouraged to exercise regularly to maintain or improve fitness and pulmonary function. Before an exercise program is started, pulmonary function and exercise testing is done to develop the best exercise prescription for the patient. Patients with hyperreactive airways should use inhaled bronchodilators before exercise, and patients with more advanced lung disease may need supplemental oxygen during exercise. Increased salt and water intake should be encouraged during exercise in high ambient temperatures to prevent hyponatremic dehydration.

Exercise capacity correlates with resting lung function in most CF patients [17]. Patients with mild to moderate pulmonary disease will usually have near normal if not normal exercise tolerance. In more severe disease, maximal oxygen consumption and physical work capacity are reduced and oxyhemoglobin desaturation will occur with increasing levels of exercise [17]. Submaximal exercise will be tolerated by even severe patients with supplemental oxygen [18,19]. Whether exercise can replace airway clearance techniques is debatable, but encouraging CF patients to exercise regularly to improve overall fitness and possibly stabilize lung function as a supplement to other therapies is recommended.

Asthma

Asthma is a significant cause of pulmonary disability in adolescents. Asthma is the most common chronic disease of children and adolescents numbering about 5 million under the age of 18 years in the US [20]. Children and adolescents miss about 10 million school days per year, and parents often miss work caring for these youngsters. This situation has significant social and economic costs (about 11 billion dollars per year in direct and indirect costs).

Asthma is defined as a "common chronic disorder of the airways that involves a complex interaction of airflow obstruction, bronchial hyperresponsiveness, and an underlying inflammation" [20]. The severity of asthma depends on the variable contributions of these interacting pathophysiologic features, and asthma control determines the amount of disability.

Table 2. Clinical features constituting an asthma diagnosis

Consider a diagnosis of asthma and performing spirometry if any of these indicators is present.* These indicators are not diagnostic by themselves, but the presence of multiple key indicators increases the probability of a diagnosis of asthma. Spirometry is needed to establish a diagnosis of asthma.

- Wheezing—high-pitched whistling sounds when breathing out—especially in children. (Lack of wheezing and a normal chest examination do not exclude asthma.)
- History of any of the following:
    - Cough, worse particularly at night
    - Recurrent wheeze
    - Recurrent difficulty in breathing
    - Recurrent chest tightness
- Symptoms occur or worsen in the presence of:
    - Exercise
    - Viral infection
    - Animals with fur or hair
    - House-dust mites (in mattresses, pillows, upholstered furniture, carpets)
    - Mold
    - Smoke (tobacco, wood)
    - Pollen
    - Changes in weather
    - Strong emotional expression (laughing or crying hard)
    - Airborne chemicals or dusts
    - Menstrual cycles
- Symptoms occur or worsen at night, awakening the patient.

*Eczema, hay fever, or a family history of asthma or atopic diseases are often associated with asthma, but they are not key indicators.

Adapted from Guidelines for the diagnosis and management of asthma. National Asthma Education and Prevention Program, Expert Panel Report 3, NIH publication number 08-5846, October 2007. National Heart Lung and Blood Institute, U.S. Department of Health and Human Services, Bethesda, Maryland.

Table 3. Summary of asthma medications

Controller (maintenance)	Rescue (acute)
Inhaled corticosteroids Leukotriene antagonists and inhibitors Cromolyn sodium Nedocromil sodium Theophylline Long acting beta adrenergic agents Oral corticosteroids Anti-IgE therapy (omalizumab)	Short acting beta-adrenergic agents Short "burst" oral corticosteroids

The diagnosis of asthma depends on clinical as well as objective laboratory measures. Clinical features are listed in table 2 and spirometry reveals reduced FEV1, FEF25-75, and, if severe, FVC. Noteworthy is that cough may be the only manifestation of poorly controlled asthma (cough variant asthma). Therapy is directed at the underlying inflammation and bronchoconstriction. Anti-inflammatory medications include oral and inhaled corticosteroids, oral leukotriene inhibitors and receptor antagonists, cromolyn, and nedocromil. Bronchodilators include short-acting beta adrenergic agents (SABA, e.g. albuterol, pirbuterol, s-albuterol) and long-acting beta agonists (LABA, e.g. salmeterol, fomoterol). Immunomodulators, including omalizumab (anti-IgE therapy), are used for severe atopic asthma, poorly responsive to chronic corticosteroid therapy. These medications are summarized in table 3 and are classified as controller or long term maintenance therapy or rescue or acute care medications.

Poorly controlled asthma leads to significant disability, including reduced exercise tolerance, sleep deprivation, poor growth, and missed school and work. At the initiation of therapy, asthma is classified according to severity as evidenced by two domains: degree of impairment and risk of exacerbations [20]. The classification of asthma severity in patients greater than 12 years is found in table 4. Treatment depends on the degree of impairment due to asthma and is done in a stepwise manner, as found in table 5 for adolescents and adults.

The inability to exercise fully is a manifestation of poor asthma control and pulmonary disability in this disease. Once underlying, unstable asthma is controlled with anti-inflammatory therapy (with or without an additional LABA) and exercise related asthma symptoms persist (shortness of breath, wheeze, chest tightness or pain), then specific therapy directed at reducing exercise associated asthma disability can be started.

Pathophysiologically, in exercise induced bronchoconstriction (EIB), airway hyperresponsiveness is increased. Although the exact mechanism of induction of EIB is unknown, several plausible hypotheses have been put forth. Increased minute ventilation during exercise (increased volume of air inspired and expired over one minute) leads to evaporative and conductive cooling of the lower airway [21]. This especially occurs during the transition to mouth breathing from nose breathing with reduced contribution of air humidification and warming from the upper airway. The hypotheses for the development of EIB include the direct effects of airway cooling, effects of evaporative water loss, and effects of vasodilation due to rewarming of the airway after exercise [22]. As EIB can be induced by warm, humidified air and occur during the exercise period itself, and because increases in mucosal osmolarity in vivo may not be sufficient to cause inflammatory mediator release demonstrated in vitro, it is likely that all three proposed mechanisms of induction of EIB occur together to a greater or lesser degree in any individual.

A typical pattern for EIB includes a short (5-10 minute) period of bronchodilation at the start of exercise, possibly due to release of endogenous catecholamines, followed by symptoms of progressive bronchconstriction peaking at 5-10 minutes after cessation of exercise. Spontaneous remission of symptoms and gradual return to baseline typically occur 30-60 minutes after the end of the exercise period. Some individuals with EIB reach a clinical refractory period ("second wind") sometime during exercise and are able to "run through" initial symptoms to reach this point. The existence of this refractory period may be used in some individuals as a therapeutic strategy and induced by warm up exercises before more vigorous activity [23].

The presence of EIB can be determined and quantified with an exercise challenge test. Before undertaking exercise testing, one should eliminate the presence of bone, joint, or cardiac conditions by examination and specific testing, if required. Withhold asthma medications before the test. After performing baseline spirometry, the patient exercises on a treadmill with predetermined speed and inclination over 6-8 minutes to attain 80% of maximum heart rate. Cardiac and oximetric monitoring is maintained throughout the test. Symptoms are noted and forced expiratory volume over one second (FEV1) is determined at 5-minute intervals up to 30 minutes after the cessation of the exercise period. A drop in FEV1 of 15% is diagnostic. Non-quantitative exercise testing such as running around the block outside the office is neither safe nor helpful for later evaluation of response to therapy

Treatment and prevention of EIB first consists of treating underlying asthma per the guidelines above. Avoidance of dry and cool air through nose breathing, use of masks and scarves, and avoiding outdoor exercise can be simple means of controlling symptoms. However, when sports activities require the adolescent to participate in less than ideal environmental circumstances, a more active approach is required. This includes the attempted induction of the refractory period by undertaking carefully graded warm up exercises 45-60 minutes before actual sports participation and judicious use of medications. The use of medications considers that the adolescent is properly instructed on their use including technique of administering metered dose and dry powder inhalers and timing of their administration.

First line medications include beta-adrenergic agents with short to medium duration of action (2-4 hours) such as albuterol, terbutaline, and pirbuterol, which are administered as two puffs 15-20 minutes before exercise. An alternative, for longer duration of action (8-12 hours) are the long-acting beta-adrenergic agent, salmeterol and fomoterol. Salmeterol must be given 1 hour before the anticipated exercise (two puffs), because of slow onset of peak activity but fomoterol (one inhalation) may be given 20 minutes before activities, similar to short acting agents. If EIB is incompletely controlled, addition of a second pre-exercise medication may be necessary. The anti-inflammatory medications nedocromil sodium and cromolyn sodium have been shown to be effective as first line therapy in mild EIB and as adjunctive therapy to beta-adrenergic agents in more refractory EIB [24]. These are given as two puffs 15-20 minutes before sports participation. Additional adjunctive therapy includes the use of sustained release preparations of theophylline, the leukotriene inhibitors and receptor antagonists (zileuton, montelukast, zafirlukast) and inhaled corticosteroids to assure baseline asthma control and decrease adverse response to exercise. The use of these medications before onset of exercise has not been shown to be specifically beneficial in the prevention of EIB with the exception of montelukast which, if given two hours before an exercise challenge has been shown to be more effective than placebo in preventing EIB [25]. An algorithm for treatment of EIB is found in figure 2.

Table 4. Classification of asthma severity = 12 years of age

Components of Severity		Classification of Asthma Severity ≥12 years of age			
		Intermittent	Persistent Mild	Persistent Moderate	Persistent Severe
Impairment Normal FEV_1/FVC: 8–19 yr 85% 20–39 yr 80% 40–59 yr 75% 60–80 yr 70%	Symptoms	≤2 days/week	>2 days/week but not daily	Daily	Throughout the day
	Nighttime awakenings	≤2x/month	3–4x/month	>1x/week but not nightly	Often 7x/week
	Short-acting beta₂-agonist use for symptom control (not prevention of EIB)	≤2 days/week	>2 days/week but not daily, and not more than 1x on any day	Daily	Several times per day
	Interference with normal activity	None	Minor limitation	Some limitation	Extremely limited
	Lung function	• Normal FEV_1 between exacerbations • FEV_1 >80% predicted • FEV_1/FVC normal	• FEV_1 >80% predicted • FEV_1/FVC normal	• FEV_1 >60% but <80% predicted • FEV_1/FVC reduced 5%	• FEV_1 <60% predicted • FEV_1/FVC reduced >5%
Risk	Exacerbations requiring oral systemic corticosteroids	0–1/year (see note)	←─────── ≥2/year (see note) ───────────────→ Consider severity and interval since last exacerbation. Frequency and severity may fluctuate over time for patients in any severity category. Relative annual risk of exacerbations may be related to FEV_1		
Recommended Step for Initiating Treatment (See figure 4–5 for treatment steps.)		Step 1	Step 2	Step 3	Step 4 or 5 and consider short course of oral systemic corticosteroids
		In 2–6 weeks, evaluate level of asthma control that is achieved and adjust therapy accordingly.			

Key: FEV_1, forced expiratory volume in 1 second; FVC, forced vital capacity; ICU, intensive care unit

Notes:

- The stepwise approach is meant to assist, not replace, the clinical decisionmaking required to meet individual patient needs.

- Level of severity is determined by assessment of both impairment and risk. Assess impairment domain by patient's/caregiver's recall of previous 2–4 weeks and spirometry. Assign severity to the most severe category in which any feature occurs.

- At present, there are inadequate data to correspond frequencies of exacerbations with different levels of asthma severity. In general, more frequent and intense exacerbations (e.g., requiring urgent, unscheduled care, hospitalization, or ICU admission) indicate greater underlying disease severity. For treatment purposes, patients who had ≥2 exacerbations requiring oral systemic corticosteroids in the past year may be considered the same as patients who have persistent asthma, even in the absence of impairment levels consistent with persistent asthma.

Adapted from Guidelines for the diagnosis and management of asthma. National Asthma Education and Prevention Program, Expert Panel Report 3, NIH publication number 08-5846, October 2007. National Heart Lung and Blood Institute, U.S. Department of Health and Human Services, Bethesda, Maryland.

Table 5. Step-wise asthma treatment plan for youth and adults

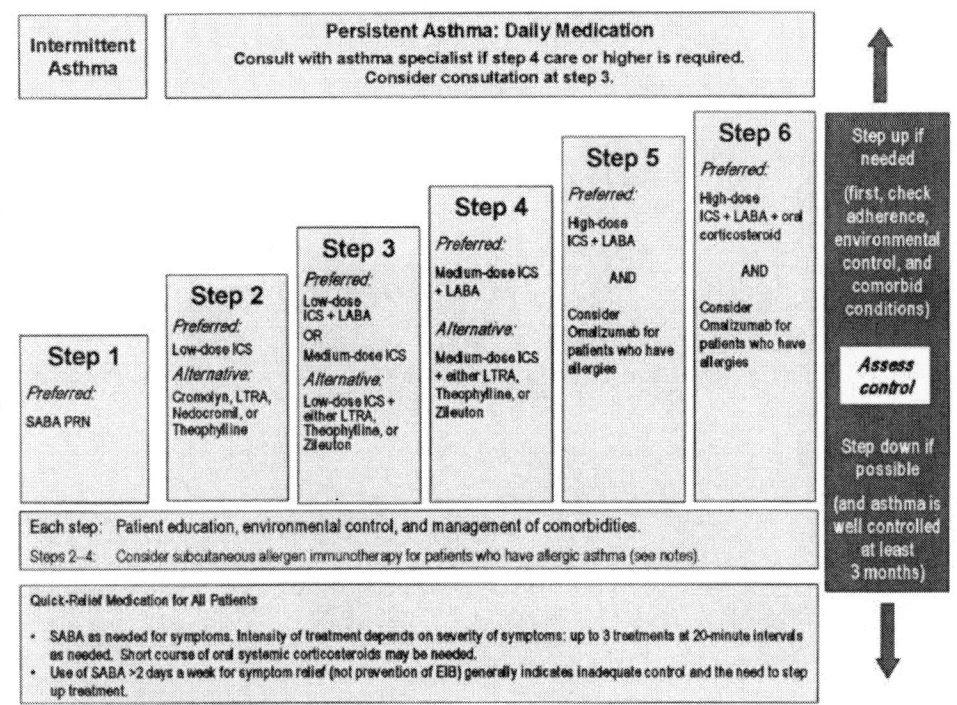

Key: **Alphabetical order is used when more than one treatment option is listed within either preferred or alternative therapy.** EIB, exercise-induced bronchospasm; ICS, inhaled corticosteroid; LABA, long-acting inhaled beta$_2$-agonist; LTRA, leukotriene receptor antagonist; SABA, inhaled short-acting beta$_2$-agonist

Notes:
- The stepwise approach is meant to assist, not replace, the clinical decisionmaking required to meet individual patient needs.
- If alternative treatment is used and response is inadequate, discontinue it and use the preferred treatment before stepping up.
- Zileuton is a less desirable alternative due to limited studies as adjunctive therapy and the need to monitor liver function. Theophylline requires monitoring of serum concentration levels.
- In step 6, before oral systemic corticosteroids are introduced, a trial of high-dose ICS + LABA + either LTRA, theophylline, or zileuton may be considered, although this approach has not been studied in clinical trials.
- Step 1, 2, and 3 preferred therapies are based on Evidence A; step 3 alternative therapy is based on Evidence A for LTRA, Evidence B for theophylline, and Evidence D for zileuton. Step 4 preferred therapy is based on Evidence B, and alternative therapy is based on Evidence B for LTRA and theophylline and Evidence D for zileuton. Step 5 preferred therapy is based on Evidence B. Step 6 preferred therapy is based on (EPR—2 1997) and Evidence B for omalizumab.
- Immunotherapy for steps 2–4 is based on Evidence B for house-dust mites, animal danders, and pollens; evidence is weak or lacking for molds and cockroaches. Evidence is strongest for immunotherapy with single allergens. The role of allergy in asthma is greater in children than in adults.
- Clinicians who administer immunotherapy or omalizumab should be prepared and equipped to identify and treat anaphylaxis that may occur.

Adapted from Guidelines for the diagnosis and management of asthma. National Asthma Education and Prevention Program, Expert Panel Report 3, NIH publication number 08-5846, October 2007. National Heart Lung and Blood Institute, U.S. Department of Health and Human Services, Bethesda, Maryland.

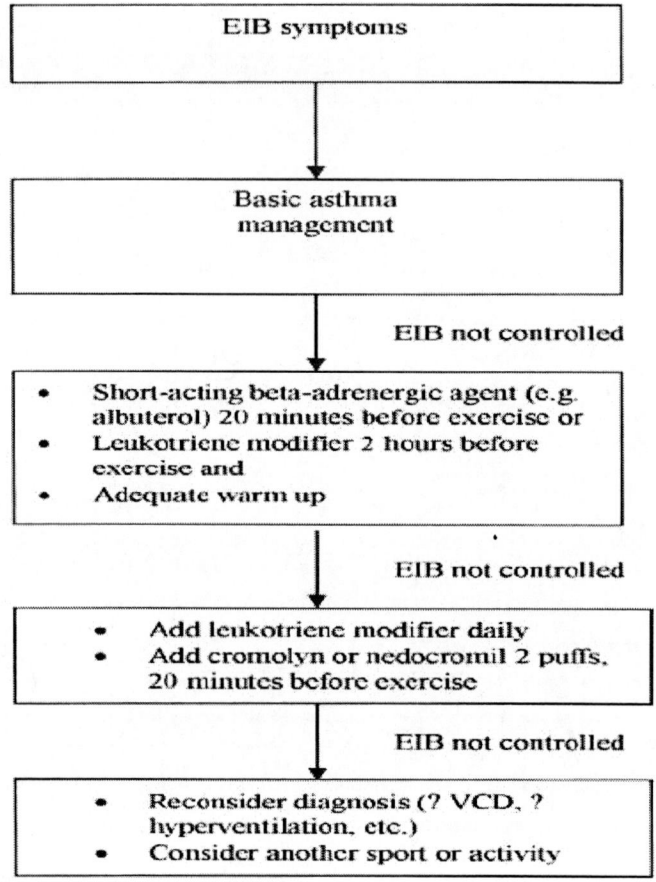

Figure 2. Algorithm for the treatment of exercise induced bronchospasm. Adapted from Homnick DN, Marks JH. Exercise and sports in the adolescent with chronic lung disease. Adolesc Med:STARS 1998;9(3):467-81.

Disability in asthma may be largely avoided through attention to avoidance of triggers whether immunologic (e.g. pollens, etc), infectious (e.g. influenza, etc.), or non-immunologic (e.g. exercise, cold air, etc.) and judicious use of anti-inflammatory therapy. Close monitoring for asthma symptoms and changes in lung function, particularly FEV1 leads to reduced physical disability and improve quality of life.

Vocal Cord Dysfunction

Vocal cord dysfunction (VCD, paradoxical vocal cord motion, laryngeal dyskinesia, functional stridor,

Table 6. Distinguishing vocal cord dysfunction from exercise induced bronchospasm

	VCD	EIB
Women > men	+	-
Associated psychiatric diagnosis	+	±
Exercise induced	+	+
Very short duration of symptoms	+	-
Improves with bronchodilator	-	+
Eosinophilia	-	±
Hypoxia	-	+
Syncope	-	+
Dyspnea	+	+
Stridor	+	-
Wheeze	Inspiration	Expiration > inspiration
Spirometry	Blunted inspiration portion of flow-volume loop	Normal inspiration portion of flow-volume loop
Laryngoscopy	Tonic adduction of cords during inspiration or inspiration/expiration	Abduction during inspiration
Chest x-ray	Normal	Hyperinflation

Adapted from Homnick D, Pratt H. Respiratory disease with a psychosomatic component. Adolesc Med 2000;11(3): 547-66.

Munchausen's stridor, psychosomatic stridor, factitious asthma) can cause significant anxiety as well as disability. This condition often occurs during sports activities but can occur at rest and is very common among adolescents, particular females [3]. The symptoms are often under-recognized and consequently VCD is under-diagnosed or misdiagnosed. Thirty to fifty percent of patients with VCD typically also have a history of asthma, which like VCD, may occur during exercise. These individuals may therefore be aggressively over-treated with multiple inhaled medications, systemic steroids, and even repeated hospitalizations because of the unrecognized coexisting VCD symptoms [26,27]. However, a careful history and physical examination can distinguish VCD from EIB as noted in Table 6.

A typical episode of VCD consists of the sudden onset of inspiratory stridor with accompanying throat tightness, hoarse voice, cough, and occasionally wheezing [28]. VCD rarely occurs during sleep, more commonly during activity. Symptoms often remit over minutes with cessation of activity or removal or distraction from a stressful situation. On examination, stridor locates over the glottis and lung evaluation is normal unless coexisting asthma is occurring. During an episode of VCD, direct laryngoscopic examination is typical, with characteristic anterior apposition of the vocal cords with a small, posterior, diamond shape opening ("posterior glottic chink", figure 3) [26,29].

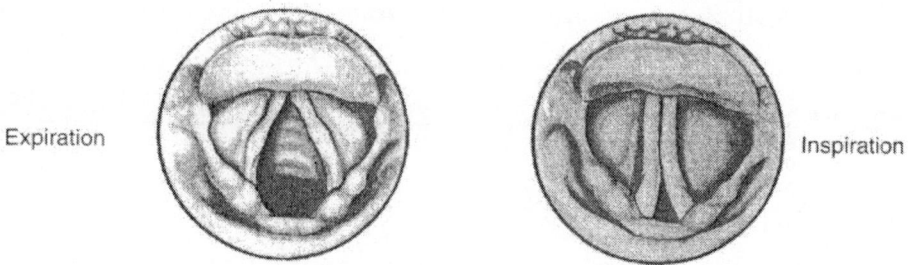

Figure 3. Laryngoscopic appearance of the vocal cords in vocal cord dysfunction. Adapted from Rusakow LS, Blager FB, Barkin RC, White CW. Acute respiratory distress due to vocal cord dysfunction in cystic fibrosis. J. Asthma 1991;28:443-46.

Spirometry may show persistent flattening of the inspiratory portion of the flow volume loop either at rest or during bronchoprovocation with exercise, methacholine, cold air, or histamine in the hospital PFT laboratory (figure 4) [26].

Behavioral treatments, particularly speech therapy for hyperfunctional voice disorders, but also including hypnosis, relaxation, breathing exercises and bio-feedback are shown to be helpful in this condition and prognosis is good [27,28,30]. If major underlying anxiety or other psychopathology is present, then more extensive evaluation and therapy for a specific psychological condition is warranted.

Pectus Excavatum

Pectus deformities (pectus excavatum and carinatum, figure 5) occur in about 1% of the population with boys affected in a 4:1 ratio to girls.31 Pectus excavatum (funnel chest) is the most common with inward indentation of the sternum readily apparent on chest inspection. With adolescent growth acceleration, the defect becomes more severe but stops progressing once one attains adult growth. Dystrophic growth of the costal cartilages appears to be the cause of the sternal depression [31]. There is often a familial tendency toward this defect. Although specific symptoms are not routinely associated with pectus excavatum, adolescents may complain of fatigue, decreased exercise tolerance, and chest and back discomfort. Mitral valve prolapse may occur in up to 20% of children with pectus excavatum and resolves about half the time with repair [32]. Pectus deformities are also seen in connective tissue disorders including Marfan and Ehlers-Danlos syndromes [31]. Embarrassment because of the cosmetic nature of the deformity most often leads to the patient seeking medical or surgical evaluation of the deformity and the psychological impact of this condition constitutes most of the disability experienced by teens.

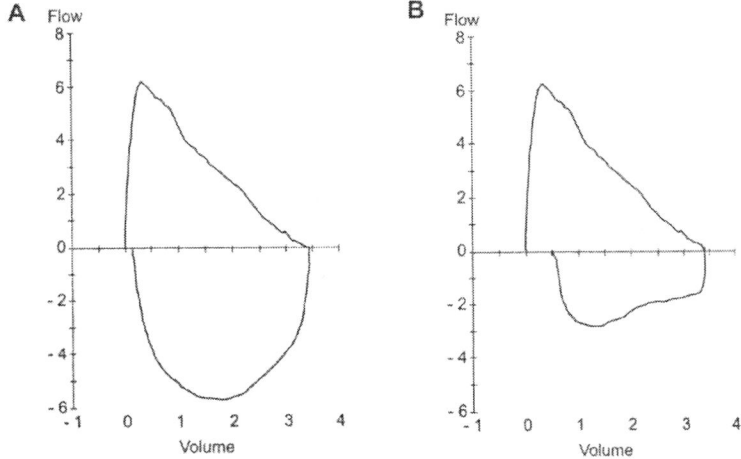

Figure 4. A normal flow-volume loop (A) and a flattened inspiratory loop (B) seen in vocal cord dysfunction. Adapted from Howenstine M, Eigen, H. Medical care of the adolescent with asthma. Adolesc Med:STARS 2000;11(3):501-519.

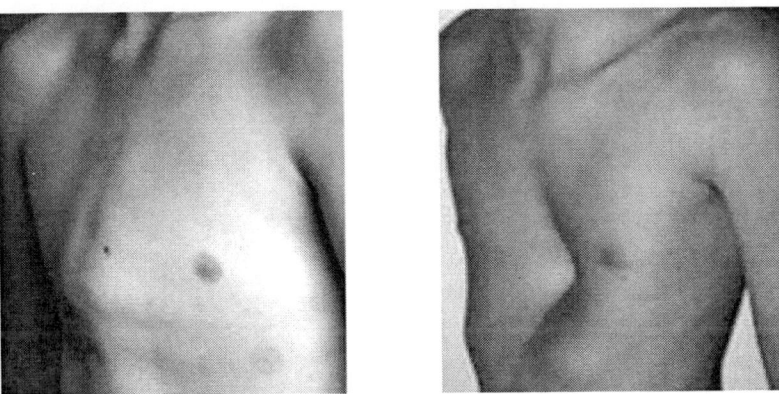

Figure 5. Pectus excavatum (right) and pectus carinatum.

Surgery is indicated primarily for cosmetic purposes. Although mild restrictive defects in pulmonary function (reduction in lung volumes) may accompany severe pectus excavatum deformities, functional improvement in lung function and exercise tolerance is quite variable after surgery [33]. The reduced exercise capacity seen in some patients with severe pectus excavatum appears to be primarily due to impaired cardiovascular performance rather than from ventilation limitation [34]. In one large study, FVC, FEV1, and the FEF25-75 (forced expiratory flow rate between 25 and 75% of vital capacity) improved postoperatively in the majority of patients [35]. Subjective improvement in exercise tolerance may be noted by patient and family.

Bronchopulmonary Dysplasia

Bronchopulmonary dysplasia (BPD), also known as chronic lung disease (CLD) of prematurity, has been recognized since 1967 [36]. In past years, the classic infant developing this inflammatory disease was premature and exposed to post natal oxygen with mechanical ventilation. With the advent of prenatal corticosteroid and the use of exogenously administered surfactant, severe cases are rarer and more common in the very small infant [37]. BPD is generally defined as the need for supplemental oxygen at one month of age or 36 weeks postmenstrual age [38,39].

The pathogenesis involves a combination of prenatal inflammation due to fetal infection or chorioamnionitis and post natal lung injury due to mechanical ventilation and oxygen inflicted on the premature lung. This condition leads to decreased pulmonary vascular growth and alveolarization [39]. A neutrophilic inflammatory response with stimulated release of proinflammatory cytokines and growth factors leads to the intense inflammation, parenchymal damage, and fibrosis [39]. Oxygen, and in severe cases, ventilatory support may be required after discharge from the neonatal intensive care unit, and significant airway hyperreactivity is common. BPD has long term effects on pulmonary mechanics, gas exchange, and the pulmonary vasculature and this often persists into childhood and beyond to adolescent years.

Although lung growth and development often improves lung mechanics in BPD, airway obstruction persists. This condition is demonstrated by a reduction in spirometric measures, measures of exercise tolerance, and persistent radiographic abnormalities in adolescents with a history of BPD but also in youths with a history of severe prematurity without BPD. Compared with normal controls, adolescents (mean age 17.7 years) with a history of severe prematurity with BPD demonstrated reductions in FEV1 that decreased in parallel to the increasing severity of neonatal lung disease [40]. In addition, a doctor's diagnosis of asthma and the use of asthma inhalers were significantly more common among youths with a history of prematurity than in controls.

Increased oxygen exposure in the neonatal period significantly predicted adolescent FEV1 [40]. Similarly, of 508 nineteen year olds with a history of prematurity, those with a history of BPD had a higher prevalence of respiratory symptoms [41]. In school age children, those with a history of BPD have a lower FEV1 than do prematures without a history of respiratory disease and children born at term [38]. Other studies have found similar results, including increased exercise disability determined during exercise testing in children with prematurity with or without BPD, although the reasons for this are not entirely clear. At 19 years old, prematurity predicted decreased exercise capacity and early attainment of anaerobic threshold (a measure of fitness) compared with normal controls [42]. In this study, no difference was found between those with a history of BPD and those without. FEV1 was lower in the premature groups compared with controls, and the authors concluded that the long-term effects of pre-maturity were increased airway obstruction and reduced exercise capacity.

Radiographic abnormalities persist into adolescence when surveyed by sensitive studies such as high resolution computerized tomography (HRCT) scans. Northway [38] described the radiographic abnormalities in BPD in 1967 as progressing through four stages from acute lung injury to structural changes of chronic lung disease. He also described the more subtle changes of hyperinflation, interstitial and pleural thickening, blebs, and peribronchial cuffing in chest radiographs at age 18 years in youths with a history of BPD. Using HRCT, Acquino et al [43] described air trapping, reticular densities, and areas of architectural distortion in 92% of 26 children (median age 10 years, range 5-18) with a BPD history. In their study, the finding on HRCT correlated with increased airway obstruction. Likewise, Aukland et al [44] found abnormal HRCT findings in 92% of 18 year olds with a history of prematurity with or without BPD.

As part of the pulmonary disability in children with a history of prematurity and BPD is due to increased airway hyperresponsiveness and asthma symptoms, treatment of these patients is much the same as for chronic asthma, including anti-inflammatory therapy with inhaled corticosteroids and long acting beta-adrenergic agents and oral leukotriene receptor antagonists and blockers. However, normalization of lung function as evidenced by persistently low FVC may not be possible. Still unclear are the effects of aging, with its natural decrease in lung volumes and flows over time, on these youths with underlying chronic lung disease.

CONCLUSIONS

The common conditions of cystic fibrosis, asthma, vocal cord dysfunction, pectus excavatum, and BPD can all lead to pulmonary disability with variable prognosis. However, optimizing lung health through the judicious use of medications, avoidance of toxic exposures (such as cigarette smoke), exercise, and occasionally surgery can slow or reverse the effects of these conditions and improve the quality of life for these patients. Monitoring of symptoms and lung function is the most rational way to determine the effects of treatment and follow the progress of these conditions to minimize the disability they cause.

REFERENCES

[1] Cystic fibrosis patient registry data. Bethesda, MD: *Cystic Fibrosis Foundation,* 2008.
[2] Rubin BK. Mucus structure and properties in cystic fibrosis. *Pediatr. Resp. Rev.* 2007;8:4-7.
[3] Treggiari MM, Rosenfeld M, REtsch-Bogart G, Gibson R, Ramsey B. Approach to eradication of initial Pseudomonas aeruginosa infection in children with cystic fibrosis. *Pediatr. Pulmonol.* 2007;42(9):751-6.
[4] Hoiby N, Frederiksen B, Pressler T. Eradication of early pseudomonas aeruginosa infection. *J. Cyst. Fibros.* 2005;4(Suppl 2):49-54.
[5] Tiddens HA. Detecting early structural lung damage in cystic fibrosis. *Pediatr. Pulmonol.* 2002; 34(3):228-31.
[6] Brody AS, Klein JS, Molina PL, Quan J, Bean JA, wilmott RW. High-resolution computed tomo-graphy in young patients with cystic fibrosis: distribution of abnormalities and correlation with pulmonary function tests. *J. Pediatr.* 2004;145(1): 32-8.
[7] Mcardle JR, Talwalker JS. Macrolides in cystic fibrosis. *Clin. Chest. Med.* 2007;28(2):347-60.
[8] Henke MO, Ratjen F. Mucolytics in cystic fibrosis. *Pediatr. Resp. Rev.* 2007;8:24-29.
[9] McIlwaine M. Chest physical therapy, breathing techniques and exercise in children with CF. *Pediatr. Resp. Rev.* 2007:8:8-16.
[10] Marks J. Airway clearance devices in cystic fibrosis. *Pediatr. Resp. Rev.* 2007;8:17-23.

[11] Freeman W, Stableforth DE, Cayton RM, Morgan MDL. Endurance exercise capacity in adults with cystic fibrosis. *Respir. Med.* 1993; 87:541-49.
[12] Strauss GD, Osher A, Wang CI, Goodrich E, Gold F, et al. Variable weight training in cystic fibrosis. *Chest.* 1987:92:273-76.
[13] Orenstein DM, Nixon PA, Ross EA, Kaplan RM. The quality of well-being in cystic fibrosis. *Chest.* 1989;95:344-7.
[14] Sawyer EH, Clanton TL. Improved pulmonary function and exercise tolerance with inspiratory muscle conditioning in children with cystic fibrosis. *Chest.* 1993;104:490-7.
[15] Orenstein DM, Franklin BA, Doershuk CF et al. Exercise conditioning and cardiopulmonary fitness in cystic fibrosis. *Chest.* 1981;80:392-8.
[16] deJong W, Grevink RG, Roorda RJ, Kaptein AA, van der Schans CP. Effect of a home exercise training program in patients with cystic fibrosis. *Chest.* 1994;105:463-8.
[17] Cropp GJ, Pullano TP, Cerny FJ, Nathanson IT. Exercise tolerance and cardiorespiratory adjust-ments at peak work capacity in cystic fibrosis. *Am. Rev. Respir. Dis.* 1982;126:211-6.
[18] Freeman W., Stableforth DE, Clayton RM, Morgan MDL. Endurance exercise capacity in adults with cystic fiborisis. *Respir. Med.* 1993; 87:541-9.
[19] Nixon PA, Orenstein DM, Curtis SE, Ross EA. Oxygen supplementation during exercise in cystic fibrosis. *Am. Rev. Respir. Dis.* 1990;142:807-11.
[20] Guidelines for the diagnosis and management of asthma. National asthma education and prevention program. Bethesda, MD: Nat. Heart Lung Blood Inst, US Dept Health Hum. Serv, *Expert Panel Report 3,* NIH 08-5846, 2007.
[21] McFadden ER, Gilbert FA. Exercise induced asthma. *N. Engl. J. Med.* 1994;330(19):1362-7.
[22] Deal EC, McFadden ER, Ingrom RH, et al. Role of respiratory heat exchange in production of exercise-induced asthma. *J. Appl. Physiol.* 1979; 46:467-75.
[23] Kyle JM, Walker RB, Hanshaw SL, Leaman JR, Frobase JK. Exercise-induced bronchospasm in the young athlete: guidelines for routine screening and initial management. *Med. Sci. Sports Exerc.* 1992;24(8):856-9.
[24] Morton AR, Ogle SC, Fitch KD. Effects of nedo-cromil sodium, cromolyn sodium, and placebo in exercise-induced asthma. *Ann. Allergy.* 1992;68: 143-8.
[25] Pearlman DS, van Adelsberg J, Phillip G et al. Onset and duration of protection against exercise induced bronchoconstriction by a single dose of montelukast. *Ann. Allergy Asthma Immunol.* 2006; 97(1):98-104.
[26] Newman KB, Mason UG III, Schmaling KB. Clinical features of vocal cord dysfunction. *Am. J. Respir. Crit. Care Med.* 1995;152:1382-6.
[27] Wood PW, Milgrom H. Vocal cord dysfunction. *J. Allergy Clin. Immunol.* 1996;98:481-5.
[28] Homnick D, Pratt H. Respiratory disease with a psychosomatic component. *Adolesc. Med.* 2000;11 (3):547-66.
[29] Landwehr LP, Wood RP II. Vocal cord dysfunction mimicking exercise-induced broncho-spasm in adolescents. *Pediatrics..* 1996;98:971-4.
[30] Wilson JJ, Wilson EM. Practical management of vocal cord dysfunction in athletes. *Clin. J. Sport Med.* 2006;16(4):357-60.
[31] Williams AM, Crabbe DCG. Pectus deformities of the anterior chest wall. *Pediatr. Resp. Rev.* 2003;4: 237-42.

[32] Shamberger RC, Welch KJ, Sanders SP. Mitral valve prolapse associated with pectus excavatum. *J. Pediatr.* 1987;111:404-7.
[33] Rowland T, Mariarty K, Banever G. Effect of pectus excavatum deformity on cardiorespiratory fitness in adolescent boys. *Arch. Pediatr. Adolesc. Med.* 2005;159:1069-73.
[34] Malek MH, Fonkalstrud EW, Cooper CB. Ventilatory and cardiovascular responses to exercise in patients with pectus excavatum. *Chest.* 2003;124:870-2.
[35] Lawson ML, Mellins RB, Tabangin M, et al. Impact of pectus excavatum on pulmonary function before and after repair with the Nuss procedure. *J. Pediatr. Surg.* 2005;4:174-80.
[36] Northway WH Jr., Rosan RC, Porter DY. Pulmonary disease following respirator therapy of hyaline-membrane disease. *N. Engl. J. Med.* 1967; 276:357-68.
[37] Bancalari E, Abdenour GE, Feller R, Gannon J. Bronchopulmonary dysplasia. Clinical presenta-tion. *J. Pediatr.* 1979;95:819-23.
[38] Bhandari A, Panitch HB. Pulmonary outcomes in bronchopulmonary dysplasia. *Semin. Perinatol.* 30;219-26.
[39] Abman SH, Davis JM. Bronchopulmonary dys-plasia. In: Chernick V, Boat TF, Wilmott RW, Bush A, eds. *Disorders of the respiratory tract in children.* Phaldelphia, PA: Saunders, 2006.
[40] Halvorsen T, Skadberg BT, Eide GE, Roksund OD, Carlsen KH, Bakke P. Pulmonary outcomes in adolescents of extreme preterm birth: a regional cohort study. *Acta Pedatr.* 2004;93:1294-1300.
[41] Vrijlandt EJ, Gerritsen J, Boezen HM, Duiverman EJ. Gender differences in respiratory symptoms in 19 year-old adults born preterm. *Respir. Rev.* 2005: 6:117.
[42] Eliane JLE, Vrijlandt LE, Gerritsen J, Boezen HM, Grevink RG, Duiverman EJ. Lung function and exercise capacity in young adults born prematurely. *Am. J. Respir. Crit. Care Med.* 2006;173:890-6.
[43] Acquino SL, Schecter MS, Chiles C, Albin DS, Chipps B, Webb WR. High-resolution expiratory CT in older children and adults with bronchopulmonary dysplasia. *AJR Am. J. Roentgenol.* 1999;173:963-7.
[44] Aukland SM, Halvorsen T, Fosse KR, Daltveit AK, Rosendahl K. High-resolution CT of the chest in children and young adults who were born prematurely: findings in a population-based study. *AJR Am. J. Roentgenol.* 2006;187:1012-8.

In: Adolescence and Chronic Illness
Editors: H. Omar et al.

ISBN: 978-1-60876-628-4
© 2010 Nova Science Publishers, Inc.

Chapter 16

CHILDHOOD ASTHMA MANAGEMENT AND CONTROL

Frank Mo[*], *Chris Robinson and Bernard C.K. Choi*

Centre for Chronic Disease Prevention and Control, , Health Promotion and Chronic Disease Prevention Branch, Public Health Agency of Canada, Ottawa, Ontario, Canada.

ABSTRACT

The objective of this chapter was to estimate the severity of childhood asthma in Canada, identify the effects of asthma interventions in different target groups, and to profile asthma management and control practices by geographic area, sex, age, and severity groups. Methods: The SLHS was conducted as a stratified and multi-staged cluster survey across Canada in 1996. It included a total of 136 public, private and separate schools in nine health units (Prince Edward Island, Halifax, Sherbrooke, Kingston, Guelph, Winnipeg, Saskatoon, Edmonton, and Kelowna). The target study population was schoolchildren aged 5 to 19 years. Descriptive analyses were used to calculate the severity of childhood asthma for the different groups. Logistic regression was then employed to measure the quality of asthma intervention and control. Multivariate logistic regression was also used to compare the severity and treatment of asthma with age, sex and lifestyle, living and housing conditions. Using existing Clinical Practice Guidelines as a reference, the study also evaluated the effectiveness of interventions such as treatment, and asthmatic education. Results: Based on the Canadian Consensus Recommendations of definition of asthma control, among all 5-19 years old students, 0.8% were well controlled, 98.7% were acceptably controlled and 0.5% were poor controlled. The rates of intermittent and mild asthma were 44.8% and 11.6% compared with moderate (15.3%) and severe (0.9%). Students with asthma reported receiving more advantaged information from a demonstration of inhaler uses (OR=37.54, 95% CI=31.65-44.54), during a medical visits (OR=26.36, 95% CI=21.97-31.63), from the pamphlet/brochures (OR=16.25, 95% CI=13.35-19.76) or from a demonstration of the correct use of medicine (OR=5.62, 95% CI=4.62-6.82). More students visited a family doctor (40.3%, OR=5.52, 95% CI=4.95-6.64) and medical specialists (31.0%,

---

[*] *Correspondence:* Frank Mo, MD, PhD, Centre for Chronic Disease Prevention and Control, Health Promotion and Chronic Disease Prevention Branch, Public Health Agency of Canada, 785 Carling Avenue, Ottawa, Ontario, Canada K1A 0K9. E-mail: Frank_Mo@phac-aspc.gc.ca

OR=3.69, 95% CI=2.58-4.78) than other specialist when they had respiratory problems. Conclusions: The results of the SLHS study demonstrated variations in the management and control of childhood asthma across Canada. The interventions and the practice guidelines for asthma control are useful for preventing and controlling asthma. These findings provide indications of interventions are being used for the control of asthma in Canada.

INTRODUCTION

Childhood asthma management and control in Canada has been significantly improved since the 1990s. However, the increase in asthma seen among children in industrialized countries in the past decades may be the results of alterations in the nature of exposures to various factors in the foetal and early childhood period, and it also remains a serious public health concern and a significant amount of national health resources have been devoted to asthma management in Canada [1]. According to the National Population Health Survey (NPHS) [2] in 1996-97, over 2.2 million Canadians have been physician-diagnosed with asthma, which were 12.2% of children and 6.3% of adults. There has been an increase in the prevalence of asthma among children in the past 15 years [3]. And the recent Canadian Community Health Survey (CCHS) reported that the prevalence of physician-diagnosed asthma in Canada was 8.5% in 2000-01, or over two million people [4]. The Physician Asthma Management Study in 1995-96 showed that physicians and paediatricians played an important role in childhood asthmatic education intervention and other behavioural change strategies that will help to improve the quality of management and control of asthma [5-6].

The Student Lung Health Survey (SLHS) was commissioned by Health Canada in 1995-1996, in order to assess the effects in asthma management and control; identify asthma interventions, improve asthma management through implementation based on the Canadian Asthma Consensus Guidelines [7-8] and to enable effective planning and implementation of measures to improve these activities by a National Asthma Prevention and Control Strategy [9].

Student Lung Health Survey (SLHS)

The SLHS was conducted as a stratified and multi-staged cluster survey across Canada in 1996. It included a total of 136 public, private and separate schools in nine health units (Prince Edward Island, Halifax, Sherbrooke, Kingston, Guelph, Winnipeg, Saskatoon, Edmonton, and Kelowna). The target study population was schoolchildren aged 5 to 19 years. Descriptive analyses were used to calculate the severity of childhood asthma for the different groups. Logistic regression was then employed to measure the quality of asthma intervention and control. Multivariate logistic regression was also used to compare the severity and treatment of asthma with age, sex, lifestyle, socioeconomic status, education levels, living and housing conditions. Using existing Clinical Practice Guidelines as a reference, the study also evaluated the effectiveness of interventions such as treatment, and asthmatic education.

WHAT DID WE FIND?

The results for female students were higher than male students in the 15-19 year age group than in the 5-9 and 10-14 age group, but the reverse was true for males in SLHS as in NPHS (see table 1).

Table 1. Prevalence of asthma by gender and age group, between NPHS and SLHS, Canada 1996

	Student Lung Health Survey (SLHS)		National Population Health Survey (NPHS)†	
	Females	Males	Females	Males
Age (years)	%*	%*	%*	%*
5-9	11.4	14.9	10.7	13.6
10-14	11.1	14.3	12.3	13.4
15-19	14.2	11.9	14.9	13.3

* Percentage weighted.
† Statistics Canada NPHS data.

Based on the Canadian Consensus Recommendations of definition of asthma control, 0.8% of all individuals with asthma were well controlled, 98.7% were acceptably controlled and 0.5% were poorly controlled. The intermittent and mild rates of asthma were 44.8% and 11.6% in comparison with moderate (15.3%) and severe (0.9%) (Table 2).

Table 2. Severity of asthma based on inhaled ß2-agonist and corticosteroids uses, SLHS, Canada 1996

Severity		Cases*	%*	Description
Intermittent	Yes	1338	44.8	Short-acting ß^2-agonists as needed
	No	1648	55.2	
Mild	Yes	346	11.6	- Inhaled corticosteroids were taken regularly at certain times of the year. - Anti-allergics were taken regularly at certain times of the year. - Oral Short-acting ß2-agonist were taken regularly at certain times of the year or throughout the year.
	No	2640	88.4	
Moderate	Yes	456	15.3	- Inhaled corticosteroids or anti-allergics were throughout the year. and - Long-acting ß2-agonists or long-acting xanthines or anti-cholinergies were taken regularly at certain times of the year or throughout the year.
	No	2530	84.7	
Severe	Yes	28	0.9	- Systemic corticosteroids were taken regularly at certain times of the year or throughout the year. - May include alpha and ß-adrenergic agonists.
	No	2958	99.1	

* Counts unweighted, Percentage weighted.

Four categories of severity (intermittent, mild, moderate and severe) for asthma showed the different Odds Ratio and 95% confidence intervals for students who had allergies, passive smoking, and smoking in home, were statistically higher than other groups. Socio-economic status, living condition and environment such as language speaking, dust mites and rugs in home, use of feather comforts, mould in wall of basement, bathroom, bedroom, and of kitchen, having animals or plants in home, or in the seasons of spring, summer, fall, and winter, also affected the morbidity of asthma (table 3).

Table 3. Adjusted Odds Ratio and 95% confidence intervals for severity of asthma by housing environments, lifestyle, and weather, SLHS, Canada 1996

Climate and housing conditions	Adjusted OR and 95% C.I. for different categories of Severity of childhood asthma†			
	Intermittent	Mild	Moderate	Severe
Allergies	1.03, 0.87-1.14	1.14, 1.07-1.22	1.34, 1.18-1.51	2.18, 1.95-2.35
Language	0.61, 0.45-0.84	0.74, 0.52-0.91	0.65, 0.47-0.86	1.30, 1.19-1.45
Passive smoking	1.12, 0.99-1.21	1.13, 1.15-1.26	1.31, 1.20-1.46	1.52, 1.31-1.97
Smoking in home	1.21, 1.13-1.22	1.38, 1.18-1.64	1.71, 1.53-1.98	4.36, 3.56-5.25
Dust mites in home	0.93, 0.80-1.16	1.12, 1.00-1.23	1.25, 1.12-1.30	2.03, 1.87-2.59
Feather covers	0.97, 0.77-1.14	1.17, 1.10-1.24	1.18, 1.11-1.25	1.19, 1.12-1.23
Mould in wall of basement	1.01, 0.85-1.18	1.33, 1.16-1.53	1.53, 1.36-1.74	1.92, 1.73-2.14
Mould in wall of bathroom	1.07, 0.92-1.25	1.26, 1.12-1.39	1.20, 1.14-1.23	1.21, 1.15-1.26
Mould in wall of bedroom	1.15, 1.06-1.24	1.29, 1.17-1.43	1.38, 1.20-1.66	1.58, 1.38-1.76
Mould in wall of kitchen	0.66, 0.48-0.94	1.13, 1.01-1.20	1.02, 0.87-1.18	3.71, 2.95-4.25
Animals in home	1.20, 1.14-1.24	1.31, 1.15-1.48	1.97, 2.16-2.68	2.24, 1.78-2.80
Plants in home	1.21, 1.12-1.23	1.29, 1.14-1.40	1.34, 1.18-1.50	1.55, 1.36-1.89
Rugs in home	1.05, 0.89-1.21	1.07, 0.86-1.25	1.04, 0.88-1.20	2.74, 2.12-2.98
Spring	1.03, 0.86-1.19	1.08, 0.94-1.27	1.17, 1.08-1.26	2.04, 1.86-2.39
Summer	1.11, 0.97-1.19	1.26, 1.11-1.40	1.41, 1.23-1.77	2.56, 1.94-2.87
Fall	0.93, 0.81-1.17	1.16, 1.09-1.21	1.39, 1.18-1.69	1.72, 1.55-1.98
Winter	1.03, 0.88-1.20	1.07, 0.91-1.22	1.22, 1.12-1.13	1.44, 1.28-1.88
Age (5-19 years)	0.87, 0.63-1.02	0.55, 0.34-0.85	0.74, 0.51-0.92	1.07, 0.91-1.23
Gender	0.93, 0.80-1.16	0.91, 0.77-1.14	0.90, 0.76-1.13	1.19, 1.12-1.26

† OR and 95% CI are based on the multivariate logistic regression.

Logistic regression results in the comparison of asthma control categories (good, acceptable, and poor), we found that 98.7% were acceptable control, good and poor control were only 0.8% and 0.6%. Their OR and 95% CI were significantly different (table 4).

Table 4. Adjusted Odds Ratio and 95% confidence intervals for asthma control categories, SLHS, Canada 1996

Asthma control Categories		Cases *	%*	Adjusted OR and 95% C.I. †	Description
Good	Yes	25	0.8	1.00 (baseline)	Based on the times spent in hospital due to asthma; sleeping times disturbed due to asthma in the last 12 months; total numbers of asthma attacks in the last 12 months; total numbers of visits to any type of doctor for asthma in the last 12 months; and total numbers of days of school missed because of asthma in the academic year.
	No	2961	99.2	1.73, 1.22-1.61	
Acceptable	Yes	2948	98.7	1.00 (baseline)	
	No	38	1.3	0.69, 0.84-1.01	
Poor	Yes	13	0.5	1.00 (baseline)	
	No	2973	99.5	2.14, 1.68-2.62	

* Counts unweighted, Percentage weighted.
† OR and 95% CI are based on the logistic regression.

More students with asthma reported receiving educative information from a demonstration of inhaler use (OR=37.54, 95% CI=31.65-44.54), during the medical visits (OR=26.36, 95% CI=21.97-31.63), from the pamphlet/brochures (OR=16.25, 95% CI=13.35-19.76), from a demonstration of the correct use of medicine (OR=5.62, 95% CI=4.62-6.82), and the demonstration of peak flow meter use (OR=1.73, 95% CI=1.34-2.24) than other sources. And over 40.3% of family doctors (OR=5.52, 95% CI=4.59-6.64), 31.0% of medical specialists (OR=3.69, 95% CI=2.85-4.78), 23.6% of pharmacists (OR=5.08, 95% CI=3.91-6.60), and 11.4% of paediatricians (OR=5.30, 95% CI=3.90-7.22), provides education information to asthmatic patients compared to other medical specialties, there is statistically significant difference between medical speciaties (Table 5).

Also, inhaled short acting β_2-agonists were used more frequently before exposure to asthma ($\chi^2=20.4$, P=0.001), and taken regularly certain times of the years ($\chi^2=22.3$, P=0.001) or throughout the year ($\chi^2=10.7$, P=0.001) than the usage of β_2-agonists as needed ($\chi^2=0.1$, P=0.826) and other short-acting β_2-agonists ($\chi^2=1.7$, P=0.188) (Table 6).

Table 5. The proportions and adjusted OR and 95% CI of asthmatic educational information sources, SLHS, Canada 1996

Sources of asthma education	Family Doctors		Medical Specialists		Pharmacists		Pediatricians		Emergency room doctors		Allergists		OR & 95%CI†
	Case	%*	Case	%*	Case	%*	Case	%*	Case	%*	Case	%*	
During a medical visits	2026	78.3	1421	57.2	1132	43.3	492	20.8	426	17.1	267	10.2	26.36, 21.97-31.63
How to live a normal life with asthma	1203	78.2	963	64.1	742	48.1	345	23.4	257	17.9	178	11.4	0.21, 0.16-0.26
From books	1253	77.6	988	64.5	787	48.2	346	23.5	275	18.5	189	12.3	0.60, 0.48-0.75
Given an asthma self management plan	180	77.3	189	84.0	112	50.6	80	36.2	60	25.9	50	21.0	0.80, 0.39-1.65
From pamphlets or brochures	1758	76.1	1290	58.0	1060	45.2	435	20.2	377	16.9	253	10.8	16.25, 13.35-19.76
How to use of peak flow meter	917	76.0	766	64.8	561	46.3	270	23.9	248	21.2	156	11.9	1.73, 1.34-2.24
How to use an inhaler	2060	75.0	1434	54.0	1192	42.5	512	20.0	459	17.4	281	10.2	37.54, 31.65-44.54
Correct use of medicine	1931	74.9	1390	56.0	1138	43.3	499	20.9	430	17.6	270	10.4	5.62, 4.62-6.82
Total	11347	40.3	8449	31.0	6732	23.6	2987	11.4	2536	9.4	1645	5.9	
OR & 95%CI†	5.52, 4.59-6.64		3.69, 2.85-4.78		5.08, 3.91-6.60		5.30, 3.90-7.22		0.85, 0.57-1.19		0.76, 0.43-1.13		

* Counts unweighted, Percentage weighted.
† OR and 95% CI are based on the multivariate logistic regression.

Table 6. Relationship between asthma prevalence and taking inhaled ß2-agonists, SLHS, Canada 1996

ß2-agonists		Prevalence of asthma			Adjusted Chi-sq (χ²)	P-Value
		Yes	No	Total		
Short-acting ß2-agonists	Yes*	2085	236	2321	5.1	0.024
	%*	89.5	9.9	99.4		
	No*	12	3	15		
	%*	0.5	0.1	0.6		
Other short-acting ß2-agonists	Yes*	919	1402	2321	1.7	0.188
	%*	41.1	58.3	99.4		
	No*	6	9	15		
	%*	0.3	0.3	0.6		
ß2-agonists before Exposure to asthma	Yes*	422	1663	2085	20.4	0.001
	%*	22.3	77.2	99.4		
	No*	1	11	12		
	%*	0.1	0.5	0.6		
ß2-agonists as needed	Yes*	1817	292	2109	0.1	0.826
	%*	83.2	16.3	99.4		
	No*	10	2	12		
	%*	0.5	0.1	0.6		
ß2-agonists taken regularly Certain times of the year	Yes*	259	1827	2086	22.3	0.001
	%*	12.4	87.0	99.4		
	No*	0	12	12		
	%*	0.0	0.6	0.6		
ß2-agonists taken regularly throughout the year	Yes*	180	1905	2085	10.7	0.001
	%*	9.4	90.0	99.4		
	No*	2	10	12		
	%*	0.1	0.5	0.6		

* Counts unweighted, Percentage weighted.

DISCUSSION

The prevalence of childhood asthma by age and gender was similar in the Student Lung Health Survey, as in the National Population Health Survey in Canada. These supported by many studies in the World [10-13] (see table 1).

Consistent use of Asthma Practice Guidelines for diagnosis, and use of appropriate medication, self-management plans, health education and follow-up would lead to improve asthma management in the children and adolescents [14]. According to the Canadian Consensus Recommendations on asthma control, the severity of asthma is based on inhaled β_2-agonist and corticosteroid uses, and asthma control is based on the times spent in hospital due to asthma, sleeping times disturbed due to asthma in the last 12 months, total numbers of asthma attacks in the last 12 months, total numbers of visits to any type of doctor for asthma in the last 12 months; and total numbers of days of school missed because of asthma in the academic year. There were 0.8% well controlled, 98.7% were acceptably controlled and 0.5% had poor control in this study. The intermittent, mild, moderate and severe rates of asthma were 44.8%, 11.6%, 15.3%, and 0.9% respectively. Table 3 and 4 show the differences between severity and control categories. Kuehni and Frey [15] reported that 18% of all asthmatics had excellent control, 33% had satisfactory, and 49% unsatisfactory in a study of 572 Swiss-German children aged 4-16 years with asthma. It is consistently different from our results.

Asthma triggers, living and environmental conditions and lifestyle such as allergy, pets or plants in home, bedding (pillow and feather comforts), mould in the walls of bathroom, kitchen, or basement, seasonality, humidity and exposure to passive smoking or smoking in home, are commonly recognised risk factors and triggers of asthma [16]. Indoor air quality is also affected prevalence of asthma, results in Table 3 of this study showed that severity of asthma is very associated to allergy (OR=2.18, 1.95-2.35), exposed to smoking (OR=1.52, 95% CI=1.31-1.97), smoking in home (OR=4.36, 95% CI=3.56-5.25) and dust mites in home (OR=2.03, 95% CI=1.87-2.59). Exposure to house dust mite (HDM) allergens is an important risk factor for childhood asthma. High exposure to house dust mite allergen during the first year of life has been found to increase the risk of subsequent asthma and mite sensitization. Environmental factors, home construction and cleaning methods used are also associated with levels of dust mites in the home [17-18]. Significantly higher allergen levels were associated with wool bedding and innerspring mattresses ($P < 0.001$), as estimated from a multiple linear regression model, up to 70% reduction in bed avoiding wool bedding and innerspring mattresses may achieve allergen levels [19]. These also appeared to be supported by the reports of Health Canada and National Academy of Sciences for the development of asthma in children [20-21]. Lau et al [22] study reported that children sensitised to any allergen early in life and sensitised to inhalant allergen by the age of 7 years were at a significantly increased risk of being asthmatic at this age (OR=10.12, 95% CI=3.81-26.88).

Sensitization to moulds is quite common among patients with allergic respiratory diseases, with a striking preponderance among children with asthma. Mould allergy could also be an important factor determining asthma severity in this environment. Among asthmatic children, severe asthma was significantly more frequent among mould-positive (51.6%) than mould-negative patients (17.5%; $p < 0.0001$) [23]. Peak flow variability (PFV) was significantly associated with smoking and visible mould. The association between visible mould and PFV was independent of season, smoking and the dose of reliever medication [24]. The presence of mould and/or mildew and use of a gas-cooking stove was a significant risk factor for schooling students in Alberta, Canada [25]. Ponsonby et al [26] reported an adverse association of current synthetic pillow and quilt use was strongly associated with frequent wheeze (Relative Risk=5.2, 95% CI=1.3-20.6). These matched the results in this study, where synthetic pillow users (OR=1.47, 95% CI=1.16-1.75), and feather comforts users (OR=1.79, 95% CI=1.21-2.68) had high Odds Ratios than other bedding users (see table 3).

Asthma education information is an important source for individuals with asthma to get knowledge in preventing and controlling asthma attacks. Table 5 showed that there are 78.3% and 78.2% of asthma educations obtained during a medical visit and how to live a normal life with asthma by family doctors; however, 84.0% given a personal asthma self management plan by a medical specialist. The differences between asthma patients visits by doctor specialty were significantly higher for family doctor (40.3%, OR=5.52, 95% CI=4.59-6.64), medical specialist (31.0%, OR=3.69, 95% CI=2.85-4.78), and paediatricians (11.4%, OR=5.30, 95% CI=3.90-7.22) than other specialties (see table 5). Our results are supported by a supplementing conventional asthma care with interactive multimedia education in the Unites States. Their study shows a significantly improve asthma knowledge and reduce the burden of childhood asthma. Their findings of increased asthma knowledge, decreased morbidity, and lowered use of emergency services have direct implications for health care providers and insurance companies [27].

Current asthma guidelines focus on self-management by the patient, in which monitoring of peak flow plays an important role. To be able to participate in self-management, the patient must be educated rigorously on pathophysiological mechanisms of the disease, such as principles of treatment, correct inhalation technique, treatment goals and the action to take when symptoms or peak flow worsen. Therefore, education is the most important component of asthma self-management, and home peak flow monitoring is not needed in the majority of asthmatic children [28].

Asthma treatment is based on the appropriate recognition and classification of children warranting treatment. corticosteroids may be combined with an inhaled long-acting bronchodilator, is the most effective in reducing symptoms and exacerbations and preventing the potential mortality from the disease [29]. Table 5 shows the variations in use of inhaled β_2 agonists. Inhaled short acting β_2-agonists were used more frequently before exposure to asthmatic stimuli (χ^2=20.4, P=0.001), and taken regularly certain times of the year χ^2=22.3, P=0.001) or throughout the year (χ^2=10.7, P=0.001) for a young child with asthma, than the usage of $\beta_2$agonists as needed (χ^2=0.1, P=0.826) and other short-acting β_2-agonists (χ^2=1.7, P=0.188). However, in a German study, Maziak et al reported only 6% of children regularly using inhaled steroids among current asthma, and reached only 21% among children with diagnosed asthma [30].

The American committee identified 11 policy recommendations in regarding improving health care delivery and financing include the development and implementation of quality-of-care standards are very useful in asthma management and control: 1) primary care, 2) self-management education, 3) case-management interventions and expansion of insurance coverage and benefit design by 4) extending continuous health insurance coverage for all children 5) developing model insurance benefits packages for essential childhood asthma services, and 6) educating health care purchasers in how to use them, 7) public health grants to foster asthma-friendly communities, 8) school-based asthma initiatives, 9) launching a national asthma public education campaign, 10) developing a national asthma surveillance system, and 11) establishing a national agenda for asthma prevention research, with an emphasis on epidemiologic and behavioral sciences, are also recommended [31].

Higgins et al [32] determined whether patient education and assignment to a primary care provider improve outcomes and cost in the management of pediatric asthma, and the results showed the favourable changes after intervention, with the decrease in the number of prescriptions of monthly-inhaled anti-inflammatory drugs and chest radiographs ordered being statistically significant ($P = 0.007$ and $P = 0.040$, respectively). Monthly admissions, emergency department visits, and clinic visits declined after intervention after 22.8 months of follow up. Annual resource savings after intervention was estimated to be $4845.29 per patient for this military hospital [32].

The limitations of our work were: 1) the three largest cities (Montreal, Toronto, Vancouver) in Canada were not included in the data and they, presumably have the greatest difficulty with air quality. 2) the environmental results to season and in home conditions without reference to air pollution and external factors. 3) the northern communities in Canada have particular problems with tobacco use and air quality and yet were excluded from the design. Furthermore, it is a cross sectional study which was susceptible to a number of biases33, it cannot randomly allocate potential effects for asthma between those who visited and those who did not visit emergency department or their family doctors. For the younger students, it was their parents or guardians who filled out the questionnaire, thus, some biases may exist.

CONCLUSIONS

The results of the SLHS study demonstrated variation in the management and control of childhood asthma in Canada. Asthma is still a serious chronic condition for children and it affects their academic performance and quality of life. The diagnostic methods and practice guidelines for asthma control are useful to prevent and control asthma.

ACKNOWLEDGEMENTS

The authors thank the Steering Committee of the Student Lung Health Survey for their assistance in the development, conduct and analysis of this study.

REFERENCES

[1] Health Canada. *Respiratory Disease in Canada.* 2001; Ottawa, Canada.
[2] Statistics Canada. The National Population Health Survey. 1996-97; Canada.
[3] The National Asthma Control Task Force. *The Prevention and Management of Asthma in Canada.* 2000; Canada.
[4] Statistics Canada. *Canadian Community Health Survey.* (CCHS), 2001.

[5] Jin RL, Choi BCK, Chan BTB, McRae L, Li F, Cicutto L, Boulet LP, Mitchell I, Beveridge R, Leith E. Physician asthma management practices in Canada. *Can. Respir. J.* 2000;7(6):456-65.

[6] Mitchell I, Choi BCK, McRae L, Chan BTB. Asthma in children: Management practices among paediatricians and family physicians. *Paediatr. Child Health.* 2001;6(6):355-60.

[7] Canadian Consensus Asthma Guidelines Dissemination and Implementation Committee. Canadian Asthma Consensus Guidelines. July, 2003.

[8] Canadian Asthma Consensus Group. Canadian asthma consensus report, 1999; *CMAJ.* 1999; 161 (11 Suppl): S1-S62.

[9] Australia National Asthma Campaign. National Asthma Strategies and Implementation. South Melbourne, Victoria, NAC: 25 Mar. 1999.

[10] Venn A, Lewis S, Cooper M, Hill J, Britton J. Questionnaire study of the effect of sex and age on the prevalence of wheeze and asthma in adolescence. *BMJ.* 1998; 316:1945–6.

[11] Sennhauser FH, Kuhni C. Prevalence of respiratory symptoms in Swiss children: is bronchial asthma really more prevalent in boys? *Pediatr. Pulmonol.* 1995; 19:161–6.

[12] Castro-Rodrigues J, Holberg C, Morgan W, Write A, Martinez F. Increased incidence of asthma-like symptoms in girls who become overweight or obese during the school years. *Am. J. Respir. Crit. Care Med.* 2001; 163:1344–9.

[13] Mo F, Robinson C, Choi B.C.K. Analysis of prevalence, triggers, risk factors and the related socio-economic effects of childhood asthma in the Student Lung Health Survey (SLHS) database, Canada 1996. *Int. J. Adolesc. Med. Health.* 2003; 15(4):00-00.

[14] The National Asthma Control Task Force. *The Prevention and Management of Asthma in Canada.* 2000.

[15] Kuehni CE, and Frey U. Age-related differences in perceived asthma control in childhood: guidelines and reality. *Eur. Respir. J.* 2002 Oct; 20(4): 880-9.

[16] Dales RE, Raizenne M, Bartlett S, El-Saadany J, Brook Burnett R. Prevalence of childhood asthma across Canada. *Int. J. Epidemiol.* 1994;23(4):775-81.

[17] Dharmage S, Bailey M, Raven J, Cheng A, Rolland J, Thien F, Forbes A, Abramson M, Walters EH. Residential characteristics influence Der p 1 levels in homes in Melbourne, Australia. *Clin. Exp. Allergy.* 1999 Apr; 29(4): 461-9.

[18] Couper D, Ponsonby AL, Dwyer T. Determinants of dust mite allergen concentrations in infant bedrooms in Tasmania. *Clin. Exp. Allergy.* 1998 Jun; 28(6): 715-23.

[19] Garrett MH, Hooper BM, Hooper MA. Indoor environmental factors associated with house-dust-mite allergen (Der p 1) levels in south-eastern Australian houses. *Allergy.* 1998 Nov; 53(11): 1060-5.

[20] Health Canada. Exposure Guidelines for Residential Indoor AIR quality: *A report of the federal-provincial advisory committee on Environmental and Occupational Health.* 1995.

[21] National Academy of Sciences, Committee on the Assessment of Asthma and Indoor Air, Division of Health Promotion and Disease Prevention, Institute of Medicine. *Clearing the Air: Asthma and Indoor Air Exposures.* National Academy Press, 2000.

[22] Lau S, Nickel R, Niggemann B, and MAS Group. The development of childhood asthma: lessons from the German Multicentre Allergy Study (MAS). *Paediatr. Respir. Rev.* 2002; 3(3): 265-72.

[23] Ezeamuzie CI, Al-Ali S, Khan M, Hijazi Z, Dowaisan A, Thomson MS, Georgi J. IgE-mediated sensitization to mould allergens among patients with allergic respiratory diseases in a desert environment. *Int. Arch. Allergy Immunol.* 2000 Apr; 121(4): 300-7.

[24] Dharmage S, Bailey M, Raven J, Abeyawickrama K, Cao D, Guest D, Rolland J, Forbes A, Thien F, Abramson M, Walters EH. Mouldy houses influence symptoms of asthma among atopic individuals. *Clin. Exp. Allergy.* 2002 May; 32(5): 714-20.

[25] Hessel PA, Klaver J, Michaelchuk D, McGhan S, Carson MM, Melvin D. The epidemiology of childhood asthma in Red Deer and Medicine Hat, *Alberta. Can. Respir. J.* 2001 May Jun; 8(3): 139-46.

[26] Ponsonby AL, Dwyer T, Kemp A, Cochrane J, Couper D, Carmichael A. Synthetic bedding and wheeze in childhood. *Epidemiology.* 2003; 14(1): 37-44.

[27] Krishna S, Francisco BD, Balas EA, Konig P, Graff GR, Madsen RW. Internet-enabled interactive multimedia asthma education program: a randomized trial. *Pediatrics.* 2003 Mar; 111(3): 503-10.

[28] Kamps AW, Brand PL. Education, self-management and home peak flow monitoring in childhood asthma. *Paediatr. Respir. Rev.* 2001 Jun; 2(2): 165-9.

[29] Stempel DA. The pharmacologic management of childhood asthma. *Pediatr. Clin. North Am.* 2003 Jun; 50(3): 609-29.

[30] Maziak W, von Mutius E, Beimfohr C, Hirsch T, Leupold W, Keil U, Weiland SK. The management of childhood asthma in the community. *Eur. Respir. J.* 2002;20(6):1476-82.

[31] Lara M, Rosenbaum S, Rachelefsky G, Nicholas W, Morton SC, Emont S, Branch M, Genovese B, Vaiana ME, Smith V, Wheeler L, Platts-Mills T, Clark N, Lurie N, Weiss KB. Improving childhood asthma outcomes in the United States: a blueprint for policy action. *Pediatrics.* 2002 May; 109(5): 919-30.

[32] Higgins JC, Kiser WR, McClenathan S, Tynan NL. Influence of an interventional program on resource use and cost in pediatric asthma. *Am. J. Manag. Care.* 1998 Oct; 4(10): 1465-9.

[33] Choi BCK, Noseworthy AL. Classification, direction and prevention of bias in epidemiological research. *J. Occup. Med.* 1992; 34:265-71.

Part X. Digestive System

In: Adolescence and Chronic Illness
Editors: H. Omar et al.

ISBN: 978-1-60876-628-4
© 2010 Nova Science Publishers, Inc.

Chapter 17

NUTRITION AND GASTROENTEROLOGY ISSUES

Arthur N. Feinberg[*,1], *Lisa A. Feinberg*[2] *and Orhan K. Atay*[2]

[1] Michigan State University College of Human Medicine,
Kalamazoo Center for Medical Studies, Michigan.
[2] Cleveland Clinic, Cleveland, Ohio, United States of America.

ABSTRACT

There are many considerations regarding the gastrointestinal tract in adolescents with disabilities. This article reviews assessment of nutritional status, the effect of disability on nutritional sufficiency, and management of common gastrointestinal problems affecting these patients.

INTRODUCTION

All adolescents have caloric requirements necessary for metabolism, growth, activity, fecal losses and specific dynamic action of protein. The basic building blocks that provide these calories are protein, including essential amino acids (~4 cal/g), fat, including essential fatty acids (~9 cal/g), and carbohydrate (~4 cal/g). In addition, it is important to consider water, trace element, and vitamin needs. To attain normal growth, both height and weight, and health, meeting all the above needs is necessary. All nutrients in children must be ingested, retained, processed, absorbed, metabolized, and excreted, the net result of which should produce nutritional sufficiency. Ingestion and retention are dependent upon the proper mechanics of sucking and swallowing as well as normal esophageal peristalsis and valve function with input from the autonomic nervous system to the 'enteric' nervous system. Processing for ultimate metabolism requires the ability to break down proteins, fats, and carbohydrates. Excretion of residual material requires proper colonic function.

---

[*] *Correspondence:* Arthur N. Feinberg, MD, Michigan State University College of Human Medicine, Kalamazoo Center for Medical Studies, 1000 Oakland Drive, Kalamazoo, MI 49008 United States. Tel: 269-337-6458; Fax: 269 337-6474; E-mail Feinberg@kcms.msu.edu

Adolescents, like children are all "works in progress" and there are changes over time in metabolic, activity, and growth needs in all of them, disabled or not. It is impossible to establish a single simple formula or equation to calculate all dietary needs. We will present a few "rules of thumb", mainly to establish a starting point for achieving nutritional goals with the understanding that monitoring is crucial and that the prescribing physician or dietician should be prepared to make several modifications to suit the needs of the individual patient. A 'rule of thumb' for daily caloric needs in normal older children and adolescents is 1,500 kcal at 20 kg; add 20 kcal/kg for each kg over 20 kg.

NEUROLOGICAL IMPAIRMENT

The Oxford Feeding Study [1,2] noted that patients with neurological impairment have inadequate caloric intake, even with the change in mind-set that those children with disabilities should not be obese. Hogan [3] discussed energy requirements of patients with cerebral palsy. Certain conditions such as tachypnea, fever, seizures, spasticity, and ambulation will alter caloric needs. Studies assessing total energy expenditure in children with cerebral palsy vary considerably. Krick et al [4] proposed a formula for energy needs of children with cerebral palsy taking the above into account. However, despite many suggested formulas, the variation among studies, ranging from 1.1 to 1.6 times resting energy expenditure, precludes establishing standards for nutritional needs of the handicapped [5].

Thus, it is necessary to estimate initially not only the patient's needs but also how to prescribe a diet that meets these needs. Some disabled adolescents will be able to thrive with a normal diet for age. Others, because of oro-motor fatigue or gastrointestinal problems may require pureed foods. In many instances, it may not be possible for the patient to meet all his/her needs orally without some modification. It is possible to increase the caloric density of standard formula feedings. This is of importance in certain conditions such as cardiac or renal failure where it may be necessary to limit fluid intake, yet provide adequate calories. If a patient cannot meet these needs orally with formula modification or supplements, it may be necessary to provide feedings through a naso- or orogastric tube or a gastro- or ileostomy tube. In addition, certain patients may require specific types of protein, fat, or carbohydrate. Special modular formulas provide these needs.

Taking measurements at every visit and following the length and weight percentile trends is important. Although Body Mass Indices (BMI) wt (in kg)/ht (in m2) are a helpful indicator for normal adolescents, no anthropometric standards have been established for many handicapping conditions. There are growth charts for conditions such as Down syndrome, prematurity, meningomyelocoele, Sickle-cell anemia, Turner and other genetic syndromes [6]. In patients with contractures or scoliosis, some investigators have proposed formulas to calculate ideal length based on tibial length. An example of such is tibial length (from medial popliteal line to bottom of medial malleolus) x 3.26 + 30.8 cm = ideal stature. Similarly, assessing the true height in a patient with spina bifida is difficult (lower extremities may be disproportionately short) and upper arm length can be a basis for growth standards [6].

To assess nutritional status, one may use another "rule of thumb" that defines mild malnutrition as < 90% of ideal weight, moderate malnutrition as < 80% of ideal weight, and severe malnutrition as < 70% of ideal weight; however, as with BMI, no anthropometric standards have been established for many handicapping conditions. Supplemental measurements of mid-arm diameter, or triceps or subscapular skinfold thickness are helpful to assess nutrition, taking into account both adipose and muscle tissue. Although no standards have been developed for bone density in children and adolescents, Chad et al [7] determined that osteopenia is worse in non-ambulatory children with spastic cerebral palsy. Duncan, Barton, and Lloyd [8] determined that poor intake played a significant role in low bone density. Cohen and Navathe [9] in 1999 delineated several factors why handicapped patients may not meet their nutritional needs.

This chapter incorporates the concepts in table 1 as an aid to diagnosis in the handicapped. Important to recognize is that all disabled adolescents are subject to the same medical conditions as their normally-developing peers. Discussing all diagnoses goes well beyond the scope of this review. We present below a framework to classify conditions and provide some scenarios that affect nutritional status of adolescents with disabilities. To approach diagnoses in the context of disability is important, but clinicians must also consider other diagnoses, some of which may not be of gastrointestinal origin. A number of conditions are now considered.

Table 1. Etiologies of feeding disorders and under-nutrition for children and adults with developmental disabilities. From Rubin IL, Crocker AC. Medical care for children and adults with developmental disabilities, 2nd ed. Baltimore, MD: Paul H Brookes, 2006

Historical perspectives	Genetic endowment
	Underlying illness
	Neurodevelopmental status
Current state	Oral motor competence
	Intercurrent illness
	Behavioral resistance
	Food-medication interaction
Nutriture	Caregiver involvement
	Food availability
	Nutrient adequacy
	Appetite/alternative sources
	Energy requirements
	Activities, expenditures, losses
	Iatrogenic
Metabolic adaptation	Digestion, absorption
	Uptake, utilization
	Storage, excretion
	Hormonal homeostasis

Congenital/Genetic/Metabolic

These derangements will lead to malnutrition a priori. For a few examples, chromosomal disorders, such as trisomies, gene deletions, and those associated with short stature regardless of the patient's weight. Cardiac disease with failure may lead to caloric deprivation for many reasons, including fatigue from feeding and increased metabolic demand secondary to tachypnea and tachycardia. Inborn errors of metabolism will cause vomiting with diminished caloric intake, acidosis, and hence poor growth. Cystic fibrosis and celiac disease will cause length and weight problems due to malabsorption. Endocrine problems, such as hypothyroidism, Cushing's disease, hypopituitarism, and rickets are associated with short stature irrespective of weight. Hyperthyroidism, on the other hand, leads to poor weight gain from a hypermetabolic state. Anatomic malformations of the gastrointestinal system, such as cleft palate, esophageal webs, fistulae, bowel atresias, malrotations, and many others will limit intake due to vomiting. There are often residual symptoms in adolescents even after surgical correction. Neurological conditions will affect oral intake. Spasticity will consistently increase the metabolic rate, thus raising maintenance caloric needs.

Traumatic/Hypoxic

Oral motor dysfunction occurs in patients with traumatic brain injuries whether occurring prenatally, at birth, or later. In such patients, there is significant vomiting, choking, and regurgitation. Injury to the gastrointestinal tract, acquired accidentally or iatrogenically (surgery, radiation) will affect nutritional adequacy.

Infection, Inflammation, Malignancy

Intercurrent illness plays a significant role when growth and weight gain are marginal in the baseline state. Specifically, intercurrent infection may cause poor intake due to lethargy and vomiting or may produce a hypermetabolic state due to fever. The immuno-compromised are more subject to any gastrointestinal infection, and it is important to consider opportunistic infections, such as gram negative, staphylococcal, and fungal infections, as well as parasitic infestations. Adolescents with disabilities may convalesce more slowly, due to their hypostatic state and inabilities to rid themselves of respiratory secretions. They also may be more subject to urinary tract infection because of a neurogenic bladder associated with central nervous system (CNS) and spinal conditions, or due to congenital urologic anomalies. Seizures will also increase caloric requirements. Other intercurrent problems include inflammatory conditions, such as collagen vascular disease, inflammatory bowel disease, malignancy, and others.

Psychosocial

Good nutrition depends upon the presence and availability of proper food and the ability of the patient to ingest and retain it with or without external help. Patients may develop secondary food-aversions because they associate the unpleasant sensations of pain, nausea, vomiting or instrumental manipulation with feeding. Feeding carries with it some of the deepest emotions between parent and child, and variations from the norm may promote significant dysfunction in this extremely sensitive dyad. When associated with vomiting, crying, and food-refusal, feeding is often prolonged and fraught with frustration. Hunt [10] discussed several psycho-social aspects of changing from oral to enteral feeding.

Iatrogenic

The composition of nutrients should meet the patient's individual metabolic and growth needs. This is contingent upon proper content, monitoring that the caregiver is following the regimen correctly. It is important to consider that medications may have a profound effect on nutritional status. Some examples are anticonvulsants that may decrease vitamin D levels, diuretics that may cause increased excretion of electrolytes, mineral oil that may interfere with absorption of fat-soluble vitamins, stimulants that may cause decreased appetite, as well as growth and corticosteroids that may cause increased appetite, fluid retention, and hyperglycemia. Tetracyclines, potassium chloride (KCl), and non-steroidal anti-inflammatory drugs (NSAIDS) may cause esophageal injury or gastric ulceration.

Other commonly-used interventions, such as total parenteral nutrition (TPN), are not without significant complications. It is important to monitor these patients for infection and for specific metabolic derangements such as abnormal glucose, electrolyte, calcium, phosphorous, magnesium, and trace element levels. Total parenteral nutrition over time is associated with hepatotoxicity and cholestasis, requiring close monitoring. Increased fat content of parenteral feedings may be associated with emboli to the lungs. Complications and malfunctions from procedures such as TPN or percutaneous gastrostomy (PEG) tubes may prevent nutrients from reaching the patient.

We will now address three major gastro-intestinal issues in adolescents with disabilities, vomiting and regurgitation, constipation, and gastrostomy tube management.

Vomiting and Regurgitation

Gastroesophageal reflux (GER) is a normal physiologic phenomenon in humans, predominantly due to transient lower esophageal sphincter relaxations (TLESR). Gastroesophageal reflux disease (GERD) is by definition GER with pathologic consequences, such as mucosal damage and/or decline in the individual's quality of life. Two basic theories exist. Increased inspiratory and expiratory effort in adolescents with chronic lung conditions (i.e., cystic fibrosis) leads to increased negative intrathoracic pressure, which may in turn predispose the adolescent to GER. Because the embryonic origin of the respiratory tract and esophagus are the same, they share autonomic innervation via the vagus nerve. In addition, esophageal irritation may lead to airway constriction due to this common nerve conduction pathway.

Other disorders of the proximal esophagus confirmed on manometric studies occur with a variety of neurodevelopmental disorders. An intricate sequence of muscle relaxation is necessary for the effective swallowing of a bolus of food. With disruption of this sequence, vomiting and dysphagia occur. Secondary causes of disorders affecting the proximal esophagus may include meningocele, Arnold Chiari malformation, cerbrovascular accidents, polymyositis, dermatomyositis, and muscular dystrophy. Disorders of the distal esophagus include achalasia, dysmotility of the esophagus and inability of the lower esophageal sphincter (LES) to relax. This, constellation of findings can occur with several other disorders, including Hirschsprung disease (aganglionosis elsewhere), diabetes mellitus, intestinal pseudo-obstruction, sarcoidoisis, and Down syndrome. Triple A, or Allgrove syndrome, is associated with adrenocorticotropic hormone insensitivity, alacrima, and achalasia. Gastroparesis associated with such conditions as type I diabetes mellitus, celiac disease, cystic fibrosis, thyroid hormone abnormality, anorexia nervosa, and medication may be associated with feeding intolerance. Hyperglycemia found in type 1 diabetics may lead to gastric hypomotility early on in the disease course.

Aspiration of gastric contents is a complication found in those with recurrent pneumonia with a history of GERD or other esophageal disorders. Bronchoscopy demonstrates lipid laden macrophages that contribute to the diagnosis of recurrent aspiration. Impedance probe testing is the diagnostic test of choice for the evaluation of GERD. This technology allows for the testing of both acidic and non-acidic fluids and gas refluxed from the stomach into the esophagus. Impedance probe testing also provides a means to correlate symptoms with reflux based on probe detection and symptom diary on the probe device. Limitations of this study exist in the adolescent population, as there is yet to be an established standard reference range.

Upper gastrointestinal series is a useful test to evaluate for gastrointestinal obstruction or malrotation. However, this test lacks adequate sensitivity and specificity for a definitive diagnosis of GERD. Gastric emptying studies can provide insight into gastroparesis, although this study also does not provide the clinician with a definitive diagnosis regarding the etiology. Gastroenterologists employ esophageal and antral-duodenal manometry as a means to confirm dysmotility. Although endoscopic and histologic evaluation is the gold standard for esophagitis, patients may still present with symptoms of GERD with unremarkable findings.

Treatment generally consists of managing the underlying systemic ailment. Dietary modification, such as reduction in high-fat containing foods and fiber are useful interventions. In severe cases, jejunostomy feedings may be necessary to bypass the stomach altogether. A gastrostomy tube may be beneficial in alleviating gastric distention by allowing venting. Medical management of GERD involves several approaches.

Prokinetics are a class of drugs that help facilitate gastrointestinal motility. Metoclopramide, a dopamine receptor blocker, is a commonly used prokinetic agent. Unfortunately, CNS effects are a documented complication. The adverse effects include extrapyrimidal signs such as dystonic reactions. Currently, there has been no definitive proof of metoclopramide's effectiveness in treating GERD. Domperidone (not available in United States) is a more tolerable prokinetic with less frequent dystonic reactions. Possible side effects include cardiac arrhythmias due to prolonged QT interval and sub-sequent ventricular fibrillation.

Erythromycin demonstrates some effect on gastric motility, but it has not been a proven treatment for GERD. There is a reported risk for development of hypertrophic pyloric stenosis in patients taking erythromycin. Cisapride is the only prokinetic drug with statistically significant effectiveness to reduce esophageal acid exposure. The United States has banned its use due to cardiac arrhythmia and prolonged QT interval. Cytochrome P4503A4 is responsible for the metabolism of cisapride. Grapefruit juice can affect the metabolism of cisapride.

Histamine-2 blockers, such as famotidine and ranitidine are common treatments for GERD. Tachyphylaxis may occur after several weeks of use. This treatment is not as effective in healing esophagitis as proton pump inhibitors (PPIs), lansoprazole, omeprazole, and esomeprazole. These compounds are "pro-drugs" as the active component is the result of an acidic environment. They bind irreversibly to the H+/K+ ATPase enzyme that inhibits acid production. Adolescents with adequate acid suppression may demonstrate healing of underlying esophagitis after 4-8 weeks of therapy. Prolonged hypochlorhydria may lead to gastric bacterial overgrowth. Vitamin B12 deficiency is another complication to acid suppression due to impaired absorption of B12 from food in an acid-suppressed environment.

Surgical intervention for GERD primarily consists of Nissen Fundoplication, which is a gastric wrap around the fundus and distal esophagus. This procedure prevents the complete relaxation of LES and reduces TLESR. Negative outcomes included GERD reoccurrence in 7.1% of the study population, gas bloat syndrome in 3.6% of the cases, and obstructive symptoms in 2.6% of the study cases [11].

Constipation

Constipation is an exceedingly common problem in healthy adolescents and is even more prevalent in those with neurological impairments. Why this subgroup of patients has this problem is unclear. A large percentage of these patients are not mobile, and this lack of ability to ambulate may contribute to delayed transit through the gastrointestinal tract. Decreased truncal tone and the inability to generate adequate intra-abdominal pressures effectively can play a role in ineffective evacuation as well. Oral motor incoordination leading to inadequate intake decreases stool bulk. Inadequate fluid intake may also cause harder stools with difficult passage. The diet of these patients is often lacking in fiber as well [12].

When first seeing an adolescent patient for constipation, a complete medical history is paramount. This history includes the size, frequency, and consistency of stools. Ask the patient about pain with passage of stools, which may lead to withholding behaviors. Also, address behaviors and postures during defecation. Typical withholding behaviors include arching, scissoring/ straightening of the legs, standing on tiptoes, or hiding. Caregivers should know what the patient's "normal" stool pattern was, and at what age the patient first developed constipation.

Constipation during infancy is more indicative of underlying pathology. Delayed passage of meconium specifically raises concerns about Hirschsprung's disease and cystic fibrosis. These diagnoses are nearly always established by adolescence. Review dietary history as well, with an emphasis on fiber and fluid intake. Growth charts should be available to assess failure to thrive and decreased growth velocity; note prior treatments and whether they were effective. A comprehensive list of medications in the history is important because several medications (particularly anti-epileptic drugs and medications used to treat spasticity) cause constipation. The presence of bright red blood with bowel movements that are large and hard is indicative of a fissure, and this may appear on physical exam as well.

The physical exam of the constipated adolescent begins with general appearance. Is the teen patient well nourished? Is his/her size appropriate for age? Is there evidence of abdominal distention? Document height and weight and plot on the appropriate growth chart. Inspect the patient's abdomen again looking for distention, poor muscle tone, or compromised abdominal musculature that could compromise the ability to generate increased intra-abdominal pressures. Auscultate bowel sounds. Hypoactive bowel sounds may be indicative of slow transit constipation. High pitched or 'tinkling' bowel sounds suggest a small bowel obstruction.

Carefully palpate the abdomen assessing for masses (fecal or otherwise). A rectal exam is essential. Inspect the external anus visually, looking specifically at placement. There may be evidence of encopresis on the exam in the toilet trained patient. Fissures may be present in the chronically constipated patient, as well as skin tags. Assess anal wink by lightly stroking the perianal area in all four quadrants. The digital examination will help to evaluate the tone of the anal sphincter and reliably determine whether the patient has a fecal impaction. Visualize the spine and palpate with attention to the sacral region. The presence of midline pigment lesions or hair tufts point to potential spinal abnormalities. Sacral dimples can be associated with tethered cord. Assess deep tendon reflexes and sensation in the lower extremities. In the ambulatory patient, always evaluate gait.

Laboratory evaluation of the constipated patient is fairly minimal. Screening for hypothyroidism is appropriate. If the patient has a history that includes failure to thrive, then celiac titers and sweat chloride testing may be in order, although cystic fibrosis is usually diagnosed during childhood.

The results of a medical history and physical should guide imaging choices. A KUB with upright may be useful in assessing the degree of fecal retention, especially if there is a limited physical exam due to the patient's body habitus or inability to cooperate. If an abdominal mass is present and is not apparently due to feces, ultrasound or CT may help to clarify its etiology.

Treatment of constipation in adolescents with medical disabilities is not significantly different from that in the otherwise healthy patient. If a fecal impaction is present, then address this first, either with enema or with high dose polyethylene glycol, and in some patients, maintenance with polyethylene glycol is adequate. Other useful medications include lactulose, magnesium hydroxide, mineral oil, and stimulants like senna or bisacodyl. An excellent guideline appears in the Journal of Pediatric Gastroenterology and Nutrition, outlining the different medications and their appropriate dosing [13].

Noteworthy is that patients with spinal cord injury or spinal cord defects often fail medical management alone. In this subset of patients, enema regimens or trans-anal irrigation systems may be beneficial in main-taining regular stooling habits and daytime continence [14]. Other options for treatment include surgical placement of either a cecostomy or a colostomy for anterograde enemas, only if medical management fails to provide adequate relief of a patient's constipation [15].

Feeding Tube Problems

Malnutrition is a major medical issue for adolescents with neurodevelopmental delays or diseases causing increased caloric demand, such as chronic cardiac or respiratory medical issues. In up to 60% of the cases, poor feeding in infancy precedes the diagnosis of cerebral palsy [16]. Nasogastric tubes may supplement short-term nutritional needs (less than 2 months), or act as a trial for gastric feedings before gastrostomy tube (GT) placement.

Percutaneous gastrostomy (PEG) is the placement of a more stable and long term means of enteral nutritional support. The initial gastrostomy tube (GT) is replaced after approximately eight weeks with a button device consisting of an internal balloon to maintain gastrostomy tube placement. Gastrostomy tubes have several risks, including infection and perforation; perforation rates may be as high as 15% [17]. Studies show that those with neurological disorders and underlying aspiration do not have a lower risk of aspiration with GT feeds, and that GT feedings in combination with Nissen fundoplication (NF) only reduce the chances of aspiration [18]. In general, a patient's tolerance of enteral feedings will determine the dietary regimen. Bolus feedings over 15-20 minutes provide nutrition throughout the day. Night time feedings are usually continuous over several hours.

Patients with neurological disabilities may require either transpyloric feedings (via gastrostomy-jejunostomy tube or direct jejunostomy tube) or an NF procedure. Patients who undergo NF may require simultaneous pyloroplasty, if they have underlying delayed gastric emptying. A trochar pierces into the stomach with endoscopic observation of internal placement. There is, however, an area between the stomach and abdominal surface that is not visible during the procedure. Immediately after the PEG placement procedure there is a critical time necessitating close observation.

Complications include perforation into an organ overlying the stomach such as the colon. Another potential for perforation is during difficult GT changes at home or in a medical office. If there is concern about proper placement of the GT, then a computed tomography (CT) scan may be helpful. In patients with GTs that present with diarrhea of unknown etiology, considering GT complications is important. In this setting, it is possible that the GT migrated into the colon and is seemingly causing diarrhea, but rather is infusing formula directly into the large bowel. A GT injection study under fluoroscopy can make this diagnosis. Another major concern is dislodgment of the GT, either by rupture of the internal balloon or by trauma. Maintaining stoma patency is imperative as the onset of closure takes relatively very little time (hours). In a medical setting, it is appropriate to insert a catheter of comparable or slightly smaller size into the stoma until performing definitive replacement of the GT. In cases in which the stoma has already begun to close, serial dilatation with caution may be helpful. GT fluoroscopy is then necessary to confirm appropriate placement of the new GT.

The occurrence of granulation tissue is common in post-GT placement. Chemical cauterization is useful to keep the surrounding skin dry to avoid burns outside of the granulation tissue. Topical steroids are also helpful. In refractory situations, surgical consultation for resection of the granulation tissue may be necessary. Gastrostomy tube occlusion can make enteral feedings difficult to impossible, depending on the degree. Stagnant formula or undissolved medications are the usual sources of occlusion. A common treatment of GT occlusion involves water flushes (up to 30 cc). Occasionally, Viokase mixed with bicarbonate may help to dissolve the obstructing agent. As a rule, infuse no more than 5 cc of water into the balloon port of the button gastrostomy tube. More than that volume can cause rupture of the balloon or ischemia of the stomach mucosa due to the pressure of the balloon against the lining of the gastric tissue.

REFERENCES

[1] Sullivan PB, Lambert B, Rose M, et al. Prevalence and severity of feeding and nutritional problems in children with impairment. Oxford Feeding Study. *Dev. Med. Child Neurol.* 2000; 42(10):674-80.

[2] Sullivan PB, Juszczak E, Lambert BR, et al. Impact of feeding problems on nutritional intake and growth: Oxford. Feeding Study. *Dev. Med. Child Neurol.* 2002;44(7):461-7.

[3] Hogan SE: Energy requirements of children with cerebral palsy. *Can. J. Diet. Pract. Res.* 2004;65(3): 124-30.

[4] Krick J, Murphy PE Markham JF, Shapiro BK. A proposed mechanism for calculating energy needs of children with cerebral palsy. *Dev. Med. Child Neurol.* 1992;34(6) 481-7.

[5] Rubin IL, Crocker AC. *Medical care for children and adults with developmental disabilities,* 2nd ed. Baltimore, MD: Paul H Brookes, 2006.

[6] Ekvall SW, Ekvall VK. *Pediatric nutrition in chronic diseases and developmental disorders*, 2nd ed. Oxford: Oxford Univ Press, 2005.

[7] Chad KE, McKay HA Zello GA, et al. Body composition in nutritionally adequate ambulatory and non-ambulatory children with cerebral palsy and a healthy reference group. *Dev. Med. Child Neurol.* 2000;42:334-9.

[8] Duncan B, Barton LL, Lloyd J, Marks-Katz M. Dietary considerations in osteopenia in tube-fed non-ambulatory children with cerebral palsy. *Clin. Pediatr.* 1999;38(3):133-7.

[9] Cohen. SA, Navanthe AS. Feeding the develop-mentally delayed child. *J. Med. Assoc. Georgia.* 1999;88:71-6.

[10] Hunt F. Changing from oral to enteral feeding: impact on families of children with disabilities. *Paediatr. Nurs.* 2007;19(7):30-2.

[11] Fonkalsrud EW, Ashcraft KW, Coran AG, et al. Surgical treatment of gastroesophageal reflux in children: a combined hospital study of 7467 patients. *Pediatrics.* 1998;101(3 Pt 1):419–22.

[12] Tse PW, Leung SS, Chan T, Sien A, Chan AK. Dietary fibre intake and constipation in children with severe developmental disabilities. *J. Paediatr. Child Health.* 2000;36(3):236-9.

[13] Constipation Guideline Committee of the North American Society for Pediatric Gastroenterology, Hepatology and Nutrition. Evaluation and treatment of constipation in infants and children: recom-mendations of the North American Society for Pediatric Gastroenterology, Hepatology and Nutrition. *J. Pediatric. Gastroenterol. Nutr.* 2006;43 (3):1-13.

[14] Christensen P, Bazzocchi G, Coggrave M, Abel R, Hultling C, et al. A randomized, controlled trial of transanal irrigation versus conservative bowel management in spinal cord-injured patients. *Gastroenterology.* 2006;131(3):738-47.

[15] Cascio S. Flett ME. De la Hunt M. Barrett AM. Jaffray B. MACE or caecostomy button for idio-pathic constipation in children: a comparison of complications and outcomes. *Pediatr. Surg. Int.* 2004;20(7):484-7.

[16] Reilly S, Skuse D, Poblete X. Prevalence of feeding problems and oral motor dysfunction in children with cerebral palsy: a community survey. *J. Pediatr.* 1996;129:877-82.

[17] Brant CQ, Stanich P, Ferrari APJr. Improvement of children's nutritional status after enteral feeding by PEG: an interim report. *Gastrointest. Endosc.* 1990;50:183-8.

[18] Bui HD, Dang CV, Chaney RH, et al. Does gastrostomy and fundoplication prevent aspiration pneumonia in mentally retarded persons? *Am. J. Ment. Retard.* 1989;94:16-9.

Part XI. Genitourinary System

In: Adolescence and Chronic Illness
Editors: H. Omar et al.

ISBN: 978-1-60876-628-4
© 2010 Nova Science Publishers, Inc.

Chapter 18

CHRONIC KIDNEY DISEASE

Timothy E. Bunchman[*]
Pediatric Nephrology, Dialysis and Transplantation,
Helen DeVos Children's Hospital, Michigan State University,
Grand Rapids, Michigan, United States of America.

ABSTRACT

Kidney disease in adolescents can leave them with physical, emotional, and intellectual disabilities. Advances in techniques for prevention of complications of chronic kidney disease (CKD) have improved survival. Ongoing research in advancements and intellectual and school performance is necessary to enhance any developmental delay, as well as intellectual delays associated with CKD. This article reviews advances in CKD, dialysis, and transplantation that have occurred in the last two decades, noting improvement in survival, yet still leaving these adolescents at risk for disabilities.

INTRODUCTION

As seen in many chronic illnesses in adolescents, those with chronic kidney disease (CKD) face a unique number of challenges in their life. This condition leaves them at risk for chronic illnesses and for having disabilities. This review identifies the unique aspects of adolescents with CKD.

---

[*] *Correspondence:* Timothy E. Bunchman, MD, Professor, Pediatric Nephrology, Michigan State University, Lansing, MI and Director, Pediatric Nephrology, Dialysis & Transplantation, Helen DeVos Children's Hospital, Grand Rapids, MI, 221 Michigan St. NE, Suite 406, Grand Rapids, MI 49503 United States. Tel: (616) 391-3788; Fax: (616) 391-7930; E-mail: timothy.bunchman@devoschildrens.org

INCIDENCE

The true incidence of CKD in pediatrics is unknown. No good epidemiologic studies have been conducted in children and adolescents to know what the true incidence is, but like adults, it is believed that the incidence is slowly rising. It is known that patients who require dialysis or transplantation (referred to as end stage renal disease or ESRD), are roughly 15-19 per million year equivalent population [1]. It is presumed that with the increased technology and survival of neonates, recipients of bone marrow transplant, and recipients of other organ transplants, the true incidence of CKD is rising [2,3]. Therefore, early recognition of CKD etiology and early interventions are important and necessary.

ETIOLOGY

The etiology of CKD in pediatrics is quite different from that in adults. For adults with CKD, 90% of the etiology is related to glomerular-based renal diseases [4]. Such diagnoses include diabetes and chronic glomerular nephritis, as well as hypertension. The commonality of glomerular-based renal disease includes active urine sediment, including blood and protein; hypertension; swelling; and often grossly bloody urine. This picture is in contrast to pediatric CKD in which more than 70% of children less than 15 years of age with CKD have tubular interstitial diseases [5]. This condition is not associated with hematuria, hypertension, or edema, and therefore is a silent process. The symptoms may be as subtle as polyuria, polydipsia, salt craving, and growth impairment. Work-up may show evidence of metabolic acidosis that may be misdiagnosed as renal tubular acidosis. The serum creatinine level, albeit the gold standard of renal dysfunction is a very poor indicator of the true glomerular filtration rate (GFR) [6]. Ongoing studies presently funded by the National Institutes of Health (NIH) have shown that one-half to two-thirds of the total renal mass has to be disrupted before changes occur in the serum creatinine. Therefore, by the time the serum creatinine becomes an obvious issue, one may have a 40% to 50% disruption of total kidney function.

The common laboratory panels used across the United States enacted by the Federal Government in 1997 include both the comprehensive metabolic panel (CMP) and the basic metabolic panel (BMP). However, both exclude the measurement of plasma phosphorous. This exclusion is very important because one of the hallmarks of CKD in adolescents and adults is phos-phorous retention with a risk of secondary hyperpara-thyroidism. As one approaches the teenage years, the incidence of tubular interstitial disease diminishes and the incidence of glomerular-based diseases increases. Glomerular-based diseases mimic those of the adult population, often related to immunologic mediated diseases, such as lupus, Wegener's Granulomatosis, focal sclerosis, and others. The metabolic consequences of CKD in adolescents and adults are identical. The outcomes include metabolic acidosis, anemia, and secondary hyperparathyroidism [7]. Additionally, pre-adolescent children with CKD are at risk for developing growth impairment. These conditions, if left untreated, will develop into significant disabilities.

METABOLIC CONSEQUENCES

Since the 1950s, metabolic acidosis has been known to impair growth [8]. Data in the 1990s showed that this has to do with an impairment of growth hormone and insulin-like growth factor axis for stimulus of growth in the face of an acidotic pH. If the CKD patient is placed on alkali (sodium bicarbonate, Bicitra), then the metabolic acidosis can be corrected. The clinical results are an improvement of growth velocity, as well as the reversal and ongoing prevention of any underlying bone damage that has occurred over time. Once dialysis commences in these patients, the bicarbonate is substituted for the alkali that is delivered by dialysis.

The anemia of CKD is multi-fold. This type of anemia has two primary two factors: iron deficiency and the loss of natural erythropoiesis [9]. Poor absorption of iron in such patients may be exacerbated because of binding with other medications, causing iron deficiency. Calcium carbonate, historically used to bind phosphorous in the diet, can also bind dietary iron. Therefore, if one is on calcium carbonate, the iron must be given independent of the calcium carbonate for maximum absorption.

In 1989, erythropoietin was first used in patients with CKD. Newer generation erythropoietin includes Epogen® (Amgen Inc, Thousand Oaks, CA), Procrit (Ortho Biotech, Bridgewater, NJ), or the long acting Aranesp® (Amgen Inc, Thousand Oaks, CA). These are subcutaneous or intravenous medications given to replace the natural loss of erythropoiesis by the patient. The complications of erythropoietin replacement include hypertension and hyperkalemia. These conditions are known complications because they increase the total red cell mass with a secondary increase of intravascular volume with an ongoing red cell turnover causing hyperkalemia.

Erythropoietin non-responsiveness is due to the inflammatory process, severe secondary hyperpara-thyroidism, and iron deficiency. Therefore, in the face of someone not responding to erythropoietin replace-ment, one has to look for these etiologies.

Secondary hyperparathyroidism is common in patients with a GFR less than 40-50 ml/min/1.73m2 [10]. The mechanism is phosphorous retention, which then lowers the calcium. Parathyroid activity will increase in response to hypocalcemia, and over time, will leach calcium from the bones. The etiology of this problem is not a lack of vitamin D, but rather phosphorous retention. Therefore, patients need either to be on a low phosphorous diet or using binding agents to lower the phosphorous. Before 1984, aluminum-based medications were commonly used as a way to bind phosphorous in the diet. Data revealed that the aluminum was retained in CKD and caused bone disease and dementia [11]. Aluminum was replaced then, in the late 1980s and early 1990s, with calcium carbonate. Calcium carbonate was given at the end of meals to bind the maximum phosphorous in the diet. Data in the late 1990s and early 2000s identified coronary calcinosis as a complication of vitamin D replacement, as well as calcium carbonate [12]. Therefore, newer generations of inert binding agents—ex. PhosLo® (Fresenius, Waltham, MA) and Renagel (Genzyme Corp., Cambridge, MA)—are medications given at the end of meals and snacks to keep the phosphorous under control. Once the phos-phorous is under control, often vitamin D replacement is necessary in such patients.

The combination of metabolic acidosis, anemia, and secondary hyperparathyroidism may cause growth impairment. The younger the patient is, the higher the risk for growth impairment. Infants with CKD have a higher nutrition requirement for maximum growth [13]. Infants may require 20% to 30% more nutrition than normal to offset negative growth impairment because of CKD. Further, patients with polyuric renal failure secondary to tubular interstitial disease often become volume and sodium depleted. Such patients may require excessive sodium and fluid back into their diet to maintain euvolemia. This high fluid intake may have a negative impact on appetite, causing a loss of interest in eating. Further, babies with CKD have a much higher incidence of gastroesophageal reflux [14]. Because they require more fluid than normal and because they have a higher incidence of gastroesophageal reflux, many of these babies will require G-tubes with Nissen fundo-plications as a way to give maximum nutrition and volume with minimal vomiting.

Growth hormone has been used in children and adolescents with CKD since the latter 1980s. This use should be done after all other factors that affect growth have been addressed. Growth hormone has been found to enhance growth during the time of CKD, but whether the final adult height is affected is unclear. One risk of growth hormone is the exacerbation of metabolic bone disease if the secondary hyperparathyroidism is not controlled [15]. The combination of sodium bicarbonate and Bicitra replacement, iron replacement, subcutaneous delivery of an erythropoietic agent, dietary phosphorous binding, vitamin D supplementation, and a phosphorous-restricted diet, have both emotional and physical impacts upon the adolescent's self-image.

School Performance

School performance has been studied in kids with CKD [16]. There are mixed messages from impaired school performance to normal school performance, depending on the study. Most of the data is really based on the era of analysis. Historically, in the face of the aluminum based binders, school performance was delayed, probably related to aluminum intoxication and dementia. Often patients with CKD have other organ abnormal-ities, including seizures, or other organ abnormalities that impair school performance. Therefore, knowing whether the CKD alone or CKD in the face of the emotional impact of all the other medications or if the CKD and the impact of the other organs is what affects school performance is difficult. Ongoing studies are in progress to look at school and intellectual performances in children and adolescents with CKD [5,17].

Dialysis

As CKD progresses through its stages, once a renal function is less than 20%, preparation for dialysis is in order. CKD level 5 is the level at which dialysis is necessary. With the use of vitamin D, erythropoietin, iron, as well as phosphorous binders, it is sometimes very difficult to know when to institute dialysis therapy. Further, because growth hormone is often used in babies and children with CKD to promote growth, such children and adolescents may have more normal growth parameters, making it more difficult to know the true indication of dialysis. Historically, dialysis was instituted at the time of poor growth, metabolic acidosis, anemia, or very difficult to control secondary hyper-parathyroidism, all of which are now easy to correct.

Dialysis can be done either as hemodialysis or peritoneal dialysis. Dialysis should be seen only as a bridge to transplantation for the patient. The mode of dialysis is often determined by the distance to center. Infants, patients that live far from center, or patients that will be listed for a deceased-donor kidney transplant are often assigned to peritoneal dialysis. Hemodialysis is more often used when patients have a short-term need for dialysis to bridge them to transplant, patients who live close to center, or older patients. The access for peritoneal dialysis is placed in the peritoneum at the time of the OR, and the access for hemodialysis can either be from a central line placed if patients will be on for less than a year, or placement of a fistula or an AV graft if greater than one year. The decision for the type of access may be related to the urgency of the institution of dialysis as well as length of time waiting for a deceased donor transplant [19].

TRANSPLANTATION

Transplant in children and adolescents is the natural outcome of CKD and ESRD. A donor source can be living or deceased. Historically, HLA typing was once important, but with the newer generation of medications that have been very effective for prevention of rejection, then really, the sources of the kidney probably are most important [20]. Over 50% of these patients receive a living-donor kidney transplant. Because children and adolescents compete in the same donor pools as adults, they are often disadvantaged based on their waiting time. There is an advantage for those less than 15 years of age to allow them to become recipients of kidney transplants much more quickly if waiting for deceased donor transplants as compared with their adult counterparts.

The outcome in CKD is related to the compliance of the patient, the compliance of the family, the underlying disease, as well as the control of the components of CKD. Children and adolescents with CKD grow poorly, have metabolic bone disease, and are often anemic with risk of rickets. Now with the newer generations of medication, it is difficult sometimes to identify the infant with CKD or the child or teen with CKD who has been well cared for. Therefore, the goal is to get these children and adolescents to transplant with 20% of children undergoing preemptive transplant without ever being on dialysis. Long-term studies in pediatric transplant are ongoing. It is thought that long-term life expectancy is still delayed compared with their non-transplant counter-parts. Advances in medical research, transplantation techniques, and growth hormone therapy have clearly improved the outcome in CKD [21].

CONCLUSIONS

The advancements in CKD, ESRD, and transplantation in children and adolescents have been significant in the last two decades. In the mid-1980s, children and adolescents with CKD and ESRD were often destined to multiple complications of diabetes, fractures, growth impairment, and early death. Advancements in nutrition, bone metabolism, correction of anemia, and immuno-suppression have now made children and adolescents with CKD and ESRD easier to care for. Whereas struggles of compliance continue to be an issue for such patients [22], their long-term prognosis is markedly improved. Newer techniques for the prevention of chronic kidney failure will rise from current studies preventing the ongoing progression [5].

REFERENCES

[1] Hogg RJ, Furth S, Lemley KV, et al. National Kidney Foundation's Kidney Disease Outcomes Quality Initiative clinical practice guidelines for chronic kidney disease in children and adoles-cents: evaluation, classification, and stratification. *Pediatrics.* 2003;111(6 pt 1):1416-21.

[2] Grönroos MH, Bolme P, Winiarski J, et al. Long-term renal function following bone marrow transplantation. *Bone Marrow Transplant.* 2007;39 (11):717-23.

[3] Klaassen I, Neuhaus TJ, Mueller-Wiefel DE, et al. Antenatal oligohydramnios of renal origin: long-term outcome. *Nephrol. Dial Transplant.* 2007;22 (2):432-9.

[4] Coresh J, Selvin E, Stevens LA, et al. Prevalence of chronic kidney disease in the United States. *JAMA.* 2007;298(17):2038-47.

[5] Furth SL, Cole SR, Moxey-Mims M, et al. Design and methods of the Chronic Kidney Disease in Children (CKiD) prospective cohort study. *Clin. J. Am. Soc. Nephrol.* 2006;1(5):1006-15.

[6] Lewis J, Greene T, Appel L, et al. A comparison of iothalamate-GFR and serum creatinine-based outcomes: acceleration in the rate of GFR decline in the African American Study of Kidney Disease and Hypertension. *J. Am. Soc. Nephrol.* 2004;15 (12):3175-83.

[7] Wong H, Mylrea K, Feber J, et al. Prevalence of complications in children with chronic kidney disease according to KDOQI. *Kidney Int.* 2006;70(3):585-90.

[8] Roderick P, Willis NS, Blakeley S, et al. Correction of chronic metabolic acidosis for chronic kidney disease patients. *Cochrane Database Syst. Rev.* 2007 Jan 24;(1):CD001890.

[9] Filler G, Mylrea K, Feber J, et al. How to define anemia in children with chronic kidney disease? *Pediatr. Nephrol.* 2007; 22(5):702-7.

[10] Salusky IB, Kuizon BG, Jüppner H. Special aspects of renal osteodystrophy in children. *Semin. Nephrol.* 2004;24(1):69-77.

[11] Sedman AB, Miller NL, Warady BA, et al. Aluminum loading in children with chronic renal failure. *Kidney Int.* 1984;26(2):201-4.

[12] Salusky IB, Goodman WG. Cardiovascular calci-fication in end-stage renal disease. *Nephrol. Dial Transplant.* 2002;17(2):336-9.

[13] Parekh RS, Flynn JT, Smoyer WE, et al. Improved growth in young children with severe chronic renal insufficiency who use specified nutritional therapy. *J. Am. Soc. Nephrol.* 2001;12 (11):2418-26.

[14] Ruley EJ, Bock GH, Kerzner B, et al. Feeding disorders and gastroesophageal reflux in infants with chronic renal failure. *Pediatr. Nephrol.* 1989; 3(4):424-9.

[15] Seikaly MG, Salhab N, Warady BA, et al. Use of rhGH in children with chronic kidney disease: lessons from NAPRTCS. *Pediatr. Nephrol.* 2007;22 (8):1195-201.

[16] Duquette PJ, Hooper SR, Wetherington CE, et al. Brief report: intellectual and academic functioning in pediatric chronic kidney disease. *J. Pediatr. Psychol.* 2007;32(8):1011-7.

[17] Goldstein SL, Gerson AC, Furth S. Health-related quality of life for children with chronic kidney disease. *Adv. Chronic Kidney Dis.* 2007;14(4):364-9.

[18] Warady BA, Bunchman TE. An update on peritoneal dialysis and hemodialysis in the pediatric population. *Curr. Opin. Pediatr.* 1996;8(2): 135-40.

[19] No authors listed. Clinical practice recommendation 8: vascular access in pediatric patients. *Am. J. Kidney Dis.* 2006;48(Suppl 1):S274-6.

[20] Davis ID, Bunchman TE, Grimm PC, et al. Pediatric renal transplantation: indications and special considerations. A position paper from the Pediatric Committee of the American Society of Transplant Physicians. *Pediatr. Transplant.* 1998;2 (2):117-29.

[21] United States Renal Data System, USRDS 2005 *Annual Data Report:* Atlas of End-Stage Renal Disease in the United States, National Institutes of Health: Table 6b, National Institute of Diabetes and Digestive and Kidney Diseases, Bethesda, MD, 2005.

[22] Bunchman TE. Compliance in pediatric transplant. *Pediatr. Transplant.* 2000;4(3):165-9.

In: Adolescence and Chronic Illness
Editors: H. Omar et al.

ISBN: 978-1-60876-628-4
© 2010 Nova Science Publishers, Inc.

Chapter 19

CHRONIC KIDNEY DISEASE AND QUALITY OF LIFE

*Jane Anne Smith and Stefan G. Kiessling**

Department of Pediatrics, Division of Nephrology, University of Kentucky, Lexington, United States of America.

ABSTRACT

Chronic disease can impair physical and cognitive function of individuals and lead to a decrease in the quality of life and disability. Decades ago, when treatment options to support children with chronic kidney disease were limited, before forms of renal replacement therapy including organ transplantation were available, the prognosis of advanced renal disease was grave. Even though the mortality rate remains high, the long-term survival rate for children has improved dramatically due to medical care advances. As the outcome continues to improve, a solid interest in disease and treatment associated morbidities and quality of life including psychosocial consequences has developed. The effect of treatment and disease related changes in child's quality of life, including disability, remain significant but might improve as we learn to understand better the involved factors. The effects on quality of life and perception of the degree of disability vary significantly, depending on the stage of kidney disease, age of the child, and support system. Quality of life, including disability, can be divided into three major domains: physical, cognitive, and psychosocial, with a variety of important sub domains that have to be assessed individually. Overall, very little data are available with regard to the perception of disability by the affected patients and their caregivers. This chapter tries to review comprehensively the etiologic factors of renal disease in children with the associated medical implications. The goal is to provide an overview of changes in quality of life that are related to the various stages of advanced renal disease in children and adolescents.

---

* *Correspondence:* Stefan G Kiessling, MD, Assistant Professor of Pediatrics University of Kentucky Children's Hospital, 740 South Limestone Street, Lexington, KY 50536 United States. Tel: 859-257-1552; Fax: 859-257-7799; E-mail: skies2@email.uky.edu

ABBREVIATIONS

NAPRTCS   North American Pediatric Renal Trials and Collaborative Study
QOL   Quality of life
HRQOL   Health related quality of life
ESRD   End stage renal disease
CKD   Chronic Kidney Disease

INTRODUCTION

Chronic kidney disease (CKD) in children is overall quite rare compared with adults. The impact for families and children living with a chronic illness has an enormous effect on daily life routines. The condition affects not only the mental and physical health of the child but also the entire support system, commonly parents. Normal function of the kidney is of extreme importance especially during the first two decades of life to allow for transition into a normal adulthood. Even though one primarily associates the kidney with water and solute balance, normal kidney function is necessary to maintain homeostasis in a variety of other body functions. Each child goes through two very vulnerable phases, infancy and puberty; in which the presence of normal kidney function is crucial for normal physical and cognitive development. Depending on the stage and type of underlying kidney disease, the daily routine of the family and child is different from healthy individuals. Unfortunately, to date, very little research has been done to assess the impact of chronic renal disease on the quality of life (QOL) in children. Even fewer data exist looking at the degree of objective and subjective disability induced by or associated with chronic renal failure, end-stage renal disease, and transplantation as somewhat separate, although connected entities. A large study by Rosenkranz et al [1] has shown the reported percentage of disabilities to be as high as 29% in children.

Children with chronic renal failure and renal transplants deal with multiple factors that can have an impact on their QOL. These factors include frequent physicians visits, sometimes with several providers; the need to routinely take multiple oral medications; and receiving injections like growth hormone or erythro-poietin. Once the disease has progressed to an advanced point and the decision to start dialysis is made, life changes even more with now the need to be connected to a machine daily with peritoneal dialysis, or at least three times per week with hemodialysis. Children receiving renal replacement therapy in the form of dialysis are dependent on a machine and probably experience the most significant disease impact when one defines disability as a condition that interferes with the person's ability to carry on his or her normal pursuits.

As for the provider, either general practitioner or specialist, who sees the child and the family for a short period of time in the office to assess medical needs, it is often easy to forget how demanding and challenging it is to live with chronic renal disease and how different life can be from what one perceives as normal.

Children who receive a kidney transplant continue to be medically fragile with ongoing extensive surveillance to optimize graft function and prevention or minimization of loss of graft function, which can be a silent process. The use of immunosuppressive medication and the related possible side effects, especially risk for infection, remain major concerns.

Spectrum of Kidney Diseases in Children and Adolescents

The etiologic factors leading to kidney disease in children are quite different from those seen in the adult population. Whereas acquired and sometimes preventable diseases like diabetes and hypertension are the leading causes of renal insufficiency in adults, congenital abnormalities of the urologic and nephrologic system or acquired diseases for which there is no prevention, dominate in children. Additionally, the incidence of chronic renal disease in children is much lower compared with adults, with an estimated number of 1.5 to 3 per million among children younger than 16 years of age [2].

The North American Pediatric Renal Trials and Collaborative Study (NAPRTCS) [3] established in 1987 is the largest registry of children in North America. The NAPRTCS includes more than 15,000 children divided into three categories: chronic renal failure, dialysis, and renal transplantation. The most recent report published in 2006 showed that renal disease is divided into five major categories:

a   Obstructive uropathy
b   Renal aplasia, dysplasia or hypoplasia
c   Reflux nephropathy
d   Focal segmental glomerulosclerosis
e   Polycystic kidney disease

These categories comprise almost 60% of all children with chronic renal disease. Other diagnoses include chronic or familial glomerulonephritis, hemolytic-uremic syndrome, or cystinosis, and each of those represent less than 3% of the total number of enrolled children. The degree of complexity of renal disease varies depending on the time of diagnosis and the underlying etiology. Children with primary renal disease are mostly managed by a team led by the pediatric nephrologist, whereas patients with associated urologic abnormalities, like posterior urethral valves, always require the expertise of a pediatric urologist to optimize care and outcomes, starting at the time of diagnosis until after successful renal transplantation. The NAPRTCS report from 2006 [3] also showed a gender distribution of 64% male versus 36% female, which is mainly due to the increased incidence of obstructive uropathy in male children. The majority of children enrolled are White (61%) with 18.8% African-Americans and 13.7% of Hispanic background.

Issues Related to Chronic Renal Failure

Chronic renal failure is commonly defined as an irreversible loss of kidney function (usually after a period greater than three months) with a glomerular filtration rate (GFR) of less than 75ml/min/1.73m [2]. Most body functions provided by the kidney are affected to a lesser degree until the GFR drops below 30ml/min/1.73m [2]. Chronic kidney disease is divided into the five categories, including end-stage kidney disease (stage V), depending on the severity and associated treatment modalities.

The kidneys are involved in a variety of important bodily functions. Loss of normal, healthy kidney tissue will affect several areas:

- Sodium and water balance as well as clearance of metabolic waste products; decline in renal function might lead to volume loading and azotemia with progression to full metabolic syndrome if left untreated
- Production of erythropoietin, stimulating bone marrow to produce red blood cells and prevention of anemia
- Homeostasis of calcium and phosphate, important for bone health and growth, with the potential for metabolic bone disease and growth deficits
- Growth related to involvement with the growth hormone axis; advanced renal disease can lead to growth failure if unrecognized and left untreated
- Normal function of the cardiovascular system; chronic and end stage renal disease are frequently associated with hypertension, potentially leading to cardiovascular dysfunction, one of the major disabling co-morbidities associated with a high morbidity and mortality rate
- Cognitive development and psychosocial adaptation; advanced renal dysfunction can lead to cognitive delay and behavioral changes. This can alter the patients academic potential and may affect employment and relationships in adulthood

Physical Health Aspects in Chronic Renal Failure

Normal kidney function is important to guarantee optimal physical health with progressive loss of renal function leading to a variety of physical health deficiencies. The previous paragraph provided an overview of the general aspects of loss of kidney function. The next two paragraphs will focus on the most important areas in a more detailed fashion.

A study by Fadrowski et al [4] recently reported a parent observed decline in health related quality of life (HRQOL) in adolescents with progressive decrease in glomerular filtration rate. As kidney function continues to decline, increased intervention becomes necessary to optimize individual care needs and hopes to improve the overall outcome for the child. Fortunately, significant progress has been made over the past few decades. Currently, several medications are available that at least partially compensate for the loss of functions related to kidney disease. Growth deficit is one of the major concerns of providers involved in the care of children with CKD. Several factors, including nutrition, metabolic acidosis, renal osteodystrophy (secondary hyperparathyroidism) and abnormalities in the growth hormone axis, play a very important role in the etiology of deficient growth. One intervention with a major impact was the start of the use of recombinant human growth hormone (rhGH) significantly increasing the final height of the child and allowing for catch-up growth, especially in pre-pubertal children [5].

Reviewing NAPRTCS study data from the time of initiation in 1987 to the early 2000s, significant progress has been made in improving the height standard deviation scores (SDS) for children at the time they receive a kidney transplant. Nevertheless, growth in children with chronic renal disease remains suboptimal despite aggressive interventions [6]. A recent review of NAPRTCS data by Seikaly et al [7] showed that younger children with a more advanced decline in GFR at the time of data entry had the highest risk for significant growth deficit. Ethnicity, underlying diagnosis, and remaining renal function are independent variables correlating with decreased height. Unfortunately, not all children are compliant with growth hormone injections. Currently, rhGH is available only in a short acting form that requires daily injections. This may at times be difficult for the child to tolerate as induced pain interferes with the child's well being. Nevertheless, the importance of optimizing growth in children with renal disease was just recently again documented as physical health has been reported to be improved with increased height in adolescents [4].

Similar to medication compliance, the optimal adherence to a restricted diet (low in phosphorus, sodium, and potassium) is also difficult to achieve as it excludes a large number of food items found in the average western diet. Children with CKD frequently crave milk products and fast food, as well as other items consumed by healthy peers and family members but not allowed to them. This state of affairs might be subjectively viewed as having a major impact on QOL.

Another area of concern is CKD-related anemia and the effects on QOL. Anemia has a known impact on exercise tolerance, the ability to complete daily activities, school performance, and sleep. The prevention and treatment of anemia, according to the Kidney Disease Outcomes Quality Initiative (KDOQI) guidelines, might minimize the effects of anemia on QOL even though few larger studies in the pediatric population have been performed and data are limited. One recently published study by Gerson et al [8] supported an increase in HRQOL (health related quality of life) in adolescents with chronic renal failure with correction of anemia in a caregiver/parent completed questionnaire.

Cardiovascular disease in children with CKD has more recently become a focus of concern, even though it has a much higher incidence in adults compared with the pediatric population. Cardiovascular disease is the major cause of mortality in adults with end stage renal disease (ESRD), but increasing evidence shows that the condition can have its origin in childhood. A recent comprehensive review by Mitsnefes [9] summarized the implications of involvement of the cardiovascular system in children with chronic renal failure. He points out that early detection and intervention of cardio-vascular pathology is the key to a decrease in the associated morbidity and mortality. However, little information is available assessing the effects of cardiovascular disease on QOL and disability in children with irreversible renal disease.

Psychosocial and Cognitive Health Aspects in Chronic Renal Failure

Advanced kidney disease starting in childhood has a profound effect on cognitive development and normal learning ability [10,11]. Several studies document that CKD in children is associated with significant neuro-cognitive and developmental delay in children. Some authors, however, have shown improved outcomes when the risk factors of malnutrition, medication side effects, inadequate dialysis, and delay in renal trans-plantation are minimized [12]. Regular school attendance is important to allow the child to learn and maximize the individual cognitive potential. School attendance is also a major concern for families and providers. Data from the NAPRTCS registry [3] showed that 59.9% of the 66.7% of school age children enrolled in the study attend school full-time; 2.6% attend school part time; and only 0.8% of children capable of attending full time school are not attending at all for unexplored reasons. The data are similar to the observed school attendance outside of the United States [1]. Although physical health aspects are reportedly affected by CKD in children and adolescents, the effects on emotion and psychosocial routines, including peer relationships, seem to be less significant [4].

Dialysis in Children and Adolescents

End-stage renal disease is defined as progression of chronic renal failure to a point, usually a GFR of less than 10cc/min/1.73m [2], at which point survival of the affected individual can no longer be guaranteed without initiation of renal replacement therapies, either a form of dialysis or a kidney transplant from a living or deceased donor. Considering the complexity of kidney disease and the involvement of this organ in such a variety of body functions, it comes as no surprise that the effects of CKD advanced to ESRD are extensive. Interestingly, due to the rather slow decline in renal function, children and adolescents do not always realize how much their health is affected until renal replacement therapy is initiated. End-stage renal disease is estimated to have a pediatric incidence of 1-2 per million with a prevalence of roughly 6,000 [11].

Physical Health Aspects in the Pediatric Dialysis Population

The initiation of renal replacement therapies in the form of either peritoneal dialysis or in-center/home hemo-dialysis is a crucial and life altering step for children with kidney disease. It is very important to realize that any form of dialysis provides only a fraction of what a normal functioning kidney is able to do, mainly clearing excess water and metabolic waste products. Therefore, supportive care and drug therapy used in children with chronic renal failure will continue more or less unchanged, focusing on the prevention of anemia, bone health, growth, and others. After the institution of dialysis, additional factors affecting the child's physical and cognitive health are introduced as the complexity of the disease increases. Peritoneal dialysis is commonly performed by connecting the patient (older children and teenagers can learn to do so themselves) to a peritoneal dialysis cycler for about 12 hours every night. Over the years, cyclers have become much smaller and more sophisticated. Because of this improvement, the patient and family are less stationary and more independent than in the past. Nevertheless, peritoneal dialysis still has significant effects on mobility and the daily life of the majority of patients.

Renal replacement therapy in the form of hemo-dialysis is most commonly performed in specialized centers within or close to a Children's Hospital. This location requires the patient and family to travel to the dialysis center three times per week. Under special circumstances, additional treatments are required to improve therapy, especially in situations when the oligo-anuric child is fluid overloaded. For hemodialysis to be performed successfully, most patients will need a surgical creation of an arterio-venous (AV) fistula—a connection of a vein and an artery building a blood reservoir, commonly on the upper non-dominant extremity. The net dialysis time for children is commonly between two and a half to four hours. This period does not include the time taken to travel to and from the dialysis center or the amount of time spent assessing the patient's vital signs; accessing the fistula; and re-infusing the blood as the patient comes off at the end of the treatment.

In addition to the time spent on each dialysis treatment, several other factors affect the ability of the child to follow a lifestyle one would consider normal. Most children on dialysis have the inability to produce normal amounts of urine and to clear metabolic waste. Due to the intensity and shortness of the dialysis treat-ments (more so with hemodialysis than with peritoneal dialysis), significant fluid and electrolyte changes occur over a rather short period. Such changes can lead to a number of side effects, including severe fatigue, cramping, nausea, and emesis; limiting the child's ability even outside of the dialysis treatment to function close to normally. Intermittent hospitalizations due to the complexity of dialysis in children and related compli-cations (peritonitis, hypotension, sepsis) also have a significant impact on the patient's daily routine.

One area of interest has been the effect of anemia on QOL. Anemic teenagers with CKD are reported by caregivers to have a lower HRQOL than non-anemic controls with kidney disease, indicating that anemia by itself has a significant impact on perception of disease. This affects a number of different areas, including decreased participation in school activities, decreased physical activities in general, and an increase in time burden from the child's illness [8]. These findings were more pronounced in the group of adolescents on dialysis versus the group of children who had received a kidney transplant.

Cardiovascular disease has become another major concern in children receiving dialysis. The major negative impact of cardiovascular disease in the dialysis population is (as in predialysis) the effect on the expected lifespan of the child. Mitsnefes et al [13] found that as many as 69% of children, at the initiation of dialysis, already had left ventricular hypertrophy indicating longer standing poorly controlled hyper-tension. The physical health aspects related to cardio-vascular disease remain largely unexplored so far.

Mental and Psychosocial Health in the Pediatric Dialysis Population

The rate of school attendance in children on dialysis is an ongoing concern. Despite the efforts to schedule hemodialysis to allow the child to attend as much school as possible, for the majority of patients, a significant time of renal replacement therapy is nevertheless spent during regular school hours. School attendance for children with chronic renal failure is overall good, but this situation changes significantly once the disease has progressed to the stage when dialysis is needed. According to NAPRTCS data from 2006 [3], 77% of children on peritoneal dialysis attended school full time, 9% part-time, and 5% of children capable of attending school did not do so at all. The results are even more concerning in the school age hemodialysis patient population with only 52% attending full time, 28% part time, and 7% capable of going to school but not attending at all.

Psychiatric disorders can have a major impact on the management of the patient with ESRD and their support system. Unfortunately, this aspect as it relates to CKD and ESRD has received little attention overall. A recent study by Bakr et at [14] found a high incidence (52.6%) of psychiatric disease in 38 children with chronic or end-stage renal disease. The leading diagnoses in this study included adjustment disorders and depression, both of which were far more prevalent in dialysis patients. These findings are very significant in that it is important for providers to recognize the presence of psychiatric disorders and institute therapy as necessary to minimize the impact of the disease on the QOL of the patient. A psychiatric evaluation is mandatory in case evidence of psychiatric pathology in a dialysis patient is apparent. In our institution, every dialysis patient and his/her family are offered a comprehensive mental health evaluation at the time dialysis is initiated. This approach has evolved from our experience that a large number of children, especially adolescents, benefit from early detection and intervention.

Disability and Quality of Life Related to Renal Transplantation

The outcome of pediatric renal transplantation has changed dramatically over the last years with a survival rate greater than 90% at 5 years post-transplantation. It was been well documented that renal transplantation is the best treatment for children who have progressed toward end-stage renal disease, regardless of the etiology. Nevertheless, it is important to remember that renal transplantation is also only a form of treatment for kidney disease and not a cure. Graft failure and loss of graft function over time will occur in virtually all patients. According to NAPRTCS data, nearly half of pediatric renal transplant recipients are teenagers or young adults at the time of transplantation. Whereas structural abnormalities of the urinary tract leading to end-stage kidney disease dominate the list of underlying etiologies in early childhood, the percentage of glomerulonephritis and focal segmental glomerulo-sclerosis (FSGS) is becoming much more prevalent in teenagers. Despite efforts to avoid prolonged treatment with dialysis and even preemptive transplantation without dialysis at all, a large number of children will end up receiving dialysis for a period of time. Given all the implications of dialysis as outlined in the previous paragraph, one might speculate that once a patient is successfully transplanted, the experienced degree of disability and perception on HRQOL might improve. However, a recent study in adult kidney transplant recipients has shown that a large number of patients feel at least partially disabled even after successful trans-plantation with a normal functioning graft [15]. The major area of concern in that study was the ability to work. In children, most studies report an improved assessed HRQOL in patients after renal transplant when compared with dialysis treatment [16].

Physical Health Aspects and Related QOL in Transplant Recipients

Several factors significantly affect the patient's ability to live a normal life after transplantation. It appears that the majority of patients report an improvement in QOL after transplantation, at least according the studies conducted in the adult population. One reason for this subjectively felt improvement in QOL might be that the time on dialysis; getting to and from the hemodialysis center, and the time connected to the cycler in peritoneal dialysis is no longer an issue. On the other hand, after transplantation, other factors affecting QOL are introduced into the daily routine. Even though late outcome studies favor transplantation over dialysis in children, transplantation is associated with the possibility of late morbidity as well, and disabling co-morbidity was reported by nearly half of transplant patients [17]. Aside from chronic bone disease, several problems were reported including headaches, tremor, and pruritus, all in direct relation to the solid organ transplant.

Most children and adolescents who have received a kidney transplant will require long term immunosup-pressive medications according to protocols that are individualized by each transplant center. The use of those drugs, usually a combination of two or three initially, bears the risk of medication-specific and other side effects, particularly the increased risk of infection. Infections can range anywhere from the increased incidence of minor viral infections to severe bacterial illnesses requiring prolonged hospitalization. Dhar-nidharka et al [18] reported the changed spectrum of post-transplant complications as infections now dominate over acute rejection episodes according to his NAPRTCS review from 2004.

Height deficit remains a major problem in children with advanced renal failure. NAPRTCS data show that over the years, significant improvement has been made in decreasing the height deficit at the time of initial transplantation. Still, overall growth improvement remains poor after renal transplantation. Younger children show some catch-up growth after transplan-tation, whereas teenagers tend to grow linearly along their percentile curve.

In our experience, parents and older patients often focus on renal transplantation as an endpoint to their kidney disease and become quite frustrated over the intensity and necessity of the post-transplant follow-up regimen. Physical examinations, careful review of each interval history, along with changes in blood work (which can be quite subtle) are key to the diagnosis of transplant rejection, organ dysfunction, and infection. This requires frequent office visits to detect abnormalities early, to review trends, and to minimize the risk for changes to be overlooked. Multiple trips to the office, especially during the first few months after trans-plantation, can take significant portions of time out of one's schedule and does not come anywhere close to allowing for what is considered a normal daily routine. This certainly decreases the chance for the individual to function as "normal" in major life activities, as defined by the American Disability Association, and might be regarded as a disability. Nevertheless, it appears that the effects of renal transplantation on health status in children are positive overall, at least in subjective reports. A small study by Krmar et al [19] that included 17 patients transplanted during an average age of 12.2 years and followed for more than 10 years showed that the majority (59%) were completely satisfied with their health status.

Psychosocial and Mental Health Aspects in the Renal Transplant Recipient

End stage renal disease in children, treated either with dialysis or by renal transplantation, can have a profound impact on quality of life and psychosocial outcome. Given improved survival of children with ESRD, the focus is shifting more toward the evaluation of the long term outcomes of these patients related to physical, cognitive and psychosocial health, even though the overall number of studies is still low. It appears that the impact of dialysis started in childhood or undergoing transplantation might not necessarily be associated with a significant difference in outcome from a pychosocial perspective. Adult follow-up data from the Dutch LERIC study (Late physical, social, and psychological Effects of Renal Insufficiency in Children) showed a statistically significant difference in involuntary unem-ployment rate in adults independent of dialysis or transplant status in former children with ESRD [20]. As outlined in the previous section, renal disease can have a significant impact on neurocognitive function even though over the years we have learned that the severity might not be as dramatic as initially reported [21]. Risk factors for decreased cognitive function include the age of onset of ESRD, time spent living with ESRD, as well as the educational level of the caregiver [22]. In a comprehensive review by Qvist et al [23], the authors comment on the dramatic improvement in QOL and psychosocial situation after transplantation in children suffering from ESRD. Nevertheless, even though some of the factors influencing psychosocial well-being will disappear after the new organ has been received, other factors become important and can affect the patients QOL. These factors include the fear of graft loss or disease recurrence, side effects of the new medications used to suppress the immunologic response to reject the graft, mental concerns about physical appearance, and financial issues [23]. In addition, such pre-transplantation factors as severity of disease, age of the child, coping strategies within the entire support system, and the presence of psychiatric disease among others affect the outcome after transplantation.

The Patient's Perspective

It seems self evident that the perception of the degree of disability one faces changes significantly with age, disease stage, and access to the health care system. Interestingly, a study by McKenna et al [24] showed that even though children with either chronic renal failure, on dialysis, or after renal transplantation rated their HRQOL lower than healthy controls, only the data of transplanted children reached statistical significance.

Sundaram et al [25] looked at adolescent renal transplant recipients and caregivers and assessed their HRQOL as a unique group going through the transition between late childhood and early adulthood. Whereas the patients themselves perceived their QOL (physical and psychological) with the exception of general health as similar to the reference population, caregivers described their children's physical, not psychological health, as poorer than the general population. Yet, the level of stress and abnormalities in daily life routine were reported to be high.

Growth has been associated with QOL with the concern that reduced height in children and adults has a negative effect [26]. A study by Busschbach et al [27] showed that a significant fraction of adult patients with chronic renal disease would have liked to be taller as a child and adult. However, the overall effect on QOL, compared with healthy short controls and sampling from the general population, was not significantly different. Another very important observation was that individuals on dialysis expressed a much higher time trade-off (percentage of years of life compared with the total expected years one would be willing to give up for living free of all symptoms associated with dialysis or a transplant) compared with patients after renal trans-plantation (47% vs. 15%). This finding might indicate that the QOL is much more negatively affected during the time on dialysis compared to the time one lives with a renal transplant. One study by Qvist et al [28] looked at self-assessed QOL in school-age children who had received their first kidney transplant at a mean of seven years before the assessment. In the assessment of 17 domains, 9 showed significant differences (ability to concentrate, friends, breathing, school and hobbies, discomfort, elimination, anxiety, sleeping and speech). Morel et al [29] assessed the long-term QOL (10 years after transplantation) in 57 patients who had undergone renal transplantation before the age of 18 years. Nine of those patients had not reached adulthood by the time they completed the questionnaire. Some of the received results were surprisingly positive with 95% of patients reporting that their health seldom or never interferes with family life. Only 3% were dissatisfied with the impact of their health on family. Fifty-five patients (96%) reported no interference of health with work life and only 3 patients (5%) were dissatisfied with their ability to perform at work, home or school.

Looking at the major categories of renal disease in children and adults, either acquired or congenital, one might speculate that children who have no health issues in the early stages of life have a different perception on HRQOL compared with children born with urologic or nephro-urologic disease. However, a recent study by Dodson et al [30] focused on HRQOL in children in their second decade of life with either congenital uronephro-logic disease or acquired primary renal disease and found overall no significant differences in mean scores.

The Caregiver's and Health Care Provider's Role

Access to a stable support system is crucial for the child with chronic renal disease to minimize the degree of disability experienced in a variety of areas. Healthcare providers, which primarily include the pediatric nephrologist, pediatrician, and adolescent health care specialist as well as nurses familiar with the child's complex medical issues, play a vital role in minimizing the degree of disability felt by providing resources for the family and patient. Optimal communication between the family and the provider team seems crucial to minimize stressors and burden of care, especially in the phase when disease complexity in maximal, which commonly is the time that the child spends on dialysis waiting for a kidney transplant. Watson [31] recommends support strategies in three distinct areas, in-hospital, home support, and in the broader community of each patient. One way to improve communication might be to assign each child to one specialized nurse providing longitudinal comprehensive care for the patient and family.

A rather unexplored area is the provider's perception on QOL and disability in families caring for children with chronic renal insufficiency (CRI) and unfortunately, very little studies that have aimed to explore this field are available. Some studies have looked at the provider perception in children with other chronic diseases [32,33]. Even though those studies might not allow drawing conclusions about the general perception of QOL from a provider perspective (given the limitations mentioned by the authors), pain/ discomfort and emotion were rated lower by treating physicians than by parents. Perhaps larger prospective studies should be conducted to assess better the effect of the health care provider team on QOL and disability in children and adolescents.

Taking care of a child with chronic disease can be associated with significant psychosocial stress factors. Studies show the family support system to be very important to balance stressors induced by CKD and that the long-term outcome of the patients with a stable support system are comparable with healthy peers [34]. A recent report by Tsai et al [35] had supporting evidence of a higher prevalence of depression in providers of children on peritoneal dialysis. Even though it seems somewhat intuitive, how and if this affects the QOL of the patient remains to be investigated. Somewhat surprisingly, there seems to be a disagreement in the perception of QOL in children with chronic disease by their providers and parents (who see a more significant impact), which does not change even after a longer relationship has been established [32,33].

Future Directions

The optimal management of children and adolescents with advanced kidney disease requires the involvement and expertise of a team of individuals, including the family, the primary care physician, and the pediatric nephrologist, urologist, nurse, dietician, and social worker. It is imperative that every member of the team understands the consequences of the disease and the implications for QOL, including the degree of disability felt by the patient and family on a daily basis.

In the health care setting, the primary focus of CKD in children is on the patient and the kidney disease related medical problems. There is limited time for a comprehensive assessment of QOL related issues. In addition, most providers have received limiting training on how to approach those issues. Even though the numbers of studies looking at overall QOL and HRQOL of the patient and caregiver have increased, the reality is that we still know little about the optimal assessment. We have learned so far that each comprehensive interval assessment should include the medical issues related to renal disease (treating anemia, optimizing growth, minimizing medication side effects); a cognitive and behavior health assessment of the patient and the caregiver; an assessment of the associated quality of life and how it could be improved. In clinical reality, this assessment is often difficult to do, as it requires a great deal of time and a solid support system that is not always readily available. As outlined by Goldstein et al [36], an integrated psychosocial assessment is especially important to optimize the transition from the pediatric to the adult patient and to maximize individual potential. Helping families and patients gain independence and providing resources might lead to empowerment maximizing individual potential.

Easier access to resources might lead to a decrease of additional stressors by increasing family and patient support. Examples include help with transportation; improved communication with the patient, the family and local providers; financial help to pay for medications; or dialysis on the weekends to avoid missed time from school. Improved assessment and understanding of the significant effects of chronic disease on quality of life, which can be affected to the level of disability, in the patient as well as the provider might improve the outcome.

CONCLUSIONS

Chronic kidney disease in children and adolescents significantly changes day-to-day life and limits the individual's ability to function comparable to age-related and accepted norms. The decrease in kidney function has numerous significant effects on body health, including growth and altered bone homeostasis, anemia, nutrition and appetite, with a decrease in overall physical well being. Chronic kidney disease and its treatment effects can lead to alterations in body image interfering with QOL, especially in teenagers. Effects on cognitive function, psychosocial well being, and psychiatric illness have been reported, but the data are scarce and there are few long term follow-up studies. Changes to QOL and HRQOL can be drastic and are frequently not the main focus of care as the assessment is time consuming and complex and requires a team of providers experienced in those areas. The perception of the degree of disability varies with the stage of kidney disease and each individual: patient, parent, and provider have different experiences. It remains important to re-assess continuously the burden of disability and the effects on overall QOL experienced by each patient and their support system. Doing so will possibly improve patient outcomes and allow children with kidney disease a chance to have some normalcy in their lives, to live a life as close to accepted normal standard as possible.

The healthcare team should always remain aware of the complexity of factors altering QOL, strive to assess comprehensively and reduce those factors, and to maximize the child's/adolescent's individual potential. This appears to be especially important in teenagers to allow a smooth transition to become productive adult citizens. Despite the improvement in supportive care and outcome of children and adolescents with all stages of CKD, a major area where data is sparse is the assessment of the QOL and the degree of disease- and therapy-related disabilities. It will be important to look at the physical, cognitive, and psychosocial health aspects in children with CKD in larger studies and to increase the pool of long-term follow-up data to improve care for children and adolescents in these areas.

REFERENCES

[1] Rosenkranz J, Bonzel KE, Bulla M, Michalk D, Offner G, Reichwald-Klugger E, et al. Psychosocial adaptation of children and adolescents with chronic renal failure. *Pediatr. Nephrol.* 1992;6:459-63.

[2] Fogo AB. Pathophysiology of progressive renal disease. In: Avner ED HW, Niaudet P: *Pediatric Nephrology,* 5th ed. Philadelphia: Lippincott Williams Wilkins 2004:1269-90.

[3] North American Pediatric Renal Transplant Co-operative Study Annual Report. *renal tranplanta-tion, dialysis, chronic renal insufficiency*. Rockville, MD, 2006.

[4] Fadrowski J, Cole SR, Hwang W, Fiorenza J, Weiss RA, Gerson A, et al. Changes in physical and psychosocial functioning among adolescents with chronic kidney disease. *Pediatr. Nephrol.* 2006; 21:394-9.

[5] Seikaly MG, Salhab N, Warady BA, Stablein D. Use of rhGH in children with chronic kidney disease: lessons from NAPRTCS. *Pediatr. Nephrol.* 2007;22:1195-204.

[6] Fine RN. Management of growth retardation in pediatric recipients of renal allografts. *Nat. Clin. Pract. Nephrol.* 2007;3:318-24.

[7] Seikaly MG, Salhab N, Gipson D, Yiu V, Stablein D. Stature in children with chronic kidney disease: analysis of NAPRTCS database. *Pediatr. Nephrol.* 2006;21:793-9.

[8] Gerson A, Hwang W, Fiorenza J, Barth K, Kaskel F, Weiss L, et al. Anemia and health-related quality of life in adolescents with chronic kidney disease. *Am. J. Kidney Dis.* 2004;44:1017-23.

[9] Mitsnefes MM. Cardiovascular complications of pediatric chronic kidney disease. *Pediatr. Nephrol.* 2008;23:27-39.

[10] Broyer M, Le Bihan C, Charbit M, Guest G, Tete MJ, Gagnadoux MF, et al. Long-term social out-come of children after kidney transplantation. *Transplantation.* 2004;77:1033-7.

[11] Gerson AC, Butler R, Moxey-Mims M, Wentz A, Shinnar S, Lande MB, et al. Neurocognitive outcomes in children with chronic kidney disease: Current findings and contemporary endeavors. *Ment. Retard. Dev. Disabil. Res. Rev.* 2006;12:208-15.

[12] Qvist E, Pihko H, Fagerudd P, Valanne L, Lamminranta S, Karikoski J, et al. Neurodevelopmental outcome in high-risk patients after renal transplantation in early childhood. *Pediatr. Transplant.* 2002;6:53-62.

[13] Mitsnefes M, Ho PL, McEnery PT. Hypertension and progression of chronic renal insufficiency in children: a report of the North American Pediatric Renal Transplant Cooperative Study (NAPRTCS). *J. Am. Soc. Nephrol.* 2003;14:2618-22.

[14] Bakr A, Amr M, Sarhan A, Hammad A, Ragab M, El-Refaey A, et al. Psychiatric disorders in children with chronic renal failure. *Pediatr. Nephrol.* 2007;22:128-31.

[15] Slakey DP, Rosner M. Disability following kidney transplantation: the link to medication coverage. *Clin. Transplant.* 2007;21:224-8.

[16] Goldstein SL, Gerson AC, Goldman CW, Furth S. Quality of life for children with chronic kidney disease. *Semin. Nephrol.* 2006;26:114-7.

[17] Groothoff JW. Long-term outcomes of children with end-stage renal disease. *Pediatr. Nephrol.* 2005;20:849-53.

[18] Dharnidharka VR, Stablein DM, Harmon WE. Post-transplant infections now exceed acute rejection as cause for hospitalization: a report of the NAPRTCS. *Am. J. Transplant.* 2004;4:384-9.

[19] Krmar RT, Eymann A, Ramirez JA, Ferraris JR. Quality of life after kidney transplantation in children. *Transplantation.* 1997;64:540-1.

[20] Groothoff JW, Grootenhuis MA, Offringa M, Stronks K, Hutten GJ, Heymans HS. Social consequences in adult life of end-stage renal disease in childhood. *J. Pediatr.* 2005;146:512-7.

[21] Rotundo A, Nevins TE, Lipton M, Lockman LA, Mauer SM, Michael AF. Progressive encephalo-pathy in children with chronic renal insufficiency in infancy. *Kidney Int.* 1982;21:486-91.

[22] Brouhard BH, Donaldson LA, Lawry KW, Mc Gowan KR, Drotar D, Davis I, et al. Cognitive functioning in children on dialysis and post-transplantation. *Pediatr. Transplant.* 2000;4:261-7.

[23] Qvist E, Jalanko H, Holmberg C. Psychosocial adaptation after solid organ transplantation in children. *Pediatr. Clin. North Am.* 2003;50: 1505-19.

[24] McKenna AM, Keating LE, Vigneux A, Stevens S, Williams A, Geary DF. Quality of life in children with chronic kidney disease-patient and caregiver assessments. *Nephrol. Dial. Transplant.* 2006;21: 1899-905.

[25] Sundaram SS, Landgraf JM, Neighbors K, Cohn RA, Alonso EM. Adolescent health-related quality of life following liver and kidney transplantation. *Am. J. Transplant.* 2007;7:982-9.

[26] Sandberg DE, Brook AE, Campos SP. Short stature: a psychosocial burden requiring growth hormone therapy? *Pediatrics.* 1994;94:832-40.

[27] Busschbach JJ, Rikken B, Grobbee DE, De Charro FT, Wit JM. Quality of life in short adults. *Horm. Res.* 1998;49:32-8.

[28] Qvist E, Narhi V, Apajasalo M, Ronnholm K, Jalanko H, Almqvist F, et al. Psychosocial adjust-ment and quality of life after renal transplantation in early childhood. *Pediatr. Transplant.* 2004;8: 120-5.

[29] Morel P, Almond PS, Matas AJ, Gillingham KJ, Chau C, et al. Long-term quality of life after kidney transplantation in childhood. *Transplanta-tion.* 1991;52:47-53.

[30] Dodson JL, Diener-West M, Gerson AC, Kaskel FJ, Furth SL. An assessment of health related quality of life using the child health and illness profile-adolescent edition in adolescents with chronic kidney disease due to underlying urological disorders. *J. Urol.* 2007;178: 660-5.

[31] Watson AR. Strategies to support families of children with end-stage renal failure. *Pediatr. Nephrol.* 1995;9:628-31.

[32] Janse AJ, Sinnema G, Uiterwaal CS, Kimpen JL, Gemke RJ. Quality of life in chronic illness: perceptions of parents and paediatricians. *Arch. Dis. Child.* 2005;90:486-91.

[33] Janse AJ, Uiterwaal CS, Gemke RJ, Kimpen JL, Sinnema G. A difference in perception of quality of life in chronically ill children was found between parents and pediatricians. *J. Clin. Epidemiol.* 2005; 58:495-502.

[34] Soliday E, Kool E, Lande MB. Psychosocial adjustment in children with kidney disease. *J. Pediatr. Psychol.* 2000;25:93-103.

[35] Tsai TC, Liu SI, Tsai JD, Chou LH. Psychosocial effects on caregivers for children on chronic peritoneal dialysis. *Kidney Int.* 2006;70:1983-7.

[36] Goldstein SL, Gerson AC, Furth S. Health-related quality of life for children with chronic kidney disease. *Adv. Chronic Kidney Dis.* 2007;14: 364-9.

PART XII. PREGNANCY AND SEXUALITY

In: Adolescence and Chronic Illness
Editors: H. Omar et al.

ISBN: 978-1-60876-628-4
© 2010 Nova Science Publishers, Inc.

Chapter 20

PREGNANCY AND YOUNG WOMEN WITH DISABILITIES

Kathy Sheppard-Jones[*,1]*, Harold Kleinert*[1]*, Cindy Paulding*[1] *and Christina Espinosa*[2]

[1] Human Development Institute, University of Kentucky.
[2] Special Education and Rehabilitation Counseling Department,
University of Kentucky, Lexington, Kentucky, United States of America.

ABSTRACT

The experience of pregnancy and disability has been referred to as "a double dose of disequilibrium". Pregnancy, on its own, can result in profound physical and psychological changes for adolescents and young women. The impact that the pregnancy has on a disability (and of disability on a pregnancy) necessitates the implementation of planning and appropriate supports. This chapter is a review of literature around family planning for adolescents and young women with disabilities. Barriers to reproductive health, including physical and societal inaccessibility, are discussed. A historical perspective is provided, along with considerations around the following stages of family planning: pre-conception, pregnancy, labor, and delivery, and post-partum care. Whereas different disabilities and syndromes can bring unique challenges, an interdisciplinary team approach can be used to promote healthy and informed family planning for adolescents and young women with disabilities. The practitioner who has been afforded continuing education opportunities, who has a desire to learn about the individual impact of a disability on a pregnancy, and who shows unconditional positive regard when working with young patients with disabilities will facilitate successful outcomes.

---

[*] *Correspondence:* Kathy Sheppard-Jones, PhD, Human Development Institute, University of Kentucky, 210 Mineral Industries Building, Lexington KY 40506-0051 United States. Tel: 859-257-8104; FAX: 859-323-1901; E-mail: Kathy.sheppard-jones@uky.edu

INTRODUCTION

The health disparities faced by young women with disabilities mirror the disparities faced by people with disabilities across many of life's domains. Women with disabilities are at a disadvantage in terms of employment, education, income, and community participation [1-3]. These overall discrepancies in quality of life are found in differences in medical care, and specifically with regard to reproductive care [4,5]. Diminished access to health care, lack of health promotion, and fewer disease prevention services can, in turn, result in decreased quality of health, as well as the introduction of secondary conditions [4]. Historically, women with disabilities have had decreased opportunities to conceive, bear children, and raise a family. Women with intellectual disabilities were being sterilized without consent well into the twentieth century [6,7], and countries around the world continue to violate the individuals' reproductive rights [7,8]. Women who did become pregnant were encouraged to abort the pregnancy. There were many reasons for this, from assumptions about lack of maternal instinct in women with disabilities to concern that a child would also have disabilities [9]. The common theme was a lack of understanding from professionals.

Currently, general practitioners report having discomfort when working with patients with disabilities [10]. The resulting negative attitudes are further heightened when the woman happens to have an intellectual disability. Other significant contributing factors toward negative attitudes included practitioners' perceptions of communication problems, lack of experience with people with disabilities, lack of time for consultation, and no training in the area of disability. Any of these concerns can result in the practitioner's conclusion that it will not be possible to conduct an examination or adequately support the person through the family planning process. Nearly one quarter of working-age adults with disabilities indicate that health care providers do not understand their disability [11]. Women with disabilities indicate that they are often refused health care because of their disability [5]. When using the health care system, women with disabilities report that the experience and interaction with the practitioner may be considered invalidating and highlight a lack of control on the part of the woman herself [12]. Practitioner training and education that addresses the health care needs of those with disabilities will go far in wiping out these misperceptions [13].

The Americans with Disabilities Act of 1990 prohibits discrimination in health care in the United States (US) and addresses physical accessibility [14]. Physical barriers that are disallowed by US law include anything that impedes a person's ability to access an establishment that may be visited by the public. Relevant examples include third-floor offices with no elevator, inaccessible examination rooms and wash rooms, lack of ramped entryways, and printed information that is not made available in alternate formats. However, physical barriers to appropriate medical care can be easier to eliminate than attitudinal ones. The final report of the National Study of Women with Physical Disabilities found that even when a gynecologist's office is physically accessible, the quality of care provided is not as good, particularly if the person has a more significant disability [15]. Attitudinal barriers can arise from a lack of knowledge or awareness of issues around safe transfer techniques, lack of people supports to aid in communication, or lack of awareness of disability and sexuality.

In fact, the very notion of females with disabilities considering sexual activity has been perceived as inappropriate by some practitioners. In a review by Valencia and Cromer [16], the risk behaviors of adolescents with chronic illnesses were examined. Although the authors anticipated that large-scale studies devised with the intent of supporting the hypothesis that adolescents with disabilities were less sexually active, in fact, the opposite was supported. This review showed that adolescents with chronic illnesses experienced increased risk behaviors, including sexual activity without contraception or an understanding of sexually transmitted diseases. Other studies echo the lack of information made available to young women with disabilities [5,15]. Further, in a comprehensive review by Rousso [9], adolescents with physical and intellectual disabilities were at a greater risk of becoming pregnant and subsequently dropping out of school.

For a young woman who is planning for her future and the future of her family, a physician must first recognize that experiences of young women with disabilities may be similar to or different from young women without disabilities. It is often expected that, either as a result of functional limitations or society's barriers, sexuality is hampered for youth with disabilities. For some young women with disabilities, the first visit to a gynecologist may be put off because of perceptions that sex and sexuality are not the "norm" for someone with a disability [15]. Reinforcing this belief, our society generally does not regard women with disabilities as a viable gynecological population, even though females with disabilities start to learn about sex around the same age as females who don't have disabilities [15]. The difference lies in the messages that these young women get from their families, communities, and social networks about sexuality and their role as sexual beings [22]. What is found is that, even though women with disabilities know of sex, they are not provided the resources related to contraception or family planning. In an interesting paradox, research shows that adolescents with disabilities are at greater risk for pregnancy [9]. Without adequate gynecological care, young women with disabilities may also not receive appropriate screening for health care conditions such as cervical or breast cancer, or instruction in such areas as breast-self examination [17,18].

Just as two young women will not have the same needs and priorities, young women with different disabilities have differing needs. Cognitive, physical, and psychiatric impairments may present different challenges for appropriate medical interventions. Although the knowledge base is increasing in this area, young women who are pregnant and disabled face additional issues as a direct result of their disability [1]. It is up to the treating physician to have adequate knowledge to advise young women of the real risks that may accompany pregnancy, as well as to dispel the myths that may arise from inaccurate perceptions shared by family, friends, service providers, and even the adolescent's religious community. Unfortunately, regardless of the type of impairment experienced, young women with disabilities may face resistance and conflict to the notion of sex and pregnancy [12,19].

INTELLECTUAL DISABILITIES

Adolescents and young women with intellectual disabilities represent a particularly vulnerable group, largely due to uncertainties around informed consent for sexual activity [18]. Supports needed to enhance outcomes are largely related to ensuring that the potential mother meets her nutritional and physical care needs during pregnancy and then has the supports to care for her newborn appropriately. Fears about labor and childbirth may be heightened until the young woman is able to understand better the process of women's health issues. This may be helped by using simple, straightforward language and multiple methods for learning (visual aids, role play, etc.) [20]. Also essential is that a woman with intellectual disabilities receives sufficient support in the care of her newborn, including feeding, infant stimulation, recognizing infant illnesses, and child safety. Hospital social workers and members of the new mother's interdisciplinary team can be especially effective in working with local and state developmental disabilities services to identify these supports before the woman leaves the hospital. Of course, when present, family members can also be a source of significant support, as they are for most women experiencing childbirth.

PHYSICAL DISABILITIES

Providers should be knowledgeable about sexuality and the impact of pregnancy and childbirth on the disabling condition. Can pregnancy exacerbate the disability? Will the continuing fetal development and enlargement impinge respiratory or cardiac function? Will birth through the birth canal be possible given the physical structure of the trunk and pelvic girdle? What are the postpartum implications? While the myriad of variable presentations can seem overwhelming, the patient can be an excellent resource on implications of her disability. It is the responsibility of the medical professional to have an understanding of the reproductive health needs for young women with disabilities. Areas to be addressed during family planning include pre-conception care, pregnancy, labor and delivery, and post-partum care.

Pre-Conception Care

Pre-conception care is correlated to improved pregnancy outcomes. Pre-conception is also the time to address screening and preventive services [17]. According to the Center for Research on Women with Disabilities, women with more significant physical disabilities receive less reproductive health care than non-disabled women [21]. When a young woman with a disability first accesses the reproductive health care system, physical accessibility is immediately addressed. Transportation to get to the appointment must be adequate. Accessible entryways and offices enable wheelchair users to participate fully at the medical visit. Examination tables that can be raised and lowered allow for transfers with or without assistance.

It is during the time of pre-conception care when practitioners dispel or solidify the perpetuation of disability stereotypes. This is the time when treatment options for care should be offered, as opposed to assuming that the young woman with a disability is an asexual being. For a young woman with a disability who is thinking about having a baby, many concerns should be addressed before conception, including medications, urologic health, physical structure (curvature of the spine, contractures), respiratory and cardiac capacity, and needed supports once the baby is born [22]. At this point, the practitioner must listen to the needs, wants and concerns of the patient and respond accordingly [23].

Pregnancy

With pregnancy and disability come various medical and psychosocial issues. Just because it occurs to a young woman with a disability, the pregnancy should not be considered unviable or unwanted [24]. As a whole, young pregnant women with disabilities may be considered a "high risk" group. This is not always the case and does not mean that pregnancy is contra-indicated [25]. Rather, care should be taken to ensure that potential complications are avoided or managed. Attention to skills needed by the new mother should be paid during pregnancy [24]. Some of the natural changes that women experience during the first trimester of pregnancy can indicate complications for a woman with a disability. As the pregnancy progresses, the risk of complications may also increase. For example, although weight gain is expected with the continuation of a pregnancy, added weight may interfere with the ability of the young woman with a disability to perform the activities of daily living, such as transferring to and from a wheelchair, keeping ones balance, or completing other tasks. A discussion may be needed about using a power wheelchair or scooter to ease the fatigue of pushing a manual chair. Secondary conditions are also a major concern [26]. For young women with mobility impairments, there must be a vigilant watch for pressure sores. A team approach, in conjunction with a physical and/or occupational therapist, can be used to determine if seating and positioning changes are needed to distribute pressure. Circulation problems can also be exacerbated as pregnancy progresses. Exercise, rest, and circulation-promoting stockings can reduce edema and improve blood flow. Smeltzer [27] provides an over-view of a variety of issues and implications that must be considered by a pregnant individual when a disability is also present.

One promising trend is that pregnant women with disabilities do access the health care system more often than do women without disabilities, but a study by Blackford and Richardson [23] showed that mothers with disabilities reported that they had received inadequate prenatal care, illustrating that quality and quantity are not synonymous. The women in this study felt that they were perceived as less than capable in terms of mothering and autonomy [23]. The literature on disability and pregnancy is expanding, but the experiences that are reflected indicate a healthcare system that is insensitive to the overall needs of young mothers with disabilities.

Labor and Delivery

Proper planning for labor and delivery can set the stage for a powerful and positive experience for both mother and baby. Labor and delivery classes can help the pregnant mother prepare for the same contingencies as all expecting mothers. The nature of the young woman's disability may necessitate additional supports to maximize knowledge gained from this experience (e.g., alternate formats of class materials, physically accessible class location, instructional aide). Participating in labor and delivery classes not only provides the patient with essential knowledge and practice for the birthing process but also "normalizes" her pregnancy experience and allows her to have the natural support of a peer group that is of such benefit to many women and their partners.

The nature of the young woman's disability may indicate the possibility for an early delivery. Planning for delivery, induction of labor, and circumstances that necessitate a caesarian section should all be discussed well before the anticipated delivery date. At the time of delivery, physical accessibility of the delivery room is a primary consideration.

Post-Partum

Recovery from labor and delivery may be increased for women with physical disabilities. For a new mother who will require additional supports in caring for their newborn, care must be taken to ensure that she retains control of the parenting activities, even if she is not physically involved in all respects. An assistive technology expert or occupational therapist may be able to provide assistance in ensuring that the woman's home is physically arranged to promote optimal care for the infant, while eliminating unnecessary physical strain in providing daily care. For example, the infant change table should be adjusted to a height easily accessible for the woman. This is also the time to ensure that present concerns around birth control and sexuality are addressed [28].

Table 1. Roles of interdisciplinary team

Team Member	Role
Primary care physician	Provide information related to women's health issues and the factors to consider in family planning and pregnancy. Discuss gynecologic issues and refer to OBGYN from an age appropriate time (i.e., at the same age in which most young women are referred). Regarding family planning, emphasize nutrition, weight control, smoking and alcohol cessation, and review medications.
Obstetrician	Provide information related to pregnancy and childbearing. Have adjustable examination tables available for the differing needs of women.
Anesthesiologist	Discuss the risks of anesthesia with each woman and develop an appropriate labor plan.
Neurologist	Consider bladder management issues as pregnancy progresses and other neurological implications as the pregnancy progresses.
Respiratory Therapist	Consider changes in respiratory capacity and function in the later stages of pregnancy and labor.
Psychiatrist	Discuss mobility and seating, provide modifications necessary to accommodate the needs of a woman throughout the stages of pregnancy.
Occupational Therapist	Discuss the changing physical requirements during pregnancy as well as post-delivery; devise strategies for how to accomplish those tasks associated with activities of daily living. Discuss assistive devices that can be used for self-care and infant care.
Physical Therapist	Consider mobility issues that might present with pregnancy.
Significant Other	Discuss relevant home and social issues that may be overlooked; provide support to the patient.
Speech language pathologist	Provide modifications necessary for the young woman to communicate with her health care providers.
Social Worker / Counselor	Provide postpartum considerations and locate community resources.
Assistive Technology Expert	Provide assistance in ensuring the woman's home is physically arranged to promote optimal care for the infant, and that assistive devices are identified to improve infant care, as well as other activities of daily living. Assist the mother in evaluating the additional mobility demands of transporting an infant, along with herself, including safe infant transport (car seats, strollers, etc.)

DISCUSSION

Practitioners are faced with a potential paradox when treating patients with disabilities. The goal of health promotion and disease prevention may initially seem an impossible challenge for a young woman with a disability. However, the mere presence of disability is not to be associated with a decreased health-related quality of life. The health-related impact that disability imposes on quality of life is an individualized experience. To be well and to flourish involve much more than one's objective level of health [29]. Therefore, the real value of disability is its meaning to the adolescent [30]. Consensus with this definition can bridge the gap between health and holistic views of quality of life [31].

Although no practitioner is expected to know everything about all disabilities and their potential impact on reproductive health, a willingness to learn must be present. Appropriate supports must also be provided to the practitioner, including adequate exam and consultation time, communication supports, and training in disability issues. A collaborative team approach can be implemented to provide comprehensive gynecological and obstetric care for young women with disabilities dependent upon the patients' specific wants, needs and disability (see table 1). The team approach is essential to ensuring that the related health conditions are adequately addressed in assisting young women with disabilities to have healthy pregnancies and appropriate aftercare for themselves and their newborn infants. Although practitioners cannot become experts in all matters related to disability and pregnancy, it is imperative to take the time to learn how pregnancy and birth can be successfully managed for the specific patients with disabilities that they do have. Also essential is that practitioners know how each member of the team contributes to ensuring a healthy outcome for the mother with a disability and her child.

A clear communication and promotion of decision-making by the young person with a disability are paramount to a positive family planning experience. This may mean making time to talk with the disabled child or adolescent about family planning options away from her family and service providers. The implicit and explicit messages that adolescents receive about sex and family planning put them more in the role of spectator than active participant. Support networks may knowingly, or unwittingly, perpetuate the myths that repress reproductive freedoms. Professionals in the health care system can take huge steps in eradicating such falsehoods. Pre-professional training, continuing education, and taking a person-centered approach that focuses on the uniqueness of the individual will ensure that the impact of the disability and of the potential pregnancy are considered before initiating a family. The mere presence of a disabling condition should not preclude the notion of a healthy pregnancy and delivery of a baby for a young woman with a disability.

REFERENCES

[1] Carty E, Conine T. Disability and pregnancy: A double dose of disequilibrium. *Rehabil. Nurs.* 1988; 13(2):85.

[2] United States Census Bureau. Census facts. National Council for Support of Disability Issues, 2005. Available: http://ncsd.org/census/census.htm. Accessed 30 October 2007.

[3] National Organization on Disability. NOD/harris survey of Americans with disabilities. New York: Author, 2000.
[4] United States Department of Health and Human Services. Disability and secondary conditions, Healthy people 2010. US Department of Health and Human Services, Office of Disease Prevention and Health Promotion, 2005. Available http://www.healthypeople.gov/default.htm. Accessed 30 October 2007.
[5] Kaplan C. Special issues in contraception: Caring for women with disabilities. *J. Midwifery Womens Health.* 2006;51(6):450.
[6] Diekema D. Involuntary sterilization of persons with mental retardation: An ethical analysis. *Ment. Retard. Dev. Disabil.* 2003; 9:21.
[7] Center for Reproductive Rights. Reproductive rights and women with disabilities. Center for Reproductive Rights, 2002. Available: http://www. reproductiverights.org. Accessed 27 October 2007.
[8] Servais L. Sexual health care in persons with intellectual disabilities. *Ment. Retard. Dev. Disabil. Res. Rev.* 2006;12:48.
[9] Rousso H. Strong proud sisters: *Girls and young women with disabilities.* Washington, DC: Center Women Policy Stud, 2001.
[10] Aulagnier M, Verger P, Ravaud J, Souville M, Lussault P, Garnier J, et al. General practitioners' attitudes towards patients with disabilities: The need for training and support. *Disabil. Rehabil.* 2005; 27(22):1343.
[11] United States Department of Health and Human Services. The 2005 surgeon general's call to action to improve the health and wellness of persons with disabilities: Calling you to action. US Department of Health and Human Services, Office of the Surgeon General, 2005. Available: http://www.surgeongeneral.gov/library/disabilities/calltoaction/whatitmeanstoyou.html. Accessed 27 October 2007.
[12] Hassouneh-Phillips D, McNeff E, Powers L, et al. Invalidation: A central process underlying mal-treatment of women with disabilities. *Women Health.* 2005;41(1):33.
[13] Center for Research on Women with Disabilities. Improving the health and wellness of women with disabilities: *A symposium to establish a research agenda,* Houston, TX: Baylor College Med, 2004.
[14] Americans with Disabilities Act of 1990. United States Public Law. 101-336. 104 Stat 327 § 12101. July 26, 1990.
[15] Nosek M, Howland C, Rintala D, et al. National study of women with physical disabilities: Final report. Center for Research on Women with Disabilities, Department of Physical Medicine and Rehabilitation. Baylor College of Medicine. *Sex Disabil.* 2001; 19(1):5.
[16] Valencia L, Cromer B. Sexual activity and other high-risk behaviors in adolescents with chronic illness: A review. *J. Pediatr. Adocesc. Gynecol.* 2000;13:53.
[17] Huff M. No need to specialize: Reproductive health is for all adolescents. *J. Pediatric Adolesc. Gynecol.* 2006;19(2):112.
[18] Sanders C, Boyd S, Kleinert H. Preservice health training modules (Version 1.0): *Carrie Case-For primary care providers-Women's healthcare.* Lexington, KY: Hum Dev Inst, Univ Kentucky, 2007.
[19] Prittentensky O. A ramp to motherhood: The experiences of mothers with physical disabilities. *Sex Disabil.* 2003;21(1):21.

[20] Carty E, Conine T, Riddell L, et al. Childbearing and parenting with a disability or chronic illness. *Midwifery Today.* 1993;28:17.

[21] Center for Research on Women with Disabilities: Improving the health and wellness of women with disabilities: *A symposium to establish a research agenda.* Houston TX: Center Res Women Disabil, Baylor College Med, 2004:1-10.

[22] Welner S. Pregnancy. In: *Welner S. Welner's guide to the care of women with disabilities.* Philadelphia: Lippincott Williams Wilkins, 2004: 209.

[23] Blackford K, Richardson H, Grieve S. Prenatal education for mothers with disabilities. *J. Adv. Nurs.* 2000;32(4):898.

[24] Welner S. Gynecologic care and sexuality issues for women with disabilities. *Sex Disabil.* 1997;15(1):33.

[25] Lipson J, Rogers J. Pregnancy, birth, and disability: Women's health care experiences. *Health Care Women Int.* 2000;21(1):11.

[26] Hershey L. Women with disabilities: Health, reproduction and sexuality. In: International encyclopedia of women: *Global women's issues and knowledge.* New York, Routledge, 2001:4-11.

[27] Smeltzer, S. Pregnancy in women with physical disabilities. *J. Obst. Gynecol. Neonat. Nurs.* 2007; 36(1):88.

[28] Grover S. Menstrual and contraceptive manage-ment in women with an intellectual disability. *Med. J. Aust.* 2002;176:108.

[29] Ryff C, Singer B. Interpersonal flourishing: A positive health agenda for the new millennium. *Pers. Soc. Psychol. Rev.* 2000;4(1):30.

[30] Coulter D. Health-related application of quality of life. In: Schalock R, ed. Quality of life: appli-cation to persons with disabilities. Washington, DC: *Am. Assoc. Ment. Retard.* 1997:95.

[31] Sheppard-Jones K. *Quality of life dimensions for adults with developmental disabilities.* Lexington KY: Univ Kentucky, 2002.

Chapter 21

DOWN SYNDROME AND SEXUALITY

Maria José Carvalho Sant'Anna[*,1], *Bruna Marques Bononi*[1],
André Chao Vasconcellos de Oliveira[1], *Tadeu Silveira Renattini*[1],
Carla Franchi Pinto[2], *Maria Lúcia Passarelli*[2],
Veronica Coates[1] *and Hatim A. Omar*[3]

[1] Adolescent Clinical Unit, Department of Pediatrics,
Santa Casa de São Paulo, Faculty of Medical Sciences, São Paulo, Brazil.
[2] Department of Pediatrics, Santa Casa de São Paulo,
Faculty of Medical Sciences, São Paulo, Brazil.
[3] Division of Adolescent Medicine, Department of Pediatrics,
University of Kentucky, Lexington, Kentucky, United States of America.

ABSTRACT

In recent years important gains and changes have been observed in the life of teenagers with Down syndrome (DS) with increased inclusion into society. This chapter will discuss adolescence and sexuality in teenagers with DS from a descriptive study of 50 patients with DS between the ages of 10 and 20 years. The mean age was 13.5 years, 50% females. 86% went to school with 62.2% in school for over six years. Of the patients that attended school, 60% went to special education school and only 10% read and wrote correctly. In evaluation of autonomy, 66% took shower, 78% performed their physiological needs, 77% intimate hygiene and 76% oral hygiene without help. 42% affirmed being able to do anything that is asked; 22% perform all tasks in the home; 10% felt they were incapable of doing anything and 4% used public transportation without help. 42% of the teenagers masturbated, 24% on a daily basis, 75% in private, and 25% in a public location. 42% had already kissed at a mean age of 12.9 years, mean age of the partner 16.1 years; 26.8% of these partners had DS. 82% found themselves attractive and 33% would not change anything in their appearance. We found that they presented normal development in the exercise of their sexuality, but with important difficulties in their autonomy and difficulties in school, needing careful interventions in order to make

---

[*] *Correspondence:* Maria José Carvalho Sant'Anna, MD, Rua Nuno Pinto 46, Jardim São Paulo, CEP-02045-030, São Paulo City, Brasil. Tel: (55+11) 69502508; Fax: (55+11) 69541577; E-mail:mjcsantanna@gmail.com

their social interaction the best possible. Their pubertal development was normal and they were satisfied with their body image with future perspectives of working, finding a partner and living a normal life getting married and having children.

INTRODUCTION

Teenagers with Down Syndrome (DS) need to be prepared for a life of limitations and possibilities. Important gains and changes have been observed in relation to these individuals and society in general is increasingly accepting and allowing their inclusion into community roles. The public is tending to see this deficiency as a natural diversity within humanity and with the advancement of the treatments devoted to chronic illnesses the life expectancy has greatly increased. Health professionals are now confronted with a new reality to provide health services for teenagers with DS and the challenge of adapting to the needs of these young adults.

As the care to special needs of these adolescents with intellectual disability improves, their quality of life improves as well, and at the same time that integration within a community structure offers great advantages, it should not be forgotten that there are also more risks, liberties and responsibilities. Therefore, during childhood and especially adolescence, it is necessary that they develop self-awareness, the ability to choose, criticize, and stimulate their own autonomy, to prepare for work, questions and acts about sexuality.

It is essential to remember that sexual desire is ever present, independent of the degree of mental/intellectual impairment. This discussion is usually handled with prejudice and discrimination, especially when dealing with patients with DS, causing various controversies. These young adults present a variety of manifestations in relation to sexuality and reproductive health, reflecting their stage of development, their experiences and circumstances of their lives. Masters and Johnson [1] also discussed the importance of recognizing that individuals with mental deficiencies differ in their ability in learning, independence, emotional stability and social abilities.

It is in this context of fear and uncertainties that health care providers (HCP) can help the teenager to develop. Often, the family is unable to answer all of the questions proposed by these individuals, offering answers that are many times incomplete or wrong. Therefore HCP should assume the role of counselor and friend, providing the necessary advice and guidance to his/her parents.

In this particular group, questions regarding sexuality (including pregnancy and contraception) are often overlooked. Several studies have demonstrated that in severely compromised patients, where social exile and negative self-image makes sexuality difficult, their actual sexuality is not different from common individuals. Sexuality is always present and may be expressed in its affective component (the feeling of good will), erotic (desire, excitement and pleasure) or affective-erotic (the association that provides a more genuine relationship).

The title of 'mentally deficient', almost entirely used indiscriminately, masks the differences and peculiarities of each case. Despite the fact that they differ in their learning capacities, independence, social stability and outlook on sexuality, almost all are able to understand some level of sexual knowledge and social behavior. The more compromised DS individuals have problems that are more centered in questions of hygiene and self-care, making it necessary most of the times, for example, to reduce or prevent menstrual flow.

There are still many beliefs and taboos in relation to the mentally challenged, ranging from being asexual to overly sexual and these people are often times treated as if they were children. The majority of the families assume an over-protective role, seeing and caring for these individuals as if they were infants and asexual. For the teenager with some type of mental limitation, the expected and progressive independence from the parents is delayed or even absent. Therefore, it is necessary that the process of transferring responsibilities should have its own rhythm for each teenager, for each family and for each limitation, with emphasis on communication and on encouraging the teen to occupy his place within society. It is up to the health professional that works with these patients to assist them, as well as their families, in the process of reaching a maximum degree of independence. Family members, HCP and teachers sometimes underestimate the abilities of these individuals, believing they will never become sexually active.

Mental deficiency alone does not determine sexual behavior. Despite the social isolation that many teenagers with DS face, studies have shown that many of these teens would like to have a sexual life, get married and have children. These teenagers have fewer opportunities to live with their peers, making it difficult to achieve their life goals. The probability of these individuals becoming isolated from society is high, in turn leading to difficulty or inability to find partners. "Different" adolescents are excluded or may feel excluded, therefore, as a way to overcome these differences and barriers, they may assume behaviors that could be of risk, each time greater, such as sexual activity without being prepared or with insufficient protection or even nonconsensual. For this teenager, sexual relations may signify being attractive, loved, chosen, even if affection is not involved.

The health professional should assist theses young adults and approach their questions in a clear and objective manner, providing the conditions for the exercise of a healthy and safe sexual life. In addition to understanding the sexual possibilities, discussions and orientations for the challenged patient and their family in relation to sexuality, the HCP should also point out the vulnerabilities these patients have (in light of their diminished capacity of self protection, victims of sexual abuse). From childhood, these individuals should understand healthy attitudes that should be taken in relation to their bodies. If integration within the community is offered, they will need orientation regarding abilities and appropriate attitudes of social behavior. It is necessary to emphasize the importance of shedding light on sexuality and contraceptive measures for these teens, their parents and educators in an individualized fashion or through educational programs [2].

The information regarding sexuality should include: relationships with others in a social context, information about the differences between genders, physiological and psychological understanding about sexual development and orientation regarding adequate social behavior. According to Elkins and Haefner [3], conversation concerning normal physical development and how to avoid sexual abuse should always be approached and Blum [4] argued that when caring for the mentally challenged, it is of utmost importance that instructions be provided about hygiene, menstruation, masturbation, STDs/AIDS, contraception and marriage. This author also discussed [4] some common beliefs concerning mentally challenged teenagers that in time has been *proven to be wrong*, like the following statements:

- Teenagers with deficiencies are not sexually active

- The social and sexual aspirations of the teenager with deficiencies and chronic illnesses are different from that of their peers
- The parents of teenagers with deficiencies provide sufficient sexual education
- Teenagers with chronic illnesses are sexually vulnerable
- Problems in relation to sexual expression are because of the chronic disease
- Individuals with chronic diseases are not satisfied with their appearance.

In a review [5] it was concluded that the pubertal development of individuals with DS is similar to that of other adolescents. Hormonal studies in proved that the hormones responsible for sexual maturation of women with DS were equivalent to those of women in the general population, with the age of the first menstruation approximately 12.5 years, while in normal women around 12.1 years. It was also shown that women with DS had regular menstrual cycles.

Pueschel and Scola [6] questioned the parents of children with DS about their perception in relation to their children's social interactions, interest in the opposite sex, sexual function and sexual education. They discovered that 40% of male teenagers and 22% of the female teenagers masturbated. Over half of the teenagers showed interest in the opposite sex and had social aspirations. Therefore, the HCP has a fundamental role since, many times, he/she is the only reference in the sexual orientation of this population and because of this, it is necessary to create space within the medical consultation, where the HCP can approach and discuss aspects about sexuality, give information about contraceptive measures and alert the patient to the risks and prevention of STDs.

One of the fundamental aspects for developing social skills is helping the teenager understand, in full, their limitations. Awareness and acceptance of this syndrome may cause suffering to the teenager and their parents, but are essential for the full development of their potential and the reformulation of their life goals given the limitations imposed.

OUR STUDY

Our study was a cross-sectional study of 50 teenagers with Down Syndrome aged between 10 and 20 years, who attended the multi-professional DS clinic of the Department of Pediatrics of the Santa Casa de São Paulo. A structured questionnaire was used, applied by the researchers along with the teenager with DS after authorization by the adolescent and his/her caretaker.

The age of the teenagers ranged between 10 and 20 years, with a mean of 13.5 years; 64% were younger than 14 years, 50% were of the male gender. 86% were enrolled in school and 62.2% were in school for over six years, 4.7% in an all day long setting. Of those who went to school, 73.3% were enrolled in public schools, 40% in traditional schools and 60% in special education schools. 28% of the teenagers considered themselves alphabetized, with only 38% being able to write their names. 10% read and wrote correctly and 6% read and wrote functionally. In analyzing the functionality of these teenagers, it was found that most were able to function independently, see table1.

Of the 25 female teenagers evaluated, 26% had already menstruated, with a mean age of menarche 11.5 years. 18% knew the date of their last menstruation, the flow was regular in 66.6% and the majority (56%) were responsible for their intimate hygiene.

Of all interviewed, 36% affirmed knowing what sexual desire was and 50% described already having felt sexual desire. When questioned about masturbation, 18% described knowing what it is and 42% answered that they frequently masturbated with 24% doing so daily, 75% in private locations and 25% in public locations. Regarding kissing, 42% affirmed that they had already kissed, being that 85.7% were simple lip kisses. The mean age for the first kiss was at the age of 12.9 years and the mean age of the partner during this first kiss was of 16.1 years. 28.6% of these partners also had DS and only two teenagers had kissed more than three partners. Of all interviewed, 18% had already dated, with 1/3 having relationships with other DS patients.

Table 1. Autonomy in the daily activity

Shower	Physiological needs	Intimate hygiene	Oral hygiene
Autonomy 66%	78%	70%	76%
With help 24%	12%	22%	14%
Totally dependence 10%	6%	8%	10%
No answer -----	4%	-----	-----

One 18 year old female teenager had sexual relations with a 15 year old partner, yet did not respond as to whether or not he had any syndrome. 34% answered that they had been given education about sexuality and that the majority (70%) were oriented by their parents. However, only 18% had discussed sexual issues with their parents and the same percentage said they discussed sex in school.

In relation to future goals of these teenagers, 58% said they intended to work, with 20.7% wanting to be teachers. When questioned about marriage, 56% showed interest and 52% intended to have children. Most subjects also showed good self-esteem, see table 2. A curious answer was given by a female teenager, saying that if she could, she would rather not have DS. Most patients were satisfied with themselves, see table 3.

Of these teenagers, 82% demonstrated aptitude in helping with tasks in their home, with the most often performed tasks related to dishes (washing, drying, putting them away) and with general cleaning (making the bed, putting away objects). On the other hand, 66% did not perform any activity outside their homes, 73% went to the grocery only for small purchases. 70% performed leisure activities: 57% of these performed some sporting activity, 20% went to parks, and 20% went to the theater and movies. 43% of those who performed leisure activities were authorized and did so by themselves. The great majority (88%) went to parties and social events. When openly questioned about what they felt capable of doing alone, 4% affirmed that they were able to do anything that is asked; 22% felt that they were capable of performing tasks of the home, 10% responded not being able to do anything and 4% were able to use public transportation without help.

Table 2. Appearance

Good looking	82%
Bad looking	2%
No answer	16%

Table 3. What would you change about yourself?

No answer	43%
Nothing	33%
Hair	
Shoulder/arms	4%
Stomach	4%
Not aware	2%
Foot	2%
Having Down syndrome	2%

DISCUSSION

If adolescence is a period of challenges and confrontations for the teenager with normal cognitive abilities, these problems can be much greater for the teenager with Down syndrome (DS). Teenagers with mental deficiencies live varying degrees of social isolation, limiting the opportunities for interaction and affective involvement that are a part of learning and sexual discovery and makes living with this disease harder. Many of these teenagers do not have the capacity to respond to the demands of their environment or own will of independence. Among the teenagers evaluated, we discovered that a great majority had been in school for a significant period. However, they had significat deficiency in learning, with only 10% being able to read and write correctly.

Concerning future perspectives of the teenagers, partically 1/3 intended to work, the majority wanted to get married and have children, demonstrating life projects, despite the great dependance they face today. On the other hand, 2/3 did not perform any activities outside their homes, confirming great dependance. It is important to emphasize that mentally challenged individuals are not similar in their learning capacity and independence, emotional stability and social abilities, yet most are capable of learning and developing some social abilities. Patients with DS with severe deficiency generally have dificulty with hygiene and self-care. Behavior training programs, such as intimate hygiene methods for the women present good results in teenagers with mild or moderate deficiencies. Siemaszko et al [7] in studying the menstrual history of teenagers with DS found that only 44% were autonomousas to menstrual hygiene, 44% needed some type of help and 12% were totally dependent.

During puberty, the teenagers are faced with an ever changing physique, and for them body image is very important and as they make themselves attractive, desired and normal. Teenagers with DS frequently have unique features, which may be a risk factor for the development of difficulties in social adaption and is even harder, when living in a society that gives such importance to body image. Merrick et al [5] found the mean age for first menstruation at 12.5 years; regular flow in the majority, which was also found in the present study. Goldstein [8] and Siemaszko [7] also did not find differences in studying the menstrual histories of teenagers with DS, while Evans [9] found the first menstruation to be 13 months later in patients with DS.

Teenagers with DS present an ample variety of manifestations in relation to sexuality and reproductive health, depending on pubertal development, on their experiences and familial and social circumstances. When evaluating the interests of teenagers with DS in the exercise of sexuality, it was found that over half of the adolescents demonstrated interest in the opposite sex. When questioned about masturbation, 18% answered that they know what it is and 42% answered that they frequently masturbated and of these, 24% did so on a daily basis, which is compatible with findings by Pueschel and Scola [6]. Another consequence of social isolation for these teenagers is the fact that they receive less information regarding sexuality, reproduction and conception. Parents, teachers and doctors do not feel comfortable discussing this theme, which impedes the patients from having adequate sexual education. Castelao et al [10] evaluated patients with DS and the health team that cared for them and discovered that the parents saw their offspring as eternal children and were afraid that they assumed a sexual life, because of the risks. Health professionals are also not prepared for the orientation of the exercise of sexuality in these adolescents. In our study, 34% of the teenagers received education about sexuality, and the majority (70%) received such education from their parents. However, only 18% had discussed sex with their parents and the same percentage discussed sex in school. Parents should be educated in relation to the existing taboos, so that in an integrated fashion and without contradiction, they can work with their children about sexual issues in a comfortable manner. They need to actively participate in the process, providing the space to expose their doubts and ask questions [11].

All of these issues indicate the necessity for sexual education for patients with mental defficiencies, and the objective should not only be the use of condoms or birth-control pills, but also the actions and attitudes of these teenagers, evaluating the particular limitations of each [12]. Teenager with DS, like other adolescents, need to express their feelings in an appropriate manner. Sexual repression can alter their internal equilibrium, lowering the possibility of psychological wellbeing. When well discussed, sexuality improves affective development, facilitating relationships, improving self-esteem and the integration within society. The information should always be repeated and have long-term attendance in order to guarantee the succes of this learning process. Whenever possible, dramatization and audio-visual material should be stimulated.

Thus, for their greater social inclusion, such patients should undergo early interventions by multidisciplinary teams, so that their development and social interaction are the best possible.

CONCLUSIONS

Teenagers with DS:

- Have normal feelings of sexuality
- Have significant difficulties in their autonomy and difficulties in school, needing careful interventions in order to make their social interaction the best possible
- Their pubertal development was normal

- Are satisfied with their body image
- Have future perspectives of working, finding a partner and living a normal life, of getting married and having children.

ACKNOWLEDGMENTS

We are grateful to the Support Center for Scientific Publications of Santa Casa de São Paulo, Faculty of Medical Sciences for the editorial assistance.

REFERENCES

[1] Masters WH, Johnson VE, Kolodny R. Sexuality in mentally retarded adolescents. In: Kolodny R, Johnson VE, Masters WH. Masters and Johnson on sex and human loving. Boston: Little Brown, 1988:500-51.
[2] Gejer D. Sexualidade e Anticoncepção no Adolescente Deficiente Mental. In: Crespin J, Reato LFN. *Hebiatria-Medicina da Adolescência*. São Paulo: Roca, 2007:457-62.
[3] Elkins TE, Haefner HK. Sexually related health care for developmentally disabled adolescents. *Adolesc. Med. State Art. Rev.* 1992;3:331-8.
[4] Blum RW. Sexual health contraceptive needs of adolescents with chronic conditions. *Arch. Pediatr. Adolesc. Med.* 1997. 151:290-7.
[5] Merrick J, Kandel I, Vardi G. Adolescents with Down Syndrome. *Int. J. Adolesc. Med. Health.* 2004;16(1):13-9.
[6] Pueschel SM, Scola PS. Parent's perception of social and sexual functions in adolescents with Down syndrome. *J. Ment. Defic. Res.* 1988;32:215-20.
[7] Siemasko K, et al. Menarche, menstrual cycles and menstrual hygiene in adolescents with Down syndrome. *Rev. Soc. Argent Ginecol. Infanto. Juvenil.* 1998;5(2):57-63.
[8] Goldstein H. Menarche, menstruation, sexual relations and contraception of adolescent females with Down syndrome. *Eur. J. Obstet. Gynnecol. Reprod. Biol.* 1988;27(4):343-9.
[9] Evans AL, McKinlay IA. Sexual maturation in girls with severe mental handicap. *Child Care Health Dev.* 1988;14(1):59-69.
[10] Castelao TB, Schiavo MR, Jurberg P. Sexuality in Down syndrome individuals. *Rev. Saude Publica.* 2003;37(1):32-9.
[11] Daquinta R. Programa de educación sexual "Venga la Esperanza"; *Sexual Education Program:* Mediciego 2004 Jun 10.
[12] Eastgate G. Sex, consent and intellectual disability. *Aust. Fam. Physician.* 2005;34(3):163-6.

Part XIII. Skin

In: Adolescence and Chronic Illness
Editors: H. Omar et al.

ISBN: 978-1-60876-628-4
© 2010 Nova Science Publishers, Inc.

Chapter 22

ACNE VULGARIS AND ADOLESCENCE

Donald E. Greydanus and Dilip R. Patel*

*Pediatrics and Human Development, Michigan State University
College of Human Medicine, Kalamazoo Center for Medical Studies,
Kalamazoo, Michigan, United States of America.*

ABSTRACT

Acne vulgaris is a common disorder of adolescents and young adults that can be very severe especially in those with concomitant hyperandrogenic conditions. The pathophysiology of acne vulgaris is reviewed along with its differential diagnosis, including acne variants. Management of acne is also reviewed including use of topical and oral anti-acne agents such as benzoyl peroxide, retinoids, and antibiotics (topical and oral). Treatment of severe acne includes management of underlying disorders (as endocrine conditions) along with oral isotretinoin. Other medications that may be useful in selective cases include oral contraceptives, low dose prednisone, antiandrogens (as spironolactone or cyproterone acetate), or gonadotropin-releasing hormone agonists.

INTRODUCTION

Acne vulgaris is a disorder of the sebaceous gland, sebaceous duct, and hair follicle with a strong genetic influence [1-4]. Acne vulgaris is found in areas of high sebaceous density such as the face, upper arms, chest, and back. Up to 80% of female adolescents and 90% of male adolescents develop some degree of acne vulgaris whereas 10% develop severe acne. Approximately 40% of children between ages 8 and 10 years develop some degree of acne as

---

* *Correspondence:* Professor Donald E Greydanus, MD, Pediatrics and Human Development, Michigan State University College of Human Medicine, Pediatrics Program, Michigan State University/Kalamazoo Center for Medical Studies, 1000 Oakland Drive, Kalamazoo, MI 49008-1284 United States. E-mail: Greydanus@kcms.msu.edu

well, as the sebaceous glands enlarge under the androgenic influence of increased levels of adrenal gland produced dehydroepiandrosterone sulfate (DHEAS).

PATHOPHYSIOLOGY

Although the precise cause of acne vulgaris is not known, the important aspects of acne pathogenesis involve sebum, a keratin plug, and effects of the microbial skin flora. Follicular keratinocytes become sticky and lead to the formation of a keratin plug that occludes the follicle with sebum trapping. The occlusion leads to formation of a comedone—closed type (also called a whitehead) or open (also called a blackhead with retained melanin) [5]. Continuing distention of the plugged follicle causes local tissue damage that is worsened by the change of sebum triglycerides to free fatty acids that are irritating to the skin. Follicle rupture allows bacterial invasion (infection) with local microbial flora (Propionibacterium acnes) that can lead to inflammatory acne lesions as erythematous papules, pustules, nodules, or cysts. Healing of severe inflammatory acne can lead to variable skin scarring.

Table 1. Classification of acne and variants. Used with permission from: Greydanus DE: Disorders of the skin. In: AD Hofmann, DE Greydanus, eds. Adolescent Medicine, 3rd ed. Stamford, CT: Appleton & Lange, 1997; ch. 18: 377

Type	Comment
ACNE VULGARIS (GROUP I)	
Comedonal acne vulgaris	Disorder of sebaceous follicles with horny impactions. Graded according to percent of face involved: I=10%; II=10%-25%; III=25%-50%; IV=more than 50%.
Papulopustular acne (inflammatory acne)	Rupture of the distended sebaceous gland with varying degrees of inflammation. Graded V-VIII.
Acne conglobata	Severe nodulocystic acne vulgaris. Described in 3% of white adolescent males, with severe scarring. Extremities and buttocks often involved, as well as groin, scalp, and axilla. Persistence into adulthood can occur. SAPHO: syndrome of acne, pustulosis, hyperostosis, and osteitis; this is classified as a seronegative spondyloarthritis.
Acne tropicalis (tropical acne)	Severe inflammatory acne vulgaris seen in young adult men exposed to tropical conditions.
Acne fulminans (acute febrile ulcerative conglobate acne)	Rare variant described in males (ulcerative conglobate acne) characterized by large nodules with scarring on trunk and sometimes face; also fever, ulcers, polyarthritis or arthralgia and leukocytosis. Sacroiliitis often noted. Osteolysis and periosteal reaction can occur.
ACNE VULGARIS VARIANTS (GROUP II)	
Infantile acne (acne neonatorum)	Comedonal acne on malar region of males during first few weeks to year of life. Occasionally noted in either sex from 1-2 years of age. Acne neonatorum refers to acne limited to the first month of life.
Premenstrual acne	Cyclical microcomedonal acne developing before the menstrual period.
Gram-negative folliculitis	Associated with long-term broad-spectrum antibiotic use. Variable patterns of facial nodules due to *Proteus*, *Pseudomonas*, *Klebsiella*, or *Enterobacter* organisms. Treat with isotretinoin or high-dose ampicillin or amoxicillin.
Excessive androgen acne	Severe acne related to high androgen levels (eg, polycystic ovary syndrome). Treatment with antiandrogens such as cyproterone acetate and ethinyl estradiol reported to be therapeutic; close medical supervision is necessary due to adverse drug effects.

Table 1. (Continued).

Type	Comment
ACNE VULGARIS (GROUP I)	
Folliculitis keloidalis	Chronic, recurrent low-grade pustular dermatitis of the occipital and posterior neck regions. May result in scarring, keloid formation, and alopecia. Most commonly noted in black males with closely shaved areas and ingrown hairs. Avoid certain shaved hairstyles and occlusive hair oils; topical or systemic antibiotics may be necessary. Intralesional corticosteroids or surgical excision of scar or keloids may be necessary.
Acne mechanica	Exacerbation of acne vulgaris by excessive rubbing to cause friction, as with overzealous face washing or even tight helmets or clothing (leotards); use of absorbent material under the occlusion can help, such as a cotton T-shirt under a leotard.
Chemical acne	Exacerbation of acne vulgaris by cosmetics, detergents, hair creams or oils, chlorinated hydrocarbons, tars, emollient skin or bath oils. Pomade acne refers to hair oil or grease inducing comedonal acne at the hair line and forehead.
Acne due to physical agents	Exacerbation of acne vulgaris by sunlight, ionizing radiation; Mallorca acne (acne aestivalis) is a sunlight-induced, winter variant with papular folliculitis of arms, shoulders, and trunk; no comedones, nodules or scarring.
Drug-induced acneform rashes	Iodides, bromides, barbiturates, rifampin, phenytoin, lithium; others may be associated. Steroid acne can occur, secondary to steroid (systemic, oral) use, and responds poorly to antibiotics. Fluorinated steroids are particularly implicated, but fluorinated creams should *never* be used on the face! Patients with acne should be screened for medications and foods that might contain high levels of "acnegenic" substances. Athletes should be warned to avoid anabolic steroid use, which has many side effects, including a drug-induced acneform disorder.
NONACNE ACNEFORM RASHES (DIFFERENTIAL DIAGNOSIS)	
Pyoderma faciale	Progressive facial inflammatory lesions (nodules, hypertrophic scars, and absence of comedones) occurring in adult females 20-40 years of age.
Acne rosacea	Facial papules and pustules associated with dilated blood vessels in the nasolabial areas in adults age 30-50
Folliculitis-associated immunologic defects	*Example*: Chronic granulomatous disease.
Periofolliculitis capitis abscendens	Diffuse, explosive scalp cellulitis associated with severe acne and hidradenitis suppurativa. Treat with antibiotics and retinoic acid
Hidradenitis suppurativa	Keratin obstruction of aprocrine ducts with secondary infection of apocrine glands in axillae, areolae, labiae, scrotum, or perineum. Fluctuant nodules with purulent drainage and sinus tract formation. Associated with obesity, severe acne vulgaris, tropical climates, poor hygiene. Unusual cases can be associated with fever, anemia, and arthralgia. Treatment is as for abscesses in general; intralesional steroid injection, exteriorization of sinus tracts, or excision of involved tissue may be required. Acne surgery is the ultimate choice for most, though oral isotretinin (40 mg, bid) is helpful to some. Oral antibiotics (tetracycline 1-2 g/day) can also help some. Avoid tight clothes over affected areas. Antibacterial soaps may help. Hygiene and aluminum chloride (6.25% in anhydrous alcohol) may help to reduce perspiration. Benzoyl peroxide and topical antibiotics may be helpful for a few patients, but not the majority. Response to all treatment measures is variable.
Pseudofolliculitis barbae	Chronic folliculitis in beard area (especially black males) aggravated by shaving. Treat by growing a beard, avoiding a close shave, clipping hairs, and systemic antibiotics if pronounced. Electric razor use is essential for most, though some may find frequent straight-edge razor changes acceptable. Multiple small keloids may form in persons predisposed to keloid formation.

Table 1. (Continued).

Type	Comment
ACNE VULGARIS (GROUP I)	
Trichostasis spinulosa	Facial eruption resembling blackheads but made up of follicular papules containing vellus hairs, keratin, and melanin and distributed over the nose and malar regions. Treat with isotretinoin
Adenoma sebaceum	Pinkish yellow sebaceous papules on face; commonly clustered in groups around the nose. One of the classic stigmata of tuberous sclerosis
Keratosis pilaris	Hereditary, self-limiting, hair follicle keratinization disorder which peaks in adolescence. Can be associated with atopic dermatitis or ichthyosis vulgaris. Flesh-colored 1-2 mm papules are noted on lateral upper arms, anterior thighs, or the face. The lesions can be red or white. Moisturizers (with lactic acid), topical keratolytics (with propylene glycol) and tretinoin may be helpful.
Neurotic excoriations	Superficial excoriation or deeper ulcer in acne areas and other generalized areas. Found in individuals with severe mental illness. Some disturbed individuals use cigarettes, knives, acids, or alkalis to produce facial injury often called factitial dermatitis. Treatment is attention to the injured skin with psychiatric treatment.

Table 1 lists types of acne and acne variants [6,7]. Androgens play a role in the pathogenesis of acne and rising levels of testosterone can contribute to acne in adolescents [8-12]. Testosterone is converted in the skin by 5-α-reductase to dihydrotestosterone leading to sebaceous gland enlargement while estrogen can inhibit sebaceous gland stimulation. Acne can worsen in females shortly before menstruation, when estrogen levels are low and androgenic progesterone is dominant. Although patients with acne usually have normal hormone levels, some can have increased free testosterone and DHEAS along with decreased levels of SHBG (sex hormone-binding globulin) [13-15].

Table 2. Causes of hyperandrogenemia in females with potential of severe acne

Genetic and familial increased androgen sensitivity
Adrenal androgens
Congenital adrenal hyperplasias
21-hydroxylase deficiency (classic or late-onset)
3-β hydroxysteroid dehydrogenase deficiency (classic or late-onset)
11β-hydroxylase deficiency (classic or late-onset)
Adrenal tumors
Adrenocortical carcinoma
Testosterone-secreting adenoma
Adrenal rest adenoma and carcinoma
Cushing's disease
Ovarian androgens
Polycystic ovary syndrome (PCOS)
Conditions associated with PCOS
PCOS with ovarian tumor
Pineal gland hyperplasia and diabetes
Congenital lipoatrophic diabetes
Hyperprolactinemia
Hyperthyroidism
Hypothyroidism
Androgen-secreting cysts and hyperplasias
Stromal hyperplasia and hyperthecosis
Solitary follicle cyst

Table 2. (Continued).

Hyperreaction luteinalis of pregnancy
Androgen-secreting ovarian tumors
Arrhenoblastoma (androblastoma)
Thecoma-fibroma group tumors
Granulosa cell tumors
Lipoid cell tumors
Gynandroblastoma
Epithelial tumor
Luteoma of pregnancy
Testicular androgens in XY females
5-α reductase deficiency
Mixed gonadal dysgenesis
True hermaphroditism
17-β hydroxysteroid dehydrogenase deficiency
Other rare intersex conditions
Exogenous androgens
Medical
Hypoplastic anemias
Growth stimulation
Adrenal replacement
Danazol
Synthetic progestins in oral contraceptives
Adrenocorticotropic hormone (ACTH) therapy
Nonmedical
Bodybuilding and athletic anabolic steroids

Source: Reprinted with permission, from: Greydanus DE, Shearin RB: Adolescent sexuality and gynecology. Philadelphia: Lea & Febiger, 1990; 177.

Acne can be severe in conditions with increased androgens, such as congenital adrenal hyperplasia, Cushing's disease, congenital adrenal hyperplasia, polycystic ovarian syndrome, metabolic syndrome (hyperlipidemia, high blood pressure, obesity, and insulin resistance), and in other states of hyperandrogenemia (see table 2) [12-16]. Acne can be worsened by a variety of medications, such as those listed in table 3. A variety of grading schemes are noted with acne, such as mild (less than 25% facial involvement with no nodules or scarring), moderate (50% facial involvement with few nodules), and severe (75% facial involvement with many nodules and possible scarring) [14].

MANAGEMENT

General

Youth with acne should be counseled that their condition does not suggest poor hygiene and that they should not pick any acne lesions because such trauma (or other injury as from athletic equipment or others) leads to increased inflammation and infection. The patient should avoid vigorous scrubbing of the face because that will worsen the overall condition. Diet in general does not worsen acne, although some patients anecdotally note worsening with specific foods (i.e., milk, fried foods, chocolate, soft drinks, nuts, others). The cautious use of cosmetics in females is important, and only water-based or oil-free (non-comedogenic) products should be applied. Pomade acne (see table 1), for example, can be improved by having the adolescent use a less oily lotion or gel on hair ends, and acne vulgaris can be improved by having reduced exposure to oils or grease in work places (as automobile repair shops or restaurant kitchens).

Table 3. Medications/chemicals that worsen acne

Androgenic steroids
Barbiturates
Bromides
Diphenylhydantoin
Glucocorticoids
Iodides
Isoniazid
Kelp and other seaweed
Lithium
Rifampin
Synthetic progestins

Anti-Acne Medications

Specific management of acne involves application of various topical and oral medications (see table 4) along with controlling underlying factors such as excess androgen production [13-18]. Table 5 outlines the management options for facial acne using medications noted in table 4. Important anti-acne medications include benzoyl peroxide and topical retinoids (tretinoin, adapalene, tazarotene). These medications may take 6-8 weeks to show visible beneficial effects, thus leading to frustration on the part of the adolescent with embarrassing acne and the need for a clinician to master the art and science of acne management. The reasons for failure of acne improvement with medication include problems with compliance (an adolescent stops using the medication after a few days or weeks), absorption (i.e., failure to take tetracycline on an empty stomach), persistent skin irritation from topicals, presence of deep nodular lesions, antibiotic resistance, presence of under-lying disorders (as hyperandrogenemic states), and misdiagnosis (see table 1) [6].

Table 4. Medications used in the management of acne vulgaris

Topicals
Benzoyl Peroxide
Topical retinoid (tretinoin, adapalene, tazarotene)
Azelaic acid
Topical Antibiotics (clindamycin, erythromycin) in combination with benzoyl peroxide
Oral Agents
Oral Antibiotics (Tetracycline, Erythromycin, Doxycycline, Minocycline)
Oral Contraceptives
Isotretinoin

The side effects of anti-acne medications should be considered at all times. For example, benzoyl peroxide can lead to skin erythema, dryness, peeling, increase in photosensitivity, pigmentary changes, phototoxicity, bleaching of towels and bed clothes, and even transient worsening of acne as the established comedones are irritated and even lead to pustules. Excessive skin irritation is especially noted in atopic, black, and fair-skinned adolescents. A slow or titrated build-up of such irritating topicals is important to minimize such adverse effects. Tretinoin can also induce severe skin irritation and redness as well as phototoxicity; 3% to 5% may have an allergic reaction with excessive erythema.

A variety of antibiotics can be used to treat acne [17,19,20]. Oral tetracycline can lead to gastrointestinal upset, photosensitivity, ulceration of the esophagus, headache, hemolytic anemia, gram-negative folliculitis, onycholysis (including photoonycholysis or nail separation from its plate after exposure to the sun), and photosensitivity; the drug should be avoided in pregnancy and in those under age 8 because it can lead to tooth discoloration with enamel defects in non-erupted teeth or to tetracycline deposition in fetal bones and teeth [6,13-15].

Erythromycin can also lead to gastrointestinal upset and resistance of P acnes. The adverse effects of oral doxycycline are similar to tetracycline, whereas minocycline can lead to tetracycline-like side effects, tissue pigmentation (skin, mucus membranes, teeth), dizziness, vertigo, photosensitivity, tooth discoloration, facial marks (dark, bluish) and rare autoimmune syndromes (hepatitis, lupus-like syndrome, hypersensitivity syndrome, and serum sickness-like reaction). The emergence of antibiotic-resistant microbiological flora is becoming a growing phenomenon.

Isotretinoin

Oral isotretinoin (13-cis retinoic acid (marketed as Accutane) is used to treat severe inflammatory (nodulocystic) acne, as well as other skin disorders, including acne rosacea, acne fulminans, psoriasis, hidradenitis suppurativa, gram-negative folliculitis, psoriasis, and various ichthyotic disorders [21]. Oral isotretinoin is an important anti-acne medication that shrinks sebaceous glands, improves abnormal keratinization, reduces sebum production, and has anti-inflammatory effects [22].

A variety of side effects noted with oral isotretinoin (see tables 6 and 7) include a major risk for teratogenicity (see table 7), and the prescription of this medication is generally under the care of dermatologists using very strict guidelines for prescription, assurance that the female patient is not pregnant, and provision for contraception while taking this medication [23].

The major teratogenic potential of oral isotretinoin has led the manufacturer to recommend the clinician follow the S.M.A.R.T. program (System to Manage Accutane Related Teratogenicity) [13,15].

Triglycerides are particularly increased in those with diabetes mellitus, obesity, alcohol abuse, and a family history positive for hyperlipidemia. Those with intestinal disorders may develop severe diarrhea or rectal bleeding on oral isotretinoin. The issue of increased depression and possible increased suicide is under research [13,24-26]. It is clear, however, that severe acne can have significant negative effects on the quality of life for adolescents with and without additional chronic illnesses [27,28].

Table 5. Management of facial acne vulgaris*

Acne severity	Lesion type	Initial treatment	If no response
Mild	Comedonal	Benzoyl peroxide or topical retinoid*	If benzoyl peroxide used initially, substitute with or add topical retinoid* once daily
	Inflammatory	Benzoyl peroxide (or topical combination preparation†)	Increase benzoyl peroxide application to twice daily, or substitute combination product† or oral antibiotic‡
	Mixed (i.e., comedones and inflammatory lesions)	Benzoyl peroxide (or topical combination product†) alone or with topical retinoid* Azelaic acid as monotherapy	If benzoyl peroxide used initially, add topical retinoid* once daily (for comedonal component) and/or substitute topical combination product† or oral antibiotic‡ (for inflammatory component)
Moderate	Comedonal	Topical retinoid*	Increase strength of topical retinoid*
	Inflammatory	Topical combination product† (or oral antibiotic‡,§)	If topical combination product† used, add or substitute oral antibiotic‡,§ and add topical retinoid*
	Mixed (i.e., comedones and inflammatory lesions)	Topical combination product† (or oral antibiotic‡,§) and topical retinoid* Azelaic acid as monotherapy)	Increase strength of topical retinoid* (for comedonal component) If combination product† used alone, substitute oral antibioic ‡,§ (for inflammatory component) and add topical retinoid
Severe	Comedonal	Topical retinoid* once daily	Increase strength of topical retinoid* or refer to dermatologist
	Inflammatory	Oral antibiotic‡,§ and topical retinoid*	Consider alternate antibiotic‡,§ or refer to dermatologist
	Mixed (i.e., comedones and inflammatory lesions)	Oral antibiotic‡,§ and topical retinoid¹	Consider increasing strength of topical retinoid* (for comedonal component) and/or beginning alternate antibiotic‡,§ (for inflammatory component), or refer to dermatologist

* For example, tretinoin cream 0.025%, Retin-A gel micro 0.04% or 0.1%; Differin; or Avita.

† For example, clindamycin or erythromycin combined with benzoyl peroxide (clindamycin and erythromycin used alone are not favored due to potential antibiotic resistance).

‡ For example, tetracycline (or possibly erythromycin) 250 to 500 mg twice daily.

§ Some experts advise the use benzoyl peroxide in patients treated with oral antibiotics to prevent the emergence of antibiotic resistant *P. acnes.**Used with permission from Krowchuk DP: "Disorders of the Skin" In: Essential Adolescent Medicine. Eds: DE Greydanus, DR Patel, HD Pratt. New York: McGraw Hill Medical Publishers, 2006; ch. 19: 413.

Table 6. Side effects of oral isotretinoin

Cheilitis (90%)
Severe dry skin and pruritus (80%)
Dry nose and mouth along with epistaxis (80%)
Conjunctivitis and difficulty with contact lenses (40%)
Increase in serum cholesterol and triglyceride levels (25%)
Musculosketal aches (16%)
Hair thinning (10%)
Photosensitivity (with decreased night vision) (5%)
Corneal opacities (5%)
Headache (5%)
Fatigue (5%)
Depression (<5%)
?Risk for suicide
Others:
  Teratogenicity (Table 7)
  Cervical spine hyperostosis
  Elevated liver enzyme and blood sugar levels
  Low back pain
  Increased sunburn susceptibility
  Peeling of palms and soles
  Pseudotumor cerebri
  Premature epiphyseal closure
  Others

Other Anti-Acne Medications

Oral contraceptives can improve acne by reducing the secretion of gonadotropin with less production of androgens from the ovaries and by raising SHBG levels that lower free testosterone levels [12-16,29-32]. Oral contraceptives are not the primary treatment for acne but can be a useful adjuvant therapy, especially in a female who is sexually active. Oral contraceptives with a low androgenic progestin are recommended, such as norgestimate (Ortho Tri-Cyclen) [14,15,18,29,30]. Females with acne should not be placed on depomedroxy-progesterone acetate or long-acting progestin implants because the acne may be worsened to a significant degree. Underlying endocrine conditions should be treated and may require low-dose prednisone, anti-androgens (as spironolactone, cyproterone acetate, or cimetidine), or gonadotropin-releasing hormone (GnRH) agonists [6,10,12,14].

Acne surgery may be helpful for severe cystic acne and includes incision and drainage, as well as the injection of steroid (as triamcinolone acetonide) into persistent cystic lesions with thick walls. Acne conglobata may improve with oral steroids, sulfone, and oral isotretinoin. Acne fulminans may improve with salicylates (for fever and muscle/joint symptoms), oral corticosteroids, oral isotretinoin, and/or Dapsone (diaminodiphenyl sulfone). Referral to the appropriate consultants in dermatology, endocrinology, and/or gynecology is necessary for severe and/or refractory acne and its variants. The website for the treatment of acne from the American Academy of Dermatology is available at www.skincarephysicians.com/acnenet.

Table 7. Teratogenic effects of isotretinoin*

Affected Area	Teratogenic Effects
Head	Microcephaly, abnormal cranium, anencephaly, seizures, psychomotor retardation.
Eyes	Microphthalmia, blindness, down-slant of palpebral fissures.
Ears	Atretic ears, hypoplastic auditory meatus, absent eighth nerve, deafness, rudimentary, or malformed pinnae.
Mouth	Cleft palate, lip micrognathia
Heart	Patent ductus arteriosus, atrial septal defects, ventricular septal defects, truncus arteriosus, others.

*With permission from: Greydanus DE: Disorders of the Skin. In: AD Hofmann, DE Greydanus, eds. Adolescent Medicine, 3rd Ed. Stamford, CT: Appleton & Lange, 1997; ch. 18:380, 1997.

CONCLUSIONS

Acne vulgaris is a common disorder of adolescents and young adults that can be very severe with considerable emotional consequences, especially in those with concomitant hyperandrogenic conditions. The pathophysiology involves sebum, a keratin plug, and effects of the microbial skin flora. The differential diagnosis of acne includes a number of acne variants, as noted in table 1. Careful management of this dermatological disorder is recommended that may include such medications as benzoyl peroxide, retinoids, and antibiotics (topical and oral). Oral antibiotics should not be used for a prolonged time (i.e., not over three months) to reduce the growing phenomenon of antibiotic resistance. Management also involves the treatment of underlying disorders as well, such as hyperandrogenic states. Treatment may also involve oral isotretinoin, oral contraceptives, low dose prednisone, antiandrogens (as spironolactone or cyproterone acetate) or GnRH agonists.

REFERENCES

[1] Hurwitz S. Acne vulgaris: its pathogenesis and management. *Adolesc. Med.* 1990;1(2):301-14.
[2] Sidbury R, Paller AS. The diagnosis and management of acne. *Pediatr. Ann.* 2000;29:17-23.
[3] Webster GF. Acne vulgaris. *Br. Med. J.* 2002; 325:475-8.
[4] James WD. *Acne. N. Engl. J. Med.* 2005;352:1463-72.
[5] Feinberg AN. The integument system. Skin, hair, nails. In: Greydanus DE, Feinberg AN, Patel DR, Homnick DN, eds. *The pediatric diagnostic examination.* Homnick, NY: McGraw-Hill, 2008:570.
[6] Greydanus DE. Disorders of the skin. In: Hofman AD, Greydanus DE, eds. *Adolescent medicine,* 3rd ed. Stamford, CT: Appleton Lange, 1997:375-407.
[7] Powell FC. Rosacea. *N. Engl. J. Med.* 2005;352:793-803.
[8] Goos SD, Pochi PE. Endocrine aspects of adolescent acne. *Adolesc. Med.* 1990;1(2):289-300.

[9] Lucky AW, McGuire J, Rosenfield RL, et al. Plasma androgens in women with acne vulgaris. *J. Invest. Dermatol.* 1983;81:70.

[10] Miller JA, Wojnarowska FT, Dowd PM, et al. Anti-androgen treatment in women with acne: A controlled trial. *Br. J. Dermatol.* 1986;114:705.

[11] Reingold SB, Rosenfield RL: The relationship of mild hirsutism or acne in women to androgens. *Arch. Dermatol.* 1987;123:209.

[12] Erkkola R, Hirvonen E, Luikku R, et al. Ovulation inhibitors containing cyproterone acetate or desogestrel in the treatment of hyperandrogenic symptoms. *Acta Obstet. Gynecol. Scand.* 1990; 69:91.

[13] Krowchuk DP. Disorders of the skin. In: Greydanus DE, Patel DR, Pratt HD, eds. *Essential adolescent medicine.* New York: McGraw Hill, 2006:411-43.

[14] Krowchuk DP, Lucky AW. Managing adolescent acne. *Adolesc. Med.* 2001;12(2):355-72.

[15] Krowchuk DP. Managing adolescent acne: A guide for pediatricians. *Pediatr. Rev.* 2005;26:250-61.

[16] Braverman PK, Braverman IM. Cutaneous manifestations of common systemic diseases in adolescents. *Adolesc. Med.* 1990; 1:199-240.

[17] Gollnick H, Cunliffe W, Berson D, et al. Management of acne: a report from the global alliance to improve outcomes in acne. *J. Am. Acad. Dermatol.* 2003;49(Suppl 1):S1-38.

[18] Haider A, Shaw JC. Treatment of acne vulgaris. *JAMA.* 2004;292:726-35.

[19] Ozolins M, Eady EA, Avery AJ, et al. Comparison of five antimicrobial regimens for treatment of mild to moderate inflammatory acne vulgaris in the community: Randomized controlled trial. *Lancet.* 2004;364:2188-95.

[20] Eady EA, Cove JH, Joanes DN, et al. Topical antibiotics for the treatment of acne vulgaris: A critical evaluation of their clinical benefit and comparative efficacy. *J. Dermatol. Treat.* 1990;1: 215-20.

[21] Abel EA. Isotretinoin (Accutane) therapy for acne in adolescents. *Adolesc. Med.* 1990;1(2):315-24.

[22] Goldsmith LA, Bologna JL, Callen JP, et al. American Academy of Dermatology Consensus Conference on the safe and optimal use of isotretinoin: summary and recommendations. *J. Am. Acad. Dermatol.* 2004;50:900-6.

[23] Medical Letter. Is Accutane really dangerous? *Med. Lett.* 2002;44:82.

[24] Lamberg L. Acne drug depression warnings high-light need for expert care. *JAMA.* 1998;279:1057.

[25] Hull PR, D'Arcy C. Isotretinoin use and subsequent depression and suicide: Presenting the evidence. *Am. J. Clin. Dermatol.* 2003;4:493-505.

[26] Wysowski DK, Pitts M, Beitz J. An analysis of reports of depression and suicide in patients treated with isotretinoin. *J. Am. Acad. Dermatol.* 2001;45:515-9.

[27] Smith JA. The impact of skin disease on the quality of life of adolescents. *Adolesc. Med.* 2001; 12(2):343-54.

[28] Mallon E, Newton JN, Klassen A, et al. The quality of life in acne. *Br. J. Dermatol.* 1999;140: 672-6.

[29] Redmond GP, Olson WH, Lippman JS, et al. Norgestimate and ethinyl estradiol in the treatment of acne vulgaris: A randomized, placebo-controlled trial. *Obstet. Gynecol.* 1997;89:615.

[30] Rosen MP, Breitkopf DM, Nagamani M. A randomized controlled rial of second versus third generation oral contraceptives in the treatment of acne vulgaris. *Am. J. Obstet. Gynecol.* 2003;188: 1158-60.
[31] Krowchuk DP. Treating acne: A practical guide. *Med. Clin. North Am.* 2000;84:811-28.
[32] Zaenglein AL, Thiboutot DM. Expert committee recommendations for acne management. *Pediatrics.* 2006;118(3):1188-99.

PART XIV. MUSCULSKELETAL SYSTEM

ACUTE MUSCULOSKELETAL SPORTS INJURY AND TOPICAL NSAID

Amit M. Deokar, Shawn J. Smith and Hatim A. Omar*
Department of Pediatrics, Division of Adolescent Medicine,
University of Kentucky, Lexington, Kentucky, United States.

ABSTRACT

The objective of this chapter is to summarize the current standards of pain management in minor sports related musculoskeletal injuries. We also address the topical form of non-steroidal anti-inflammatory drug as an effective pain management option in an out-patient setting. Design: Quantitive systematic review of randomized controlled trials. Methods: The data was obtained through literature review of articles published in the last 10 years. In addition, FDA information on non-steroidal anti-inflammatory medications was also reviewed. The patient population studied in the articles included children and adults. Conclusion: Current standards of managing pain resulting from sports injuries involve a number of analgesic drugs including non-steroidal anti-inflammatory drugs. The topical form of this class of drugs is an effective method for pain management of minor musculoskeletal sports-related injuries.

INTRODUCTION

When compared to the 1970's, there has been increased participation in sports activities. Despite an increased awareness of safety measures, the participants are still at an increased risk from sports-related injuries [1]. Various agencies are involved in the surveillance and epidemiologic data on sports-related injuries. National Health Interview Survey is one such agency that collects data for the National Center for Health Statistics (NCHS) [2]. Musculoskeletal injuries are one of the primary reasons that patients seek medical attention in

---

* *Correspondence:* Assistant professor Amit M Deokar, MD, MPH, Department of Pediatrics, Division of Adolescent Medicine (J422), University of Kentucky, Lexington, KY 40536 United States. E-mail: amit-deokar@uky.edu

the out-patient family practice setting [3]. Throughout the United States, a large portion of emergency department (ED) visits is following acute sports-related injuries [4]. Approximately 3.7 million sports-related injuries occur in people of all ages and each year about 2.5 million ED visits resulting from sports injuries occur in the pediatric population [4].

The use of nonsteroidal anti-inflammatory drugs (NSAIDs) for pain from musculoskeletal injuries is well known and extensive [3]. Musculoskeletal injuries include injuries to muscle, ligaments, tendons, and non-fracture injuries. Treatment of such injuries is generally geared toward reducing the swelling and pain by using methods such as cold compression and an anti-inflammatory agent [5]. Typically, the use of NSAIDs is due to their anti-inflammatory, analgesic, and anti-pyretic properties. The basis of the pharmacological action of NSAIDs is their ability to inhibit cylooxygenase (COX) enzymes thereby blocking the formation of certain prostaglandins (PGs). Besides reducing the inflammation, this inhibition of PG synthesis may potentially result in serious side effects such as gastrointestinal disturbance and altered renal function [3,6]. Cyclooxygenase-2 (COX-2) inhibitors such as Rofecoxib (Vioxx™) were popular analgesics especially in the last decade. This was because they do not inhibit the beneficial effects of PG's, and thus have fewer side effects on the gastric mucosal lining. They also do not affect bleeding time and platelet function [6]. Because of serious cardiovascular side effects reported with the use of COX-2 inhibitors, some of these products were withdrawn from the US markets in 2004 [7].

Due to non-availability of topical form of analgesics in the US market, and because of the negative side effects from a systemic non-steroidal anti-inflammatory drug, an alternative delivery method such as topical can be utilized. A topical route of NSAIDs has the benefit of superior local drug delivery. At the same time the systemic side effects that may arise from oral NSAIDs are reduced by using the topical route [5]. A sufficiently high concentration of the drug is necessary to penetrate the skin, muscles, and synovial fluid and this is seen when an NSAID is topically administered. In addition to this benefit, the topical form also allows a constant and slow release of the drug [5].

We conducted a literature search using PubMed and included terms such as "topical NSAIDs", "oral NSAIDs", "sports injuries", "musculoskeletal injuries", and "pain management."

Through the synopsis of articles below, this review attempts to emphasize the effectiveness of NSAIDs on pain from acute musculoskeletal sports injuries. It also addresses the use of a topical route as an effective and safe method for NSAID delivery.

DISCUSSION

Sports-related injuries that involve the ligaments, muscle, tendons, and bones are fairly common in sports activities. Some studies indicated that there has been a considerable increase in such injuries due to an increased involvement in sports activities [1,4].

Non-steroidal anti-inflammatory drugs are used frequently in pain management of musculoskeletal sports injuries [5]. In a randomized controlled trial (RCT) done in an ED setting on patients 6-17 years, who had sustained a musculoskeletal sports injury, an oral non-steroidal, Ibuprofen, was compared with Acetaminophen and Codeine [8]. Patients in the Ibuprofen group showed significant improvement compared to the other two groups, as demonstrated on the Visual Analog Scale (VAS). There was twice as much decrease in pain (24mm versus 12mm or 11 mm) on this scale (p<0.001). The effectiveness of NSAIDs is due to their mechanism of action that causes inhibition of prostaglandins at the injury site. Oral NSAIDs, when administered in such a situation achieve a relatively higher drug level systemically [3,6]. Although this may result in relief of pain symptoms, it may potentially lead to serious side effects such those on gastro protection and renal function. They may also interfere with coagulation mechanisms [9].

There are various routes by which NSAIDs can be delivered. One option is to use the topical route. Topical NSAID's when applied to an inflamed area results in local drug delivery and fewer systemic side effects from high plasma drug levels. One multicenter controlled clinical trial published in the year 2000 compared the effectiveness of the topical Diclofenac Sodium patch to a placebo in patients who had sustained a sports-related injury. Out of the two weeks of treatment, the daily pain relief on days 3, 7, and 14 was superior in the Diclofenac group (p=0.044). Another double blinded RCT conducted in Europe compared the Diclofenac patch to a placebo patch, reported significant (p<0.0001) pain relief in adult patients who sustained an acute impact sports injury and those who received the active drug [5]. This study also reaffirmed the safety and reduced systemic side effects from use of a topical form of an NSAID. Local side effects such as rash or itch occurred similarly in both active as well as inactive patch [5]. Another study (randomized double blinded, placebo-controlled) conducted in Europe concluded the efficacy of topical Ketoprofen compared to a placebo in patients who had a benign ankle sprain. This topical NSAID was also tolerated well, with only local side effects [10]. Recently, a prospective, randomized, open study compared two topical agents, Ketoprofen and Diclofenac gel in patients who sustained an acute, benign, sports-related injury. The efficacy of transdermal (TDS) Ketoprofen in relieving pain was comparable to the Diclofenac gel. The TDS Ketoprofen was found to be superior to the Diclofenac gel (64% versus 46%, p=0.004) leading to a high cure rate on day 7 of the treatment [11].

Despite growing evidence that supports the effectiveness of topical NSAID's in pain relief and minimizing the systemic adverse events, several limitations exist for the type of studies conducted thus far in this area. For example, the randomized controlled clinical trials have compared a placebo over a topical form of NSAID to examine the effectiveness and safety profile. While placebo controlled studies are usually preferred to compare the effectiveness of a new drug, it may affect the standard of care for some of the patients. In addition, not many studies have been done exclusively in the pediatric population. Data from the studies done in adults may help researchers conduct clinical trials in children.

Topical Diclofenac Sodium formulation is available for use in Europe and other countries [5]. In the United States, Dicofenac is available as an oral as well as a topical form. The topical application is a 3% gel that was FDA-approved for Actinic Keratosis in 2002. As of October 2007, the topical Diclofenac Sodium patch was in its Phase 1 clinical study, which is being conducted by Cerimon Pharmaceuticals [12]. Numerous clinical trials in the United States are currently undergoing that are looking at the use of topical NSAID for breast pain and osteoarthritis [13]. The efficacy of topical non-steroidal anti-inflammatory drugs over a placebo has been noted in various trials involving acute sprain injury as well as chronic conditions such as rheumatoid arthritis [14]. Once approved, the topical form of anti-inflammatory drugs is likely to revolutionize the standard of care in pain management of acute benign sports-related musculoskeletal injuries. The use of topical non-steroidal drugs for chronic pain will also be of particular advantage in the elderly population due to their safety profile (14).

REFERENCES

[1] www.cdc.gov. MMWR Weekly. Sports-Related Injuries Among High School Athletes-United States, 2005-06 School Year. September 29, 2006/55 (38); 1037-1040. Available from: http://www.cdc.gov/mmwr/preview/mmwrhtml/mm5538a1.htm

[2] www.cdc.gov. National Health Interview Survey. National Center for Health Statistics. NCHS-NHIS-Description. Available from: http://cdc.gov/nchs/about/major/ nhis/ hisdesc.htm

[3] Stovitz S, Johnson R. NSAIDs and musculoskeletal treatment. What is the clinical evidence? *Physician Sportsmed.* 2003;31(1). Available from: http://www.chiro.org

[4] Tamara S, Bublitz C, Hambridge S. Emergency department visits among pediatric patients for sports-related injury: Basic epidemiology and impact of race/ethnicity and insurance status. *Pediatr. Emerg. Care.* 2006;22(5):309-15.

[5] Predel HG, Pabst H, Dieter P, Gallacchi G, Giannetti B, Bulitta M, Heidecker J, Mueller E. Diclofenac patch for topical treatment of acute impact injuries: a randomised, double blind, placebo controlled multicenter study. *Br. J. Sports Med.* 2004;38:318-23.

[6] Paoloni J, Orchard J. The use of therapeutic medications for soft-tissue injuries in sports medicine. *Med. J. Aust.* 2005;183(7):384-8.

[7] www.fda.gov. Vioxx (rofecoxib) Questions and Answers. 2004. U.S. Food and Drug Administration, Center for Drug Evaluation and Research. Available from: http://www.fda.gov/cder/drug/infopage/vioxx/vioxxQA.htm

[8] Clark E, Plint A, Correll R, Gaboury I, Passi B. A randomized controlled trial of acetaminophen, ibuprofen, and codeine for acute pain Relief in children with musculoskeletal trauma. *Pediatrics.* 2007; 119(3): 460-7.

[9] Galer B, Rowotham M, Perander J, Devers A, Friedman E. Topical diclofenac patch relieves minor sports injury pain: Results of a multicenter controlled clinical trial. *J. Pain Sympt. Manage.* 2000; 19(4):287-94.

[10] Mazieres B, Rouanet S, Velicy J, Scarsi C, Reiner V. Topical ketoprofen (100 mg) for the treatment of ankle sprian: A randomized, double-blind, placebo-controlled study. *Am. J. Sports Med.* 2005;33(4):515-23.

[11] Esparza F, Cobain C, Jimenez J F, Garcia-Cota Juan, Sanchez C, Maestro A. Topical ketoprofen TDS patch versus dilofenac gel: efficacy and tolerability in benign sport related soft-tissue injuries. *Br. J. Sports Med.* 2007;41:134-9.

[12] www.cerimon.com. Cerimon Pharmaceuticals. Press Release, October 2007. Available from: http://www.cerimon.com/news/041007.html

[13] www.clinicaltrials.gov. Trial list. Search: Diclofenac Sodium. Available from: http://www.clinicaltrials.gov/ct/search;jsessionid=9343FACF0E0E3BF3AC011DA052 2316DA?term=diclofenac+sodium+&submit=Search

[14] Moore R, Tramer M, Carroll D, Wiffen P, McQuay H. Quantitive systematic review of topically applied non-steroidal anti-inflammatory drugs. *BMJ.* 1998;316:333-8.

In: Adolescence and Chronic Illness
Editors: H. Omar et al.

ISBN: 978-1-60876-628-4
© 2010 Nova Science Publishers, Inc.

Chapter 24

CHRONIC DISABILITY FROM HIP ABNORMALITIES IN ADOLESCENCE

Avinash L. Jadhav[*] and Dale E. Rowe

Department of Orthopaedic Surgery, Michigan State University/Kalamazoo
Center for Medical Studies, Kalamazoo, Michigan, United States.

ABSTRACT

Disabling mechanical hip pain in active and healthy adolescents has long been a difficult clinical problem. Our knowledge of this problem has exploded in recent years and two opposite morphological abnormalities responsible for this have been identified viz. adolescent dysplasia (AD) and femoroacetabular impingement (FAI). Recognition of the detrimental effect of these subtle morphologic abnormalities of hip has motivated development of novel joint-preserving surgeries that can relieve disability and prevent early joint degeneration; however, early intervention is key to success. Unfortunately diagnosis of these conditions is often missed because the physical signs are subtle and X-rays are often reported normal. By being aware of the classic history and typical examination as well as X-ray findings, pediatricians now have the opportunity to identify these patients early and play an important role in their management by timely referral to a specialized orthopaedic surgeon. In this chapter the distinctive pathological, clinical, radiological features and management of the two types of morphological hip abnormalities in adolescents has been described.

INTRODUCTION

By virtue of being the largest and most mobile weight-bearing joint, normal hip function is fundamental to day to day activities as well as successful sports participation. Not only it is important in running, jumping and kicking activities; it also contributes to the generation and

---

[*] *Correspondence:* Avinash Jadhav, MD, FRCS (Ortho), Associate Professor, Department of Orthopaedic Surgery, Michigan State University/Kalamazoo Center for Medical Studies, 1000 Oakland Drive, Kalamazoo, MI 49008 United States. Tel: 269-337-6250; Fax: 269-337-6444; E-mail: jadhav@kcms.msu.edu

transference of forces in upper limb dominated activities. Therefore any problem with the hip function results in significant disability. The etiology of chronic hip disability in adolescents can be divided into four groups:

- Neuromuscular causes such as cerebral palsy, myelodysplasia, spinal muscular atrophies, muscular dystrophy etc.
- Inflammatory and infective causes such as juvenile rheumatoid arthritis, septic arthritis and osteomyelitis
- Vascular problems such as avascular necrosis of femoral head
- Morphological hip abnormalities

In the past few years evidence has emerged demonstrating that subtle morphologic abnormalities resulting from mild subclinical forms or post treatment residual sequel of childhood diseases such as Perthes disease, developmental dysplasia of hip (DDH) and slipped capital femoral epiphysis (SCFE) are the commonest causes of hip disability presenting in the second or third decade of life in healthy population with increased sport activity [1]. Its importance is enormous, because it limits function in these otherwise healthy individuals at a time, which is critical for their career as well as social life. It presents as a diagnostic challenge, because the clinical as well as radiological signs are very subtle and can be easily overlooked, even by an experienced practitioner. It is also a therapeutic problem, because these patients respond poorly to symptomatic treatment and are frequently made worse by conventional physical therapy. Moreover it is now thought that the morphological hip abnormalities play an important role in the pathogenesis of primary osteoarthritis (OA) of the hip, which was up to now considered to be idiopathic in origin [2-4]. Recent realization of significance and prevalence of these morphological hip abnormalities has led to development of innovative hip surgeries in the last few years. Early studies suggest that timely correction of these morphological abnormalities not only successfully resolves the disabling symptoms in these adolescents and young adults, but may also prevent development of early osteoarthritis in the hip [5]. These inventions are of huge significance, because the conventional treatment for osteoarthritis i.e. joint replacement is inappropriate in these young patients due to their demand for high activity and long remaining life span. In this chapter the pathogenesis, classification, diagnosis and treatment of this important cause of chronic hip disability seen during late teens and early adult life will be discussed.

MORPHOGENESIS OF THE DEFORMITY

Morphological hip abnormalities can occur due to inadequate bone or excessive bone. Inadequate bone leads to instability, because of lack of support to the femoral head from the underdeveloped acetabular roof and is commonly known as adolescent dysplasia (AD). In contrast, excessive bone leads to abutment between the femoral head and the acetabulum and is commonly known as femoro-acetabular impingement (FAI).

In adolescent hip dysplasia most patients have an abnormality predominantly on the acetabular side [6] (see figure 1), where as in FAI it could be on either side. Accordingly FAI has been subdivided into two types [2]. When the excessive bone is on the femoral neck, it reduces its clearance underneath the acetabulum in flexion-internal rotation. This is called as cam impingement. When the excessive bone is on the anterior acetabular rim, it abuts with femoral neck in flexion- internal rotation. This is called as pincer impingement (see figure 2).

In cam impingement the anterior and/or lateral femoral head-neck offset and anteversion is decreased [2]. This was initially described by Stulberg in 1975 as pistol grip deformity (see figure 3). It is typically seen as a sequel of slipped capital femoral epiphysis and has been also k.a. post-slip morphology [7-9]. This deformity is also seen following Perthes disease (figure 4), avascular necrosis (AVN) of femoral head [10], malunited femoral neck fracture [11] and in idiopathic nonspherical extension of articular cartilage to the anterosuperior neck [12] (figure 5).

Pincer impingement on the other hand typically results from acetabular retroversion [13] (posteriorly orientated acetabulum) (figure 6), protrusio acetabuli (deep socket), coxa profunda (over coverage) [14-16], coxa vara, os acetabulare (figure 7) and following acetabuloplasty in DDH/Perthes disease/AD [17]. The cam and pincer impingement coexist in 86% of patients, although usually one predominates over the other [18].

As we know, current treatments of SCFE, Perthes disease and DDH may not restore normal shape of acetabulum and/or femur completely. This can result in mechanical hip pain a few years later. What is more important to note is that the unrecognized mild subclinical forms of these conditions are far more common (estimated 10 times (6)) than those that are identified and treated. These undiagnosed mild forms also leave sufficient morphological sequel which result in mechanical hip pain at a later stage. Because these mild disorders have gone undiagnosed, most patients presenting with mechanical hip pain lack a clear history of any predisposing condition [5].

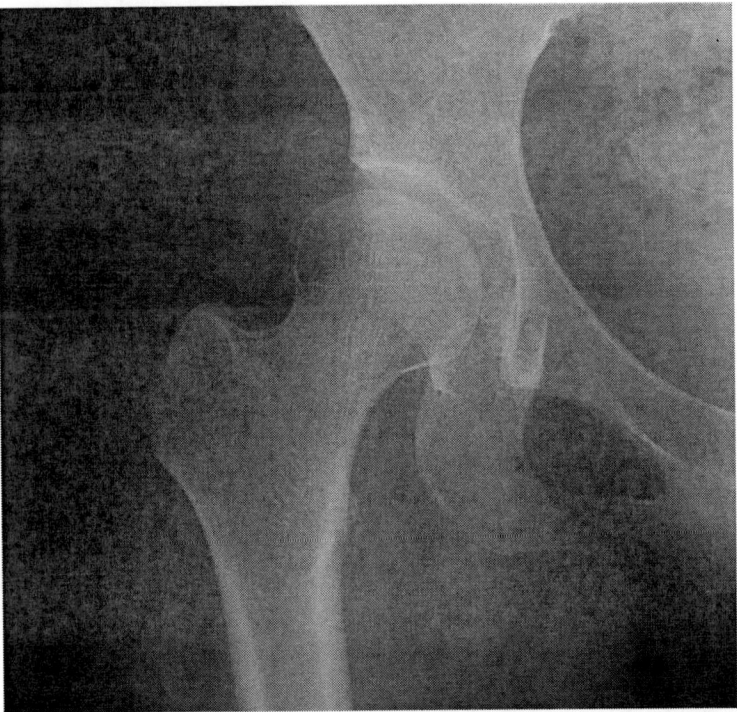

Figure 1. Adolescent hip dysplasia.

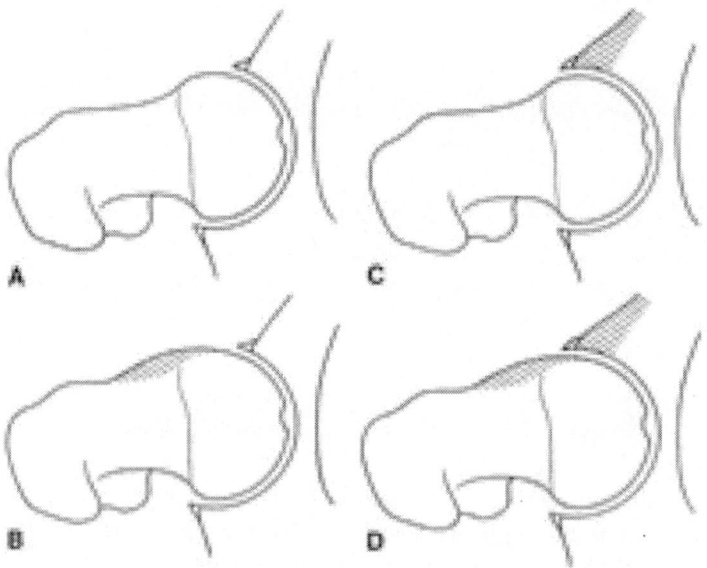

Figure 2. Types of FAI. A: normal joint; B: cam impingement; C: pincer impingement; D: mixed impingement.

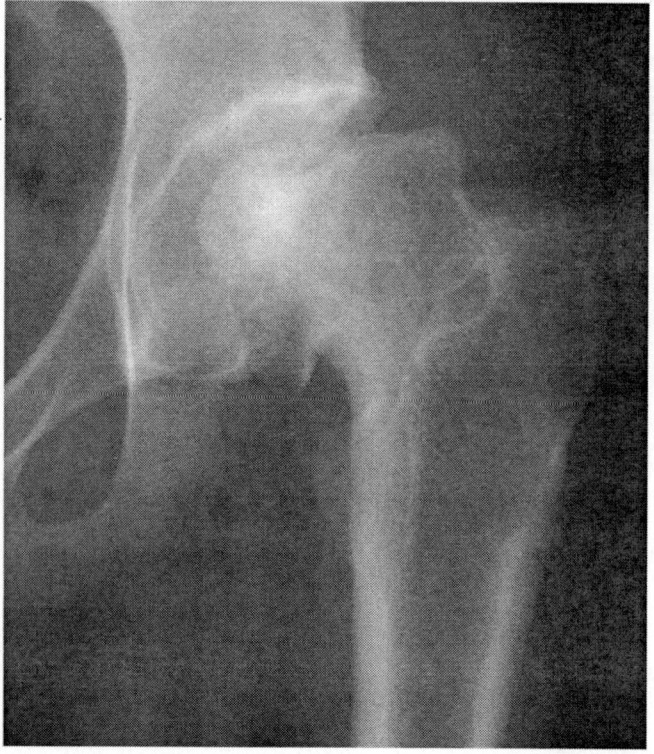

Figure 3. Sequalae of SCFE.

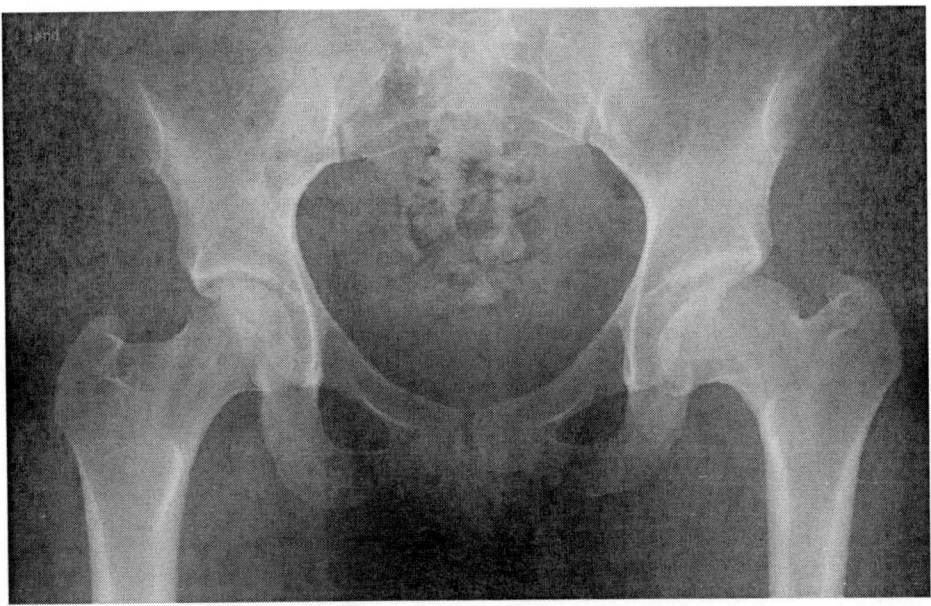

Figure 4. Post Perthes residual deformity.

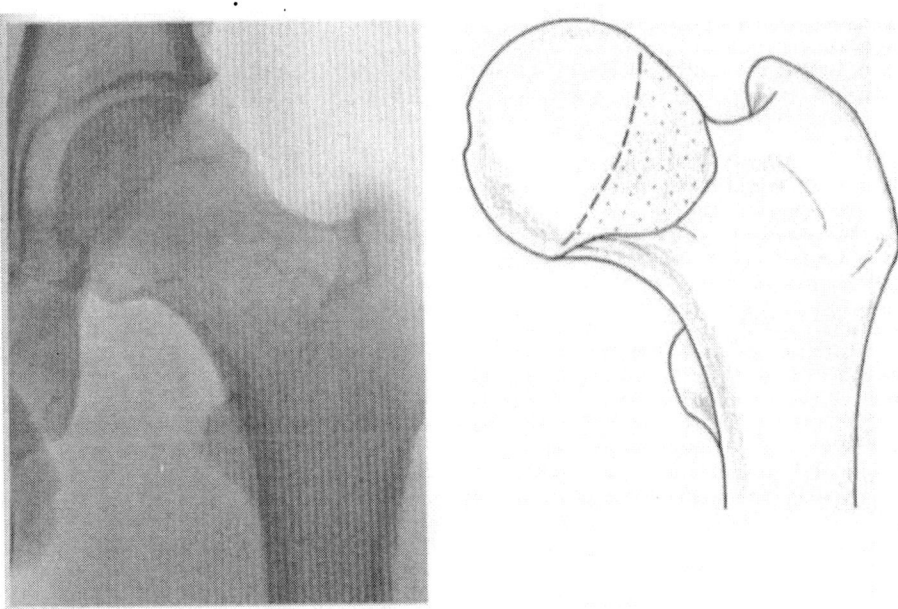

Figure 5. Non-spherical head due to abnormal anterior-lateral epiphyseal extension.

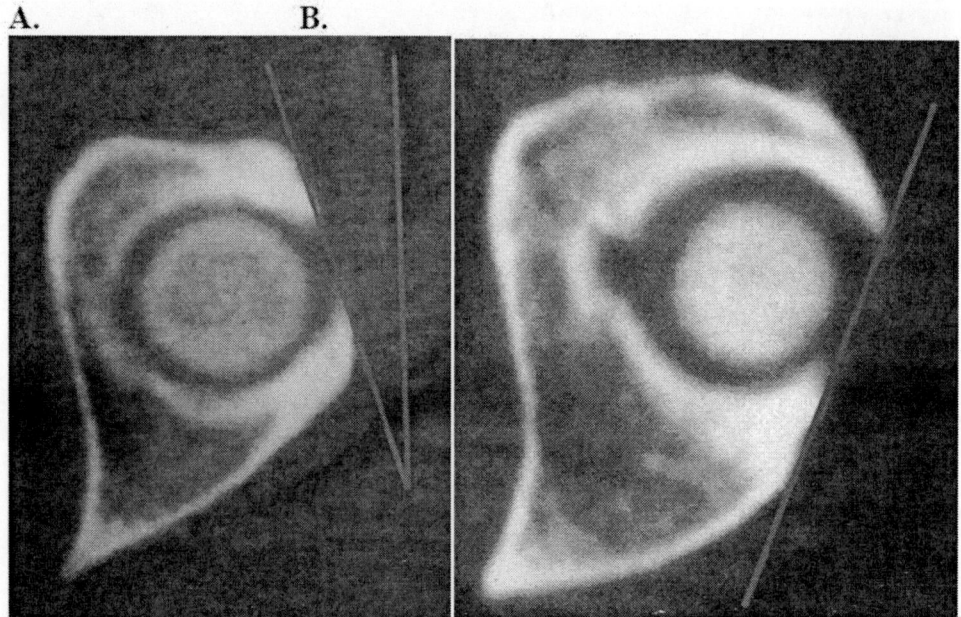

Figure 6. Acetabular retroversion. A. Normal anteverted acetabulum; B. Abnormal Retroverted acetabulum.

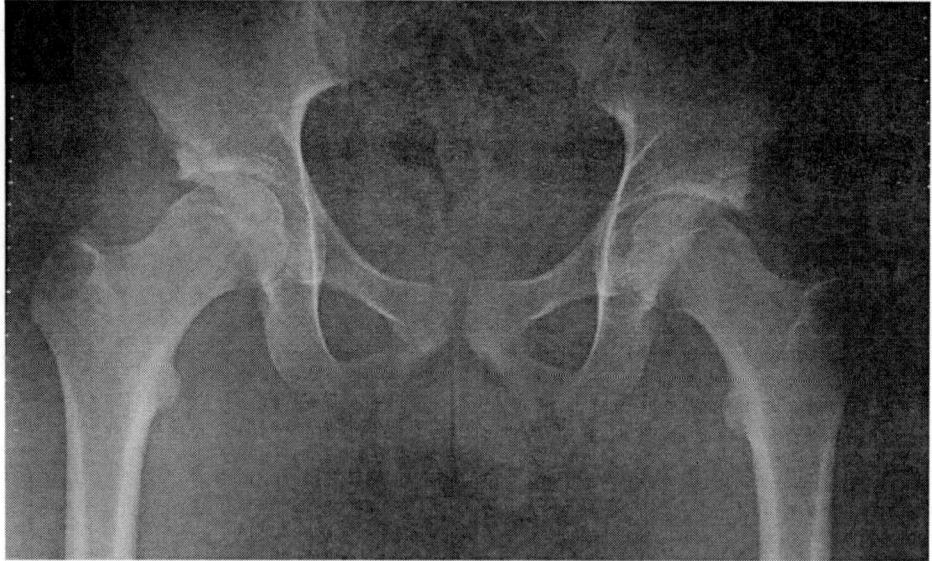

Figure 7. Os acetabulare.

PAHTOGENESIS OF MECHANICAL HIP PAIN

In both the subgroups, adolescent dysplasia as well as FAI, the pain is due to labral and chondral damage in the anterosuperior area of the acetabulum [2,19-21], although the pathogenesis is quite different. Following this initial damage osteoarthritis begins peripherally in the anterosuperior area and progresses centrally to involve the entire hip joint if the deformity is not corrected in time [1,2,22,23].

In adolescent dysplasia, due to inadequate roof, excessive stresses are placed on the labrum with weight bearing. This leads to its hypertrophy initially and mucoid degeneration later (see figure 8a). Due to relatively vertical acetabulum, the femoral head also has a tendency to slide laterally and superiorly out of the acetabulum (instability). With these repeated subclinical subluxations, the labrum is eventually sheared off inside out from the antero-lateral acetabular rim (figure 8b).

Contrary to this, in cam impingement, during flexion and internal rotation as the nonspherical (cam shaped) part of the femoral head with increased radius is jammed under the anterosuperior acetabulum, it creates an outside-in shear force separating the articular cartilage from the labrum (see figure 9).

In pincer impingement, the labrum is directly pinched between the anterosuperior aspect of the femoral neck and the acetabular rim (see figure 10). This results in fissuring rather than hypertrophy and mucoid degeneration seen in dysplasia [24] (see figure 11).

Anterosuperior osteoarthritis is also caused by opposite mechanisms in these two subgroups. In adolescent dysplasia, the weight bearing contact area of the joint is markedly reduced due to deficiency in the acetabular roof as well as the lateral subluxation of the femoral head [25]. This results in static stress concentration at the anterosuperior acetabulum (see figure 12) leading to degeneration of articular cartilage and (Pauwels theory [26]).

In contrast, in cam impingement the anterosuperior osteoarthritis is caused by motion-induced joint damage. During flexion and internal rotation as the nonspherical (cam shaped) part of the femoral head with increased radius is jammed under the anterosuperior acetabulum it creates dynamic stress concentration and outside-in abrasion of the acetabular cartilage leading to its delamination and degeneration. In contrast to impingement in total hip replacement, the natural hip is under much higher constraint, and does not allow the head to escape by subluxation or dislocation. Therefore the forceful hinging of the head against the anterosuperior part of the acetabulum during flexion, scuffs the posterior-inferior acetabular cartilage too. This is called as the countercoup injury (see figure 13).

In pincer impingement, initially the labrum is damaged due to direct pinching between the femoral neck and acetabular rim. With dysfunctional labrum, the stresses on the adjacent anterosuperior acetabulum are increased leading to cartilage degeneration, although only in the narrow peripheral strip.

From these differing mechanisms it is obvious why cartilage delamination is more predominant in cam type of FAI while labral fissuring is more common in the pincer type. Since the morphological problem is exactly opposite in AD and FAI, distinction between them is crucial to ensure appropriate treatment. Although their presentation may appear similar on the surface, they each have distinctive clinical and radiological features which help to differentiate them.

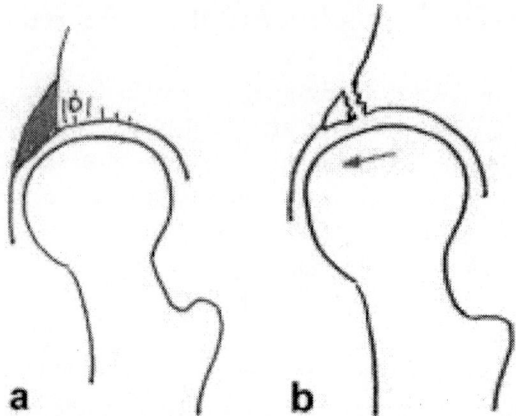

Figure 8. Mechanism of labral damage in adolescent dysplasia.

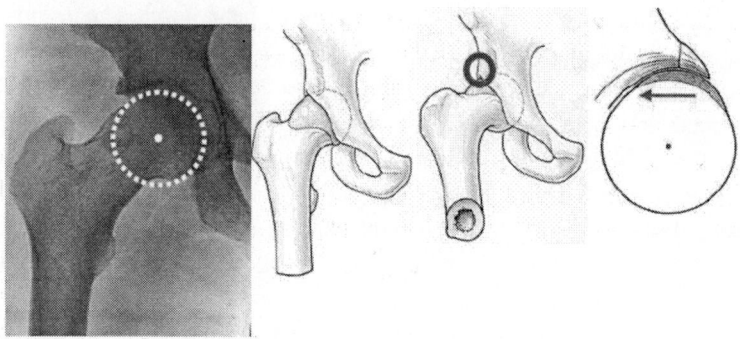

Figure 9. Mechanism of labral damage in cam impingement.

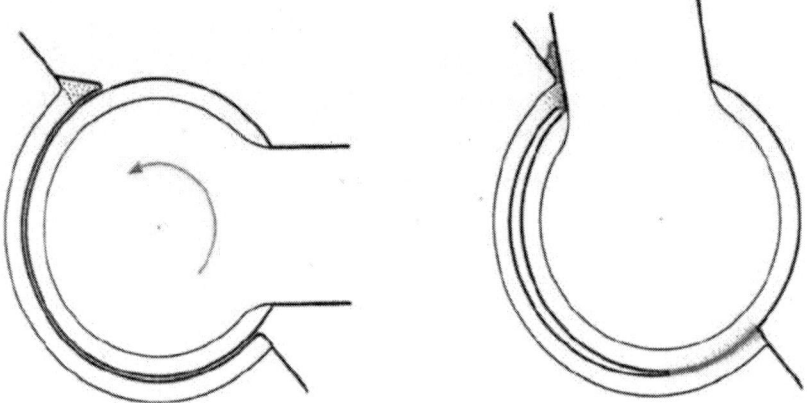

Figure 10. Mechanism of labral damage in pincer impingement.

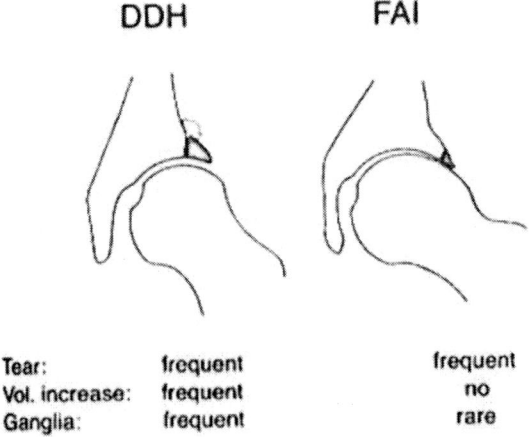

Figure 11. Difference in labral damage in adolescent dysplasia (DDH) and FAI.

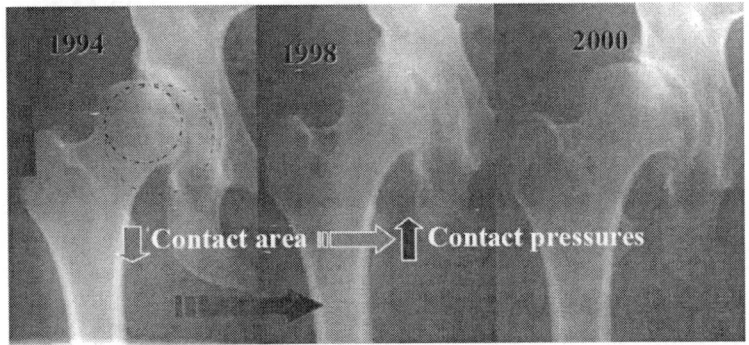

Figure 12. Mechanism of chondral damage (osteoarthritis) in adolescent dysplasia.

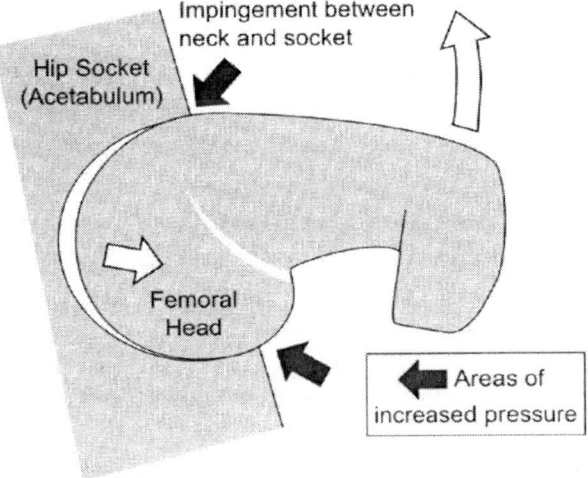

Figure 13. Mechanism of chondral damage in cam impingement.

CLINICAL PRESENTATION

The estimated prevalence of FAI is 10-15% [23]. The incidence of adolescent dysplasia is not known, but it is higher in certain ethnic groups and is bilateral in around 50% [27]. AD is more common in females, whereas cam impingement is usually seen in younger males and pincer in relatively older females [5].

HISTORY

Some patients of adolescent dysplasia report past history of treatment for DDH, while those with FAI may report history of SCFE or Perthes disease or fracture neck of femur.

Typically these are healthy, active individuals between the ages of 15 and 30 years. Many FAI patients are involved in athletic activities with extreme ranges of motion, such as ice hockey, martial arts, or track and field events that require deep hip flexion or pivoting maneuvers. Patients usually seek help, because they cannot participate in their favorite activities as they are increasingly limited by their symptoms. Often these patients have a history of extensive diagnostic workups and even inappropriate surgical treatments, such as repair of inguinal hernia, laparoscopy, and other abdominal procedures [28,29].

Limp is rare in FAI whereas in AD the typical early presentation is limp following heavy activity due to instability as well as fatigue of the abductor muscles, which are working at a mechanical disadvantage due to shortened lever arm. The common presenting feature of both the morphological hip abnormalities is activity related pain in young healthy individuals although the location, character, aggravating activities and symptoms associated with the pain differ between AD and FAI.

In adolescent dysplasia, the pain is in the form of dull ache due to predominance of chondral damage. It is generalized in location with some lateral predominance over the fatigued abductors. Occasionally trochanteric pain may develop due to secondary trochanteric bursitis and groin pain due to labral damage. The pain is worse with prolonged walking, standing and activities of daily living. Sensation of giving way may be present due to subluxations.

In FAI the pain is sharp due to impingement. It is predominantly anterior in the groin and only occasionally lateral, but without tenderness over the greater trochanter. It is worse with prolonged sitting, driving and sporting activities involving deep flexion. Sensations of aching or popping are more common due to frequent labral tears. In both the conditions, the pain is usually insidious in onset, although an occasional patient may report an inciting event. The duration of pain may vary from six months to many years. Severity of pain is proportional to the degree of morphological deformity and level of activity [23]. Rest in general relieves the pain; except that in FAI it becomes worse after prolonged periods of sitting. Patient often indicates the location of pain by gripping the lateral hip, just above the greater trochanter, between the abducted thumb and index finger. This is known as the C sign (see figure 14).

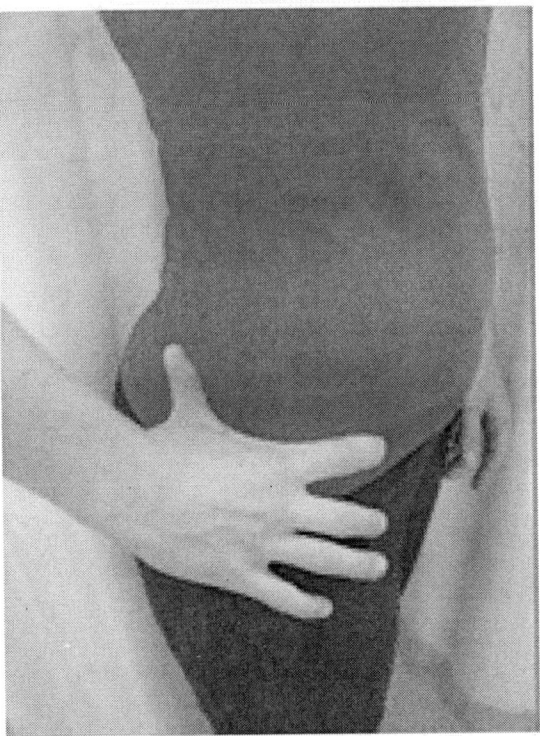

Figure 14. The C sign.

Physical Examination

Patients with dysplasia usually have full motion with more internal than external rotation, associated with limited pain. It is important to document this range of motion to ensure that the hip can cope with realignment osteotomy which will alter the arc of movement. In contrast, hip motion with impingement usually shows profound limitation of internal rotation especially in flexion with pain. Pathognomonic sign of FAI is impingement test. It is positive in all patients with FAI [2,19] and is negative in dysplasia. It has been correlated with acetabular rim lesions seen on MRI arthrogram [30]. This test is performed with the patient supine on the examination table. The hip and knee of the affected hip are flexed to 90° and then the hip is adducted and internally rotated. If this reproduces the type and location of the patient's pain, the test is considered to be positive (see figure 15A).

Although less common, Posteroinferior impingement test indicative of the countercoup injury may be positive. This test is performed with the patient lying supine with the affected leg hanging free from the edge of the bed to produce maximum hip extension. Test is positive, if external rotation of the hip in this position elicits pain (see figure 15B).

Apprehension test, although classic for instability, is not always elicitable in patients with AD. It is also performed with the patient lying supine at the edge of the exam table. With the contralateral hip flexed, the affected hip is extended over the edge of the table and then rapidly hyper-extended and externally rotated threatening anterolateral subluxation of the femoral head. The test is considered positive if it induces a feeling of dislike or discomfort with reproduction of patient's symptoms of pain/ giving way.

The Trendelenberg test is much easier to perform and is frequently positive in dysplasia, especially following a brief period of exercise which wears out the abductors working at a mechanical disadvantage. In this test, when the patient stands on the affected leg (single leg stance), the pelvis drops to the opposite side (see figure 16), as the fatigued abductors are unable to support the body weight.

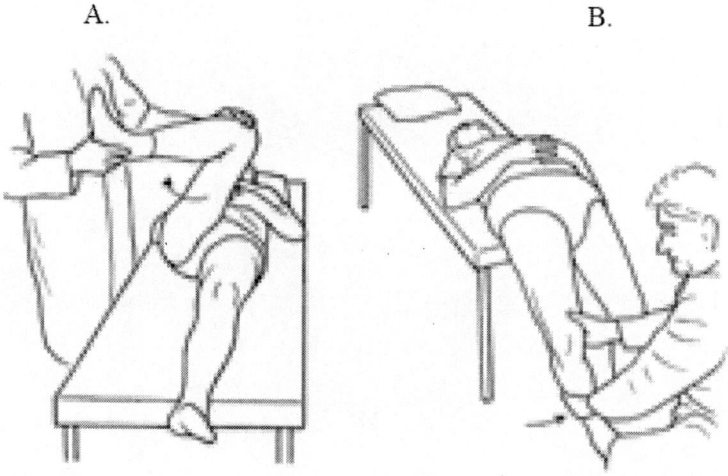

Figure 15. Impingement tests. A, Anterolateral impingement test. B, Posteroinferior impingement test.

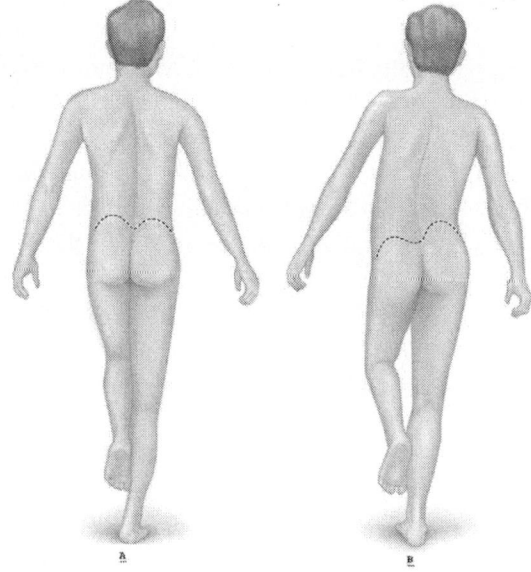

Figure 16. Trendelenberg Test:
A: Negative Test: Pelvis held horizontal in single leg stance.
B: Positive Test: Pelvis drops on opposite side during single leg stance.

DIFFERENTIAL DIAGNOSIS

Commonest causes of sports related hip pain in this age group are groin strain and trochanteric bursitis. The former can be differentiated by being an isolated episode of acute onset pain following a specific event whereas the latter by tenderness on greater trochanter and lateral hip pain with resisted adduction. Unlike FAI and AD, both of these conditions respond to conventional physical therapy

Acute labral tear is another common diagnosis made in this group of patients. However recent evidence suggests that true traumatic acetabular labral tear without underlying morphological abnormality of the hip joint is extremely rare. Therefore in all these cases covert AD or FAI should be suspected and the patient should be investigated accordingly.

Primary FAI, resulting from morphological abnormalities of the hip joint, should also be distinguished from secondary impingement which can occur due to exaggerated lumbar lordosis with pelvic tilt and to hip osteophytosis (sports or posterior hip osteoarthritis). Treatment such as osteoplasty described below will not be effective in these patients.

IMAGING

Hip X-Rays in AD and FAI are often reported to be normal. This might be because the understanding of this condition is relatively recent and the radiographic findings are subtle. Inability to recognize these subtleties should not overshadow a convincing history and physical examination findings, especially the positive impingement test.

Before referral to an orthopaedic surgeon, an anteroposterior view of the pelvis and a lateral view of the affected hip are all that is required to support the diagnosis. Basic features of AD and FAI seen on X-ray are described below. Specialized imaging and measurements to determine the extent of incongruency and degeneration should be left to the discretion of the orthopedic surgeon for surgical decision making and preoperative planning.

In adolescent dysplasia, because of the lateral and superior subluxation of the head, Shenton's line is broken. The CE angle of Wiberg (angle made by the line joining center of the head and lateral edge of the acetabulum with the vertical) is less than 25 degrees and Tonnis angle (angle made by the roof of the acetabulum with the horizontal) is more than 10 degrees (see figure 17).

In cam impingement, the head neck junction shows a bump causing the impingement (bump sign, see figure 18) or a pit resulting from the impingement (Pit sign, see figure 19). The aspherical head becomes more obvious by placing circular Mose's templates on the X-ray. In Pincer impingement the anterior lip of acetabulum is seen to cross the posterior lip (crossover sign (13), see figure 20) on AP pelvis X-ray.

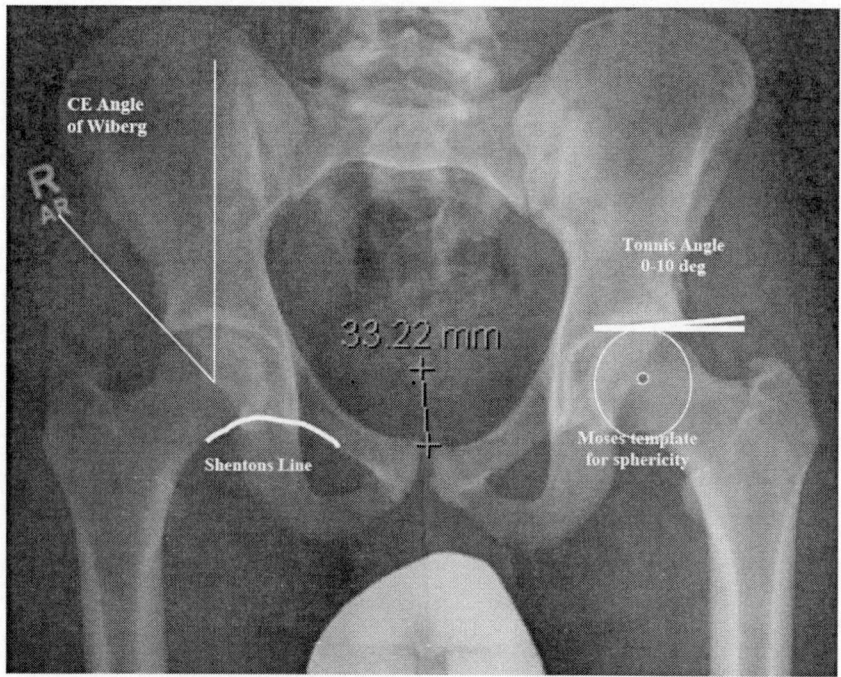

Figure 17. Radiological signs of adolescent dysplasia.

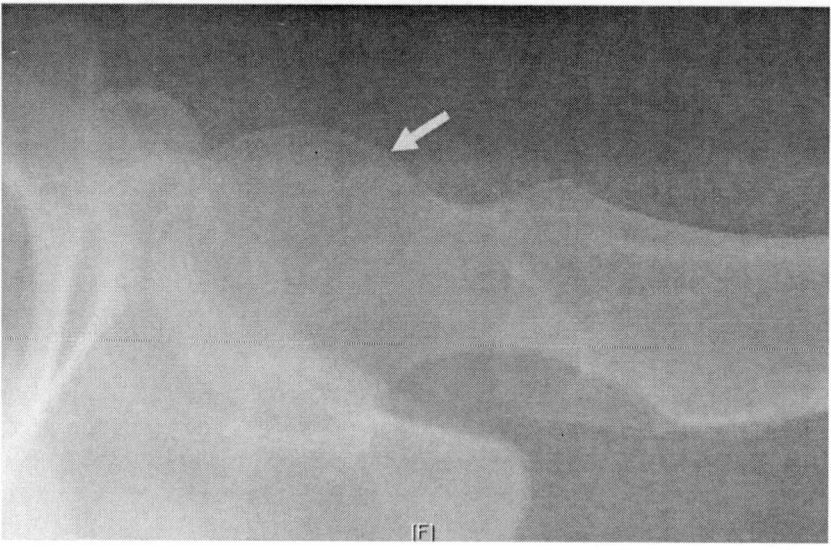

Figure 18. Pit sign.

Chronic Disability from Hip Abnormalities in Adolescence 325

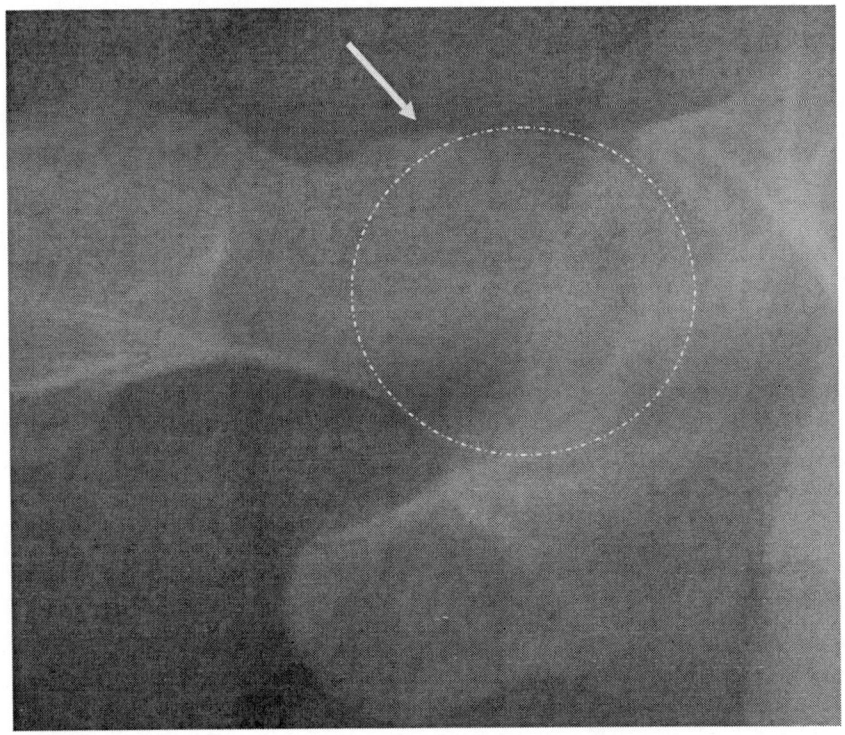

Figure 19. Bump sign.

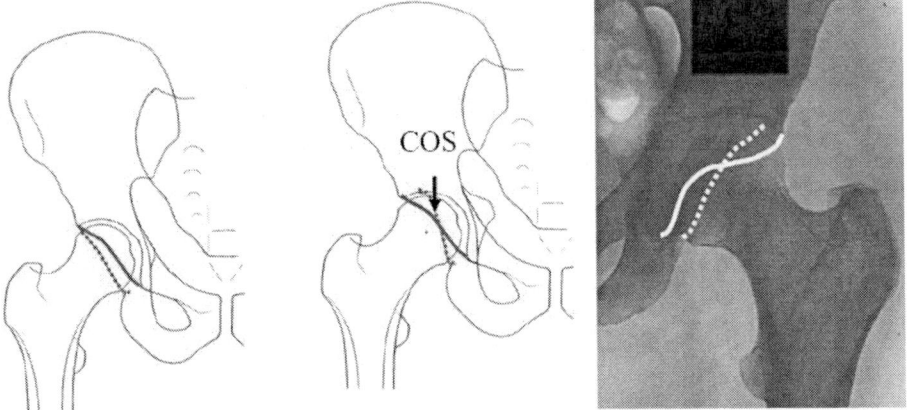

Figure 20. Cross over sign (COS).

TREATMENT

The constellation of demographic features, presenting symptoms, clinical signs and radiological findings of AD and FAI are fairly consistent and should allow the pediatricians to identify those who could benefit from a referral to an orthopaedic surgeon. As AD and FAI are still fairly new to the orthopaedic world, referral to a specialist orthopedic surgeon is required. Surgical techniques for managing these problems are highly specialized and are unlikely to be undertaken by the general orthopedist. Most orthopedic surgeons will however have knowledge of a colleague experienced with management of this condition and Pediatricians should contact a local orthopedic surgeon to inquire about appropriate referral.

NON-OPERATIVE TREATMENT

Non-operative treatment has minimal role in the treatment of morphological hip abnormalities because although it may relieve the symptoms temporarily, it cannot halt the progress of the destructive process in presence of the abnormal morphology. Pain relief is obtained with activity restriction however the young age of these patients, their high activity levels and athletic ambitions usually jeopardize their compliance. NSAIDs may be used for temporary pain relief, but their prolonged use should be avoided as they mask the symptoms of the underlying destructive process.

Conventional physical therapy with emphasis on improving range of motion and stretching is counterproductive because this actually exacerbates the instability in AD and impingement in FAI. Emphasis of physical therapy should be on isometric strength exercises to prevent muscle deconditioning rather than improving range of motion.

Nevertheless a brief trial of conservative therapy helps to differentiate groin strain and trochanteric bursitis which respond to it. It also mentally prepares the patient and the family for the surgical intervention. However it is important not to get carried away by the nonsurgical treatment and continue it for too long as it will invariably advance the destructive process and progress to arthritis. Early surgical intervention is important to successfully halt the degeneration.

SURGICAL TREATMENT

As the primary problem is a morphologic abnormality, it seems logical that correction of the morphology will cure the immediate disability and prevent future degeneration. Since the morphological problem is exactly opposite in adolescent dysplasia and FAI, their treatments are very different. Detailed description of the surgical techniques is beyond the scope of this book. However the indications, principles and results of the surgical procedures are outlined to make the reader aware of these new exciting options of hip surgery now available for their patients.

Surgical Treatment of Adolescent Dysplasia

Surgical treatment of AD is aimed at increasing the weight bearing contact area between the acetabulum and the femoral head, and shifting the centre of rotation of the hip medially. This is achieved by cutting the acetabulum out of the innominate bone without compromising its blood supply and refixing it in a more normal orientation. This is called as the periacetabular osteotomy (PAO) [30] (see figure 21). The technique in adolescents is more difficult than in toddlers because the pelvic ring is less flexible. Osteotomies performed closer to the acetabulum achieve greater correction and result in less pelvic asymmetry. Coxa valga if present, also needs to be corrected simultaneously by femoral varus osteotomy.

The outcome following PAO depends upon the quality and area of the articular cartilage placed in the weight-bearing zone. It is therefore best in patients with early symptoms and radiological evidence of 'point loading' who have not progressed to significant stiffness or degenerative change. In patients with grade 1 osteoarthritis i.e. when the joint space is still normal, symptoms are abolished and the degernerative process is halted if normal anatomy is restored by the surgery. Bernese PAO has been shown to have a better outcome than other acetabular osteotomies with 88% excellent/good results at 11 years in patients with Grade 0/1 osteoarthritis[31]

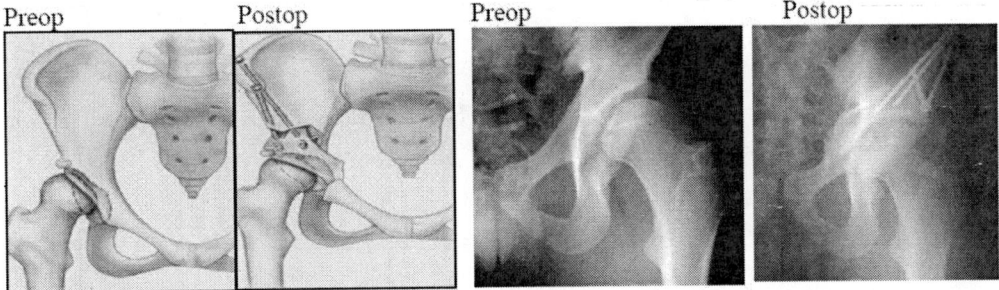

Figure 21. Bernese periacetabular osteotomy.

Surgical Treatment of FAI

In FAI the surgical goal is to excise the impinging excess bone and cartilage from the femoral head-neck junction (k.a. osteochondroplasty, see figure 22) and/or the anterior acetabular rim (k.a. acetabular recession and labral refixation, see figure 23). At the same time damaged labrum and articular cartilage is repaired or debrided. If required, trochanteric advancement and femoral neck lengthening is performed [7]. Pincer impingement from acetabular retroversion can also be treated with reverse periacetabular osteotomy [32].

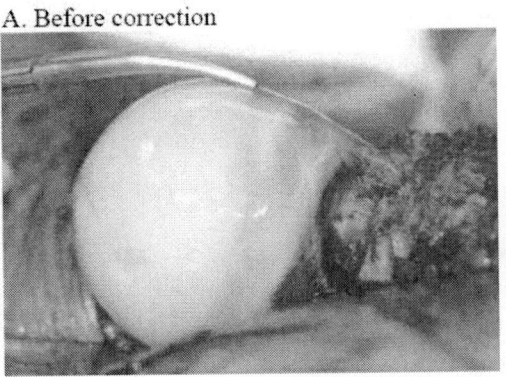
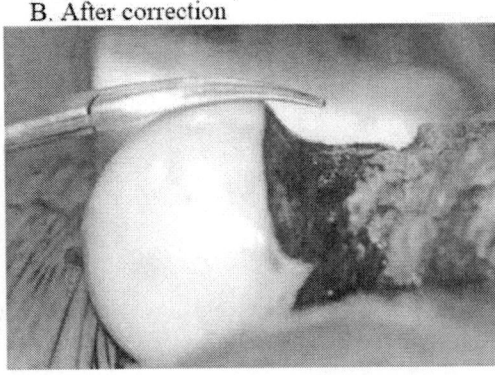

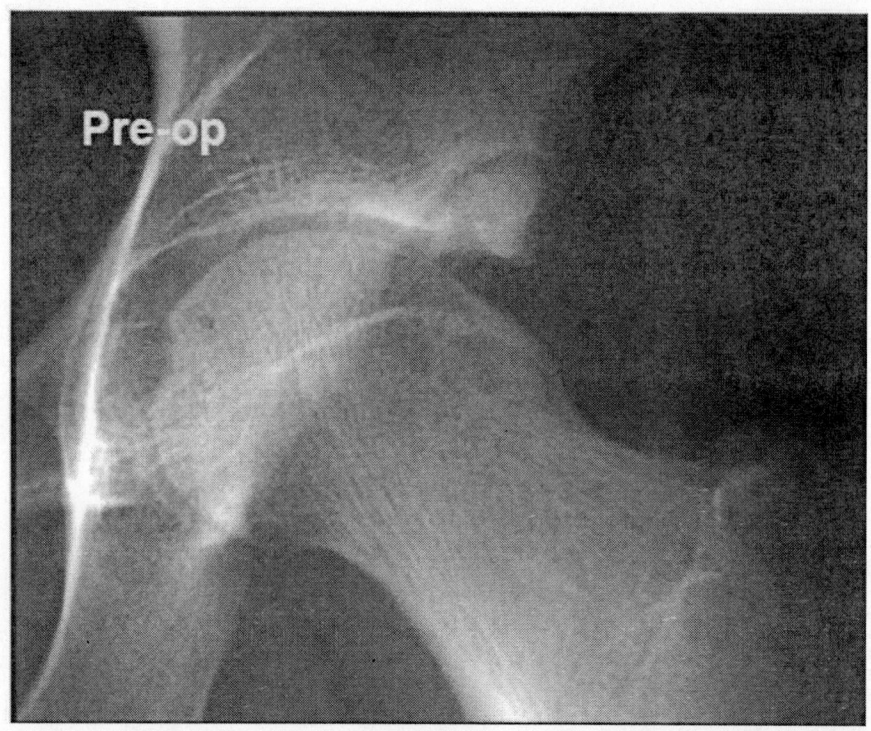
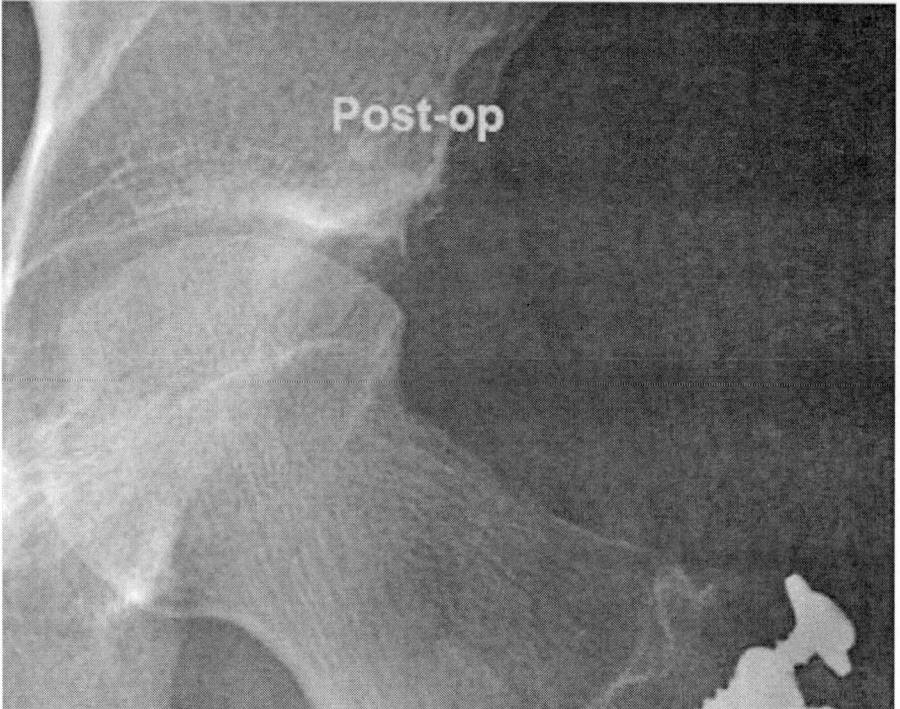

Figure 22. Osteochondroplasty.

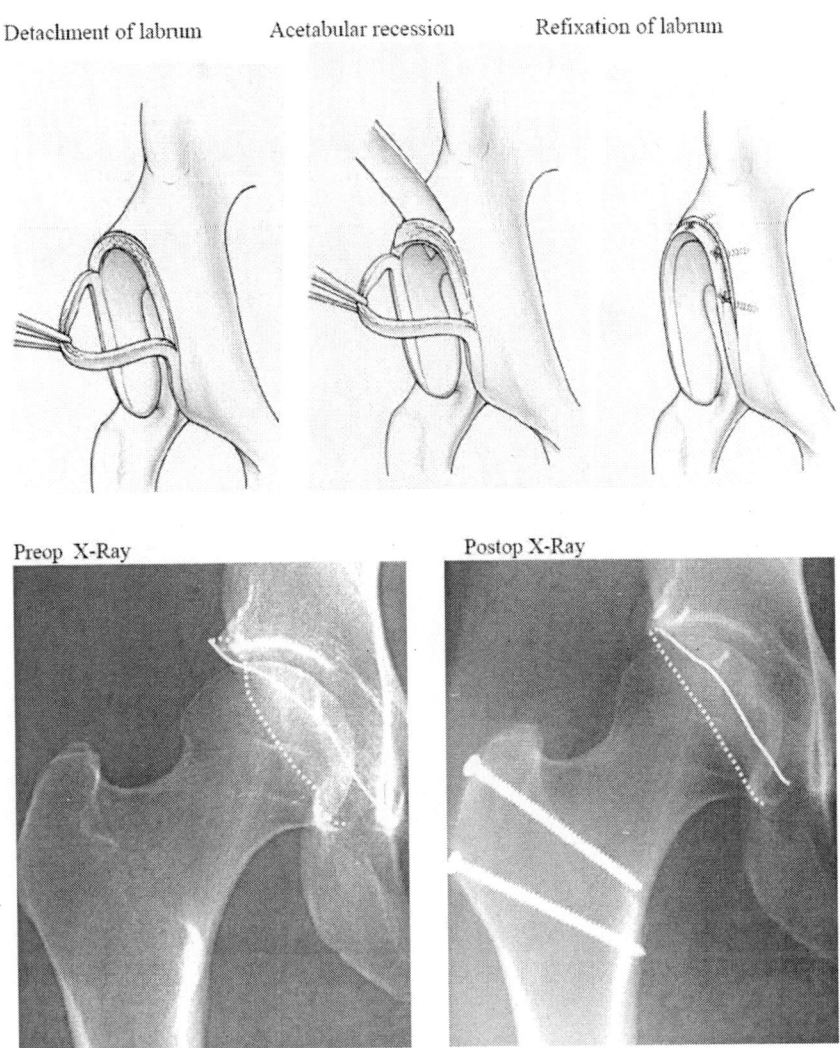

Figure 23. Surgery for pincer impingement:

Above intraarticular procedures require 360 degree visualization and access to inside of the hip joint. For this Ganz et al [22,33] developed a safe method to dislocate hip while preserving the posterior blood supply to the femoral head so as to avoid its avascular necrosis (AVN). In this technique the hip is dislocated anteriorly by using a modified trochanteric slide osteotomy and wide antero-superior 'Z' capsulotomy. This technique is called surgical hip dislocation (see figure 24). However following surgical hip dislocation, a prolonged rehabilitation period with partial weight bearing is required and trochanteric non-union is a potential complication. To avoid this and facilitate faster recovery, arthroscopic technique has been developed to treat FAI. Its obvious drawback is, due to limited space in the hip joint, visualization and access to all areas is difficult and so the debridement/ repair may be inadequate. For pincer impingement in particular, detachment of the labrum for acetabular recession and then refixation through arthroscope needs considerable expertise. Therefore more recently a combined arthroscopic with limited anterior approach has become more popular (see figure 25). Anterior mini-invasive approach alone has also been used, however its ability to address acetabular chondral lesions is limited [34]

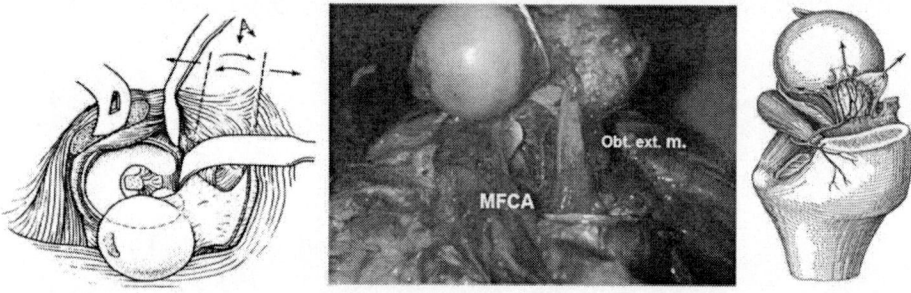

Figure 24. Surgical dislocation of hip preserving femoral head blood supply.

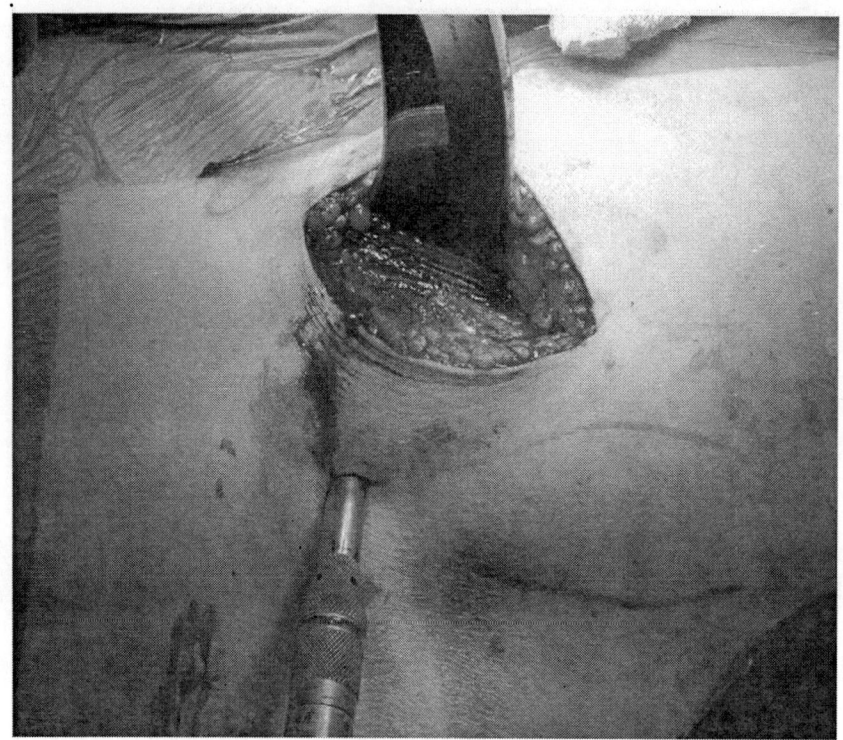

Figure 25. Combined arthroscopic and mini-open anterior surgical approach.

Like AD, outcome of FAI surgery also depends on the status of the articular cartilage. The success rate of arthroscopy in the management of the FAI is 71% in the absence of osteoarthritis and drops to 21%, when osteoarthritis is present [35]. Similarly surgical dislocation with correction of FAI yields good results without AVN of the hip or trochanteric nonunion [36], but only in patients with grade 0 or 1 osteoarthritis. Therefore these surgeries are is not recommended in patients with advanced degenerative changes and extensive articular cartilage damage [14]. Three factors indicate a favorable prognosis: preserved joint space, young age, and full correction of femoral and acetabular abnormalities. Even when there is early evidence of arthritis, reconstruction is highly desirable, as it delays the need for joint replacement by at least 20 years [37].

To prevent the morphological abnormalities leading to FAI following SCFE and LCPD, new surgical procedures using the surgical dislocation approach are being developed. In severe SCFE rather than fixation in situ which is the current standard of care, acute open reduction and internal fixation is performed [Fig. 26]. In healed Perthe's disease central collapsed part of the head is resected and the medial and lateral normal parts are joined to restore normal spherical head [Fig. 27].

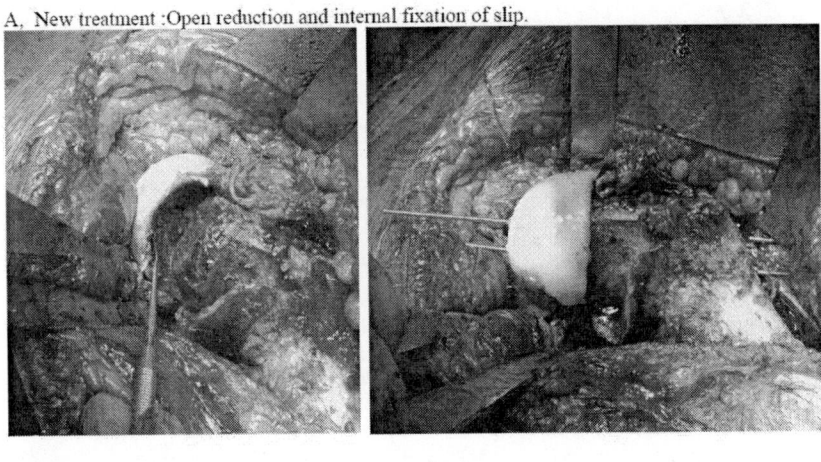

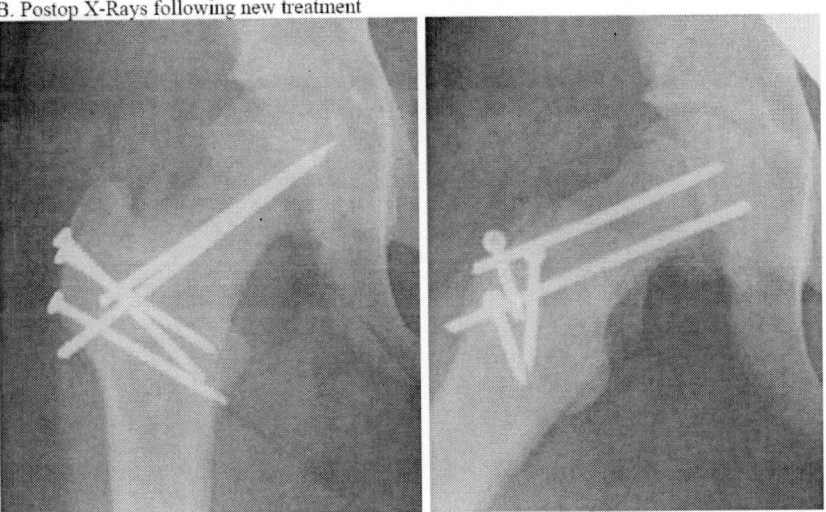

Figure 26. Continues on next page.

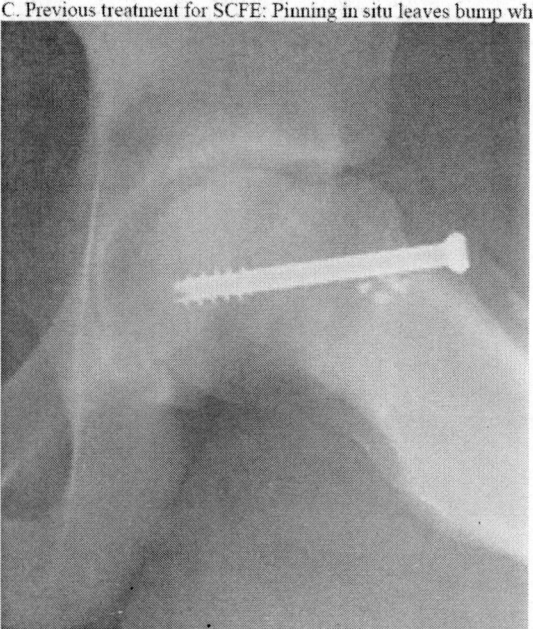

Figure 26. New approach for SCFE: Open reduction and internal fixation. A, New treatment :Open reduction and internal fixation of slip. B. Postop X-Rays following new treatment. C. Previous treatment for SCFE: Pinning in situ leaves bump which later causes FAI.

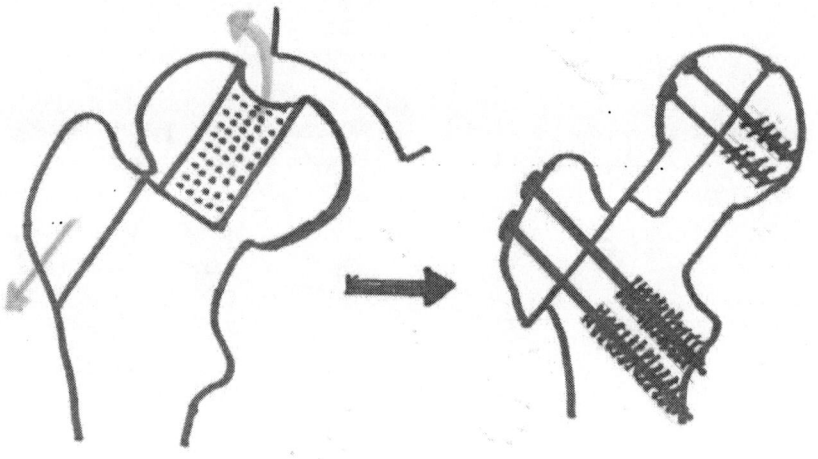

Figure 27. New treatment for correction of residual deformity following Perthes disease.

FUTURE

Although the initial clinical results of the surgical treatment of these osseous dysmorphisms have been extremely encouraging [14,38,39] prospective randomized controlled trial with long-term follow-up is needed to better define their natural history and its alteration with surgical treatment.

Further refinements of surgical procedures are required to enhance outcome and reduce rehabilitation period. With improvements in hip arthroscopy experience, technique (like intra-operative dynamic assessment of impingement) [40] and instrumentation it may become a gold standard in future, to treat these pathologies in a minimally invasive way with least morbidity.

It is well recognized that timely treatment before irreversible articular cartilage degeneration occurs is crucial for successful treatment, however accurate and early assessment of articular cartilage remains a challenge. MRI arthrograms are very sensitive and specific for detecting labral lesions, but have limitations in detecting articular cartilage degeneration [41]. Future advancements in MRI may make this possible and also enhance our understanding of the natural history of this disease which in turn will enable additional therapeutic interventions to be developed.

The difference between insufficient, adequate and excessive correction of impingement is relatively small and is influenced by many factors [31]. Excessive correction of dysplasia can result in impingement [17] and vice a versa. In future computer-navigated surgery may increase the accuracy of the positioning of the osteotomy and resection of the excess bone to improve results.

CONCLUSIONS

Recently morphological abnormalities of hip viz. AD and FAI have been identified as a common etiology of hip disability in healthy population at young age. Left untreated, these conditions cause significant pain which limits activities and leads to joint degeneration. Before its recognition these patients were misdiagnosed and mistreated expectantly. This not only affects quality of life at an important time, but also contributes to continued degeneration of the hip joint. In spite of normal reported radiograph, consistent history and a positive impingement test should alert the pediatrician to this diagnosis and warrant early referral to a specialist orthopaedic surgeon. Novel surgical treatments are now available which are effective if performed before the degeneration is advanced. They provide the patient a chance for substantial symptomatic relief, functional improvement and delay the onset of joint degeneration; although long-term results are awaited. Advances in imaging and arthroscopic surgery will make this treatment even more efficacious in future.

REFERENCES

[1] Leunig M, Ganz R. [Femoroacetabular impingement. A common cause of hip complaints leading to arthrosis]. *Unfallchirurg.* 2005;108(1):9-10,12-7. [German]

[2] Ganz R, et al. Femoroacetabular impingement: a cause for osteoarthritis of the hip. *Clin. Orthop. Relat. Res.* 2003;417:112-20.

[3] Tschauner C, Fock C, Hofmann S. [Femoro-acetabular impingement--an underestimated pathogenetic factor in coxarthrosis]. *Z. Orthop. Ihre Grenzgeb.* 2001;139(5):M88-91. [German]

[4] Tanzer M, Noiseux N. Osseous abnormalities and early osteoarthritis: the role of hip impingement. *Clin. Orthop. Relat. Res.* 2004;429:170-7.

[5] Parvizi J, Leunig M, Ganz R. Femoroacetabular impingement. *J. Am. Acad. Orthop. Surg.* 2007;15(9):561-70.

[6] Lankester BGM. Adolescent hip Dysplasia. *Curr. Orthop.* 2004;18:262-72.

[7] Rab GT. The geometry of slipped capital femoral epiphysis: implications for movement, impingement, and corrective osteotomy. *J. Pediatr. Orthop.* 1999;19(4):419-24.

[8] Goodman DA, et al. Subclinical slipped capital femoral epiphysis. Relationship to osteoarthrosis of the hip. *J. Bone Joint Surg. Am.* 1997;79(10):1489-97.

[9] Leunig M, et al. Slipped capital femoral epiphysis: early mechanical damage to the acetabular cartilage by a prominent femoral metaphysis. *Acta Orthop. Scand.* 2000;71(4):370-5.

[10] Kloen P, Leunig M, Ganz R. Early lesions of the labrum and acetabular cartilage in osteonecrosis of the femoral head. *J. Bone Joint Surg. Br.* 2002;84(1):66-9.

[11] Eijer H, Myers SR, Ganz R. Anterior femoroacetabular impingement after femoral neck fractures. *J. Orthop. Trauma.* 2001;15(7):475-81.

[12] Siebenrock KA, et al. Abnormal extension of the femoral head epiphysis as a cause of cam impingement. *Clin. Orthop. Relat. Res.* 2004;418:54-60.

[13] Reynolds D, Lucas J, Klaue K. Retroversion of the acetabulum: A cause of hip pain. *J. Bone Joint Surg.* [Br] 1999;81(B):281-8.

[14] Beck M, et al. Anterior femoroacetabular impingement: part II. Midterm results of surgical treatment. *Clin. Orthop. Relat. Res.* 2004;418):67-73.

[15] Harris WH. Etiology of osteoarthritis of the hip. *Clin. Orthop. Relat. Res.* 1986;213:20-33.

[16] Gekeler J. [Coxarthrosis with a deep acetabulum (proceedings)]. *Z. Orthop. Ihre Grenzgeb.* 1978;116(4):454.

[17] Myers SR, Eijer H, Ganz R. Anterior femoroacetabular impingement after periacetabular osteotomy. *Clin. Orthop. Relat. Res.* 1999;363:93-9.

[18] Beck M, et al. Hip morphology influences the pattern of damage to the acetabular cartilage: femoroacetabular impingement as a cause of early osteoarthritis of the hip. *J. Bone Joint Surg. Br.* 2005;87(7):1012-8.

[19] McCarthy JC, et al. The Otto E. Aufranc award: The role of labral lesions to development of early degenerative hip disease. *Clin. Orthop. Relat. Res.* 2001;393:25-37.

[20] Ito K, et al. Femoroacetabular impingement and the cam-effect. A MRI-based quantitative anatomical study of the femoral head-neck offset. *J. Bone Joint Surg. Br.* 2001;83(2):171-6.

[21] Notzli HP, et al. The contour of the femoral head-neck junction as a predictor for the risk of anterior impingement. *J. Bone Joint Surg. Br.* 2002;84(4):556-60.

[22] Ganz R, et al. Surgical dislocation of the adult hip a technique with full access to the femoral head and acetabulum without the risk of avascular necrosis. *J. Bone Joint Surg.* Br 2001;83(8):1119-24.

[23] Leunig M, et al. [Femoroacetabular impingement: trigger for the development of coxarthrosis]. *Orthopade.* 2006;35(1):77-84.
[24] Leunig M, et al. Evaluation of the acetabular labrum by MR arthrography. *J. Bone Joint Surg. Br.* 1997;79(2):230-4.
[25] Murphy SB, et al. Acetabular dysplasia in the adolescent and young adult. *Clin. Orthop. Relat. Res.* 1990;261:214-23.
[26] Pauwels F. Biomechanics of normal and diseased hip: *Theoretical foundation, technique and results of treatment.* Berlin: Springer, 1976.
[27] Li PL, Ganz R. Morphologic features of congenital acetabular dysplasia: one in six is retroverted. *Clin. Orthop. Relat. Res.* 2003;416:245-53.
[28] McCarthy JC, Lee JA. Acetabular dysplasia: a paradigm of arthroscopic examination of chondral injuries. *Clin. Orthop. Relat. Res.* 2002;405:122-8.
[29] Fricker PA. Management of groin pain in athletes. Br J Sports Med 1997;31(2):97-101.
[30] MacDonald SJ, et al. The Bernese periacetabular osteotomy for the treatment of adult hip dysplasia. *Chir. Organi. Mov.* 1997;82(2):143-54.
[31] Siebenrock KA, et al. Bernese periacetabular osteotomy. *Clin. Orthop. Relat. Res.* 1999;363:9-20.
[32] Siebenrock KA, Schoeniger R, Ganz R. Anterior femoro-acetabular impingement due to acetabular retroversion. Treatment with periacetabular osteotomy. *J. Bone Joint Surg. Am.* 2003;85(2):278-86.
[33] Gautier E, et al. Anatomy of the medial femoral circumflex artery and its surgical implications. *J. Bone Joint Surg. Br.* 2000;82(5):679-83.
[34] Jaberi FM, Parvizi J. Hip pain in young adults: femoroacetabular impingement. *J. Arthroplasty.* 2007;22(7 Suppl 3):37-42.
[35] McCarthy JC. The diagnosis and treatment of labral and chondral injuries. *Instr. Course Lect.* 2004;53:573-7.
[36] Peters CL, Erickson JA. Treatment of femoro-acetabular impingement with surgical dislocation and debridement in young adults. *J. Bone Joint Surg. Am.* 2006;88(8):1735-41.
[37] Langlais F, et al. Hip pain from impingement and dysplasia in patients aged 20-50 years. Workup and role for reconstruction. *Joint Bone Spine.* 2006;73(6):614-23.
[38] Espinosa N, et al. Treatment of femoro-acetabular impingement: preliminary results of labral refixation. *J. Bone Joint Surg. Am.* 2006;88(5):925-35.
[39] Murphy S, et al. Debridement of the adult hip for femoroacetabular impingement: indications and preliminary clinical results. *Clin. Orthop. Relat. Res.* 2004;429:178-81.
[40] Philippon MJ, et al. Arthroscopic management of femoroacetabular impingement: osteoplasty technique and literature review. *Am. J. Sports Med.* 2007;35(9):1571-80.
[41] Leunig M, et al. Magnetic resonance arthrography of labral disorders in hips with dysplasia and impingement. *Clin. Orthop. Relat. Res.* 2004;418):74-80.

Part XV. Genetics

In: Adolescence and Chronic Illness
Editors: H. Omar et al.

ISBN: 978-1-60876-628-4
© 2010 Nova Science Publishers, Inc.

Chapter 25

INTELLECTUAL DISABILITY AND GENETICS

Helga V. Toriello[*]

Spectrum Health Hospitals, Grand Rapids and Department of Pediatrics
and Human Development, Michigan State University,
East Lansing, Michigan, United States of America.

ABSTRACT

Clearly, chromosome abnormalities and single gene mutations are a significant cause of intellectual disability (ID). In many cases, however, the cause of the ID is unknown. Recently developed techniques and molecular discoveries can provide a means of diagnosing the cause of that individual's ID, thus providing that person and his/her family with prognostic and management information.

INTRODUCTION

Intellectual disability (ID) is estimated to affect 1% to 3% of the population [1,2]. Most individuals within this group have mild ID (IQ 50-70), whereas profound ID (IQ < 25) is the least common. The causes of ID include genetic conditions, prenatal exposure to teratogens, perinatal factors (e.g., hypoxia), or postnatal events (e.g., trauma). In many cases, the cause is unknown [3]. Nevertheless, because genetic factors are a significant cause of ID, with estimates between 17% and 47% [2], for an individual with ID and his or her family to be referred to a genetics clinic is not uncommon.

There are several reasons to identify the cause of the ID in an individual patient. If the cause is known, then the family can be better informed about prognosis, medical management, and recurrence risks to other family members. In many cases, however, an adolescent with ID may not have had a genetics evaluation in over 10 years, and a re-evaluation could provide a diagnosis. This article describes some of the newer diagnostic

---

[*] *Correspondence:* Helga V. Toriello, PhD, Director, Genetics Services, 21 Michigan St., Suite 465, Grand Rapids, MI 49503 United States. Tel: 616-391-2700; Fax: 616-391-3114; E-mail: Helga.toriello@spectrum-health.org

techniques, as well as some of the more recently described conditions that are a relatively common cause of ID. This paper is not meant to be a comprehensive review of all newly described conditions or causative genes, but rather to highlight those that are thought to be relatively common causes of ID of varying degrees.

METABOLIC CONDITIONS

Within this category are two groups of conditions of which the practitioner needs to be aware. Both groups have been described fairly recently, and a number of papers have been published delineating the phenotypes of these entities.

Creatine Deficiency Disorders

The group of cerebral creatine deficiency syndromes includes two autosomal recessive entities—guanidinoacetate methyl transferase (GAMT) deficiency and arginine-glycine amidinotransferase (AGAT) deficiency)—and one X-linked condition (X-linked creatine transporter defect, caused by mutations in SLC6A8). In all three conditions, the clinical phenotype can be variable and includes nonspecific ID, seizures, extrapyramidal movement disorders, speech impairment, and autistic features [4]. The GAMT deficiency affects males and females equally, and the age of onset is between early infancy to early childhood. Most have severe to profound ID. Treatment is available in the form of oral creatine supplementation and dietary restriction of arginine. An improvement in epilepsy and movement disorders occurs, but the ID is not noted to improve [5].

The AGAT deficiency also shows postnatal onset, and is characterized by ID with autistic behavior [6]. Patients with this condition also respond to creatine supplementation. The X-linked form is thought to be the most common of the three. The phenotype is similar to that of the other creatine deficiency syndromes, but with the severe expression limited to males. Carrier females might have mild ID or learning disabilities and/or behavioral disturbances. This group of conditions is thought to be relatively common; in one study, the frequency among those with ID was 2.7% [4], whereas in a second study, four families were found within one metropolitan area, leading the authors of this second report to suggest this condition is often undiagnosed [7]. Clark et al [8] estimated that X-linked creatine transporter deficiency alone accounts for 1% of males with ID of unknown etiology. Metabolic analysis yields elevated urinary creatine/creatinine ratios (in the case of XL creatine transporter defect) and elevated urinary guanidinoacetate/creatinine ratios (in the case of GAMT). Guanidinoacetate levels are low in AGAT. Further diagnostic support comes from proton magnetic resonance spectroscopy (MRS), which demonstrates an absent creatine peak. Molecular analysis of the relevant genes can confirm the diagnosis [4].

Congenital Disorders of Glycosylation (CDG)

Formerly called carbohydrate-deficiency glycoprotein syndromes, this term applies to a group of conditions that are related by abnormal assembly or processing of glycans on glycoconjugates. Glycoconjugates have diverse functions, including roles in cell recognition and adhesion, cell migration, host defense, antigenicity, and other functions. The four broad subgroups of this condition include disorders of N-glycosylation (CDGIa-Il, CDGIIa-IID), defects in O-glycosylation (4 distinct disorders), defects in both N- and O-glycosylation (6 disorders), and defects in lipid glycosylation (2 disorders). The phenotypic presentation can be extremely variable, ranging from mild to severe ID, and with or without additional organ involvement.

Some of the more common clinical manifestations include ataxia, seizures, dysmorphic features (e.g., inverted nipples, unusual fat pads), retinal abnormalities, clotting disorders (both excessive and deficient), cardiomyopathy, and liver dysfunction [9,10]. Cerebellar or cerebral atrophy are often seen, as are endocrine abnormalities, growth retardation, and hypotonia [11]. No one test will identify all disorders in this group, although most will have a defect in the isoelectric focusing of serum transferrin, and this test should be done in any individual suspected of having one of the CDGs. These conditions are inherited as autosomal recessive entities.

Cytogenetic Conditions

The field of cytogenetics has rapidly changed with first, the development of specific fluorescent in situ hybridization (FISH) probes; and more recently, the development of comparative genomic hybridization (CGH). The FISH probes can be used to diagnose a suspected syndrome (e.g., Williams syndrome, Velocardiofacial syndrome) or to determine whether small deletions or duplications are present at the ends of chromosomes, which are called the subtelomere regions. Comparative genomic hybridization is a technique recently developed to detect chromosomal deletions or duplications that are too small to be seen using classic cytogenetic techniques [12].

It has been known for a long time that cytogenetic abnormalities account for approximately 6% of cases of mild ID, and may account for as many as 28% of cases of severe ID [13,14]. The addition of subtelomere FISH studies identifies an additional 7% [15]. The yield is higher in cases of moderate to severe ID compared with mild ID. The development of CGH has added another 10% to 25% to the yield [16,17]. This technique is able to find deletions and duplications that are 5% to 10% (or less) of the size of those visualized by routine karyotype techniques [18]. It is reasonable to consider CGH studies in any individual who has eluded diagnosis, even with a normal karyotype performed in the past.

<u>Specific fluorescent in situ hybridization (FISH)</u>. Fluorescent in situ hybridization has been used for a fairly long time to confirm the clinical diagnosis of microdeletion syndromes such as Williams syndrome, velocardiofacial syndrome, Miller-Dieker syndrome, and several others. However, the use of FISH has also enabled one to identify new causes of ID based on the finding of microduplications in these regions that are associated with these microdeletion syndromes. Velocardiofacial syndrome, caused by deletions at 22q11, is a relatively common cause of learning disability or ID.

Recently it was found using interphase FISH that some individuals with variable degrees of ID have small duplications of this chromosome region. The phenotype is strikingly variable and can range from a mild learning disability to severe congenital malformations causing early death. There is overlap with the velocardiofacial syndrome phenotype, in that those patients can have cleft palate, conotruncal cardiac defects, or aplasia of the thymus. However, there is also evidence that the facial phenotype can be different, in that mild hypertelorism, downslanting palpebral fissures, superior placement of eyebrows, and a long, narrow face are commonly observed [19].

Likewise, duplications of the region responsible for Williams syndrome (caused by a deletion of 7q11) cause a distinct phenotype, which, in contrast to 22q duplications, is unlike the Williams syndrome phenotype. Individuals with this condition generally have mild to moderate ID, generally normal growth parameters, minimally dysmorphic features (prominent forehead, short philtrum, and thin lips in some, but not all), and marked speech delay. Cognitive testing generally reveals lower verbal scores than performance scores, and lower expressive language than receptive language scores [20]. Behavioral characteristics have also been described, and include anxiety, attention deficit, repetitive play/behavior, and stereotyped movements in many, but not all [20].

Subtelomere FISH. With the advent of FISH to interrogate the subtelomere regions, several new microdeletion syndromes have been described. Subtelomere FISH studies have found that deletions of the chromosome 1 short arm subtelomere (1p36 deletion) are a relatively common cause of ID. Recent estimates have suggested that as many as 1% of those with ID have this microdeletion [21]. Most individuals with this deletion have moderate to severe ID, although there are reports of individuals with smaller deletions that have mild ID. Most have postnatal growth failure and abnormal onset of puberty (both early and late have been described).

There appears to be a consistent facial phenotype, and includes deeply set eyes, straight eyebrows, narrow and/or short palpebral fissures, small mouth, pointed or prominent chin, and dysplastic ears. Palatal and digital anomalies are also often observed. Hypotonia is a consistent observation, as are seizures and aggressive or autistic behavior. Some individuals exhibit hyperphagia and develop obesity; thus, they may have a clinical diagnosis of Prader-Willi syndrome [21,22].

Another common cause of ID, usually detected by subtelomere FISH, is microdeletion 9q34, the subtelomere region of the long arm of chromosome 9. As in other microdeletion syndromes, the phenotype can be fairly variable, particularly in terms of developmental achievement. However, some degree of ID is invariably present and ranges from severe, with age of walking not until 11 years, to mild ID and the ability to attend mainstream schools with additional assistance (e.g., resource room).

Hypotonia is a common manifestation. The cranio-facial features tend to be characteristic and include microcephaly, synophrys or arched eyebrows, short nose with upturned nares, thin and tented upper lip, and protruding tongue. Some of these individuals had been suspected to have Down syndrome at or soon after birth, but a normal karyotype eliminated that diagnosis. Others have been suspected to have Smith-Magenis syndrome because of the facial phenotype, and yet others have been thought to have Prader-Willi syndrome because of food-seeking behavior and resultant obesity [23,24].

Finally, in a significant number of individuals, subtelomere FISH has identified deletions of the subtelomere region of the long arm of chromosome 22. The most characteristic findings include ID, absent or markedly delayed speech, hypotonia, high pain threshold, and autistic features. Minor facial anomalies can be present, but tend to be subtle. These anomalies include supraorbital fullness, upturned nasal tip, and dysplastic ears. Absent Cupid's bow of the upper lip and smooth philtrum are additionally described manifestations [25,26].

Comparative genomic hybridization (CGH). As noted above, CGH (also called microarray or aCGH) has revolutionized chromosome analysis in that deletions or duplications that are 5% to 10% of the size of those detectable by routine karyotyping can now be seen. The technology relies on the determination of dosage of DNA at a particular locus. The two common types of CGH testing that are available include targeted and whole genome arrays. Targeted arrays use probes aimed at regions that are known to be associated with a clinical phenotype. Whole genome arrays interrogate the entire genome, often at regularly spaced intervals. There are benefits and pitfalls to each approach [27]. However, as a result, individuals who have previously been a diagnostic puzzle to the caretakers can be diagnosed. Some of the more common microdeletions are described below.

Microdeletions at 16p11.2 have recently been described in a few individuals with autism. Kumar et al [28] surveyed a cohort of 712 patients with autism; a microdeletion at 16p11.2 was found in .6%. Individuals were said to not have any dysmorphic features and were not thought to have a distinct subtype of autism (although the authors noted that the majority tended to have aggression and overactivity as component mani-festations). Intellectual disability was not found in individuals in this group, although prior reports of larger deletions noted the presence of ID in those individuals [29].

On a different site on chromosome 16, 16p13.1 duplications and deletions have been found to be associated with autism and/or ID. Ullmann et al [30] used aCGH to study 70 autistic individuals and found 16p13 duplications in two individuals. Subsequent studies on a different cohort found the duplication in additional patients. In some cases, the duplication was found in other family members, almost all of whom had some phenotypic manifestations, albeit of variable degree. For example, in one family, the male proband's brother, sister, mother, and maternal grandmother had the same duplication. The two boys had profound ID with no speech, their sister had mild ID and learning problems in school, the mother had borderline ID, characterized by delayed speech and learning problems, and the grandmother was said to be unaffected. In yet another cohort, three individuals were found to have microdeletions of this region. All had some degree of ID, and although each was said to have minor facial anomalies, the described phenotypes appeared different among the three.

Microdeletion at 17q21.31 is another recently described chromosome condition. Individuals with this deletion are often thought to have Angelman syndrome, but with normal methylation studies. The degree of ID is described as moderate. Severe hypotonia is present in almost all, as is a characteristic facial phenotype. The face is described as long, there is ptosis and blepharophimosis, the nose is described as being pear-shaped, and the columella is long. The disposition is described as being cheerful [31,32].

Monogenic Conditions

Although there are few, if any, newly-described common monogenic syndromes, one merits mention, and two genes with expanded phenotypes are described as well.

Mowat-Wilson Syndrome

This condition is a recently described, relatively common multiple con-genital anomaly syndrome associated with speech delay and an Angelman syndrome-like phenotype. Hirschsprung disease or constipation is another common manifestation. The face is described as consisting of deeply set eyes, prominent columella, open mouth expression, and prominent jaw. An unusual configura-tion of the ears provides an excellent diagnostic clue. The earlobes are uplifted, and have a central depression. The degree of ID is thought to be in the severe range, although variability is observed. All patients have severely impaired or absent speech, although receptive language appears relatively spared. The cause is a mutation in the XFHX1B gene, and thus, the inheritance is autosomal dominant [33,34].

MECP2

Mutations in MECP2 are usually associated with Rett syndrome, a cause of severe ID in females that had exhibited normal development until the ages of 8-14 months. Historically this syndrome has been thought to be a female-limited condition, with lethality in males. Nevertheless, a number of males with MECP2 mutations have been described, with the phenotype ranging from mild ID to severe neonatal encephalopathy. Among males with ID, 1.3% to 1.7% have been estimated to have a MECP2 mutation [35]. More recently, duplications of MECP2 have been found to be a relatively common cause of ID in males. Such boys are fairly nondysmorphic, but have in common hypotonia, severe ID, absent speech, recurrent infections, and an inability to walk. Carrier females are essentially asymptomatic [36].

PTEN

PTEN mutations are associated with a number of conditions, including Cowden syndrome (CS), Bannayan-Riley-Ruvalcaba syndrome (BRRS), and Lhermitte-Duclos disease [37]. Recently Butler et al [38] and Herman et al [39] described children with a combination of macrocephaly and autism and recommended that PTEN mutation analysis be done in any child with macrocephaly and autism or ID. Buxbaum et al [37] recently reported on mutation screening in 88 individuals with autism spectrum disorders and macro-cephaly. The authors found one individual with a PTEN mutation. This individual also had some manifestations typically found in individuals with CS or BRRS, including overgrowth, motor delay, and café au lait macules. However, these authors and others [40] concluded that screening of the PTEN gene be offered to patients with autism and significant macrocephaly (> 4SD), even in the absence of other CS or BRRS findings.

CONCLUSIONS

As genetic discoveries emerge, our ability to diagnose the cause of ID will increase. The benefits for medical management and in some cases, treatment, will be tremendous. In addition, accurate genetic counseling can be provided to both the individual with ID and his/her family members. Clearly, sexual activity and reproduction occurs in individuals with ID. For example, there are numerous reports of familial Williams syndrome (41,42), familial chromosome 18p deletion (43,44) and pregnancies in women with Prader-Willi syndrome (one of which resulted in a child with Angelman syndrome) (45,46). It is therefore important to ensure that the individual has access to genetic counseling services so that unbiased, nondirective discussions around recurrence risk, reproductive options, and prenatal testing options take place. In terms of prenatal testing in particular, it is important that the individual be able to provide informed consent to the procedure.

REFERENCES

[1] Pratt HD, Greydanus DE. Intellectual disability (mental retardation) in children and adolescents. *Prim. Care Clin. Office Pract.* 2007;34:373-86.

[2] Moeschler JB, Shevell M, Committee on Genetics. Clinical genetic evaluation of the child with mental retardation or developmental delays. *Pediatr.* 2006; 117:2304-16.

[3] Yeargin-Allsopp M, Murphy CC, Cordero JF, Decouflé P, Hollowell JG. Reported biomedical causes and associated medical conditions for mental retardation among 10-year-old children, metropolitan Atlanta, 1985-1987. *Dev. Med. Child Neurol.* 1997;39:142-9.

[4] Lion-François L, Cheillan D, Pitelet G, Acqua-viva-Bourdain C, Bussy G, Cotton F, et al. High frequency of creatine deficiency syndromes in patients with unexplained mental retardation. *Neurology.* 2006;67:1713-4.

[5] Mercimek-Mahmutoglu S, Stoeckler-Ipsiroglu S, Adami A, Appleton R, Caldeira Araújo H, Duran M, et al. GAMT deficiency. Features, treatment, and outcome in an inborn error of creatine synthesis. *Neurology.* 2006;67:480-4.

[6] Battini R., Alessandri MG, Leuzzi V, Moro F, Tosetti M, Bianchi MC, et al. Arginine:glycine amidinotransferase (AGAT) deficiency in a new-born: early treatment can prevent phenotypic ex-pression of the disease. *J. Pediatr.* 2006;148: 828-30.

[7] Salomons GS, van Dooren SJ, Verhoeven NM, Marsden D, Schwartz C, Cecil KM, et al. X-linked creatine transporter defect: an overview. *J. Inherit. Metab. Dis.* 2003;26:309-18.

[8] Clark AJ, Rosenberg EH, Almeida LS, Wood TC, Jakobs C, Stevenson RE, et al. X-linked creatine transporter (SLC6A8) mutations in about 1% of males with mental retardation of unknown etiology. *Hum. Genet.* 2006;119:604-10.

[9] Jaeken J, Matthijs G. Congenital disorders of glycosylation: a rapidly expanding disease family. *Annu. Rev. Genomics Hum. Genet.* 2007;8:261-78.

[10] Coman DJ. The congenital disorders of glycosyla-tion are clinical chameleons. *Eur. J. Hum. Genet.* 2008;16:1-8.

[11] Marquardt T, Denecke J. Congenital disorders of glycosylation: review of their molecular bases, clinical presentations and specific therapies. *Eur. J. Pediatr.* 2003;162:359-379.

[12] Zahir F, Friedman JM. The impact of array genomic hybridization on mental retardation research: a review of current technologies and their clinical utility. *Clin. Genet.* 2007;72:271-287.

[13] Bundey S, Thake A, Todd J. The recurrence risks for mild idiopathic mental retardation. *J. Med. Genet.* 1989;26:260-6.

[14] Curry CJ, Stevenson RE, Aughton D, Byrne J, Carey JC, Cassidy S, et al. Evaluation of mental retardation: recommendations of a consensus conference. *Am. J. Med. Genet.* 1997;72:468-72.

[15] Knight SJ, Flint J. Screening chromosome ends for learning disability. *BMJ.* 2000;321:1240.

[16] Thuresson A-C, Bondeson M-L, Edeby C, Ellis P, Langford C, Dumanski JP, et al. Whole-genome array-CGH for detection of submicroscopic chromosomal imbalances in children with mental retardation. *Cytogenet. Genome Res.* 2007;118:1-7.

[17] Bar-Shira A, Rosner G, Rosner S, Goldstein M, Orr-Urtreger A. Array-based comparative genome hybridization in clinical genetics. *Pediatr. Res.* 2006; 60:353-8.

[18] Aradhya S, Cherry AM. Array-based comparative genomic hybridization: clinical contexts for targeted and whole-genome designs. *Genet. Med.* 2007;9:553-9.

[19] Portnoi M-F, Lebas F, Gruchy N, Ardalan A, Biran-Mucignat V, Malan V, et al., 22q11.2 duplication syndrome: two new familial cases with some overlapping features with DiGeorge/ Velocardiofacial syndromes. *Am. J. Med. Genet.* 2005;137A:47-51.

[20] Berg JS, Brunetti-Pierri N, Peters SU, Kang S-HL, Fong C, Salamone J, et al. Speech delay and autism spectrum behaviors are frequently associated with duplication of the 7q11.23 Williams-Beuren syn-drome region. *Genet. Med.* 2007;9:427-41.

[21] Slavotinek A, Shaffer LG, Shapira SK. Monosomy 1p36. *J. Med. Genet.* 1999;36:657-63.

[22] D'Angelo CS, Da Paz JA, Kim CA, Bertola DR, Castro CI, Varela MC, et al. Prader-Willi-like phenotype: investigation of 1p36 deletion in 41 patients with delayed psychomotor development, hypotonia, obesity and/or hyperphagia, learning disabilities and behavioral problems. *Eur. J. Med. Genet.* 2006;49:451-60.

[23] Cormier-Daire V, Molinari F, Rio M, Raoul O, de Blois MC, Romana S, et al. Cryptic terminal deletion of chromosome 9q34: a novel cause of syndromic obesity in childhood? *J. Med. Genet.* 2003;40:300-3.

[24] Stewart DR, Kleefstra T. The chromosome 9q subtelomere deletion syndrome. *Am. J. Med. Genet.* 2007;145C:383-92.

[25] Manning MA, Cassidy SB, Clericuzio C, Cherry AM, Schwartz S, Hudgins L, et al. Terminal 22q deletion syndrome: a newly recognized cause of speech and language disability in the autism spectrum. *Pediatr.* 2004;114:451-7.

[26] Cusmano-Ozog K, Manning MA, Hoyme HE. 22q13.3 deletion syndrome: a recognizable malformation syndrome associated with marked speech and language delay. *Am. J. Med. Genet.* 2007;145C:393-8.

[27] Shaffer LG, Bejjani BA, Torchia B, Kirkpatrick S, Coppinger J, Ballif BC. The identification of microdeletion syndromes and other chromosome abnormalities:

cytogenetic methods of the past, new technologies of the future. *Am. J. Med. Genet.* 2007;145C:335-45.

[28] Kumar RA, Mohamed SK, Sudi J, Conrad DF, Brune C, Badner JA, et al. Recurrent 16p11.2 microdeletion in autism. *HMG advance access,* 12/21/2007;1-35.

[29] Ballif BC, Hornor SA, Jenkins E, Madan-Khetarpal S, Surti U, Jackson KE, et al. Discovery of a previously unrecognized microdeletion syndrome of 16p11.2-p12.2. *Nat. Genet.* 2007;39: 1071-3.

[30] Ullmann R, Turner G, Kirchhoff M, Chen W, Tonge B, Rosenberg C, et al. Array CGH identifies reciprocal 16p13.1 duplications and deletions that predispose to autism and/or mental retardation. *Hum. Mutat.* 2007;28:647-82.

[31] Koolen DA, Vissers LELM, Pfundt R, de Leeuw N, Knight SJL, Regan R, et al. A new chromosome 17q21.31 microdeletion syndrome associated with a common inversion poly-morphism. *Nat. Genet.* 2006;38:999-1001.

[32] Shaw-Smith C, Pittman AM, Willatt L, Martin H, Rickman L, Gribble S, et al. Microdeletion encompassing MAPT at chromosome 17q21.3 is associated with developmental delay and learning disability. *Nat. Genet.* 2006;38:1032-7.

[33] Zweier C, Albrecht B, Mitulla B, Behrens R, Beese M, Gillessen-Kasebach G, et al. Mowat-Wilson syndrome with and without Hirschsprung disease is a distinct recognizable, multiple congenital anomalies-mental retardation syndrome caused by mutations in the zinc finger homeobox 1B gene. *Am. J. Med. Genet.* 2002;108:177-81.

[34] Zweier C, Horn D, Kraus C, Rauch A. Atypical ZFHX1B mutation associated with a mild Mowat-Wilson syndrome phenotype. *Am. J. Med. Genet.* 2006;140A:869-72.

[35] Villard L. MECP2 mutations in males. *J. Med. Genet.* 2007;44:417-23.

[36] van Esch H, Bauters M, Ignatius J, Jansen M, Raynaud M, Hollanders K, et al. Duplication of the MECP2 region is a frequent cause of severe mental retardation and progressive neurological symptoms in males. *Am. J. Hum. Genet.* 2005;77: 442-53.

[37] Buxbaum JD, Cai G, Chaste P, Nygren G, Goldsmith J, Reichert J et al. Mutation screening of the PTEN gene in patients with autism spectrum disorders and macrocephaly. *Am. J. Med. Genet.* 2007;144B:484-91.

[38] Butler MG, Dasouki MJ, Zhou XP, Talebizadeh Z, Brown M, Takahashi TN, et al. Subset of individuals with autism spectrum disorders and extreme macrocephaly associated with germline PTEN tumour suppressor gene mutations. *J. Med. Genet.* 2005; *J. Med. Genet.* 42:318-21.

[39] Herman GE, Butter E, Enrile B, Pastore M, Prior TW, Sommer A. Increasing knowledge of PTEN germline mutations: two additional patients with autism and macrocephaly. *Am. J. Med. Genet.* 2007; 143:589-93.

[40] Herman GE, Henninger N, Ratliff-Schaub K, Pastore M, Fitzgerald S, McBride KL. Genetic testing in autism: how much is enough? *Genet. Med.* 2007;9:268-74.

[41] Morris CA, Thomas IT, Greenberg F. Williams syndrome: autosomal dominant inheritance. *Am. J. Med. Genet.* 1993;47:478-81.

[42] Mulik VV, Temple, KI, Howe DT. Two pregnancies in a woman with Williams syndrome. *BJOG.* 2004; 111:511-2.

[43] Maranda B, Lemieux N, Lemyre E. Familial deletion 18p syndrome: case report. BMC Med Genet 2006;7:60. http://www.biomedcentral.com/ 1471-2350/7/60

[44] Velagaleti GV, Harris S, Carpenter NJ, Coldwell J, Say B. Familial deletion of chromosome 18 (p11.2). *Ann. Genet.* 1996;39:201-4.

[45] Åkefeldt A, Törnhage C-J, Gillberg C. A woman with Prader-Willi syndrome gives birth to a healthy baby girl. *Dev. Med. Child Neurol.* 1999; 41:789-90.

[46] Schulze A, Mogensen H, Hamborg-Petersen B, Græm N, Østergaard JR, Brøndum-Nielsen K. Fertility in Prader-Willi syndrome: a case report with Angelman syndrome in the offspring. *Acta Pædiatr.* 2001;90:455-9.

In: Adolescence and Chronic Illness
Editors: H. Omar et al.
ISBN: 978-1-60876-628-4
© 2010 Nova Science Publishers, Inc.

Chapter 26

DOWN SYNDROME AND ADOLESCENCE

Efrat Merrick-Kenig[1], Joav Merrick[1,2] and Isack Kandel[*3]

[1] National Institute of Child Health and Human Development, Office of the Medical Director, Division for Mental Retardation, Ministry of Social Affairs, Jerusalem, Israel.
[2] Kentucky Children's Hospital, University of Kentucky, Lexington, United States.
[3] Department of Behavioral Sciences, Ariel University Center of Samaria, Ariel, Israel.

ABSTRACT

Adolescence is a period of transition that can create stress for both adolescents and parents. Adolescents with Down syndrome (DS) go through the same stages as other adolescents, but due to lack of cognitive and behavioral factors they and their parents may find this period particularly challenging. This chapter reviews several studies, especially from the United Kingdom, of groups of adolescents with Down syndrome and their controls followed from childhood, through adolescence into adulthood. There are special medical problems for this population that require annual medical examinations and surveillance, but the focus has shifted from health problems to social maturation, developing independence, and transition from school to employment or work activity. Medical transition from a pediatric to family physician provider is mentioned with recommendations as to how that transition can be made as smooth as possible.

INTRODUCTION

Adolescence is a period of transition from childhood to adulthood associated with intense physical and psychosocial change. The period is sometimes divided into early adolescence at age 12-14 years, middle adolescence at 15-17 years, and late adolescence at 18-21 years. There is an overlap and individual differences, but an ongoing development occurs with the tasks of achieving independence from parents, adopting peer codes and life-style, realizing

---

[*] *Correspondence:* Isack Kandel, MA, PhD, Maaleh Shomron, IL-44852 Lev Shomron, Israel. Tel 972-9-7929180; Fax: 972-9-7920316; E-mail: kandelii@zahav.net.il

increased importance of body image, and establishing a sexual, egotistical, vocational, and moral identity [1].

Because of the dependence-independence struggle taking place, adolescence can be a trying period for both parents and adolescents. However, it is imortant for both parties to go through it, as it is a natural stage of development.

Adolescents with Down syndrome (DS), find themselves going through the same stages of adolescence, but due to lack of cognitive and behavioral factors they and their parents experience this period as particularly challenging.

DOWN SYNDROME

John Langdon Haydon Down (1828-96) was an English physician who described in detail the syndrome that came to bear his name [2]. While working at the Earlswood Asylum for Idiots in Surrey he tried to classify the various forms of "feeble-mindedness" and concluded that individuals with mental disabilities belonged to different ethnic varieties including, for example, the Ethiopian, Malay and Mongolian ethic groups. John Down was a promising physician and a brilliant career was predicted for him at London University Hospital, but he surprised his teachers in 1858 when he became resident physician and subsequently medical superintendent at the Earlswood Asylum for Idiots in Surrey. He wanted to work with this neglected segment of the population, and for a period of ten years (1858-1868) spent his time between the Earlswood institution and his London practice. He became lecturer in the principles and practice of medicine at the London Hospital Medical College, where he also taught about intellectual disability.

When Down in 1866 published his work on the mongoloid idiocy syndrome, he was surprised that it had not been described earlier. In fact, however, the first description had been made in 1838 by Jean Etienne Dominique Esquirol (1772-1840), a founder of modern alienism, and by Edouard Seguin (1812-1880) in 1844, who had established the Bicetre Asylum's special school for children with intellectual disability in Paris in 1840 [3]. Seguin later moved to the United States and became the first President of the Association of Medical Officers of American Institutions of Idiotic and Feeble-Minded Persons established in 1876 (today called the American Association on Mental Retardation (AAMR)).

In the middle of the 1950s new cytogenetic techniques were developed to allow researchers to visualize chromosomes in the metaphase, and in 1956 it was established that the human cell had 46 chromosomes. In 1958 a French researcher, Jerome Lejeune (1926-94), discovered an additional chromosome in the cells of a child with Down syndrome. Today we know that three genetic variations can cause Down syndrome.

In most cases, about 92%, Down syndrome is caused by the presence of an extra chromosome 21 in all cells of the individual. In such cases, the extra chromosome originates in the development of either the egg or the sperm. Therefore, when an egg and sperm unite to form a fertilized egg, three, instead of two, chromosomes 21 are present. In the development of the embryo this extra chromosome is repeated in every cell and the individual born has trisomy 21. In about 2-4% of the cases, Down syndrome is the result of mosaic trisomy 21. This condition is similar to the above, but instead of all cells in the individual having the extra chromosome 21, in the mosaic form some cells have 46 and some 47 chromosomes.

The third type of Down syndrome (3-4%) is called translocation trisomy 21. Here material from one chromosome 21 gets stuck or translocated onto another chromosome, either prior to or at conception. Cells from individuals with Down syndrome have two normal chromosomes 21, but also have additional chromosome 21 material on the translocated chromosome. Therefore, there is still too much material from chromosome 21, resulting in the features associated with Down syndrome.

STUDIES ON ADOLESCENTS WITH DOWN SYNDROME

Several studies of persons with Down syndrome have been performed using a longitudinal or cross-sectional model, mainly in the United Kingdom.

Janet Carr [4] studied a cohort of children with Down syndrome over several years (the South London Study). The 54 children (29 girls, 25 boys) were born in Surrey, England in one health district in 1963-64 and compared to a group of normal babies. They have been followed with extensive tests, interviews and questionnaires focusing on fundamental issues of development and upbringing from birth to early adulthood (age 21 years). A wide range of factors were investigated, from abilities, behaviour, discipline and independence through to effects on the family and provision of help from services.

Billie Shepperdson, affiliated with the University College of Swansea and Faculty of Medicine, University of Leicester, studied [5,6,7] two cohorts of children with Down syndrome (the South Wales Studies). One cohort (original cohort) of children, born in 1964-66 with Down syndrome (53 children, 27 girls, 29 boys) and brought up at home in South Wales, was studied and followed in 1972, in 1981, and in 1990-91. The families were interviewed about their own experiences and use of services, and about the progress of their son or daughter with Down syndrome. The children and young people were tested on language and social competence (Gunzburg Progress Assessment Charts, Reynell Language Scales, English Picture Vocabulary Test and self care skills information). A second cohort (comparative cohort) of 26 children born in 1973-75 from the same geographical area was also studied and followed in 1981 and 1990-91.

Ann Gath from Maudsley and Bethlem Royal Hospitals in London has conducted a longitudinal study (the Oxford Studies) of a group of 30 children born in Oxford during 1970-71. Development and behavior of the first two years, then again at 8-9 years, of the 22 surviving children has been described, but of interest is her study of another group of 193 children with Down syndrome and 154 children with a similar degree of handicap (but not DS) identified in the same schools [8,9]. The main purpose of her studies has been a focus on the emotional impact upon families of having a child with a disability. Families were assessed on the quality of marital relationships, physical/mental health of parents, and health/adjustment of siblings.

Cliff C Cunningham at the Hester Adrian Research Centre at the University of Manchester (Manchester Down Syndrome Cohort) has followed 181 children with Down syndrome born in 1973 and their families [10,11]. Research has been concerned with early development and intervention, maternal perceptions of family adaptation and functioning, comparison with families of non-disability children, and the issue of siblings.

Sue Buckley and Ben Sacks from Portsmouth Polytecnic started a survey of 90 families with a teenager with Down syndrome (the Hampshire study) born between 1967-74. The aim of the study was to describe the daily life of a teenager with Down syndrome [12,13].

In the United States, Marcia van Riper from Ohio State University conducted several studies on the family experience of living with a Down syndrome child [14], but the person with the biggest contribution to our understanding of Down syndrome is Siegfried M Pueschel, a pediatrician from Brown University School of Medicine at the Rhode Island Hospital Child Development Center [15].

FAMILY LIFE

Parents in a family where a child is born with Down syndrome will react differently. Some will even decide to leave the child in the hospital rather than take the child home. In the Hampshire study [12,13] one in ten left their child in the hospital, while a study in Israel showed an overall relinquishment rate of 25% during the 1970s and 1980s, but with a decrease in that number for the 1987-1991 period [16].

The South London study [4] did not find adverse effects on siblings. To the contrary, she found better sibling relationships in DS families than in the controls. When she used the Malaise Inventory by Rutter et al [17] to relate to the mother's health, she found that in the DS group these scores were higher for working class mothers, for those saying they felt depressed, and for those where their adolescents could not go outside the garden gate alone and had poor reading skills [4]. No other factors, either in the mothers themselves or in the abilities or personal qualities of DS adolescents were identified. Concerning the mother's loneliness or effect on marriage and social life, there were no significant differences between the two groups, In fact, the divorce rate for non-DS parents was higher [4]. Social class was a major factor in the experience of stress in the family. Families from working class, impoverished, unemployed, or deprived segments of the population suffered more with the burden of a DS child.

PHYSICAL DEVELOPMENT AND HEALTH

Many publications will show a higher prevalence of specific disorders for Down syndrome such as hypothyroidism, sleep apnoa or atlantoaxial instability, but the majority of children with DS reaching adolescence will be in good health [18]. It seems that most serious physical problems are present at birth and many are resolved by the time of adolescence

Concerning physical development, studies of the growth and size of persons with DS have shown that by adulthood, height is reduced by an average of about two SD (Standard Deviations). A growth chart for persons with DS can be found at the website of the United Kingdom Down Syndrome Medical Interest Group (DSMIG at http://www.dsmig.org.uk/ publications/ growthchart.html) or from the American Academy of Pediatrics [19] (http:// www.aap.org/policy/re0016.html), where guidelines for health supervision of children and adolescents with DS can also be found. A growth chart for Swedish children with DS has also been published [20]. The Hampshire study [12,13] also found that adolescents with DS were shorter, but they reached physical maturity earlier.

Concerning health, the Hampshire study [12,13] found that adolescents with DS were generally healthy, but with a higher incidence of problems concerned with vision, hearing and infections. The South London study [4] also did not find any striking differences in health between the DS group and controls. About 12% could be described as in delicate health [4]. In the adolescent years (13-21 years of age) health supervision for persons with Down syndrome should include [19,21,22]:

- annual physical examinations including CBC and thyroid function tests;
- annual audiologic evaluations;
- annual ophthalmologic evaluations;
- discussions of skin care;
- discussions of issues related to transition into adulthood.
- discussion of the appropriateness of school placement with emphasis on adequate vocational training within the school curriculum.
- explanations about the recurrence risk of Down syndrome with a patient and her family should she become pregnant;
- discussions on sexuality and socialization, including the need for and degree of supervision and/or the need for contraception; also recommendations for routine gynecologic care;
- provide information about group homes and independent living opportunities, workshop settings, and other community-supported employment.
- discussions about intrafamily relationships, financial planning, and guardianship;
- facilitation of transfers to adult medical care.

SEXUAL DEVELOPMENT AND BEHAVIOR

Secondary sex characteristics of DS adolescents are quite similar to other adolescents, and there is no significant difference between the size of the genitalia of the two groups of adolescent boys. Hormone studies have also been comparable, and studies on sexual maturation in females with DS has found the average onset of menstruation at 12.5 years compared to 12.1 years for other adolescents. Most women with DS have regular menstruation and a menstrual cycle of 27 days, and investigations of ovulatory patterns have found that 39% had a definite pattern of evulation, 15% probably ovulated, 15% possibly ovulated, and 31% had no evidence of ovulation [23,24]. About 30 pregnancies in 26 women with Down syndrome have been reported in the literature [24].

Reviews of sexual issues can be found elsewhere [18,25], but contraception is an issue that needs to be discussed with parents and the adolescent with DS. There are several methods of contraception [25] which should be considered, because in spite of a significantly impaired fertility of both sexes with DS, it is not impossible for them to bear children. One case has been reported of a male with DS, who fathered a normal male child [25]. Thirty-two pregnancies of females with DS have been reported (11 normal children, 10 with DS, two with intellectual disability, two premature non-viable, three malformed, one microcephaly, one stillborn, and two abortions)[25].

Under all circumstances sex education must be an important part of health surveillance for this population.

TRANSITION FROM CHILDHOOD TO ADULTHOOD

Life is a series of transitions where one stage must be completed in order to enter the next. For adolescents to reach adulthood they must assume responsibility for their own health care and find the physicians or health care providers who can support their health needs. This responsibility is part of growing up.

Adolescents with special needs or disability will often find this transition difficult [26]. If health care needs have been provided by a family physician throughout childhood and adolescence, there should not be a problem as the adolescent can continue with the same physician into adulthood. If that is not the case, the primary care physician can help the process of transition by

- Making a comprehensive case summary with all relevant medical information, medical events, treatment and a future plan for intervention and support by stating the strong and less strong functional aspects and care needs
- Performing a physical examination with the adolescent as a partner in the examination. Health problems and needs should be described in an unerstandable manner thus enabling the person to provide a measure of self care. Information on health problems and needs must also be conveyed to the health care provider taking over
- Providing the adolescent with the case summary and explaining its contents and relevance
- Facilitating community support groups and networks
- Providing a transition period where the physician will be available while the adolescent will get used to his/her new health care provider

Only a few years ago, children with Down syndrome were looked upon as eternal children, but with normalization, mainstreaming and de-institutionalization this has changed. Therefore the healthcare provider for the adolescent with DS should assist his client/patient in making the transition from childhood to adulthood as painless as possible, and facilitate the patient's trust in health care provision.

CONCLUSIONS

Children with Down syndrome are living longer due to medical care provided during infancy, so that today many will survive into adolescence and adulthood.

Several studies, especially in the United Kingdom, have followed groups of children with DS and controls in adolescence and adulthood. Contrary to what was expected, most adolescents with DS are quite healthy. There are special medical problems for this population that require annual medical examinations, but the focus has shifted from medical needs to social maturation, developing independence, and the transition from school to employment or work activity.

REFERENCES

[1] Neinstein LS. Adolescent health care. A practical guide. Baltimore, MD: Williams and Wilkins, 1991.
[2] Down JLH. Observations on an ethnic classification of idiots. *Clin. Lectures Reports London Hospital.* 1866;3:259-62.
[3] Braddock D. Mental retardation and developmental disabilities: Historical and contemporary perspectives. In: Braddock D, Hemp R, Parish S, Westrich J, eds. The state of the States in developmental disabilities. Washington, DC: *Am. Ass. Ment. Retard.* 1998: 3-21.
[4] Carr J. Down's syndrome. Children growing up: *A longitudinal perspective.* Cambridge: Cambridge Univ Press, 1995.
[5] Shepperdson B. Changes in the characteristics of families with Down's syndrome children. *J. Epidemiol. Community Health.* 1985;39(4): 320-4.
[6] Shepperdson B. *Growing up with Down's syndrome.* London: Cassell, 1988
[7] Shepperdson B. A comparison of the development of independence in two cohorts of young people with Down's syndrome. *Down Syndr. Res. Pract* .1994;2(1):11-8.
[8] Gath A, Gumley D. Behavior problems in retarded children with special reference to Down's syndrome. *Br. J. Psychiatry.* 1986; 149:156-61.
[9] Gath A, Gumley D. Family background of children with Down's syndrome and of children with a similar degree of mental retardation. *Br. J. Psychiatry.* 1986;149:161-71.
[10] Turner S, Sloper P, Cunningham CC, Knussen C. Health problems in children with Down's syndrome. *Child Care Health dev.* 1990;16(2):83-97.
[11] Cunningham CC. Families of children with Down syndrome. *Down Syndr. Res. Pract.* 1998;4:87-95.
[12] Buckley S, Sacks B. The adolescent with Down's syndrome. *Life for the teenager and the family.* Portsmouth, Hampshire: Portmouth Polytechnic, 1987.
[13] Buckley S, Sacks B. From adolescence to adulthood. *Portsmouth Down Syndr. Trust Newsletter.* 1996;6(5):1-5.
[14] van Riper M. Living with Down syndrome: The family experience. *Down Syndr. Quarterly.* 1999;4(1):1-7.
[15] Pueschel SM. Young people with Down syndrome: *Transition from childhood to adulthood.* Website: http://www.ndss.org/content.cfm
[16] Sadetzki S, Chetrit A, Akstein E, Keinan L, Luxenburg O, Modan B. Relinquishment of infants with Down syndrome in Israel: Trends by time. *Am. J. Ment. Retard.* 2000;105(6):480-5.
[17] Rutter M, Tizard J, Whitmore K. *Education, health and behavior.* London: Longman, 1970.

[18] Pueschel SM, Sustrova M. Adolescents with Down syndrome. *Toward a more fulfilling life*. Baltimore, MD: Paul H Brookes, 1997.
[19] Cunniff C el al. Health supervision for children with Down syndrome. *Pediatrics*. 2001;107(2):442-9.
[20] Myrelid A, Gustafsson J, Ollars B, Anneren G. Growth charts for Down syndrome from birth to 18 years of age. *Arch. Dis. Childhood.* 2002;87(2): 97-103.
[21] Merrick J. Medical concerns in Down syndrome. *Int. J. Adolesc. Med. Health.* 2000;12(1):43-51.
[22] Cohen WI, Nadel L, Madnick ME, eds. *Down syndrome*. Visions for the 21st century. New York: Wiley-Liss, 2002.
[23] Pueschel SM. Clinical aspects of Down syndrome from infancy to adulthood. *Am. J. Med. Gen.* 1990;S7: 52-6.
[24] Peuschel SM. Health concerns in persons with Down syndrome. In: Pueschel SM, Tingey C, Rynders JE, Crocker AC, Crutcher DM, eds. *New perspectives in Down syndrome*. Baltimore: Paul H Brookes, 1987:113-33.
[25] van Dyke DC, McBrien DM, Sherbondy A. Issues of sexuality in Down syndrome. *Down Syndr. Res. Pract.* 1995;3(2):65-9.
[26] Blum RW. Introduction. Improving transition for adolescents with special health care needs from pediatric to adult centered health care. *Pediatrics*. 2003;110(6Pt2):1301-3.

In: Adolescence and Chronic Illness
Editors: H. Omar et al.

ISBN: 978-1-60876-628-4
© 2010 Nova Science Publishers, Inc.

Chapter 27

RETT SYNDROME AND SNOEZELEN OR CONTROLLED MULTI-SENSORY STIMULATION

Meir Lotan[*,1,2,3] *and Joav Merrick*[3,4]

[1] Zvi Quittman Residential Center, Millie Shime Campus, Elwyn Jerusalem, Israel.
[2] School of Health Sciences, Department of Physical Therapy,
Ariel University Center of Samaria, Ariel, Israel.
[3] National Institute of Child Health and Human Development, Office of the Medical Director, Division for Mental Retardation, Ministry of Social Affairs, Jerusalem, Israel.
[4] Kentucky Children's Hospital, University of Kentucky, Lexington, United States.

ABSTRACT

Rett syndrome is a neurological disorder resulting from an X-linked dominant mutation. It is characterized by a variety of physical and perceptual disabilities, resulting in a need for constant therapy programs to be administered on a regular basis throughout life. Resistance to physical activity has driven the authors in a search for new intervention techniques which might improve the ability to cope while reducing difficulty in handling an external physical facilitator. During adolescence the person with RS goes through a stormy period that necessitates special attention and adapted care. Snoezelen, or multi-sensory environment, can provide a soothing environment appealing to the adolescent with Rett syndrome while at the same time improving physical abilities. The chapter reviews Rett syndrome typical phenotype and suggests suitable activities that might take place in the multi-sensory environment with emphasis on adolescence.

INTRODUCTION

Rett syndrome (RS) is a neurological disorder resulting from an X-linked dominant mutation [1], affecting mainly females and found in a variety of racial and ethnic groups worldwide [2]. RS is a frequent cause of neurological dysfunction in females, accounting for

---

* *Correspondence:* Meir Lotan, BPT, MSc, Rothchild 67th St. 44201, Kfar Saba, Israel. Tel: 972-9-7678588. E-mail: ml_pt_rs@netvision.net.il

the most common cause for multiple-disability among females [3], or the second most common cause for severe mental retardation in females after Down syndrome [4].

The stages of RS have been described as: Pre-regression (or stage 1); regression (or stage 2); essentially stable (or stage 3); and in some cases the term 4th stage has been utilized in circumstances when an individual becomes very handicapped [5]. This 4th stage in RS is known for its instability both in regards to emotional as well as functional realms. Childhood development in females with Rett syndrome proceeds in an apparently normal fashion during pregnancy and over the first 6-18 months, at which point development comes to a halt with regression and loss of many acquired skills [6]. Thereafter, there is a rapid deterioration and loss of acquired speech and purposeful hand use. Deceleration of head growth, along with jerky body movements of the trunk and limbs, accompany the developmental deterioration in individuals with Rett syndrome. Typically, they present with a broad base gait and swaying movements of the shoulders when walking [7]. Other physical problems such as seizures, scoliosis and breathing abnormalities may appear [8] and require constant care for the rest of the life of the person [9]. The scoliosis is a prominent feature in females with Rett syndrome, but may vary from mild to severe [10]. Apraxia (dyspraxia), inability to program the body to perform motor movements, is the most fundamental and severely handicapping aspect of Rett syndrome. It can interfere with all body movement including eye gaze and speech, making it difficult for individuals with Rett syndrome to execute what she wants to do. To sum things up, the adolescent with RS is in need of an intensive and comprehensive management program across her life span. Estimated life expectancy is at 50 years [11].

Smeets et al [12] described a survey of 30 adolescents and adults with RS and they gave the common characteristics of the person with RS at that age. Their main findings are summarized in table 1.

Table 1. The common characteristics of the adolescent and adult with RS

Function abilities			
Function	Preserved (%)	Impaired (%)	No Ability (%)
Walking abilities	42%	29	29
Sitting ability	54.1	16.6	25
Hand use	-----------	46	54
Medical conditions			
Epilepsy	79 (never developed or well controlled)		21 (uncontrolled)
Scoliosis	58 mild or absent	42 Severe scoliosis all operated	
Hand mannerisms	Less prominent than in childhood		
Breathing abnormalities	None (75)		Existing (25)
Score of manifestations common in RTT by Kerr et al., 2001(13)			
Mild condition (Score < 20)	milder- condition (Score 20- 25)	less severe clinical condition (score of 25-30)	severe clinical condition (a score of 30)
41.6	25	16.6	16.6

The diversity of functional and medical conditions of individuals with RS that is presented during childhood persists into adolescence and necessitates the application of a flexible approach that fits the individual needs of every client, such as the Snoezelen approach.

The word Snoezelen is a combination of two Dutch words: to doze and to sniff. The word doze indicates a restful activity is involved and the sniffing gives it a more dynamic/sensory aspect [14]. The multi-sensory room is a partially lit room that provides sensory stimulation to both the client and the therapist. The senses (far: hearing and sight, and near: touch, taste and smell) are provided harmoniously whether alone or combined. They are provided according to the choice of the client. The aim of the treatment is to find a balance between relaxation and activity within the framework of a safe, adapted environment by means of an enabling therapist [15].

We live our lives through our senses. It is by means of experiencing the senses that we develop an understanding about our body and through it about our environment [16]. Any medical problem which disturbs interaction with the environment may influence understanding and, as a result, disturb development. According to Longhorn [17], without sensation and awakening of the senses, people with disturbances will find it very difficult to understand the world around them and as a result, will have difficulty learning. The multi-sensory approach tries to find significance in the world by means of an adapted environment, and through the help of an enabling therapist. This environment awakens interest and the client begins to explore and discover the surroundings. This exploration acts as a stepping-stone towards learning.

Mostly, people with disabilities cannot create their own optimal environment and so it is up to us to do so. By providing a multi-sensory environment we are creating a sensory experience for the client to explore. In this presentation we will review the management of adolecents with Rett syndrome in the multi-sensory stimulation environment called Snoezelen.

When considering a suitable intervention program for the patient with RS we reviewed the suggestions of experts in the field of RS:

- Close interpersonal contact [18]
- A quiet and reassuring environment may achieve reduction in anxiety and agitation in children with RS [5]
- Music is of outmost value [19-22]
- The child will respond best to gentle loving care which encourage activity in an interesting but quiet environment [19]
- Encourage and facilitate learning without pressuring the child
- Provide face-to-face contact, talking, singing and touching
- Comfort the child and allow withdrawal during agitation
- Encourage active supervised movement in soft play
- Provide gentle movement of limbs and joints through full range [23]

All the above suggestions are integral parts of the multi-sensory environment, making it a preferred intervention method for the child and adolescent with RS.

MULTI-SENSORY ENVIRONMENT FOR PERSONS WITH RETT SYNDROME

Females with Rett syndrome (RS) present typical characteristics that might be treated in the multi-sensory environment. The problems will be screened according to typical stages of the disorder. Since the child at adolescent might be found at stage III or IV of the disorder, only these stages will be presented within this chapter

Stage III – Plateau

This stage is relatively calm. The radical physical/emotional situation now seems to be balanced. The duration of this stage is long (years) and thus enables the girl to achieve some progress, while preventing possible future problems. The variety of possible treatment goals at stage III:

1. *Relaxation:* Girls with Rett Syndrome tend to go through mood swings (not all of them and not always). This behviour was described by Smeets et al., [12] for adolescents with RS as well. At times we might see the child is extremely upset without our understanding the cause of her behavior. Since communication with RS girls is nonverbal and difficult to understand, it seems that a quiet treatment can save many hours of pain, tears, and discomfort. It is important to mention that emotional bonding between the girl and her therapist is extremely important. A loving and understanding therapist will win the girl's love and trust, and as a result, her motivation to satisfy him or her [24]. So, find the time to build an interpersonal relationship – it is worthwhile. Using the waterbed with heated water, or soft large pillows that are capable of rapping the child and enhancing a sense of security is recommended. Research has shown that deep touch pressure has been used to provide a calming effect [25] and to enhance relaxation [26]. Auditory stimulation according to the child's preference will add to building up a safe haven for the child to be treated on regular intervals or when the child seems troubled and in need of immediate relaxing intervention.

2. *Hand functions:* Stereotyped hand movements interfere and limit almost every functional movement the child can perform with her hands. These movements present during most of the girl's waking hours at childhood and together with dyspraxia and ataxia, reduce the likelihood of functional hand use are less apparent now [12]. Yet we still would like her to activate her hands, and therefore it is imperative to try using various instruments and techniques during multi-sensory environment treatments. The intervention can begin "with the therapist seated behind the child, to act as a comfortable support for the child to lean against. From this position the adult is able to play with and gently stroke the client's hands [27]. Such hand contact has been found to be effective in reducing the person with RS's stereotypic hand movements and enabling active interaction with the therapist. At this point using different interesting visual stimuli such as optic fibers, infinity, fireworks and electrical balls might be found interesting enough for the person with RS to try and use her hands. If she is able to crawl, performing such activity on thick mattresses covering the room's floor would facilitate intense proprioceptive stimulation to the hands that might pay off in functional improvement outside the multi-sensory environment. The bubbles pole creates a

visual stimulation and a vibrating feeling. At the same time, and this might be used when treatment goals are aimed at enhancing hand function.

3. *Transitions* [28]: The chief motor loss of the individual with RS is experienced in transitions. Transitions include changes from standing to sitting position, from sitting to standing, from standing to walking, and so forth. Therefore, during treatment one should include repetitive elements of movement and position changing on a regular basis [29] to assist the adolescent with RS in becoming as mobile and active as possible. Walking is very important for persons with Rett Syndrome because it stimulates the work of internal organs and the digestive system, thus reducing constipation. Standing or walking in an upright position may also delay development of scoliosis. Thick mattresses in the Snoezelen room create a rough environment for the child to handle, but at the same time allows the girl, who cannot control her body, to experience walking without risk of falling and injuring herself. Practicing transitions in the multi-sensory environment with individuals without RS, but with dyspraxia, have been found useful in enhancing functional independence. [30].

4. *Preventing potential orthopedic problems (and treating existing ones):* Individuals with RS might display the following orthopedic problems: Scoliosis (side-to-side/rotation curve of the spine), kyphosis (forward curve of the upper (thoracic) spine) and deformation of the palms and/or feet. Scoliosis can be found in 80-85% of the total cases [3, 31], especially among non-mobile children [31]. Thus, it is very important to provide motivation for walking. Kyphosis is more common among girls who can walk, but is not as severe and motorically disabling as scoliosis. In both cases, the therapist can use the waterbed in the Snoezelen room as a support system while skillfully twisting and turning the client's body. Gentle moving of the back and limbs through the full range of comfortable movements are recommended [19] in order to prevent future reduction in range of movement. The deformation that often occurs in the palms and feet and dislocation of the hips is rare and requires careful attention and specific treatments. Again, the waterbed will assist the therapist as a support system that warms and softens rigid tissues. At the same time the calm and relaxed atmosphere created wisely in the multi-sensory room can calm the child down despite disturbing and sometimes painful manipulations.

5. *Re-assembling "midline"* [32]: Some individuals with Rett Syndrome apparently lose their sense of "midline." The woman senses her midline differently from where it actually is. Sometimes they tilt so far to one side or backwards that one might easily rule out the possibility of independent seating [28]. This condition prevents her from standing straight (since standing straight seems twisted to her) and can cause damage, such as scoliosis, kyphosis, and even a loss of ability to walk and stand. Rolling on the mattresses while performing deep proprioceptive stimulation enables the therapist to work with the girl on her "midline" problem with or without the use of instruments.

6. *Equilibrium and coordination:* Among her other difficulties, the individual with RS suffers from ataxia. Ataxia is characterized by inability to control several groups of muscles at the same time in the usual coordinated manner most of us perform automatically (among them are the postural muscles). The ability to control these muscles is essential for supporting the body's posture in various positions and in movement [33]. Lacking this ability can create severe motor limitations. Knee walking across the floor of the multi-sensory environment can improve equilibrium and improve trunk control that is vital for most motor acts. Standing on all fours on the waterbed is a challenging exercise and will yield similar results.

7. *Sensation:* Adolescents with Rett syndrome are often characterized by an unbalanced sensory system. This phenomenon has been previously mentioned in the literature. Individuals with RS display decreased pain sensation and hypersensitivity to touch over their faces [34], especially around the mouth. Their fear of movement can be caused by a dysfunction of the vestibular system [35]. As a consequence, the girl is cautious and her everyday activities are interrupted, causing a distracted body scheme - a vital component in accepting and relating to the world (apraxia). The fright of movement can express itself in "gravitational insecurity" presented by a fear of external movement facilitation. The embrace of the child provides her with sensory stability. In the relaxed and familiar surroundings of the multi-sensory environment the girl, who is afraid of movement, can be moved freely and peacefully, thus enabling sensory feedback (while relaxing parts of her nervous system that is responsible for learning and executing acts), and enables an organized sense of sensory integration [16]. Constant routine visitations to the multi-sensory environment reestablishing confidence of the child or adolescent in movement might bear positive results on day-to-day independent propulsion. Girls have opened up to the experience of movement and shown lack of fear of movement by an external facilitator despite a paralyzing fear prior to intervention

Stage IV - Late Motor Deterioration

At this stage, in some girls and women, late motor deterioration that requires increased physiotherapy may be noticed. Several cases have been reported where girls with RS lost their ability to walk, but were able to improve functional mobility and regain lost ability. In one case study, rehabilitation of lost walking skill was achieved with a 43 year old individual after two decades of immobility [36]. A similar case study were a person with RS regained her walking ability after years of being in a wheelchair was recently published [37].

It is important to stress that inability to walk increases risk of secondary complications such as scoliosis, pelvic deformities, pulmonary (lung) problems, reduced bowel movements and blood flow to internal organs and lower limbs. Thus, it is extremely important to keep the adolescents with RS as active as possible.

The need for extensive intervention sometimes collides with aversion of physical intervention, but the calm and relaxing multi sensory environment can help the adolescent and adult enjoy or in some cases endure obligatory physical manipulations.

Despite new difficulties at this stage, new areas such as a decrease in repetitive hand movements and social and communicative skills are open to improvement. In stage IV, therefore, one should address problems reported in stage III and treat them more often (if necessary), but without neglecting new areas (improvements).

Most girls with RS do not communicate verbally [38]. However, they like to communicate with others, especially adults, and it is easier for them to communicate in a one-on-one situation (individual treatment). During therapy sessions in the multi sensory environment, the therapist should be in front of the person with RS, facing her and maintaining direct eye contact with her. The therapist should be attuned to non-verbal language expressed by the client's eyes and face, constantly talking to her to explain what will happen next and reinforce her activities. This is a good time to assist the individual with RS in improving her non-verbal communication. If communication is a primary treatment target, then moving across the multi-sensory environment can be performed according to preferences of the child, using a set of plastic cards (showing different areas of the room) pointed out by the eye gaze of the child or use of the hand. Such activity might have a carry-over to day-to-day situations [39].

Adolescents and woman with RS are very friendly, but communication and social skills (especially individuals that are not mobile) with friends and classmates are technically difficult. Better communicative ability can be developed during treatment in the multi-sensory environment. Reinforcing relationships with others is important at all times and in every treatment, but is highly significant at stage IV of RS. Getting friends and/or family members together in the multi sensory environment can cause joy and happiness to the child and her closest human circle. Such closeness can take the mind off daily hardships and thus recharge mental strengths for the ongoing struggle of living with RS.

At an older age, individuals with RS tend to develop high muscle tone and spasticity. Reducing this high tone requires slow and continuous movement, and this kind of movement matches the kind provided by a warm waterbed. The music bed can also be used for the same purpose, as the vibration of loudspeakers can cause muscle tone reduction. Reducing muscle tone has been found useful especially when using Vibro-acoustics [21].

CONCLUSIONS

This review has covered some of the major challenges faced by the adolescence with RS, and some possible treatment goals for weman and adolescent with Rett syndrome (RS) have been presented. One should bear in mind that individuals with RS tend to have a hypoactive para-sympathetic system [40] causing a constant high tension state of mind. Such a case necessitates regular visits to a calming environment such as the multi-sensory environment or Snoezelen room. On the other hand, it is important to stress that every person should be evaluated individually in order to understand individual problems and difficulties and create a treatment plan according to the problems and the RS stage.

It is important to realize the capacities of the adolescent with RS and its possible future achievements when planning ahead and deciding on new ways of intervention for those individuals. When we bear in mind that the two main motivational factors of individuals with RS are music [19, 20, 22] and interpersonal interaction, then the multi-sensory environment is a good place to be treated for this population. If we add the ability of the multi-sensory environment to adjust according to preferences of each client, and the empowerment it gives the user, then we add another advantage to the necessity of this environment to become a constant factor in interventions for the adolescent and woman with RS.

REFERENCES

[1]   Amir RE, Van Den Veyver IB, Schultz R, Malicki DM, Tran CQ, Dahle E, Philippi A, Timer L, Percy AK, Motil KJ, Lichtarge O, Smith EO, Glaze DG, Zoghbi HY. Influence of mutation type and X chromosome inactivation on Rett syndrome phenotype. *Ann. Neurol.* 2000;47:670-9.

[2] Hagberg B, Aicardi J, Dias K, Ramos O. A progressive syndrome of autism, dementia, ataxia, and loss of purposeful hand use in girls: Rett syndrome: report of 35 cases. *Ann. Neurol.* 1983;14:471-9.

[3] Hagberg B, ed. Rett syndrome. *Clinical and biological aspects.* London: MacKeith Press, 1993.

[4] Ellaway C., Christodoulou J. Rett syndrome: Clinical characteristics and recent genetic advances. *Disabil. Rehab.* 2001;23: 98-106.

[5] Kerr AM. Annotation: Rett syndrome: recent progress And implications for research and clinical practice. *J. Child Psychol. Child Psychiatry.* 2002;43(3):277-87.

[6] Graham JM. Rett syndrome. *Information packet.* Los Angeles, CA: Cedars-Sinai Medical Center, 1995.

[7] Kerr AM, Stephenson JBP. Rett syndrome in the west of Scotland. *BMJ.* 1985;291(6495):579-82.

[8] Budden SS. Management of Rett Syndrome: A Ten Years Experience. *Neuropediatrics.* 1995;26(2):75-7.

[9] Leonard H, Fyfe S, Leonard S, Msall M. Functional status, medical impairments, and rehabilitation resources in 84 females with Rett syndrome: a snapshot across the world from the parental perspective. *Disabil. Rehab.* 2001;23(3-4):107-17.

[10] Sponseller P. Orthopedic update in Rett Syndrome. *IRSA-Int. Rett. Syndr. Ass. Inf. Resources.* Website: www.rettsyndrome.org/main/orthopaedic-update.htm

[11] Percy AK. International research review. *IRSA-Int. Rett. Syndr. Ass. 12th Ann. Conf.* Boston, MA: 24-27 May, 1996.

[12] Smeets E, Schollen E. Moog U, Matthijs G, Herbergs J, Smeets H, Curfs L, Schrander-Stumpel C, Fryns JP. Rett Syndrome in Adolescent and Adult Females: Clinical and Molecular Genetic Findings. *Am. J. Med. Gen.* 2003:122A: 227–233.

[13] Kerr AM, Nomura Y, Armstrong D, Anvret M, Belichenko PV, Budden S, Cass H, Christodoulou J, Clarke A, Ellaway C, d'Esposito M, Francke U, Hulten M, Julu P, Leonard H, Naidu S, Schanen C, Webb T, Engerstrom I, Yamashita Y, Segawa M. 2001. Guidelines for reporting clinical features in cases with MECP2 mutations. *Brain. Dev* 2001;23:208–11.

[14] Hulsegge J, Verheul A. Snoezelen: *Another world.* Chesterfield: ROMPA, 1987.

[15] Shapiro M, & Bacher S. Snoezeling. *Controlled Multi-sensory Stimulation- A Handbook for Practitioners.* Ra'anana, Israel: Beit Issie Shapiro, 2002.

[16] Ayres JA. Sensory integration and the child. Los Angeles, CA: *Western Psychol. Serv,* 1982.

[17] Longhorn F. Planning a multi-sensory massage programme for very special people. London: *Catalyst. Educ. Resources.* 1993.

[18] Kerr AM, Belichenko P, WoodcockT, & Woodcock M. Mind and brain in Rett disorder. *Brain Dev.* 2001;23:44-9.

[19] Kerr AM. How can we help the youngest ones with Rett disorder? *A lecture presented at the annual RDAUK family weekend,* October, Northampton, England, 2002.

[20] Elefant C. Music, choice making and communication in Rett syndrome. A lecture presented at the international course on *Rett syndrome,* Ostersund, 16-18 June, Sweden, 2003.

[21] Wigram T. Vibro-acoustics. *Third Int. Conf. Developmental Disabilities.* Tel Aviv, IL: Dan Panorama Hotel, July 2-4, 2002.

[22] Wigram T. Assessment and treatment of a girl with Rett syndrome. In: Bruscia K. Case Studies in music therapy. *Gilsum,* NH: Barcelona Publ, 1991:39-53.
[23] Kerr AM. Infant development in Rett syndrome. A lecture presented at the international course on Rett syndrome, *Ostersund,* 16-18 June, Sweden, 2003.
[24] Lotan M, Hadar-Frumer M. *Hydrotherapy for individuals with Rett syndrome.* Raanana, Israel: Bcit Issie Shapira, 2002. (Hebrew).
[25] Grandin T, Scariano MM. Emegence: Labeled autistic. Novato, CA: Arena Press, 1986.
[26] Krauss KE. The effects of deep pressure touch on anxiety. *Am. J. Occup. Ther.* 1987;41:366-73.
[27] Kerr AM, Burford B. Towards a full life with Rett disorder. *Ped. Rehab.* 2001;4(4):157-68.
[28] Beuchel K. Physical therapy and gross motor skills in Rett syndrome. IRSA-Int Rett *Syndr. Ass. Annual Conf.* Washington, DC: May, 2001.
[29] Hanks SB. Physical therapy strategies. *Paper presented at the IRSA 12th Annual Conference,* Boston, MA: Tape 622-08, May 24-27, 1996.
[30] Lotan M, Burshtein S. Physical therapy intervention for senior citizens with cognitive impairment. *AAMR 127 Ann. Meeting,* Chicago, Ill: May 20-23, 2003.
[31] Rossin LK. Effectiveness of therapeutic and surgical intervention in the treatment of scoliosis in *Rett syndrome.* (Thesis). Pittsburgh, Pennsylvania: Univ. Duquesne, 1997:1-19.
[32] Hanks SB. Motor disabilities in the Rett syndrome and physical therapy strategies. *Brain Dev.* 1990;2:157-61.
[33] Brogran E. Basic mechanisms in the development of postural control. A lecture presented at the international course on *Rett syndrome,* Ostersund, 16-18 June, Sweden, 2003.
[34] Hunter K. The Rett syndrome handbook. *IRSA-Int. Rett. Syndr. Ass.* Washington, DC: 1999.
[35] Lindberg B. Understanding Rett syndrome: A practice guide for parents, teachers and therapists. *Guttingen,* Germany: Hogrefe Huber, 1990.
[36] Jacobsen K, Viken A, Von Tetzchner S. Rett syndrome and aging: a case study. *Disabil. Rehab.* 2001;23:160-6.
[37] Lotan M. Regaining waking ability in individuals with RS – A case study. (Hebrew). Isr *J. Health Intellect. Disabil.* 2008;1(1):32-43.
[38] Elefant C. Speechless yet communicative: Revealing the person behind the disability of Rett syndrome through clinical research on songs in music therapy. *V. Eur. Music Ther. Congr*, Napoli, Italy, April 20-24, 2001
[39] Gaines C. Making use of augmentative and alternative communication. *IRSA-Int. Rett. Syndr. Ass. Newsletter,* 1998.
[40] Engerstrom IW, Kerr A. Workshop on autonomic function in Rett Syndrome, Swedish Rett Center, Froson, Sweden. *Brain Dev.* 1998;20:323-6.

Part XVI. Physical Activity and Sports

In: Adolescence and Chronic Illness
Editors: H. Omar et al.

ISBN: 978-1-60876-628-4
© 2010 Nova Science Publishers, Inc.

Chapter 28

SPORTS AND ADOLESCENTS WITH DISABILITY

Dilip R. Patel[*] *and Donald E. Greydanus*

Department of Pediatrics and Human Development,
Michigan State University College of Human Medicine,
Kalamazoo Center for Medical Studies, Kalamazoo,
Michigan, United States of America.

ABSTRACT

Sport participation by children and adolescents is an integral aspect of contemporary American society and physically challenged adolescents can derive the same physical and psychosocial benefits from sport participation as those without disability. It is estimated that 12 percent of school aged children in the United States are physically challenged. Sports participation by physically challenged athletes has steadily increased over the past several years. Physically challenged athletes manifest a wide range of neuromotor impairments and disabilities that impact their sport participation. Some of the major medical concerns include increased risks for hyperthermia, hypothermia, autonomic dysreflexia, neurogenic bladder, neurogenic bowel, latex allergy, high risk for pressure sores, and osteopenia. The epidemiology of musculoskeletal injuries in physically challenged athletes is generally similar to those without physical disabilities. Management considerations for the physician include classification of athletes, preparticipation evaluation and determination of eligibility for participation. In order to illustrate some of these issues we have briefly reviewed cerebral palsy, spinal cord injury, and myelomeningocele.

INTRODUCTION

It is estimated that there are approximately 40 million physically challenged individuals in the United States [1]. Twelve percent of school-aged children and adolescents are estimated to be physically challenged [1]. Sport participation by physically challenged

---

[*] *Correspondence:* Professor Dilip R. Patel, MD, MSU/ KCMS/ Pediatrics, 1000, Oakland Drive, Kalamazoo, MI 49008 United States. E-mail: patel@kcms.msu.edu

athletes has steadily increased over past several years with an estimation of between 4,000 and 6,000 Paralympic athletes participating at various levels of competition. Just like athletes with no physical disability, physically challenged athletes also face the inherent risk of sport participation that is further complicated by associated medical complications that include problems with thermoregulation, autonomic instability, latex allergy, neurogenic bladder and bowel, and osteopenia [2-8].

The key epidemiologic findings related to musculoskeletal injuries in athletes with physical and sensory disabilities indicate that the incidence and pattern of injuries are similar to those seen in able-bodied athletes. Overuse injuries are the most common [1,4,5,9,10]. To highlight some unique aspects of sport participation by physically challenged athletes, we have reviewed three major conditions briefly here, namely, cerebral palsy, spinal cord injury, and myelomeningocele.

Cerebral Palsy

The neurologic deficits in adolescents with cerebral palsy can range from mild to severe. The child's functional abilities can be affected by motor as well as associated cognitive deficits. It is estimated that about half the athletes with cerebral palsy maintain functional ambulation, and the other half are wheelchair bound. Many factors affect the risk of injury and the ability to participate in sports by adolescents with cerebral palsy, including decreased flexibility, decreased muscle strength and endurance, spasticity, increased cost of movements, cognitive delay, sensory impairments [1,2, 3,5,8,11]. Overuse injuries are the most common type of injury reported in adolescents with cerebral palsy. Such adolescents can benefit from participating in supervised sports programs. Appropriately designed training and conditioning programs that include stretching, warm ups, strength training, and sports-specific skills not only can improve general health but also can have significant psychosocial benefits for adolescents with cerebral palsy.

Spinal Cord Injury

Although spinal cord injuries are uncommon in adolescents, such injuries can result in a lifelong negative impact for independent living and participation in sports and physical activities. The use of wheelchairs, prostheses, and other adaptive equipment increase the risk for specific musculoskeletal injuries in these athletes [12]. Lack of sensory and motor function below the level of the specific spinal cord lesion predisposes these athletes to specific medical problems. A loss of autonomic function below the level of the lesion can result in impaired thermoregulation and autonomic dysreflexia, both with significant consequences for sport participation.

Impaired thermoregulation has been reported especially in individuals with spinal cord lesions at or above T 8 [1,2,6,8,12]. Below the level of lesion, lack of active muscle contractions results in venous pooling of the blood in the lower limbs, a decreased venous return, and a decreased overall body heat loss capacity by convection or radiation. There is reduced evaporative cooling secondary to impaired sweating. These individuals may also be on certain therapeutic medications like anticholinergics that further impair thermoregulation. All these factors predispose individuals with spinal cord injury to hyperthermia.

Individuals with spinal cord injury are also pre-disposed to hypothermia when exposed to cooler ambient temperatures. Impaired vasomotor control, impaired hypothalamic temperature regulation, and lack of shiver response because of lack of active muscle contractions, all contribute to hypothermia [12]. These individuals may not be aware of wet clothes below the level of their lesion because of lack of sensation, further predisposing them to heat loss. Awareness, education, adequate hydration, and vigilance to identify these problems are essential aspects of prevention.

Autonomic dysreflexia has been reported in individuals with lesions above T6 [1,2,4,6,12]. This condition is clinically characterized by symptomatology that results from a lack of inhibition of the sympathetic response. The signs and symptoms include hyperthermia, cardiac arrhythmias, acute elevation of systemic blood pressure, chest tightness, excessive sweating above the level of the specific lesion, anxiety and apprehension, vomiting, diarrhea, and headache. Autonomic dysreflexia can be triggered by certain stimuli below the lesion of the spinal cord, including tight clothing, acute fractures, urinary tract infection, bladder or bowel distension, and decubitus ulcers. The athlete should be removed from the sport at the first signs of autonomic dysreflexia. In most cases, the condition is self-limited; however, persistent hypertension and cardiac complications can be potentially life threatening and need emergent medical care.

The term boosting refers to self-induced autonomic dysreflexia, especially reported in wheelchair athletes [1,13,14]. It is hypothesized that a heightened sympa-thetic response that characterizes autonomic dysreflexia will give the individual athlete an advantage in competition and will decrease his or her race time. Athletes trigger such self-induced response by various methods, including self-induced leg fracture, bladder distension, and drinking large amounts of fluids. Such a practice is considered an ergogenic aid and not sanctioned by official sports governing bodies.

Myelomeningocele

Open neural tube defects are closed in infancy and most children with myelomeningocele also have hydrocephalus that requires a ventriculoperitoneal shunt. There is also a high association of Arnold-Chiari type 2 malformations and tethered cord syndrome in these adolescents. Adolescents with a history of repaired myelomeningocele and shunted hydrocephalus may also have a varying degree of neurocognitive deficits. Most myleomeningocele lesions affect the lumbar region and these adolescents manifest motor and sensory deficits of the lower extremities as well as bladder and bowel dysfunction. Most adolescents with lumbosacral lesions can participate in wheelchair sports. Adolescents with myelomeningocele have lower limb paralysis and develop upper limb spasticity, and deficits of hand-eye coordination. In general, athletes with myelomeningo-cele have decreased aerobic power and, decreased peak anaerobic power [1,3,4,14].

Adolescents with myelomeningocele are also predisposed to pressure ulcers because of lack of sensation and active muscle contractions. Muscular weakness, muscle strength imbalance, and lack of weight bearing or loading activities predispose these adolescents to a significantly increased risk for musculotendonous strains, ligament sprains, osteopenia, and fractures.

Neurogenic bladder dysfunction may require intermittent catheterization. This type of regimen may often be an impediment for some athletes because it requires interruption in sports activity. Sixty to seventy percent of adolescent with myelomeningocele have latex allergy. This is an important consideration for those working with these athletes. All latex exposure must be carefully identified and avoided. The severity of hydrocephalus and the presence of the VP shunt are major factors affecting the function and sport participation for these athletes. Signs and symptoms of shunt malfunction, increased intracranial pressure, or syringomyelia must be recognized promptly with immediate evaluation and intervention initiated in consultation with a neurosurgeon. This athlete should not return to sports until fully cleared by the neurosurgeon involved in his or her care. For adolescents with myelomeningocele, certain sports that pose a relatively higher risk include football, cheerleading, scuba diving, water skiing, polo, and bob sledding.

Wheelchair Athletes

Adolescents, who have cerebral palsy, spinal cord injury, or myelomeningocele, and athletes with lower limb amputations or congenital deficiencies of lower limbs, all can be participants in various sports for wheelchair athletes. Athletes participating in wheelchair athletics are at a higher risk for upper extremity overuse injuries, shoulder and wrist being the most common injuries reported [13,14]. Peripheral entrapment or compressive neuropathies of the upper extremities are also common in wheelchair athletes, carpal tunnel syndrome being the most common one identified. Another problem developed by wheelchair athletes is pressure sores and ulcers. Injuries related to the use of equipment and prostheses are also seen at a higher rate in these athletes. Also, in athletes with lower limb amputations, common problems include an increased risk for back pain and overgrowth of the stump. Breakdown of the overlying skin and soft tissue because of friction and pressure from sport participation is common in these athletes.

Considerations for Sport Participation by Physically Challenged Athletes

The physical and mental health benefits of sport participation by adolescents with physical challenges are well recognized. The major aspects to be considered by the physician involved in providing care to adoles-cents who are physically challenges include the appropriate classification of the athletes, preparticipation assessment, and the application of sport participation guidelines [1-7].

An appropriate classification of physically challenged athletes—taking into consideration their medical condition and functional ability—is essential for fair and safe sport participation and competition. Medical classification delineates the basic disability of the athlete, whereas functional classification seeks to delineate the abilities of the athlete to perform skills and tasks of a given sport. The classification of physically challenged athletes is often a complex process done by specially trained personnel. Each sport governing body may also use its own classification system.

The physician plays a key role in the sports pre-participation evaluation (SPPE) of the physically challenged athletes. The SPPE of physically challenged athletes should ideally be done by the physician most familiar with the athlete and his or her condition. The process of this SPPE is similar to the assessment of those athletes without disability. A careful history and physical examination are the cornerstones of such an evaluation. The physician should be cognizant of the numerous disabilities and specific medical issues that might have either direct or indirect implications for sport participation by this athlete. Determination of the eligibility to participate in a particular sport is based on the findings of the SPPE, the functional classification, and specific sports offered by sport governing bodies that are especially modified for safe participation. An important aspect for the physician to consider is the use of performance enhancing drugs often noted in athletes with no disability, since the drive and motivation for the athlete with disability are the same.

CONCLUSIONS

Sports participation by all adolescents is recommended, including those who are physically challenged. Physically challenged athletes manifest a wide range of neuromotor impairments and disabilities that have an impact on their sport participation. Some of the major medical concerns include increased risks for hyper-thermia, hypothermia, autonomic dysreflexia, neurogenic bladder, neurogenic bowel, latex allergy, high risk for pressure sores, and osteopenia. Management issues for clinicians include providing a sports preparticipation examination for these athletes and helping to determine eligibility guidelines for them to allow maximum sports play with minimal risk of injury. Specific issues have been summarized with regard to athletes with cerebral palsy, spinal cord injury, and myelomeningocele.

REFERENCES

[1] Patel DR, Greydanus DE. The pediatric athlete with disabilities. *Pediatr. Clin. North Am.* 2002;49: 803-27.
[2] Chang FM. The disabled athlete, In Stanitski CL, DeLee JL, Drez D, eds. *Pediatric and adolescent sports medicine*. Philadelphia, PA: Saunders Elsevier, 1994:48-75.
[3] Wind WM, Shwend RM, Larson J. Sports for the physically challenged child. *J. Am. Acad. Orthop. Surg.* 2004;12:126-37.
[4] Winnick JP, ed. Adapted physical education and sport. Champaign, IL: *Human Kinetics,* 2000.
[5] Goldberg B. Sports and exercise for children with chronic health conditions. Champaign, IL: *Human Kinetics,* 1995.
[6] Dec KL. Challenged athletes. In: McKeag DB, Moeller JL, eds. *ACSM's primary care sports medicine,* 2nd ed. Philadelphia, PA: Lippincott Williams & Wilkins, 2007:293-304.
[7] American College of Sports Medicine. Exercise management for persons with chronic diseases and disabilities. Champaign, IL: *Human Kinetics,* 1997.

[8] Klenck C, Gebke K. Practical management: common medical problems in disabled athletes. *Clin. J. Sport Med.* 2007;17:55-60.
[9] Ferrara MS, Buckley WE, McCann BC, et al. The injury experience of the competitive athlete with a disability: prevention implications. *Med. Sci. Sports Exer.* 1991;24:184-8.
[10] Ferrara MS, Palutsis GR, Snouse S, et al. A longitudinal study of injuries to athletes with disabilities. *J. Sport Med.* 2000;21:221-4.
[11] Carroll KL, Leiser J, Paisley TS. Cerebral palsy: physical activity and sport. *Curr. Sport Med. Rep.* 2006;5:319-22.
[12] Jacobs PL, Nash MS. Exercise recommendations for individuals with spinal cord injury. *Sport Med.* 2004;34(11):727-51.
[13] Groah SL, Lanig IS. Neuromusculoskeletal syndromes in wheelchair athletes. *Sem. Neurology.* 2000;20:201-8.
[14] Wilson PE, Washington RL. Pediatric wheelchair athletics: sports injuries and prevention. *Paraplegia.* 1993;31:330-7.

In: Adolescence and Chronic Illness
Editors: H. Omar et al.

ISBN: 978-1-60876-628-4
© 2010 Nova Science Publishers, Inc.

Chapter 29

SPORTS PREPARTICIPATION EXAMINATION

Donald E. Greydanus[*] *and Dilip R. Patel*

Department of Pediatrics and Human Development,
Michigan State University College of Human Medicine,
Kalamazoo Center for Medical Studies, Kalamazoo,
Michigan, United States of America.

ABSTRACT

All youth, including those with chronic illness, need regular physical exercise, and sports participation may be the main form of exercise obtained by many youth. Clinicians should encourage these youth to play sports and as part of this process, provide a sports preparticipation evaluation (SPPE) on an annual basis to help determine what sport is best for the youth and which ones may pose eligibility problems. The SPPE includes a careful medical history and selective physical examination. Concepts of the SPPE are provided in this discussion with comments regarding sports eligibility guidelines.

INTRODUCTION

Physical exercise, including sports participation, is important for the health of all youth including those with chronic illnesses. Those involved in sports should receive a sports preparticipation evaluation (SPPE) on an annual basis and preferably 5-7 weeks before the desired sport's season begins [1-3]. The SPPE includes a careful medical history and physical examination to allow youth with or without chronic illnesses to participate in various sports activities that are best suited for them [4-6]. This chapter presents comments on the SSPE and youth with chronic illnesses.

---

[*] *Correspondence:* Donald E Greydanus, MD, Professor of Pediatrics and Human Development, Michigan State University College of Human Medicine, Pediatrics Program, MSU/Kalamazoo Center for Medical Studies, 1000 Oakland Drive, Kalamazoo, MI 49008-1284 United States. Tel: 269-337-6450; Fax: 269-337-6474; E-mail: Greydanus@kcms.msu.edu

SPPE Medical History

The clinician can obtain a thorough medical history from the adolescent as well as parents and if done well, can identify approximately 75% of problems that would interfere with sports participation by the examined youth. Table 1 provides an outline of important aspects of the SPPE medical history.

SPPE Physical Examination

The careful SPPE physical examination is based on the medical history and focuses on the pulmonary, cardiovascular, and musculoskeletal systems [1,3]. The examination should also include youth with various chronic illnesses, including asthma, cardiac conditions, diabetes mellitus, epilepsy, orthopedic disorders, and many others [1,2].

Determination of Sports Participation Eligibility

The SPPE can help determine what sports are appropriate for the adolescent with chronic illness, based on factors outlined in table 2. All athletes can be matched with appropriate sports based on such factors as age, weight, Tanner staging, and degree of sports skills. This includes youth with various handicaps, including visual or hearing impairments, cerebral palsy, amputations, traumatic brain injury, spinal cord anomalies, and others [7]. Exclusion from any sports activity should be based on the adolescent's overall health, risks of the identified sport and its intensity, maturity of the youth, and his or her fitness level. Comments on specific illnesses are now provided.

Table 1. Important aspects of the SPPE medical history. Reprinted with permission from: Patel DR, Greydanus DE, Baker R, eds. Pediatric and Adolescent Sports Medicine. New York: McGraw-Hill, 2009)

- Does the athlete have any known medical disorders? (i.e., epilepsy, diabetes, disabilities, others)
- Is there a history of heat disorders?
- Is there a history of musculoskeletal disorders? Head and/or neck injuries? Concussion or burners history?
- Is there a history of breathing problems? Asthma? Does exercise induce shortness of breath, coughing, or wheezing?
- Is there a history of cardiovascular disorders: Chest pain, murmurs, palpitations, hypertension, unexplained fatigue?
- Is there a history of syncope or pre-syncope?
- Any history of weight loss practices? Use of medications to lose weight? Abnormal eating practices?
- What is the menstrual and gynecological history?
- What medication is the athlete taking? Any nutritional supplements?
- Is there a history of allergies? Drug or environmental allergies?
- Is there a history of recent upper respiratory illnesses? Febrile illnesses?
- Is there a history of eye disorders? Does the athlete need glasses? Are there hearing problems?
- Is there a history of major or minor surgery?
- Are the immunizations up-to-date? Tetanus status normal?
- Is there any family history of medical disorders? Sudden cardiac death at an early age (i.e., under age 55). Marfan disorders? Cardiomyopathy?
- Is there a history of lipid disorders in the patient or family?

Pulmonary Disorders

Asthma (including exercise-induced asthma) is the most common chronic disorder of adolescents and is found in over 5 million children and adolescents in the United States [8,9]. The athlete with asthma should be screened for asthma triggers including smoking (tobacco or marijuana), hair sprays, strong deodorants, perfumes, and others.

Youth with asthma can participate in all sports if they receive proper medication for asthma; those with the most severe asthma may need some modification in sports play [8-10]. Though pulmonary compromise may occur in youth with cystic fibrosis, most sports can be played if they maintain satisfactory oxygenation and a graded exercise test may be used to assess specific sports participation. It is important for athletes with cystic fibrosis to have appropriate hydration to reduced risk of heat illness.

Table 2. Factors involved in establishing eligibility for sports participation (reprinted with permission from: Patel DR, Greydanus DE, Baker R, eds. Pediatric and adolescent sports medicine. New York: McGraw-Hill, 2009)

- SPPE results establishing overall health status of the athlete
- Is the desired activity a contact or non-contact sport?
- Are there static or dynamic demands of the chosen sport?
- What is the competition level of the athlete and his/her position?
- What is the SMR or Tanner Stage of the teen athlete?
- Do the athlete and the parents/guardians understand the risks involved based on the desired sport and identified conditions of the athlete (i.e., epilepsy, diabetes mellitus, single kidney, single eye, others)?
- Are the athlete and family willing to change the sport if necessary based on results of the SPPE?

Cardiac Disorders

Table 3 notes key features of a SPPE cardiovascular disorders screening to help identify cardiac problems that will compromise athletic effort and contribute to pathologic consequences while identifying what levels of exercise are appropriate for an athlete with discovered or undiscovered cardiac conditions [11-13]. Sudden cardiac death develops in 1-2 per 200,000 athletes per year in the United States and represents the cause of 95% of sudden death in adolescent and young adult athletes [14,15]. Causes of sudden cardiac death in athletes under 35 years of age include hypertrophic cardiomyopathy (36%) and anomalous or aberrant coronary arteries (24%); less common causes include aortic valve stenosis, acute myocarditis, cardiac arrhythmias, Marfan syndrome (5%), long QT syndrome, and commotio cordis (sudden precordial trauma from a baseball, hockey puck, others) [11-15]. Key aspects of the SPPE cardiovascular examination are listed in table 4.

Cardiac Disease: Sports Eligibility Criteria [11-16]

Athletes with significant primary hypertension should avoid strength training, body building, and weight as well as power lifting. Those with secondary hypertension should have a thorough evaluation before determining sports eligibility. Those with mild congenital heart disease (i.e., structural heart defects present from birth) usually have no exercise restrictions; however, those athletes with moderate or severe congenital heart disease with or without a history of corrective heart surgery need a careful evaluation before allowing any sports participation.

Table 3. Important components in the SPPE cardiovascular history (reprinted with permission from: Patel DR, Greydanus DE, Baker R, eds. Pediatric and Adolescent Sports Medicine. New York: McGraw-Hill, 2009)

- Cardiac murmur (s)
- Chest pain
- Fatigue (moderate or severe)
- High blood pressure and/or hyperlipidemia or hypercholesterolemia
- Palpations
- Syncope (or presynope) caused by physical activity
- Positive family history of hypertension, hyperlipidemia or hypercholesterolemia, Marfan syndrome or sudden cardiac death (first degree relative under 50 years of age

Those with an innocent heart murmur (i.e., no heart disease) should have no sports restrictions unless they have other (non-cardiac) disorders that require restricted sports play. If the athlete has a pathologic heart murmur, a careful evaluation is necessary by a qualified clinician. Athletes with carditis should not participate in sports because exertion may precipitate sudden cardiac death. An athlete with dysrhythmia requires a careful evaluation before allowing sports play. Those with symptomatic mitral valve prolapse (i.e., chest pain, mitral regurgitation, dysrhythmia) need further evaluation to determine specific sports participation. Those with asymptomatic mitral valve prolapse should have no restrictions in sport play.

Musculoskeletal Disorders

A thorough evaluation for musculoskeletal disorders is needed as part of the SPPE examination [7,17,18]. If there is a positive history for previous injury (i.e., knee or ankle sprain), more information is needed regarding how the injury occurred, what treatment was provided, if full recovery occurred, and whether over-training has been involved [18]. Further injury may occur if sports play occurs before full recovery from a prior injury develops. Other causes of musculoskeletal pain or injury should be considered, including infection (as arthritis or osteomyelitis) and neoplasm [19]. The criteria for sports eligibility depend on the specific orthopedic disorder that is found. For example scoliosis with curves over 20 degrees requires orthopedic evaluation. Back pain may suggest such causes as muscular strain, spondylolisthesis, or spondylolysis. Tibial tuberosity tenderness and/or swelling suggest Osgood-Schlatter disorder that usually does not require any specific sports restrictions.

Head and Neck Injuries

Any athlete who wishes to participate in sports should be screened for head and neck injuries. The trauma of sports may cause a concussion and traumatic brain injury (TBI) with resultant acute and chronic complications [20,21].

Table 4. Key aspects of the SPPE cardiovascular examination (reprinted with permission from: Patel DR, Greydanus DE, Baker R, eds. Pediatric and adolescent sports medicine. New York: McGraw-Hill, 2009)

- Blood pressure and pulse measurement (radial and femoral)
- Evaluate the femoral pulses (looking for coarctation of the aorta)
- Auscultate for pathologic heart murmurs:
  Systolic ejection murmur (consider hypertrophic cardiomyopathy: that increases with the Valsalva maneuver or with standing; the murmur decreases with squatting)
  Decrescendo diastolic murmur (consider aortic insufficiency)
  Holosystolic murmur (consider mitral insufficiency)
- Others
- Look for Marfan Syndrome [25]
  Tall (compared to first degree relatives), slender, long extremities, arm span is longer than height
  Arachnodactyly (spider fingers); dolichostenomelia (long, narrow head)
  Hyperextensible joints; joint dislocations (especially the hips); abnormal musculoskeletal examination
  Many cardiac abnormalities (abdominal aortic aneurysm, aortic dissection, aortic insufficiency, aortic root dilatation, mitral regurgitation, mitral valve prolapse, pulmonary artery dilatation, others)
  Ophthalmologic abnormalities: ectopia lentis, myopia with retinal detachment, strabismus, nystagmus, cataracts, coloboma, iris tremor, megalocornea)
  Many other defects due to this connective tissue disorder

It is important that full recovery from head or neck injuries occurs before allowing further sports play. It is necessary to know if the injury has led to any loss of consciousness and if so, for how long? Ask about a history of persistent headaches, memory difficulties, confusion, or problems in school after the head injury. Athletes who suffer a significant concussion or traumatic brain injury may develop problems in managing a chronic illness that may be present, such as diabetes mellitus, epilepsy, asthma, or other. If a neck injury occurred, ask about such potential complications as weakness of extremities, paresthesias, transient quadriplegia, or on-going numbness.

Other Chronic Illnesses and Sports Considerations

In general, athletes with chronic illness can participate in sports if their medical condition is in good control [2-4]. For example, those with diabetes mellitus can play all sports if they pay proper attention to issues related to their diet, hydration, and insulin therapy; they should be carefully taught how to regulate these issues with the physical activity, especially if the exertion lasts more than 30 minutes. Those with epilepsy that is well controlled can participate in all sports because the risk of a seizure is low; if the seizure disorder is not well controlled, however, then this individual needs an individual assessment by a qualified clinician, especially if the athlete wishes to take part in collision or contact sports. Those with poor seizure control should not take part in such sports as swimming, weight or power lifting, archery, riflery, or those that involve heights or strength training.

If the athlete has acute hepatomegaly or splenomegaly, as from infectious mononucleosis for example, sports participation should be avoided until the liver or spleen return to a normal size to reduce risk of an organ rupture. If the athlete has a disorder leading to a chronically enlarged liver or spleen, then individual assessment is needed before allowing sports play. Individual assessment by a qualified clinician is also needed if the athlete has such conditions as bleeding disorders, malignancy, obesity, eating disorders (anorexia or bulimia nervosa), or absence of an organ or structure in which there are normally two (as eyes, testicles, ovaries, others). Those who are obese need instruction in avoiding heat illness. Females who are involved in sports that emphasize a thin physique should be screened for elements of the female athlete triad with menstrual irregularities (i.e., amenorrhea, oligomenorrhea, dysfunctional uterine bleeding), eating dysfunction, and osteopenia or osteoporosis [22].

CONCLUSIONS

Physical exercise, including sports participation, is recommended for all youth, including those with chronic illnesses and disabilities. All athletes should receive a sports preparticipation evaluation (SPPE) on an annual basis and this is best if done 5-7 weeks before the desired sport's season begins. The SPPE includes a careful medical history and physical examination to allow the clinician to guide the athlete to the sport activity most appropriate for his or her skills and disability to minimize risks of this sports participation. Guidelines in this process are summarized in this article to allow all youth, including those with chronic illness or disability, the opportunity to be involved in physical and sports activities.

REFERENCES

[1] Greydanus DE, Feinberg AN, Patel DR, Homnick DN, eds. *Pediatric physical diagnosis*. New York: McGraw-Hill, 2008.

[2] American Academy of Pediatrics, American Academy of Family Physicians, American Medical Society for Sports Medicine, American Orthopedic Society for Sports Medicine, American Osteopathic Association for Sports Medicine. *Preparticipation physical evaluation*. New York: McGraw Hill, 2005.

[3] Patel DR, Greydanus DE, Luckstead EF Jr. Sports preparticipation Evaluation. In: Greydanus DE, Patel DR, Pratt HD, eds. *Essential adolescent medicine*. New York: McGraw Hill, 2006:669-75.

[4] Patel DR, Luckstead EF. Sports participation, risk taking, and health risk behaviors. *Adolesc. Med.* 2000;11:141.

[5] Pratt HD, Patel DR, Greydanus DE. Sports and the neurodevelopment of the child and adolescents. In: DeLee JC, Drez DJr, Miller MD, eds. *Orthopaedic sports medicine*. Philadelphia, PA: Saunders/ Elsevier, 2003:624-43.

[6] Patel DR, Pratt HD, Greydanus DE. Pediatric neurodevelopment and sports participation: When is the child ready to play sports? *Pediatric Clin. North Am.* 2002;49:505-31.

[7] Patel DR, Greydanus DE. The pediatric athlete with disabilities. *Pediatric Clin. North Am.* 2002; 49:803-28.

[8] Homnick DN. Disorders of the thorax and lungs. In: Greydanus DE, Patel DR, Pratt HD, eds. *Essential adolescent medicine*. New York: McGraw- Hill, 2006:103-28.

[9] Homnick DN, Marks JH. Exercise and sports in the adolescent with chronic pulmonary disease. *Adolesc. Med.* 1998;9:467.

[10] Orenstein DM. Pulmonary problems and management concerns in youth sports. *Pediatr. Clin. North Am.* 2002;49(2):709-22.

[11] 36th Bethesda Conference Report. Eligibility recommendations for competitive athletes with cardiovascular abnormalities. *J. Am. Coll. Cardiol.* 2005;45(8):1313-75.

[12] Luckstead EF, Noubani H. Cardiovascular disorders in the adolescent. In: Greydanus DE, Patel DR, Pratt HD, eds. *Essential adolescent medicine*. New York: McGraw Hill, 2006:153-5.

[13] Beckerman J, Wang P, Hlatky MC. Cardiovascular screening of athletes. *Clin. J. Sports Med.* 2004;14: 127-33.

[14] Maron BJ. Sudden death in young athletes. *N. Engl. J. Med.* 2003; 349:1064-75.

[15] Luckstead EF: Cardiac risk factors and participation guidelines for youth sports. *Pediatric Clin. North Am.* 2002;49(2):681-708.

[16] 36th Bethesda Conference. Recommendations for determining eligibility for competition in athletes with cardiovascular abnormalities. *J. Am. Coll. Cardiol.* 2005;45(8):1-64.

[17] Garrick JG. Preparticipation orthopedic screening evaluation. *Clin. J. Sport Med.* 2004;14(3):123-6.

[18] Brenner JS, Small EW, Bernhardt DT, et al. Overuse injuries, overtraining, and burnout in child and adolescent athletes. *Pediatrics.* 2007; 119(6):1242-5.

[19] Greydanus DE, Patel DR, eds. Musculoskeletal disorders. *Adolesc. Med.* 2007;18(1):1-230.
[20] Patel DR, Greydanus DE. Neurologic considerations for adolescent athletes. *Adolesc. Med.* 2002;13:569.
[21] McCrory P, Johnson K, Meeunisse W, et al. Summary and agreement statement of the 2nd International Conference on Concussion in Sport, Prague, 2004. *Br. J. Sports Med.* 2005;39:196-204.
[22] Greydanus DE, Patel DR. The female athlete: before and beyond puberty. *Pediatric Clin. North Am.* 2002;49:553-80.

In: Adolescence and Chronic Illness
Editors: H. Omar et al.

ISBN: 978-1-60876-628-4
© 2010 Nova Science Publishers, Inc.

Chapter 30

ADOLESCENTS WITH INTELLECTUAL DISABILITY AND PHYSICAL ACTIVITY

Meir Lotan[*,1,2,3] *and Joav Merrick*[3,4]

[1] Zvi Quittman Residential Center, Millie Shime Campus, Elwyn Jerusalem, Israel.
[2] School of Health Sciences, Department of Physical Therapy,
Ariel University Center of Samaria, Ariel, Israel.
[3] National Institute of Child Health and Human Development,
Office of the Medical Director, Division for Mental Retardation,
Ministry of Social Affairs, Jerusalem, Israel.
[4] Kentucky Children's Hospital, University of Kentucky,
Lexington, United States.

ABSTRACT

Numerous studies have described an association between participation in physical activity and an enhanced sense of well-being. These findings have been documented in both genders across the life span. Connections between exercise and positive physical, psychological, emotional and educational outcomes have also been found. New work indicates that is an ongoing and increasing tendency for sedentary life styles across age groups and gender in many countries. In addition, there are many factors that work together to contribute to a sedentary life style in individuals with intellectual and developmental disability (ID). These findings are concerning, and indicate that people with ID are at relatively high risk for the development of multiple negative consequences of physical inactivity. This chapter presents current literature that addresses the question of physical activity in adolescents with ID. In addition, this review presents the connection between higher levels of physical fitness and better health in youths with ID. Strategies to promote physical activity in the adolescent population with ID are presented. The available evidence base strongly supports the high need for the establishment of community based, easily accessible physical activity programs for children and adolescents with ID.

---

[*] *Correspondence:* Meir Lotan, BPT, MSc, Rothchild 67th St. 44201, Kfar Saba, Israel. Tel: 972-9-7678588. E-mail: ml_pt_rs@netvision.net.il

INTRODUCTION

The "sound body - sound mind" philosophy, although not yet scientifically established, has gained abundant empirical support. The research implications of the psychological effects of exercise on well-being are readily apparent [1]. It is generally accepted that the onset of many chronic diseases begins in early childhood. This fact, in addition to the positive effects of physical activity on the physical and mental health of participants [2], indicates that preventive fitness interventions should be implemented during childhood [3]. Coronary heart disease and risk factors such as obesity, hypertension and elevated serum cholesterol have been identified in children as young as two years of age [4], while children who are physically fit have been found to have fewer cardiovascular risk factors than less active children [5], including lower blood pressure levels [6] and lower amounts of body fat [7].

Brink [8] suggested that physical exercise stimulates brain development and enhances learning. Children who participate in daily physical education have been found to show superior motor fitness, academic performance and positive attitudes toward school compared to counterparts who are inactive [9]. Despite this and other evidence that documents the importance of physical fitness on physical and mental well-being, literature on this subject reveals that children and adolescents in many countries are becoming less active and less physically fit [10-12].

Assessments of individuals with intellectual disability (ID) consistently demonstrate extremely low levels of physical fitness [13-21]. These low levels of fitness, that are well below those in the general population [22], indicate that populations of persons with ID at relatively high risk for developing an array of future negative health outcomes. The section below addresses in detail connections between fitness in childhood and adolescence and the development of future health problems.

BENEFITS OF PHYSICAL ACTIVITY IN ADOLESCENCE

Physical activity programs in adolescents have been positively related to healthy profiles at the age of 32 years [23]. Active life styles positively correlate with predictors of good general health status in adulthood [24] and with the prevention or delay of specific adulthood diseases such as coronary heart disease [25,26] and osteoporosis [27,28]. Youths who engage in sufficient degrees of aerobic training acquire psychological benefits such as reductions in stress and the enhancement of well being and emotional health [29,30]. Physically active adolescents demonstrate increased physical performance, a lessening of total body mass and other beneficial anthropomorphic measures, and the promotion of enhanced self-image and other indicators of physical and psychological well-being [31]. More specifically, findings suggest that adolescents who regularly engaged in physical activity exhibited lower anxiety-depression scores and less social behavioral inhibition than relatively inactive counterparts [31]. The articles cited above demonstrated a positive connection between physical activity in adolescence and healthier outcomes both during adolescence and in later adult life in the general population. The section below presents evidence that younger-age physical activity confers similar health benefits in individuals with ID.

Physical Activity for Adolescents with Intellectual Disability

The literature on the subject of exercise and sports often combines individuals with ID and those who have physical disabilities [32]. Many people with cognitive impairment have concurrent physical disabilities and many studies and publications relate to both populations as one. Because of this, the present review presents evidence from populations with ID and those with significant physical impairment.

The participation in exercise and sports of children with disabilities is associated with both reductions in maladaptive behavior as well as improved physical fitness, self-esteem and social competence [33]. Adolescents and young adults with Down syndrome have shown gains in walking capacity after participating in a 10-week walking/jogging exercise training study [34].

Improved physical and psychosocial functioning are revealed in studies of both children and adults with ID, as well as in research specifically directed toward athletes enrolled in Special Olympics [33]. Young individuals with ID (mean age = 22) in Special Olympics were found to improve physical competence, social acceptance, general self-worth, adaptive behaviors [35] and social competence [36]. The results of a 20 weeks aerobic exercise demonstrated an improvement of self-concept and physical fitness in fifty-four boys with learning disabilities [37]. A daily treadmill program has revealed gains in both physical fitness as well as functional abilities of children with ID [38,39]. This current small but consistent body of knowledge supports the notion that physical activity confers physical and psychological benefits in children and adolescents with ID. These findings infer that exercise and physical activity will result in similar positive effects for the population of young people with ID. This leads to questions regarding how to motivate and in other ways encourage young people with ID to regularly participate in fitness programs.

Motivation to Participate in Activity Programs

The initiation and maintenance of regular physical activity in adults depends on a multitude of biological and socio-cultural variables that require attention across the lifespan [40]. Factors consistently associated with children's physical activity include gender (male), parental overweight status, physical activity preferences, motivational issues, perceived barriers, previous physical activity, healthy dietary practices, access to indoor facilities, and the ability to go outdoors. In adolescents, variables consistently associated with physical activity include gender (male), ethnicity (white), age (inverse), perceived activity competence, motivation, depression (inverse), previous physical activity, community sports, sensation seeking, sedentary after school and on weekends (inverse), encouragement from parents and other adults, sibling physical activity, direct help from parents, and opportunities to exercise [41].

Studies exploring motivational factors in populations of adolescents with ID were not found, but adolescents with ID are likely to face significant obstacles from engagement in regular and beneficial fitness regimens.

Barriers to Participation in Physical Activity

If participation is tailored to individual needs, the vast majority of athletes with disabilities can safely participate in a number of sports. In the recent years significant progress has been made in providing accessible sports opportunities to persons with disabilities. Unfortunately, a wide array of social and physical barriers still pevents this population from wider participation in exercise:

- inadequate facilities
- exclusion of children with disabilities
- medical professional overprotection
- lack of trained personnel and volunteers to work with children and adolescents with disabilities
- lack of public knowledge about disabilities
- lack of financial support for sport and physical education in schools [42]
- lack of supervision
- inability to walk for long distances
- equilibrium problems
- lack of health professional's knowledge about adaptive or modified physical activity techniques and opportunities [43]
- significant physiological impairments [44]

Clinical Implications

The literature on physical activity and adolescents with ID suggest that the following strategies are likely to assist health professionals in initiating physical activity programs geared towads this population:

- Gaining knowledge: There is a broad need for fitness and health clinicians to demonstrate a thorough understanding of ID (also known as mental retardation) and consequent intellectual and behavioral ramifications for persons who have this disability to help address the 'how to' of fitness evaluation and program design [45].
- Establishing the benefits of physical activity: It is necessary for physicians, therapists, people who have ID and their families to understand that participation in sports is important for the physical and emotional health of adolescents, who have physical or cognitive challenges. It is important to emphasize that sports can improve strength, endurance, and cardiopulmonary fitness while at the same time providing companionship, a sense of achievement, and heightened self-esteem [46].
- Overcoming confusion accompanying adolescence: Many adolescents spend little time thinking about their future health- and especially their health in older adulthood [47]. Anticipatory guidance strategies prepare adolescents and their parents for changes associated with puberty. Because adolescents are in many cases interested in their growth, development, and body image at this time, health supervision visits can provide an opportunity for health professionals to discuss the importance of healthy eating habits and regular physical activity.

- Setting an example: Parents and teachers can emphasize the importance of regular physical activity and show their adolescents that physical activity can be fun by role modeling. Parental encouragement and fitness lifestyles may help to promote adolescents' activity levels.
- Evaluation and assessment: Pre-participation interviews and physical examinations, including the complete medical history of the adolescent and family [48], is mandatory in order to avoid negative medical outcomes [49] and direct the young person to the appropriate physical activities that best fit his medical status, personal preferences and physical abilities. Pre and post evaluations in this population are available [50-53] and essential in order to establish program efficacy.
- Individual adjustment: Adolescents have preferences for types of physical activity. Some adolescents are primarily interested in competitive sports, but others enjoy noncompetitive activities (e.g., walking, running, swimming, biking, dancing) that provide opportunities for socialization, self expression, and accomplishment and success. Individuals' preferences and physical capabilities [40,54] can be combined with encouragement to promote enjoyable physical activity [55]. Individuals with multiple disabilities may require special environmental modifications or assistive devices to enable participation in specific physical activities.
- Using peer influence: Many adolescents with ID enjoy participating in organized programs with friends and peers. Directing adolescents to sports or other physical activities that they can enjoy with peers may enhance their participation in regular fitness activities [56].
- Promoting physically active habits: The available literature suggests that sustained physical activity needs to be incorporated into lifestyle as a habit [57]. Routine participation in activity programs needs to be promoted and maintained starting in early childhood with subsequent re-enforcements provided throughout the developmental period.
- Combined efforts: Health professionals, families, and community organizations need to work jointly to promote physical activity in adolescents with ID. Physical activity concerns and requirements should be openly discussed, with subsequent identification and utilization of community resources. Communities need to provide social and physical environments that encourage and enable safe physical activity [10] ongoing use by adolescents with ID.
- Nutritional considerations: It has been found that most children and adolescents in the US ingest a caloric intake that includes total fat and added sugars averaging 35% and 15% respectively above recommended dietary allowances [58]. It is essential to combine nutritional principles with physical activity to promote health in participants who are engaged in physical activity. Fitness incorporates both physical activity and healthy dietary choices. Fitness programs and prescriptions should include nutritional education and guidelines.
- Avoiding injury: Adolescents can engage in unsafe, impulsive behaviors: they can use poor judgment. Behaviors such as sufficient fluid intake, use of safety equipment, paced initiation of activity, safe swimming and diving practices, dangers of over-exposure to sunlight, and other potential hazards or unsafe behaviors, should be presented before and monitored during program implementation.

- A balanced program: The three primary components of physical conditioning are endurance, flexibility and strength training. It is recommended that practices that incorporate these three goals should combined in the total physical exercise program.

Suggestions for Activities

Guidelines published by the Centers for Disease Control and Prevention (CDC) propose that all Americans should have a minimum of 30 minutes a day of physical activity, preferably every day of the week [10]. These guidelines do not exempt people who have ID. An example of a regimen that implements this goal could participation in various types of physical activity such as walking, stationary cycling or climbing stairs for fifteen minutes in the morning and fifteen minutes in the evening. Other day-to-day physical activities that can be easily incorporated at residences, schools, or day programs include:

- Carrying groceries to and from the store
- Going hiking on the weekends in a local park
- Walking through malls during the winter months
- Taking the stairs at all times instead of the elevator
- Lifting light weights (or soup cans if weights are not available), while watching television
- Performing exercise video that are appropriate to individual capabilities

Previously Employed Physical Activity Programs

Over the past years individuals with ID have participated in the following exercise programs with positive results: stair climbing [59], walking, running, stretching, aerobic exercises [56], mattress and flexibility exercises [18], mile run, rowing machine, weight lifting, exercise bicycle [60,61], treadmill training [16] and walking [62,63]. The above mentioned activities present a variety of starting points for future activity programs for adolescents with ID.

CONCLUSIONS

Lack of physical activity has been repeatedly associated with higher health risks. It has been established that the low levels of physical activity in childhood and adolescence can result in obesity and a sedentary life style in adulthood. Despite such knowledge, findings from many countries suggest that increasing numbers of adults are adopting a sedentary life style [40]. In individuals with intellectual disability (ID) of all ages, we find lower levels of physical fitness and higher rates of obesity [43] and this population is thus relatively vulnerable for the later-life onset of serious health disorders.

In addition to the emotional turmoil typical of adolescence, those teens with ID have additional obstacles posed by their cognitive and physical limitations. The present review demonstrated that current literature on fitness in children and adolescents is lacking, and more evidence-based research is needed, to make solid inferences on the association between childhood and teen years sedentary lifestyles on adult-onset health disorders. In addition, more work is needed on the connection between education and implementation strategies to promote healthy lifestyles in younger people, and positive health gains in adults who have ID [3,25,55,64,65]. Despite the present paucity of knowledge, a positive connection is hypothesized to exist between physical exercise and promotion of physical, psychological, educational and cognitive status of adolescents with ID.

Due to the severe future health implications of inactive life style during childhood and adolescence, and higher rates of success that incorporate fitness activities with socialization, the authors suggest the organization of social physical exercise program models for people with ID, who constitute a population vulnerable to the health consequences of unhealthy lifestyles. This call replicates similar demands by authors around the globe [10,21,26,32,43,45,66,67].

Experts should emphasize the importance of a regular physical activity lifestyle during childhood and adolescence. To preserve health and other positive outcomes, a healthy lifestyle must continue during childhood, adolescence and throughout adulthood [68], for the health and well-being of individuals, who have ID and physical disability. Programs that correspond with an active life style should be based on clinical and research findings, centered within local community resources, and easily accessible to all individuals with disability.

REFERENCES

[1] Silvestri L. Benefits of physical activity. *Percept Motor Skills*. 1997;84(3 Pt 1):890.

[2] Leith LM. How physical education students see themselves. *Can. J. Sport Sci.* 1990;15(4):228.

[3] Twisk JW. Physical activity guidelines for children and adolescents: a critical review. *Sports Med.* 2001;31(8):617-27.

[4] Rose K. To keep the people in health. *J. Am. Coll. Health Ass.* 1973;22(2):80-3.

[5] Pate RR, Corbin CB, Simons-Morton BG, Ross JG. Physical education and its role in school health promotion. *J. School Health*. 1987;57(10):445-50.

[6] Fraser GE, Phillips RL, Harris R. Physical fitness and blood pressure in school children. *Circulation*. 1983;67(2):405-12.

[7] Sallis JF, Buono MJ, Roby JJ, Micale FG, Nelson JA. Seven-day recall and other physical activity self-reports in children and adolescents. *Med. Sci. Sports Exerc.* 1993;25(1):99-108.

[8] Brink PJ. The fattening of America. *Western J. Nurs. Res.* 1995;17(5):463-6.

[9] Myers L, Strikmiller PK, Webber LS, Berenson GS. Physical and sedentary activity in school children grades 5-8: the Bogalusa Heart Study. *Med. Sci. Sports Exercise*. 1996;28(7):852-9.

[10] Nat Center Chr Disease Prev Health Promotion, CDC. Guidelines for school and community programs to promote lifelong physical activity among young people. *J. School Health*. 1997;67(6):202-19.

[11] Tremblay A, Chiasson L. Physical fitness in young college men and women. *Can. J. Applied Physiol.* 2002;27(6):563-74.

[12] Huang TT, Harris KJ, Lee RE, Nazir N, Born W, Kaur H. Assessing overweight, obesity, diet, and physical activity in college students. *J. Am. Coll. Health.* 2003;52(2):83-6.

[13] Yoshizawa S, Ishizaki T, Honda H. Aerobic capacity of mentaly retarded boys and girls in junior high school. *J. Human Ergology.* (Tokyo) 1975;4:15-26.

[14] Pitteti KH, Jackson JA, Mays MS, Fernandez JE, Stubbs NB. Comparison of the physiological profiles of Down and non-Down syndrome mentally retarded individuals. Canada: *Proceed Ann. Conf. Human Factor Ass.* 1998:45-8.

[15] Pitteti KH, Jackson JA, Stubbs NB, Campbell KD, Battar SS. Fitness levels of adult special olympics participants. *Adapt. Physical Activity Quart.* 1989;6:254-70.

[16] Pitetti KH, Tan DM. Effects of a minimally supervised exercise program for mentally retarded adults. *Med. Sci. Sports Exercise.* 1991;23(5):594-601.

[17] King D, Mace E. Acquisition and maintenance of exercise skills under normalized conditions by adults with moderate and severe mental retardation. *Ment. Retard.* 1990;28(5):311-7.

[18] Bar-Or LJ, Skinner S, Bergsteinova V, Shearburn C, Royer D, Bell W, Haas J, Buskirk ER. Maximal aerobic capacity of 6-15 year old girls and boys with subnormal intelligence quotients. *Acta Paediatr. Scand.* 1971;Suppl 217:108-13.

[19] Fernhall B, Tymeson GT. Graded exercise testing of mentally retarded adults: A study of feasibility. *Arch. Physical Med. Rehab.* 1987;68:363-5.

[20] Fernhall B, Tymeson GT. (1988) Validation of a cardiovascular fitness field test for adults with mental retardation. *Adapt. Physical. Activity Quart.* 1988;5: 49-59.

[21] Chaiwanichsiri D, Sanguanrungsirikul S, Suwannakul W. Poor physical fitness of adolescents with mental retardation at Rajanukul School, Bangkok. *J. Med. Ass. Thailand.* 2000;83(11):1387-92.

[22] Fernhall, B., Pitetti, K.H., Rimmer, J.H., McCubbin, J.A., Rintala,P., Miller, A.L., Kittredge, J.,& Burkett, L.N. Cardiorespiratoy capacity of individuals with mental retardation including Down Syndrome. *Med. Sci. Sports Exerc.* 1996;28(3):366-71.

[23] Twisk JW, Kemper HC, van Mechelen W. The relationship between physical fitness and physical activity during adolescence and cardiovascular disease risk factors at adult age. The Amsterdam Growth and Health Longitudinal Study. *Int. J. Sports Med.* 2002;23(Suppl 1):S8-14.

[24] Van Mechelen W, Twisk JW, Kemper HC, Snel J, Post GB. Longitudinal relationships between lifestyle and cardiovascular and bone health status indicators in males and females between 13 and 27 years of age; a review of findings from the Amsterdam Growth and Health Longitudinal Study. *Public Health Nutrition.* 1999; 2(3A):419-27.

[25] Bar-Or O. Childhood and adolescent physical activity and fitness and adult risk profile. In: Bouchard C, Shephard RJ, Stephens T, eds. Physical activity, fitness, and health: *International proceedings and consensus statement.* Champaign, Ill, Human Kinetics, 1994:931-42.

[26] Merrick J, Kandel I. Physical activity, children and adolescents. *Int. J. Adolesc. Med. Health.* 2003;15(4):369-70.

[27] Janz K. Physical activity and bone development during childhood and adolescence. Implications for the prevention of osteoporosis. *Minerva Pediatr.* 2002;54(2):93-104.

[28] Khan K, McKay HA, Haapasalo H, Bennell KL, Forwood MR, Kannus P, Wark JD. (2000) Does childhood and adolescence provide a unique opportunity for exercise to strengthen the skeleton? *J. Sci. Med. Sport.* 2000;3(2):150-64.

[29] Norris R, Carroll D, Cochrane R. The effects of physical activity and exercise training on psychological stress and well-being in an adolescent population. *J. Psychosomatic Res.* 1992;36(1):55-65.

[30] Steptoe A, Butler N. Sports participation and emotional wellbeing in adolescents. *Lancet.* 1996;347(9018):1789-92.

[31] Kirkcaldy BD, Shephard RJ, Siefen RG. The relationship between physical activity and self-image and problem behaviour among adolescents. *Soc. Psychiatr. Psychiatric Epidemiol.* 2002;37(11):544-50.

[32] Rimmer JH. State of the scientific evidence in research on physical activity and intellectual disability/developmental disability. Philadelphia, PA: AAMR Conf, 2004.

[33] Dykens EM, Rosner BA, Butterbaugh G. Exercise and sports in children and adolescents with developmental disabilities. Positive physical and psychosocial effects. *Child Adolesc. Psychiatr. Clin. Neurol. Am.* 1998;7(4):757-71.

[34] Millar AL, Fernhall B, Burkett LN. Effects of aerobic training in adolescents with Down syndrome. *Med. Sci. Sports Exercise.* 1993;25(2):270-4.

[35] Weiss J, Diamond T, Demark J, Lovald, B. Involvement in Special Olympics and its relations to self-concept and actual competency in participants with developmental disabilities. *Res. Dev. Disabil.* 2003;24(4):281-305.

[36] Dykens EM, Cohen DJ. Effects of Special Olympics International on social competence in persons with mental retardation. *J. Am. Acad. Child Adolesc. Psychiatr.* 1996;35(2):223-9.

[37] MacMahon JR, Gross RT. Physical and psychological effects of aerobic exercise in boys with learning disabilities. *Dev. Behav. Pediatr.* 1987;8:274-7.

[38] Lotan M, Isakov E, Kessel S, Merrick J. Physical fitness and functional ability of children with intellectual disability: Effects of a short-term daily treadmill intervention. *Scientific World Journal.* 2004;(4):449-57.

[39] Lotan M, Isakov E, Merrick J. Improving functional skills and physical fitness in children with Rett syndrome. *J. Intellect. Disabil. Res.* 2004;48(8):730-5.

[40] Seefeldt V, Malina RM, Clark MA. Factors affecting levels of physical activity in adults. *Sports Med.* 2002;32(3):143-68.

[41] Sallis JF, Prochaska JJ, Taylor WC. A review of correlates of physical activity of children and adolescents. *Med. Sci. Sports Exerc.* 2000;32(5):963-75.

[42] Patel DR, Greydanus DE. The pediatric athlete with disabilities. *Pediatr. Clin. North Am.* 2002;49(4):803-27.

[43] Rimmer JH. The national center on physical activity and disability (NCPAD): providing web-based resources on physical activity for people with disabilities. Philadelphia, PA: AAMR Conf, 2004.

[44] Eberhard Y, Eterradossi J, Rapacchi B. Physical aptitudes to exertion in children with Down's syndrome. *J. Ment. Defic. Res.* 1989;33(Pt 2):167-74.

[45] Pitetti KH, Rimmer JH, Fernhall B. Physical fitness and adults with mental retardation. An overview of current research and future directions. *Sports Med.* 1993;16(1):23-56.

[46] Wind WM, Schwend RM, Larson J. Sports for the physically challenged child. *J. Am. Acad. Orthopedic Surgeons.* 2004;12(2):126-37.

[47] Patel DR, Pratt HD, Greydanus DE. Adolescent growth, development, and psychosocial aspects of sports participation: An overview. *Adolesc. Med.* 1998;9(3):425-40.
[48] Am Acad Fam Physicians, Am Acad Pediatr, Am Med Society Sports Med, Am. Orthopedic Society Sports Med, *Am. Osteopathic Acad. Sports Med.* (1997) Pre-participation physical evaluation, 2nd ed. Minneapolis, MN: McGraw-Hill Healthcare, 1997.
[49] Am Acad Pediatrics, Committee Sports Med Fitness. Medical conditions affecting sports participation. *Pediatrics.* 2001;107(5):1205-9.
[50] Pitetti KH, Boneh S. Cardiovascular fitness as related to leg strength in adults with mental retardation. *Med. Sci. Sports Exerc.* 1995;27(3):423-8.
[51] Aufsesser PM. Effects of repeated testing on the reliability of fitness scores of institutionalized mentally retarded individuals. *Am. J. Ment. Defic.* 1979;84(3):313-5.
[52] Graham A, Reid G. Physical fitness of adults with an intellectual disability: a 13-year follow-up study. *Res. Quart. Exerc. Sport.* 2000;71(2):152-61.
[53] Fernhall B, Pitetti KH, Vukovich MD, Stubbs N, Hensen T, Winnick JP, Short FX. Validation of cardiovascular fitness field tests in children with mental retardation. *Am. J. Ment. Retard.* 1998;102(6):602-12.
[54] Amisola RV, Jacobson MS. Physical activity, exercise, and sedentary activity: relationship to the causes and treatment of obesity. *Adolesc. Med.* 2003;14(1): 23-35.
[55] Rowland TW. Exercise and Children's Health. Champaign, IL: Human Kinetics, 1990.
[56] Halle JW, Gabler-Halle D, Chung YB. Effects of a peer mediated aerobic conditioning program on fitness levels of youth with mental retardation: two systematic replication. *Ment. Retard.* 1999;37(6):435-48.
[57] Aarts H, Paulussen T, Schaalma H. Physical exercise habit: on the conceptualization and formation of habitual health behaviors. *Health Educ. Res.* 1997;12(3):363-74.
[58] Muñoz KA, Krebs-Smith SM, Ballard-Barbash R, Cleveland LE. Food intakes of US children and adolescents compared with recommendations. *Pediatrics.* 1997;100(3):323-9.
[59] French R, Silliman LM, Ben-Ezra V, Landrien-Seiter M. Influence of selected reinforces on the cardiorespiratory exercise behavior of profoundly mentally retarded youth. *Percept. Motor Skills.* 1992;74:584-6.
[60] Tomporowski PD, Ellis NR. Effects of exercise on the physical fitness, intelligence, and adaptive behavior of institutionalized mentally retarded adults. *Applied Res. Ment. Retard.* 1984;5:329-37.
[61] Tomporowski PD, Ellis NR. The effects of exercise on the health, intelligence, and adaptive behavior of institutionalized severely and profoundly mentally retarded adults: A systematic replication. *Applied Res. Ment. Retard.* 1985;6:465-73.
[62] Bauer D. Aerobic fitness for the severely and profoundly mentally retarded. *Practical Pointers.* 1981;5(4):1-41.
[63] Bauer D. Aerobic fitness for the moderately retarded. *Practical Pointers.* 1981;5(5):1-33.
[64] Bar-Or O. Pediatric sports medicine for the practitioner: *From physiologic principles to clinical applications.* New York, NY: Springer, 1983.
[65] Malina RM. Physical activity and fitness: pathways from childhood to adulthood. *Am. J. Human Biol.* 2001;13(2):162-72.

[66] Yoshinaga M, Shimago A, Koriyama C, Nomura Y, Miyate K, Hashiguchi J, Arima K. Rapid increase in the prevalence of obesity in elementary school children. *Int. J. Obesity Rel. Metabol. Disord.* 2004;28(4):494-9.

[67] Huang TT, Harris KJ, Lee RE, Nazir N, Born W, Kaur H. Assessing overweight, obesity, diet, and physical activity in college students. *J. Am. Coll. Health.* 2003;52(2):83-6.

[68] Malina RM. Tracking of physical activity and physical fitness across the lifespan. *Res. Questions Exerc. Sport.* 1996;67(3 Suppl):S48-57.

Part XVII. Dental Aspects

In: Adolescence and Chronic Illness
Editors: H. Omar et al.

ISBN: 978-1-60876-628-4
© 2010 Nova Science Publishers, Inc.

Chapter 31

DENTAL CARE NEEDS

Joseph D'Ambrosio[*]
Michigan State University College of Human Medicine,
Kalamazoo Center for Medical Studies, Kalamazoo,
Michigan, United States of America.

ABSTRACT

Special needs patients of all ages are among the dental underserved population in the United States. Within this group of special needs individuals, the subgroup of pediatric and adolescent patients find access to dental care most difficult. The factors responsible for this lack of dental care are multiple but relate to three general issues. The first of these issues is the low rate of reimbursement provided by public assistance programs that pay for dental services in low income recipients. This factor has significant impact on the willingness-if not the ability-of dentists to provide services for which they may be losing money. The second factor is the lack of training and experience in the care of special needs patients during undergraduate dental education. Most general dentists do not feel that they have received adequate training to care for such special needs patients comfortably and safely. Finally, the large debt service incurred by most dental school graduates makes "public service" dentistry impossible.

INTRODUCTION

A decade ago, the United States (US) Census Bureau reported that ~20% of the American population experienced some degree of disability, and that 12% of the population were indeed severely disabled [1]. For many reasons, the disabled and special needs population has had, and continues to experience, difficulty in accessing dental care. The issues are numerous but

---

[*] ***Correspondence:*** Joseph D'Ambrosio, MD, DMD, Assistant Professor, Internal Medicine and Pediatrics & Human Development, Michigan State University College of Human Medicine, Program Director, Combined Medicine-Pediatrics Program, Michigan State University/Kalamazoo Center for Medical Studies, 1000 Oakland Drive, Kalamazoo, MI 49008-1284 United States. Tel: 269-337-6350; Fax: 269-337-6374; E-mail: Dambrosio@kcms.msu.edu

have been reasonably well defined and discussed over the last several decades. In addition to the physical challenges of actually getting the disabled into a dental office, the ever-present question remains of who will pay for these services and will the payment actually cover the cost of delivering care.

Finally, there is the issue of finding a dentist who is properly trained and capable of dealing with the multiple, complex needs of the patient at hand. This issue has received great attention in recent years, but questions about whether dental schools have made appropriate changes in undergraduate education remain unanswered. Finally, there is the issue of the cost of dental education, which is undoubtedly having a significant impact on the willingness and ability of the general dentist to provide care to the special needs population.

PROBLEMS IN PROVIDING DENTAL CARE

Social change in America has certainly contributed in some manner to the problem of dental care delivery to the physically and mentally handicapped of all ages. In the 30 years before 1997, the number of disabled adults living in institutions decreased by 75% [2]. Although the arguments for a more normalized existence are quite moving, one negative result has been the loss of central access to dental care that was at one time provided by resident dental providers in the larger institutions. It must be remembered that the provision of dental services is quite costly and exhibits more parallels to surgical care than to primary medical care. Special needs patients frequently need sedation and/or general anesthesia to receive safe, quality dental services. In the surgical setting, the "overhead" is paid for by the hospital or outpatient surgery center and is not at all the concern of the individual provider. In the dental office, this overhead and the issue of appropriate reimbursement is the immediate and urgent concern of the dental provider.

By the very nature of their disability, special needs patients require frequent, complicated, and often difficult to perform dental service. The normal development of the teeth and supporting structures—in particular the mandible—is influenced by forces applied from the tongue and perioral musculature. These forces are delivered in a normal, healthy individual during speech, swallowing, and mastication; such activities frequently are lacking in the severely or even moderately handicapped individual. In addition, many genetic syndromes associated with mental and physical handicap are also associated with significant deformity of the orofacial structures, producing crowding and malocclusion. In addition, many of these patients have a lack of manual dexterity, which makes routine oral hygiene difficult or impossible. Such individuals are thus dependent on caretakers who may or may not have the time and or the training to provide adequate preventive care.

As long as Medicaid reimbursements for dental care remain low, it will be impossible in any way to insure enough providers to care for the special needs population. The situation is further complicated in the adolescent population because as such individuals move from childhood to adulthood, they frequently lose the insurance benefits that are granted selectively to the pediatric age group. Certain disabled or chronically youths may be covered under the Medicare program, but this program specifically excludes payments for dental treatment with but a few uncommon exceptions. The oral cavity seems somehow and strangely not to be a part of the human body in much the same way that mental illness has been dismissed and demeaned by insurers for decades.

In 2000 a report was produced by the Institute of Medicine at the request of Congress to evaluate the possibility of extending Medicare coverage to include "medically necessary dental services" [3]. This report concluded that the scientific evidence was sufficient to recommend payment for a few isolated dental treatments that could have an impact on underlying medical conditions. In several other instances, the report concluded that the evidence was insufficient to support or deny a recommendation for the coverage of dental services. Unfortunately this report did not make any attempt to evaluate improvements in the quality of life associated with the preservation of a healthy, natural dentition. Neither did it adequately evaluate the long-term costs of dental extractions and tooth replacement resulting from failure to treat caries and periodontal disease.

The importance of adequate financial reimbursement for dental services to special needs individuals cannot be ignored; nevertheless, most experts now recognize that the lack of training of the general dentist to care for such individuals is the main barrier to care. Several states—most notably Pennsylvania—over the last decade, have significantly increased the reimbursements for dental services to children and adolescents, with little impact on the access to care for such individuals. The disparity between oral health status and access to dental care of special needs patients and their healthy counterparts was outlined in the US Surgeon General's report on oral health released in 2000 [4]. Subsequently, the Commission on Dental Accreditation in 2004 adopted new standards for both dental and dental hygiene education programs with the intent to ensure that dental providers are more prepared and ready to care for special needs patients. It is yet too early to know whether such changes have been made or will make an impact on the availability of care in a positive manner.

Data published in 2005 from a survey at the University of Michigan showed that few general dentists have received adequate training in or feel comfortable with providing care to special needs children and adults [5]. Those respondents who reported a positive feeling about their undergraduate dental training and experience in regard to the treatment of special needs children also reported treating significantly more such patients in private practice than did those respondents who reported that undergraduate dental education did not prepare them well for such individuals. It is essential that dental school administrators and faculty initiate such changes as mandated and monitor the results to ensure their effectiveness.

ROLE OF THE PHYSICIAN

The role of the physician in dental care has never been clearly defined. As a trained dentist and physician, I am convinced that pediatricians and adult medicine colleagues as well, must take an increasingly active role in providing at least preventive services to both healthy and special needs patients. Although this article focuses on the special needs adolescent, dental care for low income children and adults is universally difficult to obtain in the US. In our pediatric residency program in Kalamazoo, Michigan, we have begun to provide some basic training in dental examination and basic preventive care to our residents. We must particularly focus on training parents and caretakers to provide daily effective dental hygiene and must educate families on the need for topical and systemic fluoride and noncariogenic diets. Such efforts in the medical office should reduce caries and dental disease and allow the dental provider more time to deal with those unfortunate cases that have failed prevention measures. Clearly when it comes to actually treating established dental disease, a trained dental provider will be required. The undergraduate dental program must prepare the general dentist to provide the majority of such services, thus leaving the dental specialists to deal with the more severe cases, in particular those requiring surgical services with general anesthesia.

Conclusions

Adolescents with special needs make up a largely underserved population with regard to dental care. Although public assistance programs funded through State and Federal governments generally cover the pediatric and adolescent population, the low reimburse-ment rates of these programs result in correspondingly low participation rates by providers. The Medicare program, which covers certain disabled adolescents, specifically excludes coverage for virtually all dental services. Finally, the lack of training in dental school in the care and management of the special needs patient has produced a shortage of general dentists who feel capable of dealing with the needs of this population.

References

[1] McNeil J. Americans with disabilities: 1997. Current population reports, series P70-73. Washington, DC: US Dept Commerce, Bureau Census, 2001. www.census.gov/prod/2001pubs/p70-73.pdf

[2] Anderson LL, Lakin KC, Mangan TW, Prouty RW. State institutions: Thirty years of depopu-lation and closure. *Ment. Retard.* 1998;36(6):431-43.

[3] Patton LL, White BA, Field MJ. Extending Medicare coverage to medically necessary dental care. *JADA.* 2001;132:1294-9.

[4] Oral health in America: A report of the Surgeon General. Rockville, MD: *U.S. Dept. Health Hum. Serv.* 2000.

[5] Dao LP, Zwetchkenbaum S, Ingelhart MR. General dentists and special needs patients: Does dental education matter? *J. Dent. Educ.* 2005;69: 1107-15.

Part XVIII. Transition

In: Adolescence and Chronic Illness
Editors: H. Omar et al.

ISBN: 978-1-60876-628-4
© 2010 Nova Science Publishers, Inc.

Chapter 32

ADOLESCENTS WITH SICKLE CELL DISEASE AND TRANSITION TO ADULT CARE

Joseph Telfair[*], *John E. Ehiri*, *Penny S. Loosier* and *Monica L. Baskin*

Department of Maternal and Child Health, School of Public Health, University of Alabama at Birmingham, Behavioral Science Core Center for AIDS Research and Department of Health Behavior, University of Alabama at Birmingham, United States.

ABSTRACT

Cross-sectional data were collected by means of structured questionnaire interviews, using standard instruments. A volunteer sample of 172 adolescents with SCD (sickle cell disease) aged 14 years and older still in pediatric care within community-based and medical center SCD programs across the United States was recruited. Statistically significant results indicated the top concerns of adolescents were: lack of information relating to their transition to adult care; fear of leaving the healthcare provider with whom they were already familiar; fear that adult care providers might not understand their needs; belief that an SCD transition program was needed and that it should focus on provider support; information provision about adult care programs; ways to meet adult care providers; and ways to help healthcare providers understand their needs. We conclude that many adolescents with SCD have concerns and fears about their transition to adult care. Based on findings from this study, it is recommended that transition programs address structural and interpersonal issues of adolescents and providers if they are to be successful. Strategies by which this can be achieved are recommended, including the need to encourage, support and provide assistance for peer education, outreach programs and peer-led instructions, since these hold great promise as approaches that are adolescent-centered and adolescent-delivered.

---

[*] *Correspondence:* Professor Joseph Telfair, DrPH, MSW, MPH, Director, Division of Public Health Genetics and Evaluation, Department of Public Health Education, School of Health and Human Performance, University of North Carolina at Greensboro, 437 HHP Building, 1408 Walker Avenue, POBox 26170, Greensboro, NC 27402-6170 United States. Tel: (336) 334 – 4777; Fax: (336) 334 – 3238; E-mail: j_telfai@uncg.edu

INTRODUCTION

Sickle cell disease (SCD) refers to a group of disorders in which 'sickling' of the red blood cells due to loss of oxygen gives the cell a thin, elongated crescent-like shape, resulting in chronic anemia and obstruction of the smaller vessels of the circulatory system [1]. In the United States, there are about 75,000 individuals with SCD, mostly (but not exclusively) African-Americans [2]. Unexpected, intermittent, and at times life-threatening complications characterize the course of SCD (1). As recently as twenty-five years ago, it was characterized as a disease of childhood, with relatively few patients reaching adult life [3,4]. However, due to advancements in and the wider availability of healthcare, the life of an individual with SCD can now extend into the fourth and fifth decades and longer [4,5-10]. However, survival into adolescence and adulthood is associated with a number of health problems, including predisposition to infections, chronic lung disease, cardiac failure, stroke, vaso-occlusive crises, life-threatening anemia, delayed growth, high morbidity associated with pregnancy and psychosocial issues such as self-care, coping, readiness for independence and the process of transitioning from adolescent to adult centered care [11,12]

Because an increasing number of adolescents with SCD are surviving into adulthood and ready for transfer from pediatric to adult care, transition has become a critical issue [11]. Given the chronicity of SCD, this transition encompasses both medical and life transition, and is defined as the process involved in the movement of adolescents from a focus on pediatric life skill issues to adult life skill issues, including transfer from pediatric or child-centered care to adult health care services [11]. Transition readiness is defined as the specific decisions made and actions taken in building the capacity of the adolescent and those in his/her primary medical microsystems (parental caretakers/family and providers) to prepare for, begin, continue, and finish the process of transition [11].

Transition from pediatric to adult health care is identified as "the most difficult and potentially traumatic passage faced by adolescents with SCD" [13,14] and many adolescents and young adults with chronic conditions [15], such as diabetes [16], cystic fibrosis [17], spina bifida [18], congenital heart disease [19], and chronic arthritis [20], lack the self-advocacy, independent living and vocational skills, and sense of self-efficacy that would allow them to smoothly transition into adult life [15].

Thus, transition to adult care is a challenge for adolescents with SCD, as well as those with other chronic conditions. Improved survival of young people with chronic diseases is associated with participation in appropriate child to adult care transition programs, though there is little evidence to suggest that this is happening at a rate commensurate with clinical requirements [21]. A study by Crosnier and Tubiana-Rufi [16] evaluating the conditions in which diabetic adolescents were transferred from pediatric to adult care revealed a number of challenges, including problems of information exchange: a quarter of the diabetologists were visiting for the first time without any information on the adolescent; only half of the referring pediatricians received feedback information from the internist after the first visit; medical relationships were poor; the adolescents expressed the view that their expectations were not being met; and 80% of the pediatricians and diabetologists felt that the transfer of diabetic adolescents to adult care deserved better planning in order to assure coherence in medical follow-up and minimize the psychological effects of transition.

There is evidence that interventions aimed at addressing the life skill needs of late adolescents with chronic conditions are effective in decreasing many of the difficulties associated with transitioning into adult life and medical systems [22-24]. Despite this, the provision of these and other long-term comprehensive care services has been and remains limited [25]. As a result, late adolescents and young adults do not receive much medical care on a regular basis [26,27]. A national survey of Directors of Maternal and Child Health (MCH) and other state health programs from fifty US States by Blum and Okinow [28], found that the directors recognized that late adolescents are at risk for many psychosocial and long-term life skill difficulties. Nonetheless, they expressed the view that this population group "was not a priority" for services, because in most children's health initiatives and programs, priority is given to those under five years of age. Where crucial services for adolescents do exist, they are relatively few and often fragmented. The quality and availability of comprehensive health, social, vocational, and educational services can have a powerful impact on the ability of adolescents with chronic conditions to master many of the challenges they face [29-31].

The study reported here is an expansion of an earlier pilot study involving a small sample of adolescents from one local SCD center [11]. Based on our experience it was realized that prior to launching a more rigorous longitudinal study, we needed to determine, through the use of a much larger sample, whether or not the findings from the pilot were similar or different from the views of adolescent across centers in the United States.

The objective of the current chapter was to present the 'voice' of the adolescent with SCD as part of the discussion of transition issues by answering the following research questions: 1) Do adolescents with SCD believe a program for transition into adult care should exist?; 2) What are the expressed concerns of adolescents with SCD about transition into adult care?; 3) What are the expectations of adolescents with SCD with regard to the priorities of a transition program? While much has been learned in the last ten years regarding the process and issues of transition for adolescents with special needs, it is rare for their voices to be heard as part of the development and implementation of research on them. In addition, little is known about these issues of transition to adult care in regard to adolescents with SCD.

OUR STUDY

This was a cross-sectional survey of a volunteer national sample of adolescents with sickle cell disease, aged 14 years and over, who were still receiving care in pediatric community-based and medical center sickle cell disease programs. Respondents came from community-based and medical center sickle cell programs from 18 centers in the US. Each site collected data for an average of six months. This allowed for a larger sample to be gathered and for each site to exhaust their eligible participant base. Given the low prevalence of SCD, it was rare for a center to have more than 40 adolescents, ho met the inclusion criteria on its active patient list. The total number of adolescents in the centers, who met the inclusion criteria was 264. All 264 adolescents were invited to participate in the study. One hundred and seventy-two of these consented, giving a response rate of 65%. At the time of data collection for the various sites, none had an active transition program.

Development of the study instrument, the adolescent sickle cell transfer questionnaire (SCTQ), was based on: (i) observational experiences of clinicians serving pediatric and adult persons with SCD; (ii) interviews with multidisciplinary providers serving adolescents and young adults with SCD and other chronic conditions; (iii) review of the literature regarding transition issues faced by this population group; (iv) open-ended responses from adolescents with SCD on potential items and the planned data collection methodology; and (v) results of a pilot study of adolescents, young adults and parental caretakers [11].

The first author and a team of multidisciplinary providers wrote the first draft. Three Delphi32 (expert) review rounds were completed to identify and clarify pertinent questions, verify the purpose of the questionnaire, and discuss appropriate responses. The results of the Delphi review were used to generate a checklist of items for the questionnaire. Provision was made for open-ended items to provide participants with opportunities for elaboration if necessary. After the third revision, the final draft of the questionnaire was developed and piloted with 36 adolescents. Results of this pilot are reported elsewhere [11]. The Delphi and pilot processes allowed for the validation of the final version of the SCTQ. The final version of the SCTQ, consisting of the domains listed below, was administered to the adolescents participating in the current study. Only sections applicable to this study will be discussed.

Demography

This section covered the basic sociodemographic characteristics of the respondents, including hemoglobinopathy status, race, gender, marital status, employment, health insurance status, geographic location, school education, household size, and type of care program received.

Concerns About Transition

This section queried factors that influence and may predict successful transition to adult care for adolescents with SCD. Respondents were asked if they had any concerns about moving from a child or adolescent medical care program to an adult care program, and if so, were directed to a checklist of sixteen potential concerns. The responses were divided into two main categories: (i) items related to independent management of health care included assessment of assumption of responsibility by the young adult and mature/adult treatment by others, and (ii) items related to transfer from pediatric to adult medical care. Each main category was further divided into subsections included assessment of the health care provider's perception/treatment of the young adult patient, transition-related anxieties, and practical considerations.. An open-ended "Other" response was included to allow addition of any potential concerns not listed. Respondents chose as many response options as they felt were applicable.

Feelings About Moving to an Adult Care Program

This section was designed to elicit information about the adolescent's feelings regarding transfer from pediatric to adult care. Thirteen response options were used to explore four constructs pertaining to the adolescent's feelings: positive/optimistic, negative/pessimistic, anxious/fearful, and neutral. An open-ended "Other" response was included to allow addition of any potential feelings not listed. Respondents chose as many options as they felt were applicable.

Reasons for a Transition Program

This section was designed to query whether or not respondents felt a program that helps people with sickle cell disease go from a children and adolescent treatment program to an adult program was needed. The checklist of nine responses were divided into two sections: (i) reasons why a transition program is needed and, (ii) reasons why a transition program is not needed. An open-ended "Other" response option was included, which allowed for inclusion of options not provided. Respondents chose as many options as they felt were applicable.

Adolescent's Perceptions About Content of Transition

This section was designed to elicit the adolescent's perception of which kinds of things a transition program should offer. The 11 response options were divided into two main sections: (i) information/education regarding independent management of care and (ii) information/education to facilitate transition to adult medical care. An open-ended "Other" response option was added to capture features transition programs should offer which were not represented in the list. Respondents chose as many options as they felt were applicable.

Human subjects approval was obtained from the Institutional Review Boards at the relevant agencies before commencement of the study. Signed consent was sought from the parent(s) or legal guardian(s) and the assent of the eligible adolescent was obtained. Parents/guardians and adolescents were informed by mail about the purpose and procedures of the study. They were told participation in the project was completely voluntary and they could refuse to participate, discontinue participation at any point, or refuse to answer questions they did not feel comfortable answering. Participants were reassured that if they chose not to participate in the study, they would not lose any benefits from their healthcare providers. Thus, participation in the study was voluntary and no incentive was provided to respondents. A stamped postcard was included for parents and adolescents to sign and return if they did not want to participate in the study. The adolescent sickle cell transfer questionnaire (SCTQ) was mailed to the 264 eligible adolescents from all participating centers. After two reminders, one hundred and seventy-two adolescents returned their questionnaire, giving a response rate of 65%.

Data were analyzed using the Statistical Package for the Social Sciences (SPSS), Version 11.0 [33]. Consistent with standard practice, univariate statistics were used to assess patterns of responses to the questionnaire items in order to facilitate identification of concerns and opinions that were most important to the adolescents, while chi-square tests were used to assess differences between categories. Ninety-five percent confidence intervals were calculated for the proportions using the Confidence Interval Analysis (CIA) for proportions and their differences (single sample) version 1.0 [34]. P-values of less than 0.05 were considered significant.

WHAT DID WE FIND?

Characteristics of Respondents

For a summary of the sociodemographic characteristics of the respondents, see table 1. As indicated, a majority were single, African-American women, with a mean age of 17 years (SD =2.45). Most were high school students, and had the sickle-cell genotype SS. Many (n=118; 69%) expressed concern regarding their transition from pediatric to adult care programs. Less than a third (n=54; 31%) had no transition-related concerns (p=0.001; Chi-square=27.38). The respondents were asked to indicate how they paid for their healthcare. As table 1 indicates, over half paid for some of their healthcare through Medicaid (n=94; 55%), while a relatively sizeable proportion (n=20; 14%) paid for health care through school or employment-related health insurance. Although household income was not specifically measured, these findings suggest that a majority of the respondents have a family income at or below poverty, which qualifies them for this type of assistance. A majority (94%) of those who paid for their healthcare through health insurance reported that their insurance caters for care at a SCD clinic.

Table 1. Sociodemographic characteristics of respondents

Parameters	N = 172	
Gender	No (%)	Mean (SD)
Female	109 (63)	
Male	63 (37)	
Race or ethnic background		
African-American	168 (98)	
Other	2 (2)	
Marital status		
Single	170 (99)	
Married	2 (1)	
Age of respondent		
14-17	115 (67)	
18-20	45 (26)	
21-23	9 (5)	
24+	3 (2)	
		16 ± 2.45
Genotype		
SS	104 (61)	
SC	33 (19)	
S-B Thal.	13 (8)	
Unknown	21 (12)	
Highest school grade completed		
Middle school (6-8th grade)	7 (4)	
High school (9-12th grade)	152 (88)	

Table 1. (Continued)

Parameters	N = 172	
1-4 year college+	13 (8)	
Employment		
Full-time students	135 (78)	
Disabled	5 (3)	
Employed	14 (8)	
Unemployed	12 (7)	
Student & Employed	6 (4)	
Average household size		
1-3	71 (41)	
4-6	86 (50)	
7-9	13 (8)	
10+	2 (1)	
		3 ± 1.8
Method of financing healthcare		
Self	7 (4)	
Health Insurance (through employment or school)	20 (12)	
Private Health Insurance	12 (7)	
HMO/PPO	1 (1)	
CHAMPUS	2 (1)	
Medicaid	94 (55)	
SSI	11 (6)	
SCD Program	11 (6)	
Other	14 (8)	
Expressed transition concerns		
Yes	118 (69)	
No	54 (31)	

Concerns About Transition

As shown in table 2, the top five concerns expressed by the adolescents were (i) lack of information relating to their transition to adult care (n=63; 53%), (ii) fear of leaving the healthcare provider with whom they were already familiar (n=56; 47%), (iii) fear that adult care providers might not understand their needs (n=53; 45%), (iv) fear of being treated as an adult (n=50; 42%), and (v) concern about payment for cost of care (n=43; 36%). Based on other statistical analyses, no differences were found regarding concerns about transition to adult care when gender, age, education and hemoglobin types were examined.

Table 2. Respondent's concerns about their transition to adult care

Respondents' concerns	N=118 No. (%)
Did not have adequate information	63 (53)
Do not want to leave the health care provider that I already know	56 (47)
Adult health care providers might not know me and my circumstance	53 (45)
Worried about being treated as an adult	50 (42)
Wondered if I would know how to ask for information	43 (36)
Worried about how to pay for my medical care	43 (36)
Afraid new staff would not believe me when I am in pain	43 (36)

Table 2. (Continued).

Respondents' concerns	N=118 No. (%)
Concerned about being seen as 'drug seeking' when in crisis	42 (35)
Wondered if I would be able to make decisions on my own	40 (34)
Wondered if health care people would talk to me, not my parents	39 (33)
Worried about my ability to discuss my health with others	39 (33)
Scared about getting to know new care providers	39 (36)
Would have to take responsibility of self	36 (31)
Concerned about transportation to and from care program	28 (24)
Worried if parents will let me talk to care providers myself	14 (12)
Other Concerns	11 (9)

Note: Totals exceed 118 because some respondents had multiple concerns.

Feelings About Moving to an Adult Care Program

The adolescents were asked to state what their feelings would be if they were asked to move to an adult care program. As seen in table 3, although some felt it was the right time to move on, most had reservations. These range from those who felt unsure (n=77; 45%); nervous (n=75; 44%), afraid (n=44; 26%), or angry (n=25; 15%), to those who felt they had no control over the decision (n=48; 28%).

Table 3. Feelings about transitioning to an adult treatment program

Respondents' feelings about transition to adult care		N=172 No. (%)		
	Yes	No	95% CI	P-value
Right time to move on	49 (28)	123 (72)	.217-.352	0.001
Unsure	77 (45)	95 (55)	.373-.522	0.16
Worried	57 (33)	115 (67)	.261-.402	0.001
Have no feelings one way or the other	31 (18)	141 (82)	.123-.238	0.001
Nervous	75 (44)	97 (56)	.362-.510	0.12
Afraid	44 (26)	128 (74)	.191-.321	0.001
Anxious	33 (19)	139 (81)	.133-.251	0.001
Angry	25 (15)	147 (85)	.0927-.198	0.001
Deserted/ Abandoned	15 (9)	157 (91)	.0496-.140	0.001
I had no control over the decision	48 (28)	124 (72)	.212-.346	0.001
Is a program to prepare adolescents for transition needed?	159 (92)	13 (8)	.874-.959	0.001

Reasons for a Transition Program

When asked if they thought a program to help young people with SCD transition from pediatric to adult care was needed, a majority (n=159; 92%) answered in the affirmative. Only a few (n=13; 8%) did not think that such a program was important (p=0.001; c2= 137.78). Those admitting that a transition program was needed were asked to indicate what the benefits of such a program might be (see table 4). The four most common reasons cited were that such a program would make transition easier since: (i) it would enable them to know what to expect; (ii) it would provide them with support in meeting care needs; (iii) it would help them become acquainted with being treated as adults, and (iv) it would give them the chance to meet with other adult SDC patients.

Table 4. Reasons for a transition program for adolescents with SCD

Reason for advocating a transition program		N=159 No. (%)		
	Yes	No	95% CI	P-value
Would make transition easier	99 (62)	60 (38)	.547-.698	0.002
Would know what to expect	110 (69)	49 (31)	.620-.764	0.001
Would provide more support in meeting care needs	94 (59)	65 (41)	.515-.668	0.02
Would help become used to being treated as adults	92 (58)	67 (42)	.502-.655	0.03
To give them a chance to meet other SCD adults	92 (58)	67 (42)	.502-.655	0.03
To give them more control health decisions/ life	88 (55)	71 (45)	.476-.631	0.2
It would help focus attention to SCD	15 (9)	144 (91)	.0538-.151	0.001

Adolescent's Perceptions About Content of Transition

All respondents were asked to indicate specific forms of help they believe a transition program could offer. As shown in table 5, most (n=131; 70%) were of the opinion that an effective transition program should provide information about adult programs, as compared to few (n=51; 30%), who did not think that information was an issue (p=0.001; c2= 30.42). Well over half (n=100; 58%) would like to see a transition program that creates a forum for the adolescents to meet adult care, while others believe that the content of a transition program should include helping providers understand new patients' needs (n=103; 60%). Finding ways to help parents "let the adolescents grow up" was considered important by 45% (n=78) of the adolescents, while 55% (n=94) did not consider this to be important.

The one hundred and seventy-two adolescents who responded to this survey (out of a sample of 264) represented a response rate of 65%. In an effort to understand whether those who did not respond to the survey were different from those who did respond, we followed up a random sample of fifteen non-responding adolescents through direct interviews at five randomly selected study sites. Results of this follow-up did not highlight any marked difference between the non-respondents and the study respondents in terms of age, gender, education, genotype, or transitional concerns. Thus, there is no reason to believe that non-respondents were different from the study participants and the results can thus be taken with confidence.

Table 5. Adolescents perceptions about content of transition program

Parameters	Yes	N=172 No. (%) No	95% CI	P-value
Information about adult care programs	121 (70)	51 (30)	.635-.772	0.001
Ways to help me care for my own health needs	112 (65)	60 (35)	.580-.722	0.01
Ways to help me solve health care problems	106 (63)	66 (37)	.544-.689	0.004
Ways to help me be on my own	105 (61)	67 (39)	.538-.683	0.002
Ways to meet adult health care providers	100 (58)	72 (42)	.508-.655	0.03
Ways to help educate others about my condition	104 (60)	68 (40)	.532-.678	0.01
To help providers understand new patients needs	103 (60)	69 (40)	.526-.672	0.01
Ways to help me learn more about my condition	99 (58)	73 (42)	.502-.649	0.03
Provide someone to talk to when I need it	90 (52)	82 (48)	.449-.598	0.6
How to deal with other health provider/ situations	96 (56)	76 (44)	.484-.632	0.2
Ways to help parents let adolescents grow up	78 (45)	94 (55)	.379-.528	0.3

DISCUSSION

Many adolescents with SCD transitioning from pediatric to adult care have a number of concerns that merit the attention of those responsible for planning their health care provision (see table 2). Of the 172 who responded, 118 (69%) expressed one or more concerns about their transition. The most common concerns were lack of information about transition to adult care, fear of leaving the healthcare provider with whom they were already familiar, fear that adult care providers might not understand their needs, fear of being treated as adults, and concern about payment for cost of care. Although specific to adolescents with SCD, these primary findings are consistent with recent work by others [57-60], who describe similar concerns among other chronic conditions. Repeated concerns include: inadequate patient education, patients' difficulty terminating established and trusting relationships with pediatric teams, concerns about forming new relationships with adult care team members, questions about the competence of adult care providers, anxiety about becoming the responsible person for his/her care, and distress over payment for health care services [57-60]. Given similar findings in this study, it is not surprising a majority (92%) of respondents believed a program that supports them in their transition to adult care is needed.

Our study addressed an important, but largely neglected component of SCD management among adolescents. While many studies have been conducted on SCD, very few have focused on transitional concerns of adolescents and young adults and the implications of such concerns for service delivery. The emergence of chronic conditions or disability like SCD as a problem for healthcare systems to address is becoming more obvious, and research indicates that adolescents with chronic conditions have opinions and expectations about their future health care and health management [11,36]. Since it is accepted that care for persons affected by SCD would improve, if their views were considered in service planning and delivery [35], the expressed concerns and feelings of adolescents transitioning from pediatric to adult care, particularly from their point of view, should be a subject of considerable importance to healthcare planners and providers. Insights gained from the work presented here can assis providers in structuring programs that are congruent with the beliefs and expectation of these adolescents, increasing the potential success of the programs.

It is germane to mention that there are currently no official policies regarding the management of transitional healthcare issues for adolescents with chronic conditions or disability. Many pediatric providers extend their care of young adults for a number of reasons and attempt to work with adult providers to begin the transition process. To facilitate coherence with regard to transition policy and practice, the American Academy of Pediatricians, working in collaboration with the American Academy of Family Physicians, the American College of Physicians and the American Society of Internal Medicine, recently produced a consensus statement on healthcare transitions for young people with special health care needs [56]. The consensus statement examines why planning for transition is important and puts forth a set of recommendations for the facilitation of transition that addresses both structural and intrapersonal issues relevant to working with adolescents and young adults with SCD. Other recommendations to ensure effective transition policy and practice can be found in a recent publication by Reiss and Gibson [57]. Rapid advancements in the treatment and care of persons affected by SCD have not been matched by development of effective programs focusing on the acquisition of the needed personal, interpersonal and social life skills, independent living, self-advocacy, medical self-management and system negotiation, educational, and vocational readiness for young people [52]. As a result, many adolescents with SCD and their primary caretakers have a difficult time transitioning into adult care [30,41,53,54]. Results of our study and anecdotal observations by those in the Multi Site Study of Transition of Adolescents and Young Adults with Sickle Cell Disease Collaborative Group suggest that adolescents recognize that their relationships with medical providers and with those in their social environment play a critical role in the realization of a successful transition process. The following recommendations are consistent with the implications of this study and are believed to be achievable by practitioners planning and implementing such a program for adolescents with SCD.

Transition planning is ideally constructed by a multidisciplinary team consisting of the pediatric and proposed adult physician, pediatric and adult nursing staff, a psychologist skilled in clinical and developmental psychology, a vocation specialist, an adult care social worker, the patient, and the patient's parent/guardian. Each of these individuals is needed to help assess the unique needs of the SCD transitioning young adult and develop a developmentally and culturally responsive program that builds upon the youth's skills, strengths, and resources. Based on current study findings and similar findings of others [57-60], it is recommended that specific elements of the transition plan include patient and provider education, orientation to adult care, psychosocial services, vocational training and support, and assistance with social services.

Patient and provider education. Appropriate and on-going education for patients and medical staff is essential to successful transition. Lack of adequate information about adult care was the top concern listed by respondents in this study. Others have noted that SCD youth often lack basic knowledge about their disease and treatment, including hemoglobin type and the fact that SCD is a hereditary disease [14]. Education should include information about the patient's condition (e.g., disease type, currently prescribed treatment regimen), current research findings, preventive health care strategies, and recognizing when medical intervention is needed. Formal structured education programs administered by health educators or providers can be developed [55] for provision in small groups or education can be provided by providers to individual patients during regularly scheduled medical appointments.

On-going training of medical personnel is also critical to facilitate smooth transition. Providers should participate in regular continuing education to alert them to new research findings related to SCD sequelae and treatment. This is particularly the case for medical staff who may have limited knowledge of SCD (e.g., emergency room staff). Another area of provider education includes training on how to successfully terminate or "let go" of pediatric patients who are ready for transition. Pediatric providers have acknowledged that they often are not adequately prepared to "say goodbye" to their patients and this may inadvertently prolong transition [57]. Adult providers, on the other hand, may need training on how to active engage shy and concerned adolescents with SCD in the development of new relationships.

ORIENTATION TO ADULT CARE

Many study respondents expressed an interest in meeting adult care staff in advance to transition. Ideally, this may start as early as six months to a year in advance and would include joint appointments with the pediatric and adult provider, meetings with adult psychosocial support staff (e.g., social worker, vocation specialist), and a tour of the facility and auxiliary units (e.g., blood bank, emergency room). Other basic information concerning policies (e.g., privacy, communication, payment for services), scheduling appointments, contacting adult care team members, etc., should be provided to the transitioning patient prior to his/her initial adult care appointment. A discussion with the patient and parent/guardian of how the adult-centered care system differs from the pediatric-centered care system may facilitate more realistic expectations of the transition [14]. Such discussions should begin early and include both pediatric and adult providers.

Psychosocial Services

Psychologists and social workers on the multidisciplinary transition team are well-suited to provide valuable feedback on the patient's psychological and emotional maturity and relay informed hypotheses on how the patient may be impacted by premature transition [55]. In addition, they can assist in the development of interventions to help transitioning adolescents with SCD achieve empowerment, enhance self-efficacy, and acquire life skills that will assist them in becoming self-sufficient and independent, and provide them with the capacity to manage the physical, psychological, and financial challenges of SCD.

Through individual, group, and/or family interventions, youth can be coached on how to participate in effective communication with providers, become more comfortable talking about their condition to peers and social support members, apply effective coping techniques, mobilize and utilize effective social and family support, and negotiate new responsibilities regarding assumption of control over their health care. Multidisciplinary providers must understand, support, and encourage the critical role independent decision-making by the adolescent with SCD plays in assuring the success of the transition process. Thus, the goal of transition would be to assist youth in becoming more autonomous and less dependent on providers and parents to manage their disease.

Vocational training and support. Prior to transitioning an adolescent with SCD, a post high-school employment and/or educational plan should be formulated [14]. Many adolescents and young adults with SCD are ill-prepared for post-secondary education or participation in vocational activities due to psychosocial maladjustment and/or excessive school absence due to frequent hospitalizations [62]. As such, a systematic assessment of the patient's academic and vocational functioning is helpful in developing a realistic plan for once he/she completes high school or a GED. Counseling on viable school/work options, skills training (e.g., resume writing, basic computer skills, job interview skills, etc.), and job referral services may increase the likelihood that the adolescent with SCD matriculates to an academic or vocational setting that will support his/her ability to function more independently and maintain good health.

Social Support

Transition planners must understand, encourage, and support the critical role played by families and significant others in the transition process. As such, efforts to utilize peer and family networks as well as community services in the planning, promotion and implementation of transition activities is paramount. A number of forums including support groups, advocacy organizations, and peer outreach and mentoring can serve to foster the positive impacts of social support on the health care of SCD patients.

During the orientation to adult care, patients and parents should be introduced to current adult care patients and caregivers and informed about local and regional support groups (if they exist). Ideally, family members would begin attending support group meetings prior to transition to gain insight about issues typical for adult patients and family members of adult patients. If no groups exist, it would behoove providers to encourage, support and provide assistance for the development of such programs. Groups for youth would promote the opportunity for peer support, mentoring, recognition that others are experiencing "their problems," and opportunities to practice newly acquired skills (e.g., assertiveness) and receive feedback on these skills [55]. Groups for parents may be beneficial to help them to process their changing role from caretaker to support person and assist them to relinquish the role of gatekeeper of information from the provider and allow youth to have direct communication without censorship [14]. Like teens, they would also be able to hear others with stories similar to theirs and benefit from peer support.

Advocacy and outreach efforts are also ways to enhance social support for transitioning youth and families. Patients and parents should be informed about existing local and national SCD advocacy groups and encouraged to become active in advocating for increased public awareness of SCD and monitoring of health care delivery to patients with SCD [14]. Similarly, adolescents with SCD might become involved in the training of peers in schools, in community health settings, and in other 'natural environments.' Peer outreach programs empower young people by placing them in leadership roles which build their self-esteem and advance self-efficacy enhancement and empowerment. Taking responsibility for others will go a long way in helping adolescents take responsibility for their selves.

Negotiation of Medical Systems

The shift from pediatric to adult care carries significant financial ramifications and should be considered when making a decision about when to transfer. Changes in health insurance coverage, such as denied coverage to individuals over a certain age, limitations of Title V Programs for Children with Special Health Care Needs, limitations of Medicaid eligibility, and age-limit policies of pediatric hospitals and clinics are a reality for transitioning adolescents with SCD [57]. Many youth will lack the health care coverage necessary to ensure the receipt of adult health care comparable to that received when they were enrolled in pediatric care [57]. Many adult patients with SCD must rely exclusively on Medicaid for medical coverage and often utilize emergency departments as the primary source of care [61]. Social work staff play an essential role in assessing the financial resources and limitations of transitioning patients. They can also provide education and instruction on securing all services to which the individual is entitled. Conclusion

CONCLUSIONS

Although health care providers and policy planners' interest in and concern about adolescents and young adults with chronic conditions has increased significantly in the last decade [55], empirical studies of the most rudimentary issues of transition, especially from the point of view of the adolescent, remain rare. Further research is needed to gain more understanding of transition needs of young adults in order to facilitate development of policies and programs that are relevant and effective in meeting their transition needs. Given the increase in the number of adolescents and young adults with chronic and disabling conditions and the comparable rise in concern about this population, this statement is truer today than it has ever been. By following these structural, intrapersonal relationship and social environmental guidelines, medical providers, institutions and programs can make great strides toward ensuring a successful transition process for adolescents with chronic conditions, and those with SCD in particular.

ACKNOWLEDGEMENTS

This work was supported by funds from the National Heart, Lung, and Blood Institute, and the Maternal and Child Health Bureau. The authors are eternally grateful to the former member of the Multi-Site Study of Transition of Adolescents and Young Adults with Sickle Cell Disease Collaborative Group (Duke/UNC Comprehensive Sickle cell center, Medical University of South Carolina Adult Sickle Cell program (SC) Children's Hospital of Alabama

Pediatric Sickle Cell program (AL), Kansas Children's Mercy Hospital Sickle Cell Program (MO), Children's Hospital of Oakland Sickle Cell Program (CA), Douglas Community health Center (MI), Jimmy Everest Sickle Cell Center (OK), Sickle Cell Disease Parent and Family Network of Cincinnati (OH), West Central Ohio Sickle Cell Center (OH), Minneapolis Children's Hospital Sickle Cell program (MN), Sickle Cell Disease Association of the Piedmont (NC), International Black Women's Congress (NJ), Brent Sickle Cell and Thalassemia Centre (UK), Marion County Health Department Sickle Cell program (IN), Cordellia Martin Health center (IN), UAB Kirkland Clinic Adult hematology program (AL), University of Tennessee-Memphis Adult Sickle Cell program (TN), Medical College of Georgia Adult Sickle Cell Program (GA), St. Agnes Pediatric Sickle cell program (CA), Cooper Green Hospital Adult Hematology/Oncology program (AL), and Maine Children's Hospital (ME). Without their partnership, this research would not have been possible. Preparation of this work has been facilitated in part by the infrastructure and resources provided by the NIH CFAR Core Grant P30 AI27767.

REFERENCES

[1] Vichinsky EP, Hurst D, Lubin BH. Sickle cell disease: basic concepts. *Hosp. Med.* 1983;128:158.

[2] Charache S, Lubin BH, Reid CD, eds.. Management and therapy of sickle cell disease, *US Department of Health and Human Services. Public Health Service Publication,* No. 92-21177. Washington, D.C., National Institutes of Health, 1992.

[3] Diggs LM. Anatomic lesions in sickle cell disease. In Abramson H, Bertles JF, Whethers DL. (eds.). *Sickle cell disease diagnosis, management, education and research*. St. Louis: Mosby, 1973.

[4] Platt OS. The natural history of sickle cell disease: life expectancy. *Proceedings of the Bone Marrow Transplantation for Hemoglobinopathies Workshop*. National Heart, Lung and Blood Institute, NIH, Bethesda, MD, 1992.

[5] Serjeant GR. The role of preventive medicine in sickle cell disease. *J. Royal Coll. Physicians London*. 1996;30(1):37-41.

[6] Scott RB. Advances in the treatment of sickle cell disease in children. *Am. J. Dis. Children*. 1985;139(12):1219-22.

[7] Thomas R, Holbrook T. Sickle cell disease: ways to reduce morbidity and mortality. *Postgraduate Med.* 1987;81(5):273-80.

[8] Platt OS, Brambrilla DJ, Rosse WF, Milner PF et al. Mortality in sickle cell disease: life expectancy and risk factors for early death. *New Engl. J. Med.* 1994;330(23):1639-44.

[9] Smith JA. Management of sickle cell disease: Progress during the past 10 years. *Am. Postgrad. Med.* 1983;81(5):265-80.

[10] Platt OS, Thorington BD, Brambilla DJ, Milner PF, Rosse WF, Vichinsky E, Kinney TR. Pain in sickle cell disease: Rates and risk factors. *New Engl. J. Med.* 1991;325(1):11-6.

[11] Telfair J, Myers J, Drezner S. Transfer as a component of the transition of adolescents with sickle cell disease to adult care: adolescent, adult, and parent perspectives. *J. Adoles. Health*. 1994;15(7):558-65.

[12] Adolescent Health Care and Transitions. In: National Institutes of Health, National Heart, Lung, and Blood Institute. *The Management of Sickle Cell Disease.* NIH Publication, 2002:35-40.

[13] Kinney TR, Ware RE. The adolescent with sickle cell anemia. *Hematol. Oncol. Clin. North Am.* 1996;10(6):1255-64.

[14] Hauser ES, Dorn L. Transitioning adolescents with sickle cell disease to adult-centered care. *Pediatr. Nurs.* 1999;25(5):479-88.

[15] Wagner M. A second Look. In: Wagner, M., D'Amico R, Marder C, Newman L, Blockorby J. *What happens next? Trends in post-school outcomes of youth with disabilities.* The second comprehensive Report from the National Longitudinal Transition Study of Secondary Special Education Students. Menlo Park, CA: SRI International, 1992:1-15.

[16] Crosnier H, Tubiana-Rufi N. Transition from pediatric to adult care for diabetic adolescents in the Paris-Ile-de-France area. *Arch. de Pediatrie.* 1998;5(12):1327-1333.

[17] Landau LI. Cystic fibrosis – transition from pediatric to adult physicians care. *Thorax.* 1995;50(10):1031-2.

[18] Sawyer SM, Collins N, Bryan D et al. Young people with spina bifida: transfer from pediatric to adult health care. *J. Pediatr. Child Health.* 1998;34(5):414-417.

[19] Dore A, de Guise P, Mercier LA. Transition of care to adult congenital heart centers: what do patients know about their heart condition? *Can. J. Cardiol.* 2002;18(2):141-6.

[20] Ansell BM, Chamberlain MA. Children with chronic arthritis: the management of transition to adulthood. *Baillieres Clin. Rheumatol.* 1998;12(2):363-74.

[21] Sawyer SM, Blair S, Bowes G. Chronic illness in adolescents: transfer or transition to adult services? *J. Pediatr. Child Health.* 1997;33(2):88-90.

[22] White P, Shear ES. Transition/job readiness for adolescents with juvenile arthritis and other chronic illness. *J. Rheumatol.* 1992;33(19 suppl):23.

[23] Richardson SA. Transition to adulthood. In: Stein REK. (ed.). *Caring for children with chronic illness: issues and strategies.* New York, NY: Springer, 1989.

[24] Rojewski J. A rural based transition model for students with learning disabilities: a demonstration. *J. Learn Disabil.* 1989;22(10):613-20.

[25] Perrin JM, Guyer B, Lawrence JM. Health care services for children and adolescents. In: The future of our children: *U.S. Health Care Children.* 1992;2(2):58-77.

[26] Schidlow D, Fiel S. Life beyond pediatrics: transition of chronically ill adolescents from pediatric to adult health care systems. *Med. Clin. North Am.* 1990;74(5):1113-20.

[27] Carroll G, Massarelli E, Otzoomer A. Adolescents with chronic disease: Are they receiving comprehensive health care? *J. Adoles. Health Care.* 1983;4(4):261-5.

[28] Blum RW, Okinow NA. Teenagers at Risk - A national perspective of state level services for adolescents with chronic illness of disability: Executive Summary. In *Connections: The Newsletter of the National Center for Youth with Disabilities.* 1993;3(suppl 3):1-8.

[29] Magrab PR, Millar HEC. (eds.). Growing up and getting medical care: youth with special health care needs. *Proceedings of the Surgeon General's Conference.* Washington, DC: Georgetown Univ Child Dev Center, 1987.

[30] Garrison MT, McQuiston S. *Chronic illness during childhood and adolescence: psychological aspects.* Newbury Park, CA: Sage, 1989.

[31] Rosen DS. Transition from pediatric Care: barriers still exist. In: *Connections: The Newsletter of the National Center for Youth with Disabilities.* 1992;3(2):1-2.

[32] Denzin NK, Lincoln YS. H*andbook of qualitative research.* Newbury, CA: Sage, 2000.

[33] Statistical Package for the Social Sciences, Inc. SPSS Version 11.0. Chicago, Ill: SPSS, 2002.

[34] Gardner SB, Winter PD, Gardner MJ. Confidence interval analyses version 1.0. London: *BMJ.* 1989.

[35] Clare, N. Management of sickle cell disease would improve if doctors listened more to patients. *BMJ.* 1998;316(7135):935.

[36] Court, J.M., (1993). Issues of transition to adult care. *J. Pediatr. Child Health.* 1993;29(suppl 1):S53-5.

[37] McArnarney, E. (1985). Social maturation: a challenge for handicapped and chronically ill adolescents. *Adoles. Health Care.* 1985;6:90-101.

[38] Kellerman J. Psychological effects of illness in adolescence. I. Anxiety, self-esteem, and perception of control. *J. Pediatrics.* 1980;97(1):126-31.

[39] Hurtig AL, Koepke D, Park KB. Relation between severity of chronic illness and adjustment in children and adolescents with sickle cell disease. *J. Pediatr. Psychol.* 1989;14(1):117-32.

[40] Hurtig AL, White LS. Psychological adjustment in children and adolescent with sickle cell disease. *J. Pediatr. Psychol.* 1986;11(3):411-27.

[41] Thompson RJ Jr., Gil KM, Gustafson KE, George LK, Keith BR, Spock A, Kinney TR. Stability and change in the psychological adjustment of mothers of children and adolescents with cystic fibrosis and sickle cell disease. *J. Pediatr. Psychol.* 1994;19(2):171-88.

[42] Committee on Child Health Financing. Guiding principles for managed care arrangements for the health care of infants, children, adolescents, and young adults. *Pediatrics.* 1995;95(4):613-5.

[43] Jessop DJ, Stein REK. Providing comprehensive healthcare to children with chronic illness. *Pediatrics.* 1994;93(4):602-7.

[44] Ballas SK. Managed care and sickle cell disease. *Blood.* 1998;92(10 Part 2 suppl 1):3093

[45] Palfrey JS, Samuels RC, Haynie M, Cammisa ML. Health care reform: what's in it for children with chronic illness and disability. *J. Sch. Health.* 1994;64(6):234-7.

[46] Betz CL. Adolescent transitions: a nursing concern. *Pediatr. Nurs.* 1998;24(1):23-30.

[47] Callahan ST, Feinstein R, Keenan P. Transition from pediatric to adult-oriented health care: a challenge for patients with chronic disease. *Curr. Opin. Pediatr.* 2001;13(4):310-6.

[48] Scal P, Evans T, Blozis S, Okinow N, Blum R. Trends in transition from pediatric to adult health care services for young adults with chronic conditions. *J. Adolesc. Health.* 1999;24(4):259-64.

[49] Chamberlain MA, Rooney CM. Young adults with arthritis: meeting their transitional needs. *Br. J. Rheumatol.* 1996;35(1):84-90.

[50] Maternal and Child Health Bureau. *Moving-on.* 1992.

[51] Blum RW, Garel D, Hodgman CH, Jorissen TW, Okinow, NA, Orr D, Slap GB. Transition from child-centered to adult health-care systems for adolescents with chronic

conditions: a position paper of the Society for Adolescent Medicine. *J. Adoles. Health.* 1993;14:570-6.

[52] Reinholt PM, Oberg C. Teens can't get by with status quo. In: *Connections: Newsletter Nat. Center Youth Disabil.* 1993:3(1).

[53] Thompson R, Gil K, Abrams M, Phillips G. Stress, coping and psychological adjustment of adults with sickle cell disease. J Consult Clin Psychol 1992;60(3):433-40.

[54] Wallander JL, Varni JW, Babani L, Banis HT, Dehagan CB, Wilcox KT. Disability parameters, chronic strain, and adaptation of physically handicapped children and their mothers. *J. Pediatr. Psychol.* 1989;14(1):23-42.

[55] Baskin ML, Collins MH, Brown F. et al. Psychosocial considerations in sickle cell disease (SCD): the transition from adolescence to young adulthood. *J. Clin. Psychological. Med.* 1998;5(3):315-41.

[56] American Academy of Pediatrics. A consensus statement on health care transitions for young adults with special health care needs. *Pediatrics.* 2002;110(6):1304-6.

[57] Reiss J, Gibson R. Health care transitions: destinations unknown. *Pediatrics.* 2002;110(6):1307-14.

[58] Betz CL. Facilitating the transition of adolescents with chronic conditions from pediatric to adult health care and community settings. *Iss. in Ped. Nurs.* 1998;21: 97-115.

[59] Betz CL. Adolescents with chronic conditions: Linkages to adult service systems. *Ped. Nurs.* 1999;25(5):473-4.

[60] Shultz AW, Liptak GS. Helping adolescents who have disabilities negotiate transitions to adulthood. *Iss. Comp. Ped. Nurs.* 1998;21:187-201.

[61] Woods KF, Karrison TG, Koshy M., Patel A, Friedmann R, Cassel CK. Hospital utilization patterns and costs for adult sickle cell patients in Illinois. *Pub. Health Reports.* 1997;112:44-51.

[62] Utsey SO. Vocational rehabilitation and counseling approaches with sickle cell anemia. *J. Applied Rehab. Couns.* 1991;22:29-31.

In: Adolescence and Chronic Illness
Editors: H. Omar et al.

ISBN: 978-1-60876-628-4
© 2010 Nova Science Publishers, Inc.

Chapter 33

THE TRANSITION OF CARE FOR YOUNG PEOPLE WITH CHRONIC DISEASE

Katherine S. Steinbeck[*1], *Lynne Brodie*[2] *and Susan J. Towns*[3]

[1] Director, Youth Consultancy, Sydney South West
Area Health Service, Sydney, Australia.
[2] Program Manager for Transition in Chronic Illness and
Disability Program, GMCT, Macquarie Hospital, Ryde, Sydney, Australia.
[3] Head, Department of Adolescent Medicine,
The Children's Hospital at Westmead, Sydney, Australia.

ABSTRACT

Young people with a chronic illness or disability originating in childhood ultimately need transition to adult care. The process of leaving a familiar paediatric service and effectively engaging in appropriate adult health care can be challenging and complex. The process often occurs, when there are other significant transitions in a young person's life. Australia has a number of state wide transition initiatives, which aim to address the consistent themes of transition including health care equity, information transfer between health services, consumer participation and the engagement of adult services. What is apparent is the need for the development of transition models, ideally by collaboration between paediatric and adult services, which can be trialed and evaluated in order to best inform how resources need to be distributed. It is also clear that there will be a number of models, defined by the specific disease process. There should always be an emphasis on the needs and wellbeing of young people with chronic illness and the acknowledgement that they should be supported in their quest to lead a normal life.

---

[*] *Correspondence:* Katherine S Steinbeck, Endocrinology and Adolescent Medicine, Royal Prince Alfred Hospital, Missenden Road, Camperdown 2050 Sydney, Australia. Email: kss@email.cs.nsw.gov.au

INTRODUCTION

Transition has been defined as 'the purposeful, planned movement of adolescents and young adults with chronic physical conditions from child-centred to adult- orientated health care systems' [1]. Transition has been much discussed and written about, but much of this output is less scientific evidence and more conjecture and expert opinion with a call for trials and evaluation of clinical programs [2,3]. With advances in health and medical care the life expectancy of children and adolescents with chronic illness continues to increase.

There is also evidence that the prevalence of some chronic illnesses is increasing [1,4]. Thus young people with chronic illness look forward to adult life with expectations that they will lead a life similar to that of their non-illness peers. Young people with chronic illness need an adult health care system which is able to meet their adult health care needs. Sexual health, fertility and reproduction, lifestyle including alcohol and other drugs, nutrition and physical activity, capacity around education and employment and conditions associated with physical aging are all relevant [5]. Even if pediatricians were willing to continue with long term care they do not have the expertise to provide that care and to provide it in the context of independence from families. Most pediatricians acknowledge this but also raise concerns that there may not be a suitable or equivalent service in the adult health care system. Limited evidence would suggest that the majority of adult physicians have no particular opinion on transition and see themselves as peripheral to the transition issue [6]. In this review transition as a process not an event, data capture, health care equity, information transfer between health services, consumer participation, the engagement of adult services, and delineation of models which can be trialed and evaluated will be considered.

THE AUSTRALIAN CONTEXT

The Australian Bureau of Statistics records the current Australian population at 20,250,000 million. Children aged 0–14 years account for four million and young people aged 15–24 for 2.8 million. Three percent of the population is indigenous. In the Australian Institute of Health and Welfare study (2004) on the health of 15-24 year olds, 70% rated their health as excellent or very good and 7% fair or poor with the rest falling somewhere in between. Nine percent (about 250,000) were living with a disability. Sixty percent of males and 72% of females had a long term condition (lasting for more than 6 months) with asthma the most prevalent [7]. In Australia, universal health insurance, Medicare, is funded by general taxation and a Medicare levy. This is a federal initiative, but the individual states are responsible for health care budgets, creating a duality in the system. Access to bulk billing (that is no additional patient payment above the federally determined amount per consultation) is dependent on practitioner discretion. There are additional funding packages related to the care of chronic illness in general practice. Access to public hospital in-patient, emergency and out-patient services is free-of-charge for Medicare patients. Many people with chronic illness may be eligible for further concessionary benefits via health care cards. However medical equipment may become more costly after 18 years, when the young person is considered adult.

While the majority of Australians live in the coastal band of the continent, the majority of the continent is rural or remote. The issues of rural and remote health are complex and challenging [8]. Young people with chronic illness often travel to the major tertiary paediatric hospitals for medical care, or access care through country outreach services. By 18 years of age these options are no longer available and local adult specialist care may be absent or limited. Health care equity needs to be addressed in transition care from a number of psychosocial perspectives, and for Australia the rural and remote perspective is a vital one.

The NSW Centre for the Advancement of Adolescent Health, a public health initiative of the Department of Adolescent Medicine (funded by the New South Wales Department of Health) has pioneered studies into what young people want from the health care system [9]. This ACCESS Study, Phase 1 identified confidentiality, understanding, straightforward answers and tolerance as important qualities desired in heath professionals. It also identified barriers to young people accessing services, including concerns around confidentiality and trust, being made to feel ashamed or stupid, not knowing about the service or what it offers and unfriendly services. Some of these barriers relate to the maturity and developmental stage of the young person and are thus of great importance when considering transition services.

AUSTRALIAN TRANSITION CARE INITIATIVES

There are identified transition programs in the states of New South Wales, Victoria and Western Australia. In New South Wales, NSW Health has funded since 2004 the Greater Metropolitan Clinical Taskforce (GMCT) Transition Care Program for young people with chronic illness and disability arising in childhood. GMCT is a clinician driven program based on the principles of equity of access and equity of outcome, services based on clinical need, and clinician and consumer involvement. Twenty specialty-based clinical networks, chaired by clinicians and involving doctors, nurses, allied health professionals, scientists, managers and consumers, identify how and where improvements can be made in the particular specialty and implement these changes in association with NSW Health and the Area Health Services [10].

The Transition Care Program in Chronic Illness was initiated by clinicians concerned about the transition difficulties experienced by young people with thalassaemia major when moving from paediatric to adult care. It was acknowledged that these transition difficulties were relevant to a wide range of young people and hence the establishment of the Transition Care Program. A Transition Care Program Manager and three Transition Coordinators were appointed, under the guidance of a clinical executive group and supported by a larger working party of health care professionals and consumers. The transition co-ordinators are individually responsible for the three Child Health Networks which cover the state of New South Wales. Each of these Networks is related to one of three tertiary paediatric hospitals (The Children's Hospital at Westmead (Western Sydney), the Sydney Children's Hospital (Eastern Sydney) and the John Hunter Hospital (North of Sydney in Newcastle)). The transition co-ordinators are based in adult hospitals, an important signal about the importance of transition to adult health services. Mental health conditions, including eating disorders, are not included in the Transition Care Program as these are addressed elsewhere through the statewide Child and Adolescent Statewide Acute Mental Health Network. However young people with a dual diagnosis of chronic illness and mental health problems are included. Oncological disorders are also included, not because transition occurs during definitive oncological therapy, but because the need for long term surveillance raises transition issues. The Transition Care Program website has been developed to provide patient and clinician resources relevant to transition and continuing information on the program [11].

In the state of Victoria the Centre for Adolescent Health and the Royal Children's Hospital in Melbourne have contributed to the understanding of transition in Australia, including self management in chronic disease [12] and the prolonged retention of young people with chronic illness in the paediatric system [13]. The Victorian Transition project based at The Royal Children's Hospital (RCH) has been in place since November 2004 [14]. The first aim of the project is to establish adult multidisciplinary clinics in tertiary hospitals to receive the many young adults surviving to adulthood with conditions such as cerebral palsy and spina bifida [15]. Secondly, the project works with all departments at RCH caring for patients with any chronic illness and assists them to develop effective and appropriate transition programs including preparation of patient and family, and policy development and implementation with hospital staff. Outcomes include an increase from one transition clinic in January 2005 to 10 transition clinics in December 2006. There has also been a 30% reduction in 'over-age' inpatient (> 20 years) attendances at RCH between January 2004 and December 2006 and a 24% reduction in over-age outpatient attendances between January 2004 and December 2006 for the same age group. (Personal communication, Felicity Sloman, Transition Co-ordinator, RCH)

There is a Five Year Transition Plan in Western Australia which has dual roles. firstly, to provide appropriate transition education for young people with chronic disease moving to adult care; and secondly, to encourage recognition of the need for and development of services appropriate for adolescents and young adults within the adult health sector, particularly in hospitals. The plan has a three tiered approach that identifies and addresses the generic issues [16], the disease specific issues and the individual's issues and needs. Work is underway with the State's Department of Education to develop education modules addressing the skills and knowledge required by all young people to access adult health care facilities. The modules will be available for use in school as well as accessible in multi-media format to provide the widest possible access for the community. These will also be aligned with health education provided in schools and dovetail with disease specific and individual specific education packages. The transition program will commence as the young person turns thirteen, starts secondary school or at diagnosis, if this occurs during adolescence. It will progress over a period of approximately five years with transfer to adult care being planned to coincide with leaving school.

There are common themes to transition programs and an acknowledgement that there are generic issues in transition that transcend specific disease processes. However it is important to acknowledge that at the clinical level, disease specific modifications will need to be made to transition programs [17].

PEDIATRIC SERVICES

Transition is a process not an event. The starting point is within paediatric services. Children and adolescents with chronic illness are largely managed by general or subspecialty paediatricians supported by good communication with local general practitioners and other services. Tertiary children's hospitals provide comprehensive care in multidisciplinary clinics so that the disruption caused by chronic illness can be minimized. Recent research has been reassuring; demonstrating that adolescents with Cystic Fibrosis appear to be a psychologically well functioning and well-adjusted group [18]

Paediatric services are generally perceived to be family centred and indeed strong bonds are often formed between the paediatric team and the children and families in their care. From diagnosis however, whether it is at birth or throughout childhood or adolescence it is important to be providing education and support for the progression to adult care. This process begins in the early years with comprehensive education and support for parents at diagnosis. Cohesive, communicative families who are able to promote structure and routine around management plans appear to help children and teenagers to accept and manage their illness [18].Within The Childrens Hospital at Westmead, a tertiary Childrens Hospital of 235 beds transition to adult care has been acknowledged as an important process involving all clinicians to ensure continuity of care. From about the age of 12 years self management can be more actively promoted by establishing Adolescent Clinics and seeing the young person by themselves initially with subsequent discussion with parents or carers. This also provides an opportunity for the young person to ask questions and address other general issues that may be impacting adversely on their illness. The timing of transition is individualized, however usually coincides with the end of high school (normally 18 years) when the young person has completed growth and pubertal development and is making informed future orientated decisions. From the age of 16 years the transition process therefore becomes more active; focusing on informing the young person and family about adult care options. Ideally, an individual Transition plan is discussed with each young person and family and reviewed 6-12 monthly. An opportunity to meet adult care providers in joint clinics is felt to be most beneficial by both parents and teenagers as is having their first appointment made and the provision of comprehensive referral information to the adult service(Craig S, Moving on from Paediatric to Adult Health Care: University of Sydney, Honours Thesis 2005).

Surveys of adolescents and families who have transitioned to adult care indicate that good preparation and a transition program are most important [19,20] however also acknowledged the barriers to successful transition; funding and access to adult health care providers. The transition process is completed when the young person is actively engaged with the adult service evidenced by verbal and written feedback. The process is more complex and difficult for the large numbers of adolescents and families where developmental delay is significant as in these circumstances the young person will continue to require the support and involvement of their families [21]. This becomes another challenge for the adult health system where there is an expectation of emerging independence.

This process, of course, requires substantial systemic support within the paediatric hospital setting provided within CHW by the establishment of Transition Care Support Services and a Transition Project Manager networking with Transition Co-coordinators in the adult hospitals. Within the paediatric setting this enables the Transition Clinical Practice

Guidelines and Policy to be implemented. Transition resources, an intranet site for clinicians and internet website for young people and their families have been developed. With early diagnosis and intensive management of childhood complex chronic illness resulting in significant improvements in long term survival the adult health services are faced with increasing challenges and demands for provision of long term care.

DATA CAPTURE AND INFORMATION TRANSFER

Data capture on transition is vital to ensure transition efficacy and to enable argument for additional resources. The quality of data capture for specific disease processes is likely to vary widely in both content and format (electronic or hard copy). In Australia there are specific registries for some chronic disease conditions but none have been set up specifically to consider transition to adult care. The GMCT Transition Care Program has identified diabetes, other endocrinology, general neurology, spina bifida and gastroenterology as the five most prevalent clinical areas in New South Wales which have specialist to specialist transition, followed by cystic fibrosis and hemophilia/thalassemia [22]. Cerebral palsy and other developmental disabilities have higher numbers than diabetes, but transition is often not to specialist adult care. Specific working groups have been set up with both paediatric and adult clinicians for the top five conditions. These working groups will identify the transition issues that are of most concern to young people, their families and the clinicians managing them, to develop effective transition models and a proposal to trial the model/s using a collaborative framework. The working groups also aim to establish a registry of services and key transition resources such as transition checklists for specific chronic illnesses and a discharge summary from the paediatric service that meets the needs of adult clinicians.

A minimum dataset which enables tracking of young people with chronic illness between paediatric and adult care has been developed by the GMCT Transition Care Program and is now under trial. The dataset is voluntarily completed by the tertiary paediatric service and passed to one of the three transition co-ordinators, who then becomes responsible for ascertaining the efficacy of transition. There are data from one young adult diabetes service in Australia showing that active follow up of young people with Type 1 Diabetes after their discharge from paediatric services improves their attendance at the adult service, improves diabetes control and reduces hospitalisation rates for diabetic keto-acidosis [23].

Related to data capture is the information transfer between health services. In the future the fully electronic medical record will facilitate such transfer. In a consumer forum targeted at young people aged between 16 and 25 years with a chronic illness or disability who were preparing to move or had already moved from paediatric to adult health services, consistent suggestions included: being provided with a summary of their personal medical history, centralised medical records and personal handover of health information so that 'you don't have to repeat everything to all the new people' [24]. Anecdotally, summarizing the information from the medical record is time consuming, not re-imbursable for paediatricians and may be handed on to someone else to do who does not have the full knowledge of the patient. The use of a template system to ensure uniformity and inclusion of essential information is a potential solution. It is clearly adaptable to electronic completion and transfer, using memory sticks.

CONSUMER PARTICIPATION

Consumer participation is an integral part of the three transition programs described above. It allows an increase in the health professionals' understanding of what young people see as the issues around moving from paediatric to adult health services and their health priorities, particularly where institutional health care falls in their priorities [24]. Consumer participation also provides an opportunity for young people to learn about and contribute to transition programs, and perhaps develop new friendships and support networks. The ChIPS (Chronic Illness Peer Support) program has been developed by the Centre for Adolescent Health in Victoria and is now implemented in other parts of Australia [25]. The program is run by illness peers with some health professional support. The aims of the program are to empower adolescents to gain control over their health status, encourage a positive attitude towards living with chronic illness using other young people as positive role models, decrease social isolation and loneliness, and importantly, to create leadership opportunities for young people to speak about youth health.

ENGAGING ADULT SERVICES

Engagement of adult services is necessary in the continuum of transition. There is little if any evidence to inform how best to undertake this engagement. Liaison between paediatric and adult services will allow an understanding of the cultural differences between paediatric and adult services, but understanding and education do not guarantee behaviour change in health professionals. There is evidence that the introduction of young people to the adult service prior to transition enhances medium term engagement in the adult system [26]. Young people often represent a small percentage of an adult clinician's patient load. They are 'diluted' in the health care system. Routine follow up of non-attendance for all ages has recently been initiated in some adult services as part of the duty of patient care, but resources may limit such follow up. Adult clinicians may also lack the resources to provide the multi-disciplinary care that is common in paediatrics. A new and unfamiliar system may encourage early attrition from the adult service, thus promoting the stereotype of unreliability in young patients. Adult clinicians may also lack knowledge of specific age related issues and make no therapeutic distinctions on the basis of developmental stage and age.

For the hospitalised young person with chronic illness the use of a youth specific clinical care plan has the potential to both enhance clinical care and improve staff knowledge about developmental issues [27]. The attitudes and practices of adult services cannot be expected to change quickly but there are potential levers for change. Transition care should be included in medical, nursing and allied health curricula. The addition of transition to scientific meeting programs, where there is joint attendance by paediatric and adult specialists, could occur. The collaborative development of management protocols by paediatric and adult medicine sub-specialists should be fostered as the gold standard for care.

Policy related to transition with associated performance indicators should form part of Health Area Service plans and NSW Health has invited GMCT to review and comment on the Draft Healthcare Services Plans (Memo 06/585 – Strategic Development Division of Statewide Services Development Branch, NSW Health). In observational clinical practice, the identification of one youth friendly health professional in an adult team has the capacity to enhance that whole team's approach to young people.

The delineation of transition models which can be trialed and evaluated is clearly important. The available literature is generally theoretical and needs testing to develop an evidence base. There is unlikely to be one 'best fit' model of care for young people with chronic illnesses [3, 28]. Rare and complex chronic conditions demand an adult tertiary service for safe and effective care. Admission to hospital for even routine procedures usually requires expert management and the number of clinicians able to provide the necessary care will be few. For such conditions a single service or co-ordinated limited tertiary network may be necessary [29].

A collaborative tertiary shared care model i involving paediatric and adult services may be applicable to some conditions [30]. Multiple tertiary care centres are likely to be the most common model. Expert review and assessment at tertiary adult centres at regular intervals may be required, but other parts of the health care system might be delivered by general practitioners and other local services. This model implies the early engagement of general practitioners well before transition occurs. Community shared care models are also attractive and could make use of both designated youth health services and general practitioner care.

CONCLUSIONS

Young people with chronic illness need to travel the pathway between their familiar paediatric service and the new adult health care service, with its cultural differences. Over the past decade or so, as more and more young people with chronic illness have survived into adult life, interest in and action on the transition process have increased in Australia, as in many other countries. Australia has a number of transition initiatives, which function at a state level, mainly due to the way health services are funded in this country. However, the themes of transition transcend state and indeed country barriers. Equity in health care, the ability to transfer complex patient information, consumer participation and working with adult services to increase their capacity to respond in a developmentally appropriate manner are all important aspects of the process. Data collection on the numbers of young people with chronic illness who are transitioning is important, as is an understanding of their needs and perspectives as they enter adult healthcare and of the gaps in these services. The formal trialing and evaluation of transition services will enhance an evidence base to inform training and allocation of health care professionals and resources. In this process the needs and wellbeing of young people with chronic illness are paramount as is the support of their quest to lead a normal life.

ACKNOWLEDGEMENTS

The authors would like to thank Ms Penny Shannon, Princess Margaret Hospital for Children, Perth, Western Australia who provided information on the Western Australian Transition Program and Ms Felicity Sloman who provided information on the Transition Program initiatives at the Royal Children's Hospital, Melbourne, Victoria.

REFERENCES

[1] Blum RW, Garell D, Hodgman CH et al. Transition from child-centred to adult healthcare. A position paper of the Society for Adolescent Medicine. *J. Adolesc. Health.* 1993;14:570-6.

[2] Rosen DS, Blum RW, Britto M et al. Society for Adolescent Medicine. Transition to adult health care for adolescents and young adults with chronic conditions: position paper of the Society for Adolescent Medicine. *J. Adolesc. Health.* 2003;33:309-11.

[3] Viner R. Barriers and good practice in transition from paediatric to adult care. *J. Royal Soc. Med.* 2001;94(Suppl 40):2-4.

[4] Onkama P, Vaananen S, Karvonen M, Tuomilehto J. Worldwide increase in the incidence of Type 1 diabetes – the analysis of the data on published incidence trends. *Diabetologia.* 1999;42:1395-1403.

[5] Report of the British Cardiac Society Working Party. Grown-up congenital heart disease (GUCH) disease: current needs and provision of service for adolescents and adults with congenital heart disease in the UK. *Heart.* 2002;88:i1-i14.

[6] Flume P A, Anderson DL, Hardy KK, Gray S. Transition programs in cystic fibrosis centers: perceptions of pediatric and adult program directors. *Pediatr. Pulmonol.* 2001;31:443-50.

[7] http://www.aihw.gov.au/publications/index.cfm/title/10321

[8] Gregory AT, Armstrong RM, Van Der Weyden MB. Rural and remote health in Australia: How to avert the deepening health care drought. *Med. J. Aust.* 2006;185:654-60.

[9] Booth ML, Bernard D, Quine S, Kang MS, Usherwood T, Alperstein G, Bennett DL. Access to health care among Australian adolescents young people's perspectives and their sociodemographic distribution. *J. Adol. Health.* 2004;34:97-103.

[10] Stewart GJ, Dwyer JM, Goulston KJ. The Greater Metropolitan Clinical Taskforce: an Australian model for clinician governance. *Med. J. Aust.* 2006;184:597-8.

[11] www.health.nsw.gov.au/gmct

[12] Sawyer SM, Aroni RA. Self-management in adolescents with chronic illness. What does it mean and how can it be achieved. *Med. J. Aust.* 2005;183:405-9.

[13] Lam P-Y, Fitzgerald BB, Sawyer SM. Young adults in children's hospitals: why are they there? *Med. J. Aust.* 2005;182:381-4.

[14] http://www.rch.org.au/transition

[15] Sloman F. Transfer of young adults with complex medical needs project. www.health.vic.gov.au/subacute/transfer_young.pdf

[16] Bennett DL, Towns SJ, Steinbeck KS. Smoothing the transition to adult care. *Med. J. Aust.* 2005;182:373-4.

[17] McDonagh JE, Shaw K, Southwood TR. Growing up and moving on in rheumatology: development and preliminary evaluation of a transitional care programme for a multicentre cohort of adolescents with juvenile, idiopathic arthritis. *J. Child Health.* 2006;10:22-42.

[18] Szyndler JE, Towns SJ, van Asperen PP, McKay KO. Psychological and family functioning and quality of life in adolescents with cystic fibrosis. *J. Cystic Fibrosis.* 2005; 4:135-44.

[19] Por J et al. Transition of care: health care professionals view. *J. Nurs. Manag.* 2004;354-361.
[20] Telfair J, Alexander L, Loosier P, Alleman-Velez, Summons J. Providers' perspective and beliefs regarding transition to adult care for adolescents with sickle cell disease. *J. Health Care Poor Underserved.* 2004;15:443-63.
[21] Reiss JG, Gibson RW, Walker LR. Health care transition: youth, family, and provider perspectives. *Pediatrics.* 2005;115(1):112-20.
[22] Steinbeck KS, Brodie LS. The state of transition care for young people with chronic illness in NSW. *Proceed Ann. Sci. Meet Royal Australasian College Physicians,* 2006.
[23] Holmes-Walker DJ, Llewellyn AC, Farrell K. A transition care program which improves diabetic control and reduces hospital admission rates in young adults with Type 1 diabetes aged 15-25 years. *Diabetic Med.* (in press)
[24] Steinbeck K, Brodie L. Bringing in the voices: a transition forum for young people with chronic illness or disability. *Neonatal Paed. Child Health Nurs.* 2006;9:22-6.
[25] www.rch.org.au/chips
[26] Kipps S, Bahu T, Ong K et al. Current methods of transfer of young people with Type 1 diabetes to adult services. *Diabetic Med.* 2002;19:649-54.
[27] Sturrock T, Masterson LM, Steinbeck KS. Adolescent Appropriate Care in an Adult Hospital - The use of a Youth Care Plan. *Aust. J. Adv. Nurs.* (in press)
[28] Betz, CL. Adolescents with chronic conditions: Linkages to adult service systems. *Pediatr. Nurs.* 1999;25:473-6.
[29] Report of the NIH Consensus Development Conference. Phenylketonuria (PKU): *Screening and Management.* 2000;17:1-33.
[30] Cole CH. Doing better with cancer in adolescents and young adults. *Med. J. Aust.* 2004;180:52.

Part XIX. Acknowledgements

ABOUT THE EDITORS

Hatim A Omar, MD, FAAP, Professor of Pediatrics and Obstetrics and Gynecology and Director of the Section of Adolescent Medicine, Department of Pediatrics, University of Kentucky, Lexington. Dr. Omar has completed residency training in obstetrics and gynecology as well as Pediatrics. He has also completed fellowships in vascular physiology and adolescent medicine. He is the recipient of the Commonwealth of Kentucky Governor's Award for Community Service and Volunteerism He is the recipient of the Commonwealth of Kentucky Governer's Award for community service and volunteerism in 2000, KY teen Pregnancy Coalition Award for outstanding service 2002, Awards for suicide prevention from the Ohio Valley Society for Adolescent Medicine and Kentucky Pediatric Society in 2005 and 2007, Sexual Abuse Awareness Month Award for his work with sexual abuse victims from the KY association of sexual assault professionals in 2007, Special Achievement Award from the American Academy of Pediatrics 2007 and the Founders of Adolescent Medicine Award from the AAP in 2007. He is well known internationally with numerous publications in child health, pediatrics, adolescent medicine, pediatric and adolescent gynecology. Email: haomar2@uky.edu
Website: https://weblink.ukhealthcare.uky.edu/weblink/phyPro.do?poid=161106&ofid

Donald E Greydanus, MD, FAAP, FSAM, FIAP (H) is Professor of Pediatrics and Human Development at Michigan State University College of Human Medicine (East Lansing, Michigan, USA) and Director of the Pediatrics Residency Program at Michigan State University/ Kalamazoo Center for Medical Studies (Kalamazoo, Michigan, USA). Received the 1995 American Academy of Pediatrics' Adele D. Hofmann Award for "Distinquished Contributions in Adolescent Health", the 2000 Mayo Clinic Pediatrics Honored Alumnus Award for "National Contributions to the field of Pediatrics," and the 2003 William B. Weil, Jr., M.D. Endowed Distinguished Pediatric Faculty Award from Michigan State University College of Medicine for "National & International Recognition as well as Exemplary Scholarship in Pediatrics." Received the 2004 Charles R. Drew School of Medicine (Los Angeles, CA) Stellar Award for Contributions to Pediatric Resident Education and awarded an honorary membership in the Indian Academy of Pediatrics—an honor granted to only a few pediatricians outside of India. Was the 2007 Visiting Professor of Pediatrics at Athens University, Athens, Greece and received the Michigan State University College of Human Medicine Outstanding Community Faculty Award in 2008. Past Chair of the National Conference and Exhibition Planning Group (Committee on Scientific Meetings) of the

American Academy of Pediatrics and member of the Pediatric Academic Societies' (SPR/PAS) Planning Committee (1998 to Present). Member of the Appeals Committee for the Pediatrics' Residency Review Committee (RRC) of the Accreditation Council for Graduate Medical Education (Chicago, IL) in both Adolescent Medicine and General Pediatrics. Numerous publications in adolescent health and lectureships in many countries on adolescent health. E-mail: Greydanus@kcms.msu.edu

Dilip R Patel, MD, FAAP, FSAM, FAACPDM, FACSM, is professor in the Department of Pediatrics and Human Development at the Michigan State University College of Human Medicine, East Lansing, Michigan, USA. He is a full time teaching faculty member in the Pediatric Residency Program at the Michigan State University Kalamazoo Center for Medical Studies, Kalamazoo, Michigan, USA. Dr Patel has subspecialty training and interests in neurodevelopmental disabilities, developmental-behavioral pediatrics, adolescent medicine and sports medicine. He has published numerous papers on a wide ranging topics in these areas and has edited several special symposia and books. E-mail: patel@kcms.msu.edu

Joav Merrick, MD, MMedSci, DMSc, is professor of pediatrics, child health and human development affiliated with Kentucky Children's Hospital, University of Kentucky, Lexington, United States and the Zusman Child Development Center, Division of Pediatrics, Soroka University Medical Center, Ben Gurion University, Beer-Sheva, Israel, the medical director of the Division for Mental Retardation, Ministry of Social Affairs, Jerusalem, the founder and director of the National Institute of Child Health and Human Development. Numerous publications in the field of pediatrics, child health and human development, rehabilitation, intellectual disability, disability, health, welfare, abuse, advocacy, quality of life and prevention. Received the Peter Sabroe Child Award for outstanding work on behalf of Danish Children in 1985 and the International LEGO-Prize ("The Children's Nobel Prize") for an extraordinary contribution towards improvement in child welfare and well-being in 1987. E-Mail: jmerrick@zahav.net.il; Website: www.nichd-israel.com; Home-page: http://jmerrick50.googlepages.com/home

About the Division of Adolescent Medicine at the University of Kentucky, Lexngton, Kentucky, United States

The Division of adolescent medicine was founded in 1998 to provide state of the art care for adolescent patients from all areas of the commonwealth of kentucky, to serve as a state wide resource for education and training for local providers on adolescent issues, to study specisifc factors on the local level affecting youth in the state, to help teach medical students and residents and to provide community service to help improve teen future in the commonwealth.

The division provides comprehensive, holistic team approach to adolescents, where teans receive all aspects for care from mental health to routine care from a team of professionals including physicians, mental health providers, social workers, nutritionists and nursing staff. One unique program within the division is the Young Parent Program, where pregnant teens are cared for throughout pregnancy then they and their babies are cared for together in the program.

The division is active in research with more than 10 peer reviewed articles published each year as well as several books and special journal editions.

In the community, the program has founded several grass route programs to help prevent youth suicide, teen pregnancy, accidental death and substance abuse among adolescents in Kentucky.

The division has provided more than 300 lectures, worshops, media events and teaching for community providers, parents, teachers and school counselors. It also provides adovocacy work on behalf of teens with active work at the state legislative and executive government as well as local governments to help improve the lives of teens.

Collaborations

The division collaborates locally with school boards, youth service centers, state and local goverments, other universities and child advocacy centers as well as with regional adolescent medicine programs.

Internationally with the Institute for Child Health and Human Development in Israel, the Division of Adolescent Medicine at Santa Casa University, Brazil, Quality of Life Research

Center and Nordic School of Holistic Health, Copenhagen, Denmark, School of Social Work, Chinese University, Hong Kong.

THE VISION

The vision of the Division of Adolescent Medicine is to improve the health and long term wellbeing of Kentucky Youth to grow into productive adults. We also invision global work to help positive youth development world wide.

TARGET AREAS OF INTERESTS

The interest areas of the division are all aspects of youth development and adolescent health with focus on prevention and community involvement in colloboration on the local, national and global level with programs having the same goal.

Contact

Hatim Omar, MD, FAAP
Professor of Pediatrics and Obstetrics/Gynecology
Director of Adolescent Medicine & Young Parent programs
J422, Kentucky Clinic
Department of Pediatrics, Kentucky Children's Hospital
University of Kentucky College of Medicine
Lexington, KY 40536
Tel. 859-323-6426 ext. 311
Fax. 859-257-7706
E-mail: haomar2@uky.edu
Website://www.mc.uky.edu/

About the Department of Pediatrics and Human Development, Michigan State University College of Human Medicine, MSU/Kalamazoo Center for Medical Studies, Kalamazoo, Michigan, United States

The Department of Pediatrics and Human Development (PHD) at Michigan State University College of Human Medicine (MSUCHM) was developed in 1968 with the formation of the College of Human Medicine (CHM) at Michigan State University (MSU) in East Lansing, Michigan. It is a nationally-recognized Department of PHD that involves four Michigan State University (MSU) campuses including East Lansing and Kalamazoo, Michigan. Michigan State University/Kalamazoo Center for Medical Studies (MSU/KCMS) is a nationally recognized university/community based residency program with over 170 residents in over 12 disciplines including Pediatrics that is located in Kalamazoo, Michigan, USA.

Mission and Service

The MSUCHM PHD has a unique balance between behavioral science, basic biological research, and clinical pediatrics. The Department has a commitment to a comprehensive approach to the health and development of the child, adolescent, and the family. PHD has a unique blend of community integrated medical training centers with a unified educational mission that serves medical students, pediatric residents, and four communities in Michigan, USA.

The mission is to "advance the healthy development and well being of children and adolescents through innovative medical education, research, clinical care, and advocacy, emphasizing community-based partnerships." To this end, the department offers a broad range of clinical and laboratory services to the children and adolescents of Michigan. PHD draws on the talents of over 100 faculty members and over 500 volunteer teaching faculty members. The mission of the Kalamazoo, Michigan program (MSU/KCMS Pediatrics Program) is to train both medical students in their 3rd and 4th year as well as many residents in the field of Pediatrics. MSU/KCMS Pediatrics is a fully accredited, three year program preparing physicians for board-certification in Pediatrics.

Values of MSU/KCMS include compassionate service, leadership training, commitment to lifelong learning, emphasis on teamwork, and commitment to excellence in health care. Trainees at MSU/KCMS become skilled at providing patient care that is compassionate, appropriate, and effective for the treatment of health problems and the promotion of health. They learn to demonstrate interpersonal and communication skills that result in the effective exchange of information and collaboration with patients, their families, and health professionals. They are taught to develop a commitment to carrying out professional responsibilities and an adherence to ethical principles throughout their training with a goal of these values becoming a lifelong habit that reveals professional compassion, integrity, and respect for others. Kalamazoo is the home of the Kalamazoo Promise, a truly unique program that funds college education for students who graduate from the Kalamazoo public schools.

RESEARCH ACTIVITIES

MSU/KCMS has a variety of research projects in adolescent medicine, neurobehavioral pediatrics, adolescent gynecology, pediatric diabetes mellitus, asthma, cystic fibrosis, and pediatric oncology. MSU/KCMS Pediatrics is involved with a number of studies with the Children's Oncology Group in the United States.

MSU/KCMS Pediatrics has recently published a number of medical textbooks: Essential adolescent medicine (McGraw-Hill Medical Publishers), The pediatric diagnostic examination (McGraw-Hill), Pediatric and adolescent psychopharmacology (Cambridge University Press), Behavioral pediatrics, 2nd Edition (iUniverse Publishers in New York and Lincoln, Nebraska), and Pediatric practice: Sports medicine (McGraw-Hill).

MSU/KCMS Pediatrics has edited a number of journal issues published by Elsevier Publishers covering Pulmonology (State of the Art Reviews: Adolescent Medicine—AM:STARS), Genetic disorders in adolescents (AM:STARS), Neurologic/neurodevelopmental disorders (AM:STARS), Behavioral pediatrics (Pediatric Clinics of North America), Nephrologic disorders in adolescents (AM:STARS), College health (Pediatric Clinics of North America), Adolescent medicine (Primary Care: Clinics in Office Practice), Behavioral pediatrics in children and adolescents (Primary Care: Clinics in Office Practice), and Developmental disabilities (Pediatric Clinics of North America). The Department has also edited a journal issue on musculoskeletal disorders in children and adolescents for the American Academy of Pediatrics' AM:STARS.

The department has developed academic ties with a variety of international medical centers and organizations, including the Queen Elizabeth Hospital in Hong Kong, National Taiwan University Hospital (Taipei, Taiwan), Indian Academy of Pediatrics (New Delhi, India), the University of Athens Aghia Sophia Children's Hospital (First and Second Departments of Paediatrics) in Athens, Greece and the National Institute of Child Health and Human Development in Israel.

Contact

Professor Donald E Greydanus, MD and Professor Dilip R. Patel, MD
Pediatrics and Human Development
Michigan State University College of Human Medicine PHD Department
Michigan State University/Kalamazoo Center for Medical Studies
1000 Oakland Drive, Kalamazoo, MI 49008-1284 United States
E-mail: Greydanus@kcms.msu.edu and Patel@kcms.msu.edu
Website: http://www.kcms.msu.edu/ and http://phd.msu.edu

About the National Institute of Child Health and Human Devlopment in Israel

The National Institute of Child Health and Human Development (NICHD) in Israel was established in 1998 as a virtual institute under the auspicies of the Medical Director, Ministry of Social Affairs and Social Services in order to function as the research arm for the Office of the Medical Director. In 1998 the National Council for Child Health and Pediatrics, Ministry of Health and in 1999 the Director General and Deputy Director General of the Ministry of Health endorsed the establishment of the NICHD.

Mission

The mission of a National Institute for Child Health and Human Development in Israel is to provide an academic focal point for the scholarly interdisciplinary study of child life, health, public health, welfare, disability, rehabilitation, intellectual disability and related aspects of human development. This mission includes research, teaching, clinical work, information and public service activities in the field of child health and human development.

Service and Academic Activities

Over the years many activities became focused in the south of Israel due to collaboration with various professionals at the Faculty of Health Sciences (FOHS) at the Ben Gurion University of the Negev (BGU). Since 2000 an affiliation with the Zusman Child Development Center at the Pediatric Division of Soroka University Medical Center has resulted in collaboration around the establishment of the Down Syndrome Clinic at that center. In 2002 a full course on "Disability" was established at the Recanati School for Allied Professions in the Community, FOHS, BGU and twice a year seminars for specialists in family medicine. In 2005 collaboration was started with the Primary Care Unit of the faculty and disability became part of the master of public health course on "Children and society". In the academic year 2005-2006 a one semester course on "Aging with disability" was started as part of the master of science program in gerontology in our collaboration with the Center for Multidisciplinary Research in Aging.

Research Activities

The affiliated staff has over the years published work from projects and research activities in this national and international collaboration. In the year 2000 the International Journal of Adolescent Medicine and Health and in 2005 the International Journal on Disability and Human development of Freund Publishing House (London and Tel Aviv), in the year 2003 the TSW-Child Health and Human Development and in 2006 the TSW-Holistic Health and Medicine of the Scientific World Journal (New York and Kirkkonummi, Finland), all peer-reviewed international journals were affiliated with the National Institute of Child Health and Human Development. From 2008 also the International Journal of Child Health and Human Development (Nova Science, New York), the International Journal of Child and Adolescent Health (Nova Science) and the Journal of Pain Management (Nova Science) affiliated.

National Collaborations

Nationally the NICHD works in collaboration with the Faculty of Health Sciences, Ben Gurion University of the Negev; Department of Physical Therapy, Sackler School of Medicine, Tel Aviv University; Autism Center, Assaf HaRofeh Medical Center; National Rett and PKU Centers at Chaim Sheba Medical Center, Tel HaShomer; Department of Physiotherapy, Haifa University; Department of Education, Bar Ilan University, Ramat Gan, Faculty of Social Sciences and Health Sciences; College of Judea and Samaria in Ariel and recently also collaborations has been established with the Division of Pediatrics at Hadassah, Center for Pediatric Chronic Illness, Har HaZofim in Jerusalem.

International Collaborations

Internationally with the Department of Disability and Human Development, College of Applied Health Sciences, University of Illinois at Chicago; Strong Center for Developmental Disabilities, Golisano Children's Hospital at Strong, University of Rochester School of Medicine and Dentistry, New York; Centre on Intellectual Disabilities, University of Albany, New York; Chandler Medical Center and Children's Hospital, Kentucky Children's Hospital, Section of Adolescent Medicine, University of Kentucky, Lexington; Chronic Disease Prevention and Control Research Center, Baylor College of Medicine, Houston, Texas; Division of Neuroscience, Department of Psychiatry, Columbia University, New York; Institute for the Study of Disadvantage and Disability, Atlanta; Center for Autism and Related Disorders, Department Psychiatry, Children's Hospital Boston, Boston; Department of Pediatrics and Human Development (PHD) at Michigan State University College of Human Medicine (MSUCHM), Kalamazoo, Michigan; Centre for Chronic Disease Prevention and Control, Health Canada, Ottawa; Department of Paediatrics, Child Health and Adolescent Medicine, Children's Hospital at Westmead, Westmead, Australia; International Centre for the Study of Occupational and Mental Health, Düsseldorf, Germany; Centre for Advanced Studies in Nursing, Department of General Practice and Primary Care, University of

Aberdeen, Aberdeen, United Kingdom; Quality of Life Research Center, Copenhagen, Denmark; Centre for Quality of Life of the Hong Kong Institute of Asia-Pacific Studies and School of Social Work, Chinese University, Hong Kong.

TARGETS

Our focus is on research, international collaborations, clinical work, teaching and policy in health, disability and human development and to establish the NICHD as a permanent institute at one of the residential care centers for persons with intellectual disability in Israel in order to conduct model research and together with the four university schools of public health/medicine in Israel establish a national master and doctoral program in disability and human development at the institute to secure the next generation of professionals working in this often non-prestigious/low-status field of work. For this project we need your support. We are looking for all kinds of support and eventually an endowment.

Contact

Professor Joav Merrick, MD, MMedSci, DMSc
Medical Director, Division for Mental Retardation
Ministry of Social Affairs, POBox 1260
IL-91012 Jerusalem, Israel
E-mail: jmerrick@internet-zahav.net
Website: www.nichd-israel.com;

INDEX

A

AAP, 433
abdomen, 71, 87, 91, 241, 242
abnormalities, 13, 15, 19, 29, 35, 49, 52, 53, 60, 66, 75, 78, 113, 153, 189, 204, 216, 217, 242, 250, 257, 258, 262, 263, 264, 311, 312, 320, 323, 326, 331, 333, 334, 339, 341, 346, 358, 379, 381
absorption, 43, 237, 239, 241, 249, 298
academic performance, 25, 73, 230, 384
academic success, 181
acceleration, 214, 252
accessibility, 274, 276, 278
accidental, 435
accidents, 76, 100, 114, 167, 170, 239
accommodation, 181
accounting, 69, 357
accuracy, 114, 333
acetabulum, 312, 313, 316, 317, 323, 326, 334
acetaminophen, 310
acetate, 41, 293, 294, 301, 302, 303
achalasia, 239
achievement, 25, 68, 69, 99, 100, 342, 386
acid, 14, 19, 58, 59, 240, 295, 296, 298, 299, 300
acidic, 240
acidosis, 60, 237, 248, 249, 426
acidotic, 249
acne, 103, 293, 294, 295, 296, 297, 298, 299, 300, 301, 302, 303, 304
acne fulminans, 299
acne vulgaris, 293, 294, 295, 298, 300, 303, 304
ACTH, 39, 47, 297
activity level, 326, 387
acute, 15, 25, 30, 35, 36, 39, 44, 45, 46, 47, 58, 59, 74, 75, 76, 77, 79, 81, 82, 83, 85, 92, 93, 94, 109, 123, 133, 140, 159, 191, 196, 208, 216, 263, 268, 294, 308, 309, 310, 323, 331, 371, 377, 379, 380

acute leukemia, 47
acute lung injury, 216
acute lymphoblastic leukemia, 25, 30, 45
acute myeloid leukaemia, 46
acute rejection, 263, 268
acute stress, 123, 140
adaptation, 101, 104, 118, 155, 237, 258, 267, 268, 351, 420
adaptive functioning, 100, 101
addiction, 75, 147
adduction, 213, 323
adenoma, 296
adenosine, 16, 61
adenosine triphosphate, 16, 61
ADH, 41
ADHD, 68, 112, 114, 115, 118, 120
adhesion, 66, 341
adipose, 237
adiposity, 190
adjunctive therapy, 209
adjustment, 6, 9, 10, 73, 79, 104, 107, 119, 158, 184, 261, 269, 351, 387, 419, 420
administration, 39, 49, 59, 83, 205, 209
administrators, 399
adolescent behavior, 176
adolescent boys, 219, 353
adolescent female, 117, 169, 290
adolescent patients, 119, 174, 182, 397, 435
adrenal gland, 294
adrenal hyperplasia, 296, 297
adrenal insufficiency, 39, 41
adrenocorticotropic hormone, 239
adult obesity, 200
adult population, 248, 257, 262
adult providers, 414
adverse event, 309
advocacy, 180, 182, 404, 413, 415, 434, 435, 437
aerobic, 15, 191, 204, 206, 371, 384, 385, 388, 390, 391, 392

aerobic exercise, 191, 385, 388, 391
aetiology, 125
affective disorder, 111, 123, 125, 126, 131, 133, 136
Africa, 110, 115
African American, 5, 67, 82, 252, 257, 404, 408
African Americans, 82
agent, 29, 209, 240, 243, 250, 308
agents, 16, 18, 29, 40, 44, 109, 206, 208, 209, 217, 249, 293, 295, 309
aggression, 115, 123, 130, 132, 133, 134, 136, 143, 343
aggressive personality, 128
aggressive therapy, 203
aging, 52, 61, 100, 217, 365, 422
aging process, 100
agonist, 223, 228
aid, 41, 195, 237, 274, 371
aiding, 182
AIDS, 121, 152, 285, 403
air, 206, 208, 209, 212, 214, 216, 228, 230, 295, 377
air pollution, 230
air quality, 228, 230
airflow obstruction, 207
airway hyperreactivity, 216
airway hyperresponsiveness, 208, 217
airways, 203, 206, 207
alcohol, 113, 160, 278, 295, 299, 422
alcohol abuse, 299
aldosterone, 194
alendronate, 45
alertness, 153, 155
alexithymia, 147
algorithm, 210
alkali, 249
alkylating agents, 40
ALL, 25
allergens, 228, 232
allergic reaction, 299
allergy, 228, 369, 370, 372, 373
allograft, 27
allografts, 267
alopecia, 295
alpha, 72, 73, 132, 206, 223
alternative, 93, 161, 209, 237, 308, 365
aluminum, 249, 250, 252, 295
alveolar macrophages, 15
alveoli, 204
amenorrhea, 44, 380
American Academy of Pediatrics, 352, 381, 420, 433, 438
American Diabetes Association, 44
American Psychiatric Association, 68, 77, 124, 146
Americans with Disabilities Act, 274, 280

amino acids, 59, 235
amputation, 27, 28
AMR, 391
anabolic, 295, 297
anabolic steroid, 295, 297
anabolic steroids, 297
anaerobic, 204, 216, 371
analgesia, 83, 84, 91, 92, 94, 95
analgesic, 74, 91, 94, 95, 307, 308
analgesics, 178, 308
anatomy, 15, 327
androgen, 294, 296, 298, 303
androgens, 296, 297, 301, 303
anemia, 5, 71, 72, 74, 236, 248, 249, 251, 252, 258, 259, 260, 261, 266, 267, 295, 404
anencephaly, 302
anesthesiologist, 278
aneurysm, 379
anger, 132, 138, 145, 157, 158
anger management, 157, 158
animal models, 15
animal studies, 15
animals, 133, 224
ankles, 69
anomalous, 377
anorexia, 39, 44, 49, 59, 114, 124, 125, 126, 127, 128, 129, 130, 131, 133, 134, 145, 146, 147, 148, 155, 193, 196, 200, 240, 380
anorexia nervosa, 37, 44, 49, 103, 114, 124, 125, 126, 127, 128, 129, 131, 133, 134, 145, 146, 147, 148, 155, 193, 200, 240
antagonists, 208, 209, 217
antibacterial, 72
antibiotic, 17, 115, 206, 294, 298, 299, 300, 302
antibiotic resistance, 298, 300, 302
antibiotics, 16, 18, 293, 295, 299, 300, 302, 303
anticholinergic, 16
anticonvulsants, 239
antidiuretic, 41
antidiuretic hormone, 41
antigenicity, 341
anti-inflammatory drugs, 85, 230, 308, 309
anti-inflammatory medications, 209, 307
antineoplastic, 29
antineoplastic agents, 29
anti-retroviral medications, 115
antisocial behavior, 27
anus, 242
anxiety, 27, 79, 100, 105, 106, 107, 110, 111, 112, 113, 114, 115, 116, 117, 118, 120, 125, 126, 127, 128, 130, 131, 132, 133, 138, 139, 144, 152, 169, 197, 213, 214, 264, 342, 359, 365, 371, 384, 412, 419

anxiety disorder, 107, 110, 111, 114, 115, 117, 118, 125, 126, 129
aorta, 379
aortic aneurysm, 379
aortic insufficiency, 379
aortic valve, 377
APA, 77
aplasia, 257, 342
appetite, 43, 125, 239, 250, 266
application, 119, 184, 281, 298, 300, 309, 358, 372
apraxia, 362
aptitude, 287
arabinoside, 25
arginine, 41, 340
argument, 426
arrhythmia, 240
arrhythmias, 240, 371, 377
arteries, 70
arteriography, 194
artery, 260, 335, 379
arthralgia, 294, 295
arthritis, 4, 48, 112, 118, 184, 326, 331, 378, 404, 418, 419, 429
arthrogram, 321
arthroscope, 329
arthroscopy, 330, 333
articular cartilage, 313, 317, 327, 330, 333
ascites, 71
ASD, 115
asexual, 276, 285
aspiration, 14, 15, 19, 203, 240, 243, 244
aspiration pneumonia, 14, 15, 19, 244
assault, 184, 433
assertiveness, 415
assessment, 39, 40, 72, 79, 99, 101, 103, 116, 118, 129, 145, 146, 162, 193, 196, 197, 235, 264, 266, 267, 269, 333, 372, 373, 380, 387, 406, 415, 428
assignment, 177, 230
assistive technology, 278
assumptions, 274
asthma, 4, 43, 100, 106, 107, 110, 117, 156, 163, 203, 204, 205, 207, 208, 209, 210, 211, 212, 213, 215, 216, 217, 218, 221, 222, 223, 224, 225, 226, 227, 228, 229, 230, 231, 232, 376, 377, 379, 422, 438
asthma attacks, 110, 225, 228, 229
asthmatic children, 228, 229
asymmetry, 327
asymptomatic, 15, 197, 344, 378
ataxia, 168, 341, 360, 361, 364
ATC, 82, 84
atelectasis, 14

athletes, 107, 218, 335, 369, 370, 371, 372, 373, 374, 376, 377, 378, 380, 381, 382, 385, 386
athletic competence, 113
athleticism, 128
atmosphere, 361
atopic asthma, 208
atopic dermatitis, 296
ATP, 61
ATPase, 240
atrial septal defect, 115, 120, 302
atrophy, 28, 168, 341
attachment, 148, 152
attacks, 110, 225, 228, 229
attention problems, 118
attitudes, 148, 194, 200, 274, 280, 285, 289, 427
attractiveness, 124
augmentative and alternative communication, 365
Australia, 6, 24, 231, 421, 422, 423, 424, 426, 427, 428, 429, 442
autism, 53, 55, 168, 343, 344, 346, 347, 364
autoimmune, 42, 47, 53, 299
autoimmune manifestations, 53
autonomic nervous system, 235
autonomy, 26, 103, 127, 152, 277, 283, 284, 289
autosomal dominant, 344, 347
autosomal recessive, 16, 72, 340, 341
availability, 125, 237, 238, 308, 399, 404, 405
avascular necrosis, 74, 75, 79, 312, 313, 329, 334
averaging, 387
aversion, 362
avoidance, 126, 185, 212, 217
avoidant, 126, 128
awareness, 25, 274, 284, 307, 415
axilla, 294
azotemia, 258

B

babies, 16, 60, 250, 351, 435
back, 73, 87, 175, 178, 179, 214, 250, 293, 301, 361, 372
back pain, 184, 301, 372
bacteremia, 17, 18
bacteria, 14, 15, 16, 18
bacterial, 17, 18, 19, 20, 59, 206, 241, 263, 294
bacterial infection, 206
banking, 41
barbiturates, 295
barrier, 399
barriers, 104, 106, 274, 275, 285, 385, 386, 419, 423, 425, 428
basketball, 179
BED, 111

bedsore, 17
behavior, 27, 62, 67, 73, 77, 85, 103, 104, 112, 119, 129, 133, 148, 155, 156, 157, 160, 161, 162, 176, 195, 197, 266, 340, 342, 351, 355, 360, 385, 392
behavior modification, 195
behavior therapy, 148
behavioral assessment, 200
behavioral change, 258
behavioral disorders, 115, 169
behavioral problems, 85, 101, 107, 109, 113, 114, 115, 195, 346
behavioral sciences, 230
behaviours, 127
beliefs, 160, 285, 413, 430
benchmarking, 131
beneficial effect, 298, 308
benefits, 8, 206, 229, 343, 345, 369, 370, 372, 384, 385, 386, 398, 407, 410, 422
benign, 168, 184, 309, 310
benzoyl peroxide, 293, 298, 300, 302
beverages, 190
bias, 143, 232
bicarbonate, 243, 249, 250
binding, 38, 44, 49, 54, 249, 250, 296
binding globulin, 296
binge eating disorder, 103, 07, 125
bingeing, 103
biological processes, 174
birth, 10, 52, 53, 58, 100, 128, 131, 133, 134, 137, 144, 147, 148, 219, 238, 276, 278, 279, 281, 289, 342, 348, 351, 352, 356, 378, 425
birth control, 278
births, 58, 66, 113, 115
bisphosphonate treatment, 45
bladder, 17, 170, 238, 278, 369, 370, 371, 372, 373
blaming, 195
bleaching, 299
bleeding, 24, 66, 67, 69, 70, 77, 299, 308, 380
bleeding time, 308
blindness, 169, 302
blood clot, 66, 67
blood flow, 67, 277, 362
blood glucose, 6
blood group, 67
blood pressure, 91, 189, 191, 192, 194, 195, 196, 197, 198, 371, 378, 379, 384, 389
blood stream, 18
blood supply, 326, 329, 330
blood transfusion, 76
blood vessels, 295
body fat, 384

body image, 6, 69, 102, 103, 111, 112, 124, 144, 145, 147, 153, 154, 193, 199, 266, 284, 288, 290, 350, 386
body language, 174
body mass index (BMI), 48, 102, 107, 124, 190, 191, 192, 193, 196, 236
body shape, 107
body size, 102, 107, 153, 198
body weight, 103, 124, 127, 191, 199, 322
bolus, 239
bonding, 360
bonds, 425
bone age, 39
bone density, 42, 44, 45, 49, 75, 237
bone marrow, 25, 46, 47, 73, 248, 252, 258
bone marrow transplant, 25, 46, 47, 248, 252
bone mass, 44
bone mineral density, 75
bone tumors, 26, 27, 29
borderline, 196, 343
oston, 290, 364, 365, 442
bowel, 119, 170, 238, 241, 243, 244, 362, 369, 370, 371, 373
bowel obstruction, 241
bowel sounds, 241
boys, 68, 73, 77, 102, 114, 184, 192, 199, 214, 231, 343, 344, 351, 385, 390, 391
bradycardia, 85
brain, 24, 25, 26, 28, 29, 37, 38, 45, 46, 47, 53, 58, 60, 61, 68, 114, 153, 155, 167, 168, 170, 238, 364, 384
brain damage, 58
brain development, 384
brain injury, 114, 120, 167, 168, 170, 376, 379
brain tumor, 24, 25, 26, 29, 45, 46, 47
Brazil, 115, 283, 435
breakdown, 60
breast cancer, 275
breathing, 132, 206, 208, 209, 214, 217, 264, 358, 376
bronchial asthma, 231
bronchial hyperresponsiveness, 207
bronchiectasis, 206
bronchioles, 204
bronchoconstriction, 208, 218
bronchodilator, 205, 213, 229
bronchopulmonary dysplasia, 203, 204, 219
bronchospasm, 212, 213, 218
bronchus, 15
brothers, 128, 134
bubbles, 360
building blocks, 57, 58, 235

bulimia, 124, 125, 126, 128, 129, 131, 145, 147, 148, 193, 196, 380
bulimia nervosa, 103, 124, 125, 126, 128, 129, 145, 147, 148, 149, 193, 380
bullying, 153
Burkholderia, 16
burn, 61
burning, 92
burnout, 381
burns, 83, 243
bursitis, 320, 323, 326
buttocks, 294
bypass, 15, 240

C

calcinosis, 249
calcium, 44, 239, 249, 258
calcium carbonate, 249
caliber, 204
caloric intake, 236, 237, 387
calorie, 206
Canada, 173, 174, 221, 222, 223, 224, 225, 226, 227, 228, 229, 230, 231, 390, 442
cancer, 23, 24, 25, 26, 27, 29, 30, 31, 36, 38, 39, 40, 45, 46, 47, 61, 95, 106, 112, 113, 118, 119, 174, 430
cancer treatment, 30, 40
capillary, 15
carbohydrate, 235, 236, 341
carbohydrates, 57, 58, 235
carbon, 204
carbon dioxide, 204
carcinoma, 296
cardiac arrest, 129
cardiac arrhythmia, 240, 371, 377
cardiac function, 276
cardiac surgery, 115, 120
cardiomyopathy, 59, 341
cardiopulmonary, 218, 386
cardiovascular disease, 189, 194, 199, 259, 261, 390
cardiovascular risk, 192, 198, 384
cardiovascular system, 258, 259
care model, 428
caregiver, 72, 110, 239, 259, 264, 266, 268
caregivers, 103, 104, 105, 255, 261, 264, 269, 415
caretaker, 286, 415
caries, 399, 400
carpal tunnel syndrome, 372
cartilage, 313, 317, 327, 330, 333, 334
case study, 184, 362, 365
catabolism, 36, 48, 58
cataracts, 379

catecholamines, 209
category a, 29, 340
catheter, 17, 243
catheterization, 17, 372
catheters, 71
cation, 281
Caucasian, 16, 67, 107, 175
Caucasian population, 16, 67
Caucasians, 113, 205
causal relationship, 110
causality, 128
cauterization, 243
CDC, 52, 68, 190, 191, 388, 389
Celiac disease, 42, 47
cell, 5, 37, 41, 43, 46, 61, 72, 74, 76, 79, 82, 83, 92, 93, 117, 236, 249, 297, 341, 350, 404, 405, 408, 416, 417
cell transplantation, 37, 72
cellulitis, 18, 295
censorship, 415
Centers for Disease Control, 52, 68, 114, 120, 388
central nervous system, 25, 36, 53, 60, 70, 238
central retinal vein occlusion, 78
cerebral palsy, 13, 59, 113, 119, 167, 170, 171, 236, 237, 242, 244, 312, 369, 370, 372, 373, 376, 424
cerebrovascular, 73, 77, 167, 170, 191, 197
cerebrovascular accident, 167, 170
cerebrovascular disease, 191, 197
certification, 438
chemicals, 154, 298
chemotherapy, 24, 26, 28, 36, 37, 39, 40, 46, 47, 71, 156
chest, 16, 74, 76, 87, 91, 203, 204, 206, 208, 214, 216, 218, 219, 230, 293, 371, 378
chest radiograph, 216, 230
Child Behavior Checklist, 196, 200
child benefit, 4
child rearing, 162
child welfare, 434
childbearing, 278
childbirth, 275, 276
child-centered, 404, 419
child-rearing practices, 133
China, 52
Chi-square, 408
chloride, 16, 239, 242, 295
chlorinated hydrocarbons, 295
chocolate, 297
cholestasis, 239
cholesterol, 301, 384
chorea, 168
chorioamnionitis, 216

chromosome, 19, 43, 339, 342, 343, 345, 346, 347, 350, 351
chromosomes, 341, 350, 351
chronic disease, 13, 68, 76, 99, 100, 162, 163, 207, 244, 265, 266, 286, 373, 384, 404, 418, 419, 424, 426
chronic diseases, 13, 163, 244, 265, 286, 373, 384, 404
chronic disorders, 71, 203
chronic kidney disease (CKD), 247, 252, 255, 269
chronic kidney failure, 252
chronic pain, 71, 74, 75, 94, 173, 174, 179, 180, 181, 182, 183, 185, 310
chronic renal failure, 252, 256, 257, 259, 260, 261, 264, 267, 268
chronic stress, 159
chronically ill, 79, 99, 100, 101, 102, 104, 105, 106, 109, 116, 156, 158, 159, 161, 181, 269, 418, 419
CIA, 408
cigarette smoke, 217
cigarette smoking, 27
cigarettes, 113, 296
cimetidine, 301
circadian, 44
circadian rhythm, 44
circulation, 277
cisplatin, 31, 41
citizens, 267, 365
CKD, 247, 248, 249, 250, 251, 256, 258, 259, 260, 261, 265, 266, 267
classes, 191, 277
classification, 3, 79, 208, 229, 252, 312, 355, 369, 372, 373
classroom, 176
classrooms, 110
cleaning, 228, 287
cleft palate, 238, 342
clinical diagnosis, 140, 341, 342
clinical disorders, 129, 136, 143
clinical presentation, 14, 15, 36, 70, 346
clinical symptoms, 124
clinical trial, 43, 94, 309, 310
clinical trials, 309
clinically significant, 112
clinician, 40, 53, 115, 157, 158, 240, 298, 299, 376, 378, 380, 423, 424, 427, 429
clinics, 107, 131, 182, 416, 424, 425
clonidine, 169
closure, 243, 301, 400
CNS, 25, 26, 27, 28, 36, 39, 59, 70, 238, 240
Co, 125, 184, 267, 331, 424, 425
coagulation, 66, 67, 77, 78, 309
coagulation factor, 66

coagulation factors, 66
coagulopathy, 77
coarctation, 379
cocaine, 160
Cochrane, 232, 252, 391
codes, 349
coding, 175
coeliac disease, 48
co-existence, 35
cognition, 25, 26, 28, 77, 162
cognitive abilities, 153, 288
cognitive behavior therapy, 148
cognitive capacity, 152
cognitive deficit, 68, 76, 370
cognitive deficits, 68, 76, 370
cognitive development, 25, 256, 259
cognitive dysfunction, 85
cognitive effort, 174
cognitive flexibility, 160
cognitive function, 120, 255, 263, 266
cognitive impairment, 19, 25, 68, 73, 174, 365, 385
coherence, 404, 413
cohesion, 161
cohort, 26, 52, 54, 68, 71, 192, 219, 252, 343, 351, 429
cold compress, 308
collaboration, 7, 413, 421, 438, 441, 442
collagen, 238
college students, 107, 125, 390, 393
colon, 243
colonization, 15, 16, 20
colonizers, 18
colostomy, 242
coma, 59
communication, 6, 25, 28, 74, 85, 123, 127, 130, 131, 133, 140, 141, 144, 159, 161, 265, 266, 274, 279, 285, 360, 362, 363, 364, 365, 414, 415, 424, 425, 438
communication skills, 127, 161, 438
communities, 162, 177, 181, 230, 275, 437
community, 7, 16, 55, 57, 61, 100, 104, 107, 124, 146, 152, 193, 232, 244, 265, 274, 275, 278, 284, 285, 303, 353, 354, 383, 385, 387, 389, 403, 405, 415, 416, 420, 424, 433, 435, 436, 437
community service, 415, 433, 435
community support, 354
co-morbidities, 258
comorbidity, 107, 110, 116, 126, 147, 198
compartment syndrome, 70
compassion, 438
compensation, 7
competence, 104, 110, 113, 119, 237, 385, 412
competency, 391

competition, 370, 371, 372, 377, 381
competitive sport, 387
complexity, 14, 100, 120, 145, 257, 260, 261, 265, 267
compliance, 76, 110, 111, 157, 197, 251, 252, 298, 326
complications, 6, 13, 14, 16, 18, 23, 24, 27, 30, 53, 75, 79, 85, 121, 129, 167, 168, 170, 189, 190, 191, 192, 197, 239, 243, 244, 247, 249, 251, 252, 263, 267, 277, 362, 370, 371, 379, 380, 404
components, 39, 40, 107, 154, 177, 251, 378, 388
composition, 239, 244
compounds, 36, 58, 240
compulsion, 132
computed tomography, 206, 243
computer skills, 415
concentration, 26, 72, 82, 132, 133, 308, 317
conception, 273, 276, 289, 351
conceptual model, 119
conceptualization, 29, 392
conceptualizations, 105
concordance, 128
concrete, 157
concussion, 379
conditioning, 204, 205, 218, 370, 388, 392
conductance, 43
conduction, 239
conductive, 208
confidence, 58, 105, 153, 155, 159, 224, 225, 362, 408, 411
confidence interval, 58, 224, 225, 408
confidence intervals, 224, 225, 408
confidentiality, 423
conflict, 275
conformity, 145
confusion, 179, 379, 386
congenital adrenal hyperplasia, 297
congenital heart disease, xi, 3, 115, 120, 203, 378, 404, 429
congenital malformations, 342
congestive heart failure, 29
conjecture, 422
connective tissue, 214, 379
consensus, 196, 231, 346, 390, 413, 420
Consensus Development Conference, 430
consent, 29, 85, 174, 274, 275, 290, 345, 407
consolidation, 15
constipation, 20, 85, 239, 241, 242, 244, 344, 361
construction, 131, 228
consultants, 301
consumers, 423
consumption, 92, 94, 106, 204, 207
continuity, 7, 425

contraceptives, 44, 67, 68, 169, 293, 297, 301, 302, 304
contractions, 370, 371
control group, 138, 193
controlled studies, 115, 309
controlled trials, 307
convection, 370
cooking, 229
cooling, 208, 370
coping, 10, 104, 107, 174, 182, 184, 185
coping strategies, 6, 104, 113, 264
coping strategy, 182
coronary arteries, 377
coronary heart disease, 384
corpus callosum, 168
correlation, 68, 114, 193, 217
corticosteroid therapy, 208
corticosteroids, 156, 208, 209, 217, 223, 229, 239, 295, 301
corticotropin, 44
cortisol, 39, 44
cosmetics, 295, 298
costs, 93, 124, 148, 156, 192, 207, 399, 420
cotton, 295
cough, 14, 15, 206, 208, 213
coughing, 169, 376
counseling, 26, 59, 157, 192, 197, 345, 420
couples, 154
course work, 195
covering, 360, 438
COX-2 inhibitors, 308
coxa vara, 313
craniopharyngioma, 36
cranium, 302
craving, 248
creatine, 340, 345
creatinine, 248, 252, 340
creativity, 131
CRH, 44
crisis intervention, 130, 131
critical period, 147
cross-sectional, 48, 113, 127, 162, 286, 351, 405
cross-sectional study, 286
crying, 89, 169, 238
cryopreservation, 29, 41
cultural differences, 427, 428
cultural factors, 125
cultural norms, 159
cultural practices, 125
culture, 124, 194, 206
curriculum, 353
CVD, 194
cyanotic, 115

cycles, 103, 286, 290
cycling, 40, 388
cyclophosphamide, 29, 40, 46
cyproterone acetate, 293, 294, 301, 302, 303
cyst, 296
cystic acne, 301
cystic fibrosis, xi, 3, 13, 16, 19, 43, 48, 113, 119, 120, 182, 203, 204, 214, 217, 218, 239, 240, 241, 242, 377, 404, 419, 426, 429, 438
cysts, 294, 296
cytogenetics, 341
cytokines, 76, 206, 216
cytoplasm, 61
cytosine, 25

D

daily care, 278
daily living, 28, 170, 206, 277, 278, 320
data collection, 68, 83, 405, 406
data set, 9
database, 231, 267
deafness, 302
death, 68, 93, 112, 116, 130, 132, 148, 190, 197, 251, 342, 376, 377, 378, 381, 417, 435
death rate, 130
deaths, 191
debridement, 18, 20, 329, 335
debt, 397
debt service, 397
decision making, 323
decisions, 105, 153, 160, 191, 404, 410, 411, 425
decubitus ulcer, 17, 20, 371
deductive reasoning, 153
defecation, 241
defects, 13, 20, 58, 59, 61, 71, 120, 215, 242, 295, 299, 341, 342, 371, 378, 379
defense, 341
deficiency, 29, 36, 38, 39, 41, 42, 43, 44, 45, 58, 59, 60, 66, 67, 74, 241, 249, 284, 285, 288, 296, 297, 317, 340, 341, 345
deficit, 26, 27, 28, 37, 46, 68, 77, 112, 168, 169, 258, 259, 263, 342
deficits, 26, 28, 35, 36, 37, 39, 45, 52, 68, 70, 71, 76, 162, 167, 170, 206, 258, 370, 371
definition, 3, 4, 9, 181, 221, 223, 239, 279
deformation, 361
deformities, 214, 215, 218, 362
dehydration, 60, 71, 74, 207
dehydroepiandrosterone (DHEA), 44, 294
dehydrogenase, 296, 297
delayed gastric emptying, 243
delayed puberty, 42, 43, 44

delinquency, 123, 138, 139, 143
delivery, 19, 76, 105, 229, 250, 273, 276, 277, 278, 279, 308, 398, 412, 415
dementia, 15, 19, 61, 249, 250, 364
demographic data, 130
demographics, 72
denial, 7, 110
Denmark, 4, 436, 443
density, 42, 43, 44, 45, 49, 75, 79, 236, 237, 293
dental treatments, 399
dentist, 398, 399
dentistry, 397
dentists, 397, 399, 400
Department of Education, 424, 442
Department of Health and Human Services, 19, 200, 207, 210, 211, 280, 417
deposition, 76, 299
depressed, 157, 193, 352
depressive disorder, 117, 126
depressive symptoms, 79, 110, 111, 193, 199
deprivation, 41, 208, 237
dermatitis, 295, 296
dermatologic, 52
dermatologist, 300
dermatologists, 299
dermatology, 301
dermatomyositis, 239
desert, 232
destruction, 43, 204, 206
destructive process, 326
detachment, 329, 379
detection, 41, 57, 59, 60, 61, 195, 240, 259, 262, 346
detergents, 295
developed countries, 109, 116, 189
developing countries, 116
developmental delay, 59, 61, 85, 101, 247, 259, 345, 347, 425
developmental disabilities, 55, 62, 161, 203, 237, 244, 276, 281, 355, 391, 426
developmental disorder, 244
developmental factors, 163
developmental process, 106, 127
developmental psychology, 127, 413
deviant behaviour, 133, 141
diabetes, 6, 42, 43, 44, 48, 52, 53, 54, 61, 76, 100, 106, 111, 117, 118, 155, 156, 180, 192, 197, 206, 239, 248, 251, 257, 296, 299, 376, 377, 379, 380, 404, 426, 429, 430, 438
diabetes mellitus, 42, 43, 44, 53, 111, 117, 118, 155, 197, 239, 299, 376, 377, 379, 380, 438
Diagnostic and Statistical Manual of Mental Disorders, 124
diagnostic criteria, 43

dialysis, 247, 248, 249, 250, 251, 253, 256, 257, 259, 260, 261, 262, 263, 264, 265, 266, 267, 268, 269
diarrhea, 59, 60, 243, 299, 371
diet, 3, 42, 48, 59, 60, 125, 156, 192, 236, 241, 249, 250, 259, 380, 390, 393
dietary, 42, 59, 111, 124, 191, 236, 241, 243, 249, 250, 340, 385, 387
dieting, 107, 111, 125, 153, 196
diets, 400
differential diagnosis, 293, 302
diffusion, 205
DiGeorge Syndrome, 37
diphenhydramine, 85, 89
direct cost, 124
disabled, 4, 5, 6, 7, 59, 236, 237, 262, 275, 276, 279, 290, 373, 374, 397, 398, 400
discipline, 351
discomfort, 180, 214, 264, 265, 274, 322, 360
discriminant analysis, 140
discrimination, 156, 274, 284
diseases, xi, 3, 13, 14, 57, 59, 60, 61, 65, 66, 67, 69, 71, 72, 119, 169, 189, 190, 191, 205, 232, 242, 244, 248, 257, 265, 286, 303, 312, 373, 384, 404
disequilibrium, 273, 279
dislocation, 317, 329, 330, 331, 334, 335, 361
dislocations, 170, 379
displacement, 7
disposition, 343
dissatisfaction, 102, 103, 111, 124
distortions, 102
distraction, 179, 182, 213
distress, 6, 15, 60, 132, 214, 412
distribution, 15, 85, 91, 131, 133, 175, 217, 257, 429
diuretics, 103, 239
diversity, 284, 358
diving, 168, 372, 387
division, 435, 436
divorce, 352
dizygotic, 128
dizygotic twins, 128
dizziness, 85, 90, 92, 299
DNA, 343
doctors, 159, 225, 226, 229, 230, 289, 419, 423
dogs, 67
donor, 251, 260
dopamine, 240
Doppler, 72, 76, 80, 194
dosage, 94, 343
dosing, 17, 44, 82, 93, 94, 242
Down syndrome, 5, 52, 53, 54, 56, 168, 236, 239, 283, 288, 290, 342, 349, 350, 351, 352, 353, 354, 355, 356, 358, 385, 390, 391
draft, 406

drainage, 206, 295, 301
drinking, 113, 371
drought, 429
drowsiness, 85, 90, 92
drug addict, 75
drug addiction, 75
drug delivery, 308, 309
drug therapy, 260
drug withdrawal, 75
drug-induced, 295
drugs, 17, 54, 72, 112, 160, 168, 240, 241, 263, 307, 309, 373, 422
drying, 16, 287
DSM-IV, 77, 121, 124, 162
duality, 422
ductus arteriosus, 302
duplication, 343, 346
duration, 3, 4, 15, 114, 128, 129, 131, 137, 209, 213, 218, 320, 360
dust, 224, 228, 231
dysarthria, 170
dyskinesia, 212
dysphagia, 239
dysplasia, 203, 204, 215, 219, 257, 311, 312, 313, 317, 318, 319, 320, 321, 322, 323, 324, 326, 333, 334, 335
dyspnea, 71, 74
dysthymia, 114
dystonia, 168
dystonic reactions, 240

E

E. coli, 14, 17, 18
ears, 61, 302, 342, 343, 344
Eastern Europe, 110
eating behavior, 103, 111
eating disorder, 103, 107, 117, 119, 123, 124, 125, 127, 130, 139, 145, 146, 147, 193
eating disorders, 49, 103, 114, 123, 124, 125, 126, 127, 128, 129, 130, 131, 133, 134, 136, 137, 138, 139, 140, 141, 142, 143, 144, 145, 146, 147, 148, 193, 195, 380, 423
eating disturbances, 144
echolalia, 169
economic status, 133, 224
eczema, 100
edema, 70, 248, 277
educational attainment, 195
educational programs, 285
educational services, 4, 405
educational system, 7
educators, 285, 414

Einstein, Albert, 3
egg, 350
Ehlers-Danlos syndrome, 214
elaboration, 406
elbows, 69
elderly, 310
elderly population, 310
electrolyte, 129, 239, 261
electrolyte imbalance, 129
electrolytes, 43, 194, 239
elementary school, 393
email, 255, 421
emancipation, 153, 154, 156, 159
emboli, 67, 239
embolism, 78
embolization, 67
embryo, 29, 350
emergency department, 86
emergency departments, 416
emission, 31
emotion, 101, 137, 181, 260, 265
emotional disorder, 101, 116, 131, 134, 138
emotional health, 162, 193, 384, 386
emotional reactions, 6, 152
emotional responses, 152
emotional stability, 284, 288
emotional well-being, 72, 107, 145
emotionality, 131, 132
emotions, 155, 156, 238
empathy, 126
employment, 26, 29, 258, 274, 349, 353, 355, 406, 408, 409, 415, 422
employment status, 26
empowerment, 105, 266, 363, 414, 416
encephalitis, 168
encephalopathy, 344
encopresis, 242
encouragement, 385, 387
endocrine, 16, 35, 36, 37, 43, 44, 45, 46, 49, 51, 52, 53, 54, 55, 189, 293, 301, 341
endocrine disorders, 45, 52
endocrinological, 53
endocrinology, 45, 46, 49, 301, 426
end-stage kidney disease, 258, 262
end-stage renal disease, 107, 252, 256, 261, 262, 268
endurance, 206, 370, 386, 388
enemas, 242
energy, 43, 44, 45, 49, 53, 57, 58, 60, 61, 101, 105, 154, 191, 192, 236, 244
engagement, 176, 385, 421, 422, 427, 428
England, 55, 351, 364
enlargement, 276, 296
enrollment, 90

entrapment, 372
enuresis, 20, 41, 111, 117, 169
environment, 7, 36, 101, 152, 153, 154, 155, 195, 224, 228, 232, 240, 288, 357, 359, 360, 361, 362, 363
environmental conditions, 228
environmental factors, 116, 128, 231
enzyme induction, 169
enzymes, 58, 308
epidemic, 121, 189, 190, 198, 200
epidemics, 8
epidemiologic studies, 102, 248
epidemiology, 8, 20, 30, 118, 119, 146, 147, 183, 232, 310, 369
epidermis, 18
epilepsy, 100, 111, 112, 113, 118, 167, 168, 169, 170, 340, 376, 377, 379, 380
epiphysis, 334
epistaxis, 301
epithelial transport, 43
equilibrium, 289, 361, 386
equity, 421, 422, 423
erythematous, 294
erythropoietin, 249, 250, 258
esophagitis, 240
esophagus, 239, 240, 241, 299
essential fatty acids, 235
estradiol, 294, 303
estrogen, 39, 40, 44, 296
ethical principles, 438
ethnic background, 72, 408
ethnic groups, 320, 357
ethnicity, 72, 102, 310, 385
etiologic factor, 255, 257
etiology, 36, 79, 189, 240, 242, 243, 248, 249, 257, 258, 262, 312, 333, 340, 345
Europe, 4, 5, 9, 19, 309
European Commission, 9
European Union, 113, 119
evacuation, 241
evening, 388
examinations, 263, 349, 353, 355, 387
excess demand, 104
excision, 27, 295
exclusion, 248, 386
excretion, 237, 239
excuse, 179
executive function, 127
executive functions, 127
exertion, 378, 380, 391
exocrine, 16
expenditures, 5, 8, 10, 237
expertise, 182, 257, 266, 329, 422

exposure, 16, 18, 29, 40, 41, 69, 152, 153, 154, 161, 168, 216, 225, 227, 228, 229, 231, 240, 298, 299, 339, 372, 387
expressivity, 72
eye, 169, 358, 362, 371, 376, 377
eye contact, 362
eyes, 61, 342, 344, 362, 380

F

factor analysis, 132
factor VIII, 66, 69
factorial, 132
FAI, 311, 312, 314, 317, 319, 320, 321, 323, 325, 326, 327, 329, 330, 331, 332, 333
failure, 17, 26, 39, 40, 42, 44, 47, 59, 101, 237, 241, 242, 258, 262, 298, 342, 399, 404
failure to thrive, 39, 42, 44, 59, 241, 242
familial, 125, 128, 140, 144, 214, 257, 289, 296, 345, 346
family environment, 160
family functioning, 429
family history, 130, 194, 196, 299, 376, 378
family income, 408
family life, 130, 264
family medicine, 441
family members, 104, 133, 156, 259, 276, 339, 343, 345, 363, 415
family physician, 7, 231, 349, 354
family planning, 273, 274, 275, 276, 278, 279
family relationships, 102, 123, 129, 141, 155
family structure, 128
family support, 160, 265, 415
family therapy, 162
fast food, 259
fasting, 125, 194
fat, 14, 124, 199, 200, 235, 236, 239, 240, 341, 387
fatalities, 129
fatigue, 74, 159, 214, 236, 237, 261, 277, 320, 376
fats, 235
fatty acid, 58, 59, 235, 294
fatty acids, 294
fear, 69, 103, 115, 132, 157, 158, 264, 284, 362, 403, 409, 412
fears, 102, 113, 120, 157, 403
fecal impaction, 242
feces, 18, 242
feedback, 105, 214, 362, 404, 414, 415, 425
feeding, 15, 19, 169, 170, 237, 238, 240, 242, 243, 244, 276
feelings, 113, 124, 126, 128, 132, 161, 181, 289, 407, 410, 413
feet, 175, 361

femoral neck, 312, 313, 317, 327, 334
femur, 313, 320
fertility, 29, 31, 41, 42, 47, 353, 422
fertilization, 41
fetal, 72, 216, 276, 299
fetus, 53, 169
fever, 15, 60, 85, 236, 238, 294, 295, 301
fiber, 240, 241
fibers, 28, 360
fibrinogen, 69
fibroma, 297
fibromyalgia, 181, 182, 184, 185
fibrosis, xi, 3, 5, 13, 16, 19, 29, 37, 43, 48, 113, 119, 120, 152, 182, 203, 204, 205, 214, 216, 217, 218, 237, 239, 240, 241, 242, 377, 404, 418, 419, 425, 426, 429, 438
filtration, 248, 257, 258
financial distress, 159
financial planning, 353
financial resources, 416
financial support, 386
financing, 229, 409
fine tuning, 154
Finland, 4, 442
first degree relative, 148, 378, 379
FISH, 341, 342
fitness, 206, 207, 216, 218, 219, 376, 383, 384, 385, 386, 387, 388, 389, 390, 391, 392, 393
fixation, 331, 332
flank, 70
flatulence, 42
flexibility, 152, 370, 388
flora, 15, 294, 299, 302
flow, 66, 67, 205, 206, 213, 214, 215, 225, 226, 228, 229, 232, 277, 285, 287, 288, 362
flow rate, 215
fluid, 15, 41, 206, 236, 239, 241, 250, 260, 261, 308, 387
fluoride, 399
fluorinated, 295
fluoroscopy, 243
focus group, 173, 174, 175, 176
focusing, 179, 182, 260, 341, 351, 413, 425
follicle, 294, 296
follicles, 294
follicular, 296
folliculitis, 294, 295, 299
food, 42, 57, 58, 61, 103, 126, 190, 196, 238, 239, 241, 259, 342
Food and Drug Administration (FDA), 42, 43, 307, 309, 310
food intake, 58, 103
football, 372

forgiveness, 158
fractionation, 36
fracture, 308, 313, 320, 371
fractures, 27, 28, 42, 48, 54, 75, 251, 334, 371, 372
France, 418
freedoms, 159, 279
friction, 18, 295, 372
friendship, 103, 184
fruit juice, 190
fruits, 190
frustration, 156, 238, 298
FSH, 41
functional approach, 182
functional aspects, 354
funding, 422, 425
funds, 416, 438
fundus, 241
fungal, 238
fungal infection, 238
fusion, 144

G

gait, 170, 242, 358
galactorrhea, 54
gallbladder disease, 206
games, 168
gametes, 29, 39
gangrene, 70
gas, 204, 205, 216, 229, 240, 241
gas exchange, 204, 205, 216
gases, 205
gastric, 14, 206, 239, 240, 241, 242, 243, 308
gastric mucosa, 308
gastric ulcer, 239
gastroesophageal reflux, 15, 203, 244, 250, 252
gastroesophageal reflux disease, 203
gastrointestinal, 15, 59, 60, 61, 235, 236, 237, 238, 240, 241, 299, 308
gastrointestinal tract, 235, 238, 241
gastroparesis, 240
gastrostomy, 242, 243
gel, 298, 300, 309, 310
gels, 40
gender, 25, 85, 102, 128, 131, 133, 138, 142, 144, 154, 182, 190, 223, 228, 257, 286, 383, 385, 406, 409, 411
gender differences, 138, 142
gender role, 154
gene, 19, 43, 60, 61, 72, 110, 237, 339, 344, 347
gene therapy, 60, 61
general anesthesia, 398, 400
general practitioner, 256, 274, 425, 428

general practitioners, 274, 425, 428
generalized seizures, 168
generation, 249, 251, 304, 311
genes, 340, 343
genetic defect, 57, 58
genetic disease, 205
genetic disorders, 59
genetic factors, 116, 339
genetic syndromes, 236, 398
genetics, 29, 339, 346
genome, 61, 343, 346
genomic, 341, 343, 346
genotype, 72, 78, 85, 408, 411
genotypes, 72, 75
Germany, 123, 129, 130, 365, 442
germline mutations, 347
gerontology, 441
girls, 39, 40, 44, 46, 60, 68, 73, 114, 169, 184, 192, 199, 214, 231, 290, 351, 360, 361, 362, 364, 390
gland, 36, 293, 294, 296
glasses, 376
globulin, 296
glomerulonephritis, 257, 262
glottis, 213
glucagon, 47
gluconeogenesis, 58
glucose, 6, 43, 53, 111, 157, 194, 239
glucose tolerance, 43, 53
glycans, 341
glycine, 340, 345
glycoconjugates, 341
glycol, 242, 296
glycoprotein, 60, 341
glycosylation, 341, 345, 346
goal setting, 161
goals, 6, 25, 26, 100, 229, 236, 285, 286, 287, 360, 361, 363, 388
going to school, 261
gold, 240, 248, 333, 427
gold standard, 240, 248, 333, 427
gonadal dysgenesis, 297
gonadotropin, 40, 44, 293, 301
gonadotropin-releasing hormone (GnRH), 301
gonads, 47
governance, 429
government, 400, 435
grades, 75, 116, 177, 389
grading, 297
gram negative, 17, 238
Gram-negative, 14, 15, 294
Gram-positive, 14
grants, 229
grass, 435

Graves disease, 53
Greece, 433, 438
group activities, 177
growth factor, 38, 48, 49, 216, 249
growth factors, 49, 216
growth hormone, 36, 38, 44, 45, 46, 47, 48, 49, 55, 249, 250, 251, 256, 258, 259, 268
growth spurt, 37, 153
guardian, 85, 407, 413, 414
guidance, 151, 284, 386, 423
guidelines, 49, 193, 195, 209, 218, 222, 229, 230, 231, 252, 259, 299, 352, 372, 373, 375, 381, 387, 388, 389, 416
guilt, 69, 132, 158
gynecologist, 274, 275

H

H_2, 142
hair cells, 28
hair follicle, 293, 296
half-life, 84
haloperidol, 169
handicapped, 236, 237, 358, 398, 419, 420
handling, 357
hands, 175, 360
hanging, 321
happiness, 363
hardships, 102, 363
hate, 178
hazards, 387
head injuries, 114
head injury, 114, 120, 379
headache, 299, 371
healing, xi, 18, 20, 240
Health and Human Services, 19, 200, 207, 210, 211, 280, 417
health care professionals, 159, 178, 180, 181, 182, 183, 198, 423, 428, 430
health care system, 77, 264, 274, 276, 277, 279, 418, 422, 423, 427, 428
health education, 228, 424
health expenditure, 5
health information, 426
health insurance, 5, 229, 406, 408, 416, 422
health problems, 102, 192, 197, 200, 349, 354, 384, 404, 438
health services, 55, 124, 284, 421, 422, 423, 426, 427, 428
health status, 8, 55, 99, 263, 377, 384, 390, 427
healthcare, 29, 101, 109, 115, 192, 267, 277, 280, 354, 403, 404, 407, 408, 409, 412, 413, 419, 428

hearing, 28, 29, 31, 61, 113, 116, 121, 132, 169, 353, 359, 376
hearing impairment, 113, 376
hearing loss, 29, 31, 116, 121, 169
heart, xi, 3, 4, 5, 29, 53, 61, 76, 91, 100, 106, 115, 120, 152, 198, 199, 203, 207, 209, 210, 211, 218, 302, 378, 379, 384, 389, 404, 416, 417, 418, 429
heart disease, xi, 3, 4, 5, 53, 61, 100, 106, 115, 120, 378, 384, 404, 429
heart murmur, 378, 379
heart rate, 91, 209
heat, 218, 370, 371, 376, 377, 380
heat illness, 377, 380
heat loss, 370, 371
height, 37, 39, 42, 45, 46, 48, 85, 103, 191, 192, 235, 236, 241, 250, 258, 263, 264, 278, 352, 379
helmets, 295
hemarthrosis, 69
hematocrit, 75
hematological, 65, 66, 68, 69, 76
hematology, 83, 85, 92, 417
hematomas, 69, 70
hematopoietic, 46
hematopoietic stem cell, 46
hematuria, 70, 71, 248
hemisphere, 24
hemodialysis, 251, 253, 256, 260, 261, 262
hemodynamic, 198
hemoglobin, 65, 66, 72, 76, 85, 86, 409, 413
hemoglobinopathies, 65, 66, 71, 72, 76
hemoglobinopathy, 406
hemolytic anemia, 299
hemophilia, 66, 68, 69, 70, 77, 78, 426
hemophilia a, 78
hemophiliacs, 68, 77
hemorrhage, 67, 68, 77
hemorrhages, 69, 70, 71, 78
hemostasis, 65, 66
hemostatic, 68
hepatitis, 299
hepatomegaly, 380
hepatotoxicity, 239
heroin, 160
heterogeneity, 124, 125
heterogeneous, 58, 60
hidradenitis suppurativa, 295, 299
high blood pressure, 67, 191, 192, 198, 297
high density lipoprotein, 53
high resolution, 206, 216
high risk, 25, 28, 40, 67, 73, 114, 115, 192, 197, 277, 369, 373, 383, 384
high school, 26, 177, 180, 390, 408, 415, 425
high-fat, 240

high-risk, 110, 268, 280
hip, 170, 311, 312, 313, 317, 320, 321, 323, 326, 329, 330, 333, 334, 335, 360
HIP, 83
hip joint, 317, 323, 329, 333
hip replacement, 317
hips, 69, 75, 335, 361, 379
hirsutism, 303
Hispanic, 72, 107, 257
histamine, 214
HIV, 37, 77, 115, 121
HIV infection, 115, 121
HIV/AIDS, 37, 115, 121
HIV-1, 121
HLA, 42, 251
hockey, 320, 377
holistic, 76, 279, 435
holistic approach, 76
homeostasis, 237, 256, 266
homosexuality, 125
honesty, 160
hopelessness, 132
hormonal therapy, 45
hormone, 29, 36, 38, 39, 40, 41, 42, 43, 44, 45, 46, 47, 48, 49, 54, 55, 76, 240, 249, 250, 251, 256, 258, 259, 268, 293, 296, 297, 301
hormones, 38, 52, 53, 55, 286
hospital, 17, 74, 81, 82, 83, 86, 91, 92, 101, 104, 105, 173, 177, 178, 179, 180, 214, 225, 228, 230, 244, 265, 276, 352, 398, 422, 424, 425, 428, 430
hospitalization, 4, 7, 73, 82, 86, 87, 88, 89, 90, 91, 92, 106, 114, 115, 116, 120, 263, 268
hospitalizations, 7, 74, 82, 93, 121, 213, 261, 415
hospitalized, 17, 70, 83, 93, 94, 110, 206
hospitals, 83, 416, 423, 424, 425, 429
host, 341
hostility, 6, 132, 138, 139
house dust, 228
household, 406, 408, 409
household income, 408
housing, xi, 3, 221, 222, 224
HPA, 39
HSCT, 37, 40
human, 16, 38, 42, 47, 49, 52, 57, 59, 61, 71, 121, 147, 258, 290, 350, 363, 399, 434, 441, 443
human development, 57, 61, 434, 441, 443
human genome, 61
human immunodeficiency virus, 121
human kinetics, 373, 390, 392
human leukocyte antigen, 42
humanity, 284
humans, 59, 66, 67, 239
humidity, 228

hyaline, 219
hybridization, 341, 343, 346
hydration, 371, 377, 380
hydro, 295
hydrocephalus, 20, 371, 372
hydrops, 73
hydroxide, 242
hygiene, 15, 109, 283, 285, 287, 288, 290, 295, 297, 398, 399
hyperactivity, 68, 77, 112, 131, 168, 169
hypercholesterolemia, 192, 378
hypercoagulable, 67
hyperglycemia, 111, 239
hyperinflation, 216
hyperkalemia, 249
hyperlipidemia, 297, 299, 378
hypernatremia, 41
hyperparathyroidism, 248, 249, 250, 258
hyperplasia, 69, 75, 296, 297
hyperprolactinemia, 42
hyperreactivity, 216
hypersensitivity, 299, 362
hypertelorism, 342
hypertension, 53, 76, 152, 189, 191, 192, 193, 194, 195, 196, 197, 198, 199, 248, 249, 252, 257, 258, 268, 371, 376, 378, 384
hypertensive, 193, 197
hyperthermia, 369, 371
hyperthyroidism, 38
hypertonic saline, 206
hypertriglyceridemia, 53
hypertrophic cardiomyopathy, 377, 379
hypertrophy, 261, 317
hypnosis, 214
hypoglycemia, 39, 53, 111, 156
hypogonadism, 39, 40, 41, 44, 76
hypopituitarism, 238
hypoplasia, 257
hypotension, 39, 85, 261
hypothalamic, 36, 41, 44, 47, 371
hypothalamus, 36, 38, 39, 41
hypothermia, 369, 371, 373
hypothesis, 142, 143, 144, 193, 275
hypothyroidism, 37, 38, 44, 46, 52, 53, 55, 76, 238, 242, 352
hypotonia, 60, 341, 343, 344, 346
hypoxemia, 15
hypoxia, 339
Hypoxia, 213

I

IASP, 93

IBD, 114
ibuprofen, 85, 206, 310
ICD, 124, 142
ice hockey, 320
ICU, 115
identification, 72, 111, 125, 127, 131, 346, 387, 407, 428
identity, 6, 69, 102, 154, 182, 350
idiopathic, 112, 118, 312, 313, 346, 429
idiosyncratic, 173, 182
IFG, 43
IgE, 208, 232
IGF, 38, 42, 43, 44, 49, 55
IGF-1, 38, 42, 43, 44, 49
IL-4, 349
IL-8, 51
ileostomy, 236
imagery, 182
images, 103, 155
imaging, 39, 40, 194, 242, 323, 333
imbalances, 346
immigration, 110
immunosuppressive, 257
impaired glucose tolerance, 43, 53
impairments, 25, 28, 67, 69, 73, 83, 85, 119, 167, 168, 170, 176, 241, 275, 277, 364, 369, 373, 386
implants, 301
implementation, 52, 222, 229, 273, 387, 389, 405, 415, 424
impulsive, 112, 130, 387
impulsivity, 126, 127, 129
in situ, 189, 260, 331, 332, 341
in situ hybridization, 341
in transition, 361, 419, 423, 424, 429
in utero, 73
in vitro, 208
in vivo, 208
inactivation, 54, 363
inactive, 309, 384, 389
inattention, 115
incentive, 59, 192, 407
inclusion, 145, 283, 284, 289, 405, 407, 426
income, 5, 274, 397, 399, 408
incurable, 205
independence, 6, 26, 101, 103, 104, 106, 127, 153, 155, 160, 161, 266, 284, 285, 288, 349, 350, 351, 355, 361, 404, 422, 425
independent variable, 259
India, 24, 115, 433, 438
indication, 42, 128, 144, 145, 195, 250
indicators, 4, 9, 384, 390
indigenous, 422
individual development, 162

individual differences, 349
individuality, 181
induction, 169, 208, 209, 277
industrialized countries, 24, 115, 222
inert, 249
infancy, 20, 190, 241, 242, 256, 268, 340, 354, 356, 371
infant care, 278
infants, 19, 59, 62, 79, 101, 183, 244, 250, 251, 252, 279, 285, 355, 419
infarction, 29, 78
infection, 14, 15, 16, 17, 18, 19, 20, 24, 27, 60, 73, 82, 83, 115, 121, 203, 206, 216, 217, 238, 239, 242, 257, 263, 294, 295, 297, 371, 378
infections, 16, 17, 20, 44, 48, 116, 167, 170, 238, 263, 268, 344, 353, 404
infectious, xi, 3, 13, 14, 18, 52, 212, 380
infectious disease, xi, 3, 18, 52
infectious diseases, 52
infectious mononucleosis, 380
inferences, 389
inferiority, 132
infertility, 29, 43
infestations, 238
inflammation, 16, 19, 67, 206, 207, 208, 216, 294, 297, 308
inflammatory, 14, 69, 76, 85, 114, 119, 120, 206, 208, 209, 212, 216, 217, 230, 238, 239, 249, 294, 295, 299, 300, 303, 307, 308, 309, 310
inflammatory bowel disease, 114, 119, 120, 238
inflammatory cells, 206
inflammatory disease, 216
inflammatory response, 14, 206, 216
inflation, 143
influenza, 212
information exchange, 404
informed consent, 275, 345
infrastructure, 417
ingest, 238, 387
ingestion, 18
inguinal, 320
inguinal hernia, 320
inhalation, 209, 229
inhaler, 156, 221, 225, 226
inheritance, 344, 347
inherited, 57, 59, 62, 66, 67, 68, 71, 72, 82, 116, 341
inherited disorder, 59, 67, 82
inhibition, 59, 123, 126, 130, 132, 138, 139, 143, 144, 308, 309, 371, 384
inhibitor, 69
inhibitors, 29, 208, 209, 240, 303, 308
inhibitory, 39

initiation, 27, 35, 41, 45, 84, 92, 189, 192, 208, 258, 260, 261, 385, 387
injection, 243, 295, 301
injections, 256, 259
injuries, 100, 114, 143, 156, 238, 307, 308, 309, 310, 335, 369, 370, 372, 374, 376, 379, 381
injury, 15, 17, 18, 19, 28, 39, 66, 68, 114, 120, 132, 136, 143, 167, 168, 170, 197, 216, 239, 242, 296, 297, 308, 309, 310, 317, 321, 369, 370, 371, 372, 373, 374, 376, 378, 379, 387
innervation, 17, 239
innominate, 326
insecurity, 123, 138, 143, 144, 362
insight, 7, 240, 415
inspection, 214
inspiration, 213
instability, 27, 312, 317, 320, 321, 326, 352, 358, 370
instinct, 274
institutionalization, 354
institutions, 55, 398, 400, 416
instruction, 175, 275, 380, 416
instrumental support, 105
instruments, 76, 83, 196, 360, 361, 403
insulin, 16, 38, 43, 44, 48, 49, 111, 117, 156, 249, 297, 380
insulin dependent diabetes, 156
insulin resistance, 297
insulin-like growth factor, 38, 48, 49, 249
insulin-like growth factor I, 48
insurance, 5, 8, 229, 310, 398, 406, 408, 416
insurance companies, 229
integration, 49, 174, 284, 285, 289, 362, 364
integrity, 204, 438
integument, 302
intellectual development, 157
intellectual disabilities, 55, 247, 274, 275, 280
intellectual flexibility, 161
intellectualization, 7
intelligence, 25, 123, 130, 131, 133, 134, 143, 152, 160, 390, 392
intelligence quotient, 123, 130, 131, 134, 143, 390
intensive care unit, 216
interaction, 7, 104, 207, 237, 274, 284, 288, 289, 359, 360, 363
interactions, 100, 159, 177, 178, 286
interdependence, 204
interdisciplinary, 273, 276, 278, 441
interference, 35, 36, 265
internal fixation, 331, 332
internalizing, 110, 115
internet, 232, 426, 443
internist, 404

interpersonal contact, 359
interpersonal relations, 126, 144, 360
interpersonal relationships, 126, 144
interphase, 342
intersex, 297
interstitial, 216, 248, 250
interval, 83, 84, 91, 263, 266, 419
intervention, 60, 145, 157, 196, 221, 222, 230, 241, 258, 259, 262, 311, 326, 351, 354, 357, 359, 360, 362, 363, 365, 372, 391, 414
interview, 4, 7, 116, 130, 131, 132, 173, 175, 415
interviews, 6, 115, 351, 387, 403, 406, 411
intimacy, 154
intoxication, 250
intracranial, 47, 68, 77, 372
intracranial pressure, 372
intramuscular, 40, 70
intramuscular injection, 40
intravascular, 249
intravenous, 25, 77, 83, 249
intrinsic, 74
introversion, 131, 132
invasive, 330, 333
inventions, 312
inversion, 347
iodine, 38
ionizing radiation, 295
IQ, 123, 127, 133, 134, 137, 339
iris, 379
iron, 73, 74, 76, 249, 250
iron deficiency, 249
irradiation, 25, 28, 37, 38, 39, 40, 41, 45, 46, 47
irrigation, 242, 244
irritability, 116
irritation, 239, 298, 299
ischaemic heart disease, 106
ischemia, 67, 68, 243
ischemic, 53
ischemic heart disease, 53
isolation, 24, 58, 104, 126, 128, 132, 154, 169, 181, 285, 288, 289, 427
Israel, x, 4, 9, 24, 51, 52, 54, 55, 56, 57, 59, 349, 352, 355, 357, 364, 365, 383, 434, 435, 438, 441, 443
Italy, 148, 365

J

JAMA, 19, 118, 197, 198, 252, 303
jaw, 344
Jews, 24
jobs, 195
joining, 323

joint damage, 317
joints, 28, 67, 69, 70, 359, 379
Jordan, 117
judgment, 153, 387
jumping, 19, 311
Jun, 121, 231, 232, 290
junior high, 390
junior high school, 390
juvenile idiopathic arthritis (JIA), 112, 118
juvenile rheumatoid arthritis, 42, 48, 312

K

K^+, 240
karyotype, 341, 342
karyotyping, 343
Kentucky, x, 8, 51, 57, 99, 189, 190, 191, 198, 255, 273, 280, 281, 283, 307, 349, 357, 383, 433, 434, 435, 436, 442
keratin, 294, 296, 302
keratinocytes, 294
ketamine, 93
kidney, 61, 70, 180, 247, 248, 251, 252, 253, 255, 256, 257, 258, 259, 260, 261, 262, 263, 264, 265, 266, 267, 268, 269, 377
kidney transplant, 251, 256, 258, 260, 261, 262, 263, 264, 265, 267, 268
kidney transplantation, 267, 268
kidneys, 61, 258
killing, 156
kinship network, 105
Kirchhoff, 347
knee, 78, 87, 175, 321, 378
knees, 69, 87
kyphosis, 361

L

labor, 273, 275, 276, 277, 278
lack of control, 274
lactic acid, 58, 296
lambda, 138, 139, 140
language, 94, 116, 131, 153, 174, 196, 224, 276, 278, 342, 344, 346, 351, 362
language delay, 346
laparoscopy, 320
large-scale, 275
late-onset, 296
latex, 369, 370, 372, 373
laughter, 176
law, 274
laxatives, 103

leach, 249
leadership, 416, 427, 438
learning, 6, 25, 26, 61, 68, 69, 71, 106, 112, 160, 162, 168, 169, 259, 276, 284, 288, 289, 340, 341, 342, 343, 346, 347, 359, 362, 384, 385, 391, 418
learning disabilities, 25, 61, 168, 169, 340, 346, 385, 391, 418
learning environment, 160, 169
learning process, 289
left ventricular, 261
leg, 75, 321, 322, 371, 392
leisure, 287
lens, 176
lenses, 301
lesion, 300
lesions, 17, 18, 28, 242, 294, 295, 296, 297, 298, 300, 301, 321, 330, 333, 334, 370, 371, 417
lethargy, 28, 39, 59, 60, 238
leukaemia, 46, 47
leukemia, 5, 24, 25, 26, 29, 30, 38, 45, 47
leukemias, 36
leukocyte, 42
leukocytosis, 294
Leydig cells, 40, 41
life changes, 256
life expectancy, xi, 3, 43, 71, 190, 198, 251, 284, 358, 417, 422
life experiences, 104
life satisfaction, 27, 31
life span, 312, 358, 383
life style, 29, 162, 383, 384, 388, 389
lifelong learning, 438
lifespan, 261, 385, 393
lifestyle, 154, 159, 221, 222, 224, 228, 261, 387, 389, 390, 422
lifestyle changes, 159
lifestyles, 387, 389
life-threatening, 35, 75, 77, 106, 110, 404
lifetime, 110, 114
ligament, 372
likelihood, 73, 111, 130, 193, 195, 360, 415
Likert scale, 131
limitation, 3, 5, 27, 92, 102, 215, 285, 321
limitations, 6, 74, 101, 155, 159, 160, 162, 230, 265, 275, 284, 286, 289, 309, 333, 361, 388, 416
linear, 42, 43, 113, 138, 140, 228
linear regression, 140, 228
lipid, 60, 194, 240, 341, 376
lipid profile, 194
lipids, 57, 58
lipoprotein, 53
listening, 159, 174, 179
lithium, 295, 298

liver, 58, 59, 60, 61, 71, 76, 206, 268, 301, 341, 380
liver disease, 59
loading, 252, 258, 327, 371
local community, 389
local government, 435
localization, 16
location, 27, 67, 81, 82, 85, 91, 93, 94, 175, 260, 277, 283, 320, 321, 406
locus, 107, 343
loneliness, 352, 427
long distance, 386
longevity, 35, 36
longitudinal study, 193, 351, 374, 405
lordosis, 323
loss of consciousness, 14, 379
losses, 235, 237
love, 360
low back pain, 184
low risk, 23, 24
lower esophageal sphincter, 239
low-income, 5
lumbar, 323, 371
lumen, 17
lung, 15, 16, 19, 44, 48, 203, 204, 205, 206, 207, 212, 213, 215, 216, 217, 239, 362, 404
lung disease, 16, 204, 205, 206, 212, 215, 216, 217, 404
lung function, 19, 44, 48, 203, 205, 206, 207, 212, 215, 217
lungs, 16, 43, 67, 71, 203, 239, 381
lupus, 248, 299
lying, 17, 298, 321
lymphoma, 26
lymphomas, 24

M

macrophages, 15, 240
macules, 344
magical thinking, 101
magnesium, 239, 242
magnetic resonance spectroscopy, 340
mainstream, 181, 342
maintenance, 27, 39, 104, 125, 129, 153, 208, 238, 242, 385, 390
major depression, 147
malabsorption, 16, 42, 59, 206, 237
maladaptive, 123, 126, 130, 141, 144, 161, 385
malaria, 110
male infertility, 43
males, 41, 52, 66, 74, 78, 81, 86, 123, 125, 128, 131, 133, 135, 137, 142, 143, 153, 154, 191, 193, 223, 294, 295, 320, 340, 344, 345, 347, 390, 422

malignancy, 27, 29, 238, 380
malignant, 25, 168
malnutrition, 45, 155, 236, 237, 259
malocclusion, 398
management practices, 231
mandible, 398
manipulation, 238
manufacturer, 299
mapping, 147
Marfan syndrome, 377, 378
marijuana, 160, 377
marital status, 406
market, 308
markets, 308
marriage, 195, 285, 287, 352
marrow, 60, 72
MAS, 231
masculinity, 128
mask, 37, 326
mass spectrometry, 52, 59
mastery, 101, 105
mastication, 398
maternal, 79, 274, 343, 351
mathematics, 68
maturation, 40, 109, 154, 155, 163, 286, 290, 349, 353, 355, 419
maxillary, 75
meals, 249
measurement, 39, 194, 248, 379
measures, 8, 27, 35, 81, 82, 83, 153, 191, 196, 203, 205, 208, 216, 222, 285, 286, 295, 307, 384, 400
mechanical ventilation, 216
meconium, 241
media, 424, 435
median, 16, 206, 216
Medicaid, 398, 408, 409, 416
medical care, 4, 5, 45, 109, 255, 274, 353, 354, 371, 398, 405, 406, 407, 409, 418, 422, 423
Medical Expenditure Panel Survey, 5
medical services, 56
medical student, 435, 437
Medicare, 398, 399, 400, 422
medication, 38, 54, 83, 89, 93, 101, 102, 103, 110, 111, 157, 175, 179, 209, 228, 229, 237, 240, 251, 257, 259, 263, 266, 268, 298, 299, 376, 377
medication compliance, 259
medicine, 7, 13, 18, 60, 65, 66, 67, 77, 162, 170, 191, 203, 221, 225, 226, 302, 303, 310, 350, 373, 377, 379, 381, 392, 399, 417, 427, 433, 434, 435, 438, 441, 443
Medline, 15
melanin, 294, 296
melanoma, 24

membership, 103, 433
membranes, 299
memory, 25, 379, 426
men, 106, 107, 124, 125, 213, 239, 294, 390
menarche, 287
meningitis, 168
menopause, 29, 40
menorrhagia, 77
menstrual cycle, 286, 290, 353
menstruation, 67, 285, 286, 287, 288, 290, 296, 353
mental development, 154
mental disorder, 68, 77, 121
mental health, 5, 54, 68, 99, 100, 101, 102, 103, 104, 105, 106, 107, 116, 121, 169, 170, 190, 193, 195, 196, 197, 262, 351, 372, 384, 424, 435
mental health professionals, 99, 100, 116
mental illness, 100, 133, 195, 200, 296, 399
mental retardation, 55, 59, 62, 112, 168, 169, 170, 280, 345, 346, 347, 355, 358, 386, 390, 391, 392
mentally retarded adolescents, 290
mentoring, 415
messages, 250, 275, 279
meta-analysis, 120, 128
metabolic, 52, 55, 57, 58, 59, 60, 61, 62, 204, 205, 236, 237, 239, 248, 249, 250, 251, 252, 258, 260, 261, 297
metabolic acidosis, 248, 249, 250, 252, 258
metabolic disorder, 60, 62
metabolic pathways, 57, 58
metabolic rate, 238
metabolic syndrome, 258, 297
metabolism, 49, 57, 58, 59, 235, 237, 240, 251
metaphase, 350
methotrexate, 28
methylation, 343
metropolitan area, 340
metyrapone test, 39
mice, 19
microarray, 343
microbial, 294, 302
microcephaly, 342, 354
midbrain, 36, 39
migraine, 184
migraines, 75
migration, 15, 72, 341
mild asthma, 221
mildly depressed, 157
military, 230
milk, 14, 259, 297
mimicking, 218
mineral oils, 14
minority, 125
mirror, 274

mites, 224, 228
mitochondria, 61
mitochondrial, 58, 61
mitral, 378, 379
mitral insufficiency, 379
mitral regurgitation, 378, 379
mitral valve, 378, 379
mitral valve prolapse, 378
mobility, 6, 25, 27, 28, 54, 65, 68, 71, 112, 169, 260, 277, 278, 362
modalities, 25, 28, 35, 36, 42, 44, 71, 73, 75, 258
modality, 27
modeling, 387
models, 15, 146, 152, 153, 389, 421, 422, 426, 427, 428
moderators, 199
modules, 280, 424
molecules, 57, 58
Møller, 46, 47, 48
money, 397
monogenic, 343
monotherapy, 300
montelukast, 209, 218
mood, 77, 115, 118, 125, 128, 193, 199, 360
mood disorder, 125, 128
mood swings, 360
moral development, 6
moral identity, 350
morbidity, xi, 3, 16, 23, 24, 25, 29, 35, 36, 45, 58, 69, 72, 76, 106, 110, 115, 121, 190, 197, 200, 224, 229, 258, 259, 262, 333, 404, 417
morning, 388
morphine, 81, 82, 83, 84, 85, 86, 89, 90, 91, 92, 93, 94, 95
morphological, 311, 312, 313, 317, 320, 323, 326, 331, 333
morphological abnormalities, 311, 312, 323, 331, 333
morphology, 313, 326, 334
mortality, 19, 23, 24, 29, 35, 45, 58, 71, 72, 76, 112, 115, 128, 129, 144, 148, 195, 197, 200, 229, 255, 258, 259, 417
mortality rate, 129, 144, 255, 258
mosaic, 350
motherhood, 280
mothers, 6, 119, 128, 144, 277, 280, 281, 352, 419, 420
motion, 212, 317, 320, 321, 326
motivation, 127, 147, 360, 361, 373, 385
motives, 157
motor function, 25, 28, 370
motor skills, 365
motor tic, 169

motor vehicle accident, 114
mouth, 208, 301, 342, 344, 362
movement, 27, 59, 70, 153, 167, 170, 321, 334, 340, 358, 359, 360, 361, 362, 363, 404, 422
movement disorders, 167, 170, 340
MRA, 194
MRI, 321, 333, 334
MRS, 340
MSW, 403
mucoid, 317
mucosa, 243
mucus, 299
multidimensional, 125
multidisciplinary, 15, 18, 75, 76, 115, 116, 170, 289, 406, 413, 414, 424, 425
multidrug resistance, 18
multi-ethnic, 198
multimedia, 229, 232
multiple factors, 115, 256
multivariate, 5, 224, 226
murmur, 378, 379
muscle, 17, 28, 58, 61, 69, 70, 78, 199, 204, 206, 218, 237, 239, 241, 301, 308, 326, 363, 370, 371
muscle contraction, 370, 371
muscle relaxation, 239
muscle strength, 206, 370, 371
muscle tissue, 237
muscle weakness, 61
muscles, 61, 69, 70, 308, 320, 361
muscular dystrophy, 13, 239, 312
musculoskeletal, 27, 28, 52, 307, 308, 309, 310, 369, 370, 376, 378, 379, 438
musculoskeletal pain, 378
musculoskeletal system, 376
music, 179, 363, 365
music therapy, 365
mutation, 67, 71, 110, 344, 347, 357, 363
mutations, 16, 43, 339, 340, 344, 345, 347, 364
mutual respect, 154
myasthenia gravis, 168
myelodysplasia, 312
myeloid, 46
myelomeningocele, 369, 370, 371, 372, 373
myocardial infarction, 106
myocarditis, 377
myocardium, 58
myopia, 379
myotonic dystrophy, 13

N

narcissistic, 154
narcolepsy, 168
narcotic, 74, 75
nares, 342
nasal polyp, 16
Nash, 374
nation, 200
National Academy of Sciences, 228, 231
National Health Interview Survey (NHIS), 4, 5, 7, 8, 307, 310
National Institutes of Health (NIH), 30, 118, 207, 210, 211, 218, 248, 253, 417, 418, 430
nationality, 131
natural, 78, 217, 249, 251, 277, 284, 317, 333, 350, 399, 416, 417
natural environment, 416
nausea, 24, 42, 85, 89, 90, 92, 132, 238, 261
neck, 25, 26, 29, 31, 38, 112, 169, 175, 295, 313, 317, 320, 323, 327, 334, 376, 379
neck injury, 379
necrosis, 18, 28, 74, 75, 79, 312, 313, 329, 334
negative attitudes, 112, 194, 274
negative body image, 125
negative consequences, 383
negative emotions, 126, 145
negative experiences, 178
negative outcomes, 155
neglect, 105, 127
negotiation, 413
neonatal, 52, 53, 58, 59, 60, 216, 344
neonatal intensive care unit, 216
neonate, 53, 71
neonates, 248
neoplasm, 378
neoplasms, 21, 46, 167, 168, 170
nephritis, 248
nephrologist, 257, 265, 266
nephropathy, 257
nephrotic syndrome, 71
nerve, 239, 302
nerves, 61, 70
nervous system, 60, 77, 162, 235, 362
network, 7, 159, 161, 162, 428
networking, 425
neurobehavioral, 167, 170, 438
neurobiological, 127
neuroblastoma, 26
neurodegenerative diseases, 167, 170
neurogenic, 17, 238, 369, 370, 372, 373
neurogenic bladder, 17, 238, 369, 370, 373
neurological condition, 167, 170
neurological deficit, 167
neurological disease, 169
neurological disorder, 167, 168, 170, 243, 357
neuromotor, 170, 369, 373

Index 465

neuromuscular diseases, 167, 170
neuropsychiatry, 162
neurotic, 123, 131, 133, 134, 136, 137, 138, 139, 140, 141, 142
neurotoxicity, 28
neutrophil, 14
Newton, 303
next generation, 443
NHL, 116
NHS, 124
Nielsen, 348
Niemann-Pick disease, 60
Nissen fundoplication, 243
Nobel Prize, 434
nocturia, 41
nodules, 38, 294, 295, 297
non-clinical, 143
non-Hodgkin lymphoma, 26
nonsmokers, 110
non-steroidal anti-inflammatory drugs (NSAIDs), 85, 239, 307, 308, 309, 310, 326
non-union, 329
nonverbal, 360
normal children, 353
normal development, 162, 283, 344, 398
normalization, 217, 354
norms, 138, 159, 266
NOS, 103
nose, 208, 209, 296, 301, 342, 343
novelty, 145
novelty seeking, 145
nuclei, 41
nurse, 82, 84, 92, 265, 266
nurses, 265, 423
nursing, 19, 94, 184, 413, 419, 427, 435
nursing home, 19
nutrient, 43
nutrients, 42, 235, 239
nutrition, 19, 36, 44, 109, 206, 237, 238, 239, 243, 244, 250, 251, 258, 266, 278, 422
nutritional supplements, 376
nuts, 297
nystagmus, 379

O

obese, 76, 103, 107, 190, 191, 192, 193, 194, 195, 196, 197, 198, 199, 200, 231, 236, 380
obese patients, 195, 198
obesity, 54, 56, 67, 100, 156, 189, 190, 191, 192, 193, 194, 195, 196, 197, 198, 199, 200, 295, 297, 299, 342, 346, 380, 384, 388, 390, 392, 393
observations, 413

obsessive-compulsive, 126, 132, 138, 139
obsessive-compulsive disorder (OCD), 126
obstruction, 14, 17, 67, 216, 239, 240, 295, 404
obstructive sleep apnea, 192
obstructive uropathy, 257
occlusion, 78, 82, 243, 294, 295
occupational, 67, 129, 277, 278
Odds Ratio, 224, 225, 229
oil, 239, 242, 295, 298
oils, 14, 295, 298
older adults, 19, 55, 70
oligomenorrhea, 380
olympics, 390
omeprazole, 240
oncological, 424
oncology, 23, 29, 30,31, 65, 77, 81, 9, 417, 438
online, 55
onycholysis, 299
oocyte, 39, 40, 47
ophthalmic, 59
opioid, 84, 94
opioids, 93, 95
optimal health, 7
optimism, 27
oral, 15, 16, 19, 41, 44, 49, 67, 68, 94, 206, 208, 217, 238, 244, 256, 283, 293, 295, 297, 298, 299, 300, 301, 302, 304, 308, 309, 340, 398, 399
oral antibiotic, 300
oral antibiotics, 300
oral cavity, 398
oral contraceptives, 44, 67, 68, 293, 297, 302, 304
oral health, 399
oral hygiene, 283, 398
organ, 25, 27, 28, 29, 43, 61, 65, 68, 70, 71, 73, 74, 76, 190, 191, 192, 197, 243, 248, 250, 255, 260, 262, 263, 264, 268, 341, 380
organic, 58, 59, 189, 191, 193
organic disease, 189, 193
organism, 206
orientation, 69, 285, 289, 326, 413, 415
orthopaedic, 311, 323, 325, 333, 364
orthopedic surgeon, 323, 326
osteoarthritis, 309, 312, 317, 319, 323, 327, 330, 333, 334
osteomyelitis, 18, 312, 378
osteopenia, 43, 49, 237, 244, 369, 370, 372, 373, 380
osteoporosis, 29, 43, 44, 54, 75, 380, 384, 390
osteosarcoma, 31
osteotomies, 327
osteotomy, 321, 327, 329, 333, 334, 335
ototoxicity, 31
outpatient, 398, 424
outreach programs, 403, 416

ovarian tumor, 296, 297
ovaries, 39, 40, 41, 301, 380
ovary, 40, 294, 296
overeating, 54
overload, 76, 206
overnutrition, 190
overproduction, 36
overtraining, 381
overweight, 102, 107, 189, 190, 191, 192, 193, 194, 196, 197, 198, 231, 385, 390, 393
ovulation, 353
ownership, 180
oxidation, 58
oxygen, 18, 61, 66, 85, 204, 206, 207, 216, 218, 404
oxygen consumption, 204, 207
oxygen saturation, 85
oxygenation, 204, 377
oxyhemoglobin, 207

P

pacing, 178, 182, 183, 185
pain care, 180, 182
pain clinic, 174, 175, 176, 182, 183
pain management, 75, 83, 93, 94, 175, 307, 308, 309
palate, 5, 302
palpebral, 302, 342
palpitations, 376
pancreas, 43, 61, 76
pancreatic, 16
pancreatic insufficiency, 16
PAO, 327
paradox, 13, 275, 279
paradoxical, 212
paralysis, 17, 371
paranoia, 132
parasitic infestation, 238
paraventricular, 41
parenchyma, 206
parenchymal, 216
parental care, 404, 406
parental consent, 29
parenteral, 239
parenting, 278, 281
paresthesia, 28
paresthesias, 70, 380
Parkinson, 61
partial seizure, 168
partnership, 129, 417
partnerships, 437
passive, 128, 224, 228
pathogenesis, 20, 190, 216, 294, 296, 302, 312, 317
pathogenic, 125, 153, 184

pathogens, 14, 16, 17, 18, 69
pathologist, 15, 278
pathology, 35, 39, 107, 241, 259, 262
pathophysiological, 58, 76, 229
pathophysiological mechanisms, 229
pathophysiology, 71, 203, 204, 293, 302
pathways, 57, 61, 163, 392
patient care, 427, 438
patterning, 199
pay off, 360
PCA, 81, 82, 83, 84, 85, 91, 93
pediatric patients, 94, 115, 253, 310, 414
pediatrician, 7, 115, 265, 333, 352
peer, 6, 7, 27, 75, 101, 102, 103, 104, 125, 153, 154, 155, 156, 158, 160, 161, 182, 183, 184, 260, 277, 349, 387, 392, 403, 415, 435, 442
peer conflict, 27
peer group, 7, 102, 103, 277
peer influence, 387
peer rejection, 104, 153, 156
peer relationship, 6, 75, 101, 103, 104, 155, 161, 182, 184, 260
peer review, 435
peer support, 7, 182, 415
peers, 3, 24, 79, 99, 101, 102, 104, 106, 117, 119, 128, 152, 153, 154, 155, 156, 157, 159, 160, 161, 173, 174, 176, 177, 178, 180, 181, 182, 193, 237, 259, 265, 285, 286, 387, 415, 422, 427
pelvic, 17, 29, 39, 40, 47, 175, 276, 323, 327, 362
pelvic ultrasound, 39
pelvis, 322, 323
penicillin, 15, 72
Pennsylvania, 68, 365, 399
percentile, 190, 191, 192, 194, 196, 236, 263
perception, 74, 102, 110, 120, 182, 255, 261, 262, 264, 265, 266, 269, 286, 290, 406, 407, 419
perceptions, 112, 113, 157, 269, 274, 275, 351, 412, 429
perfectionism, 126, 132, 143
perforation, 242, 243
performance indicator, 427
perfusion, 204
perinatal, 339
perineum, 18, 295
periodontal, 399
periodontal disease, 399
peripheral, 372
peripheral nervous system, 204
peristalsis, 235
peritoneal, 251, 253, 256, 260, 261, 262, 265, 269
peritoneum, 251
peritonitis, 261
peroxide, 295, 300

personal identity, 154
personal qualities, 352
personal relations, 73
personal relationship, 73
personality, 101, 113, 114, 123, 125, 126, 129, 133, 136, 139, 140, 142, 143, 145, 148, 152, 162, 196
personality characteristics, 101, 143, 152
personality disorder, 125, 126, 129, 133, 136, 142, 143
personality disorders, 147
personality factors, 126, 145
personality scales, 139, 140
personality traits, 126
persons with disabilities, 280, 281, 386
pets, 159, 228
pH, 249
pharmacists, 225, 226
pharmacokinetics, 17, 19, 93, 94
pharmacological, 308
phenomenology, 124
phenotype, 86, 126, 340, 342, 343, 344, 346, 347, 357, 363
phenotypes, 61, 72, 340, 343
phenotypic, 72, 75, 341, 343, 345
phenylalanine, 59, 62
phenylketonuria, 52, 58, 60, 62, 168
phenytoin, 295
philosophy, 384
philtrum, 342, 343
phobia, 126
phobic anxiety, 132
Phoenix, 94
phosphate, 258
phosphorous, 248, 249, 250
phosphorus, 259
photosensitivity, 298, 299
PHS, 223
physical activity, 27, 29, 54, 126, 191, 198, 357, 374, 378, 380, 383, 384, 385, 386, 387, 388, 389, 390, 391, 393, 422
physical aging, 422
physical diagnosis, 381
physical education, 176, 177, 191, 373, 384, 386, 389
physical environment, 181, 387
physical exercise, 191, 375, 384, 388, 389
physical fitness, 383, 384, 385, 388, 390, 391, 392, 393
physical health, 27, 68, 189, 193, 197, 256, 258, 259, 260, 261
physical therapy, 75, 217, 312, 323, 326, 365
physicians, 124, 192, 222, 231, 253, 256, 265, 354, 381, 386, 392, 413, 417, 418, 422, 430435, 438

physiological, xi, 127, 134, 155, 283, 285, 386, 390
physiology, 16, 204, 433
physiotherapy, 16, 175, 176, 206, 362
pilot study, 405, 406
pituitary, 36, 37, 38, 39, 41, 44, 47, 49, 52, 76
pituitary gland, 36, 39, 41
placebo, 19, 49, 210, 218, 303, 309, 310
planning, 222, 273, 274, 275, 276, 277, 278, 279, 323, 353, 363, 404, 412, 413, 415
plants, 224, 228
plasma, 41, 248, 309
plastic, 363
platelet, 66, 76, 308
platelet count, 76
platelets, 66
play, 101, 104, 127, 179, 189, 190, 193, 241, 258, 265, 276, 296, 311, 312, 342, 359, 360, 373, 375, 377, 378, 379, 380, 381, 413, 416
pleasure, 284
pleural, 216
pneumonia, 14, 15, 16, 19, 240
pneumonitis, 14, 19
pollution, 230
polycystic ovarian syndrome, 297
polycystic ovary syndrome, 294
polydipsia, 41, 248
polyethylene, 242
polymorphonuclear, 15
polymorphonuclear cells, 15
polymyositis, 239
polyuria, 248
pools, 251
poor, xi, 3, 6, 14, 16, 26, 27, 28, 36, 37, 38, 42, 43, 44, 60, 61, 71, 73, 75, 103, 111, 116, 129, 155, 191, 208, 221, 225, 228, 237, 238, 241, 242, 248, 250, 263, 295, 297, 352, 380, 387, 404, 422
poor health, 6
population group, 405, 406
portal vein, 71
positive attitudes, 384
positive correlation, 76
positive mental health, 99, 100, 104, 105
postoperative, 94, 95
postpartum, 276, 278
post-stroke, 15, 19
posttraumatic stress disorder, 110, 120
posture, 361
potassium, 239, 259
potatoes, 190
poverty, xi, 3, 6, 152, 195, 408
poverty line, 6
powder, 209
power, 277, 371, 378, 380

PPO, 409
Prader-Willi syndrome, 53, 55, 342, 345, 348
pragmatic, 117
precocious puberty, 37, 39, 55
predictive validity, 196
predictor variables, 140
predictors, 106, 107, 120, 129, 140, 148, 384
predisposing factors, 14
prednisone, 293, 301, 302
preference, 102, 360
pregnancy, 60, 73, 169, 273, 274, 275, 276, 277, 278, 279, 284, 297, 299, 358, 404, 435
pregnant, 60, 274, 275, 277, 299, 353, 435
pregnant women, 277
prejudice, 284
prematurity, 204, 215, 216, 217, 236
prenatal care, 277
press, 119, 430
pressure, 14, 17, 18, 20, 67, 70, 89, 91, 189, 191, 192, 194, 195, 196, 197, 198, 239, 243, 277, 297, 360, 365, 369, 371, 372, 373, 378, 379, 384, 389
pressure sore, 277, 369, 372, 373
prevention, 20, 59, 60, 73, 197, 198, 209, 218, 230, 232, 247, 249, 251, 252, 256, 257, 258, 259, 260, 274, 279, 286, 371, 374, 384, 390, 400, 433, 434, 436
prevention of infection, 73
preventive, 15, 276, 384, 398, 399, 414, 417
priapism, 73, 74
primary care, 125, 200, 229, 230, 266, 280, 354, 373, 413
primary medical care, 398
privacy, 160, 178, 414
private, 5, 124, 221, 222, 283, 287, 399
private practice, 399
probability, 70, 190, 285
proband, 343
probands, 148
probe, 195, 240
problem solving, 152, 153
problem-focused coping, 181
production, 36, 39, 40, 45, 58, 60, 66, 218, 241, 298, 299, 301
professions, 105
progesterone, 40, 44, 296, 301
progestins, 297, 298
prognosis, 7, 48, 59, 61, 118, 125, 129, 145, 214, 217, 252, 255, 330, 339
prognostic factors, 149
proinflammatory, 216
prolapse, 214, 219, 378, 379
prophylactic, 69, 70
prophylaxis, 72

propulsion, 362
propylene, 296
prostaglandins, 308, 309
prostheses, 370, 372
prosthesis, 27
protection, 5, 163, 218, 285, 309
protective factors, 104
protective role, 285
protein, 38, 44, 45, 48, 49, 60, 66, 67, 71, 78, 235, 236, 248
proteins, 49, 54, 57, 58, 67, 235
prothrombin, 67, 69, 71, 78
protocol, 92, 94
protocols, 263, 427
proton pump inhibitors, 240
pruritus, 85, 262, 301
pseudo, 239
Pseudomonas, 14, 16, 17, 206, 217, 294
Pseudomonas aeruginosa, 16, 206, 217
psoriasis, 152, 299
psychiatric diagnosis, 130, 213
psychiatric disorder, 59, 79, 107, 111, 114, 115, 116, 120, 121, 126, 128, 147, 148, 199, 261
psychiatric disorders, 79, 107, 111, 114, 115, 116, 120, 121, 126, 128, 148, 199, 261
psychiatric illness, 266
psychological development, 26, 104, 152, 154, 160
psychological distress, 73, 196
psychological health, 132, 264
psychological pain, 175
psychological problems, 73, 110, 151, 158, 196
psychological stress, 99, 100, 391
psychological well-being, 129, 384
psychologist, 157, 175, 195, 196, 197, 413
psychology, 7
psychopathology, 113, 114, 115, 116, 118, 121, 125, 128, 214
psychopharmacology, 438
psychosis, 114
psychosocial development, 102, 169
psychosocial factors, 189, 195
psychosocial functioning, 30, 99, 120, 129, 267, 385
psychosocial stress, 265
psychosocial support, 414
psychosomatic, 124, 133, 145, 213, 218, 391
psychotherapeutic, 124
psychotherapy, 148
psychoticism, 132
psychotropic medications, 54
PTA, 86
ptosis, 343
pubertal development, 39, 40, 284, 286, 289, 425

puberty, 39, 41, 42, 43, 44, 45, 53, 73, 75, 102, 103, 114, 127, 153, 154, 157, 160, 256, 288, 342, 382, 386
public, 5, 156, 160, 182, 189, 198, 221, 222, 229, 274, 283, 284, 286, 287, 386, 397, 400, 415, 422, 423, 438, 441, 443
public awareness, 415
public education, 230
public health, 189, 198, 222, 229, 423, 441, 443
Public Health Service, 417
public schools, 286, 438
public service, 397, 441
pulmonary edema, 15
pulmonary embolism, 71, 78
pulmonary function test, 204, 205, 217
pulse, 379
pulses, 379
pupils, 133, 176
P-value, 408, 410, 411, 412
pyloric stenosis, 240
pyloroplasty, 243
pylorus, 15
pyretic, 308

Q

QOL, 256, 259, 261, 262, 264, 265, 266, 267
QT interval, 240
qualitative research, 183, 184, 419
quality of life, 8, 24, 26, 27, 29, 71, 74, 76, 79, 199, 203, 204, 206, 212, 217, 230, 239, 253, 255, 256, 258, 259, 263, 266, 267, 268, 269, 274, 279, 281, 284, 299, 303, 333, 399, 429, 434
Quality of life, 31, 255, 256, 268, 269, 281
query, 407
questioning, 178
questionnaire, 3, 9, 27, 107, 116, 130, 132, 139, 175, 195, 230, 259, 264, 286, 403, 406, 407
questionnaires, 121, 131, 144, 351

R

race, 199, 310, 371, 406
radiation, 24, 25, 26, 28, 29, 36, 38, 39, 40, 45, 46, 47, 238, 295, 370
radiation therapy, 36, 38, 46
radio, 15
radioactive iodine, 38
radiography, 15
radiological, 311, 312, 317, 325, 327
radiotherapy, 31, 39, 46, 47, 112
radius, 317

rales, 15
random, 177, 411
randomized controlled clinical trials, 309
range, 27, 38, 59, 61, 65, 66, 76, 83, 86, 92, 93, 103, 110, 113, 114, 130, 131, 132, 154, 167, 168, 170, 216, 240, 263, 321, 326, 342, 344, 351, 359, 361, 369, 370, 373, 410, 423, 437
rash, 309
rating scale, 85
ratings, 82, 85, 86, 87, 88, 91, 92, 123, 130, 132
reading, 112, 175, 352
reading skills, 352
reaffirmation, 55
reality, 114, 231, 266, 284, 416
reasoning, 153, 161
reasoning skills, 161
rebelliousness, 126
recall, 155, 389
recession, 327, 329
recognition, 59, 112, 153, 182, 192, 229, 248, 333, 341, 415, 424
recombinant DNA, 16
reconstruction, 27, 331, 335
recovery, 49, 82, 92, 123, 129, 130, 144, 146, 329, 378, 379
recreational, 25, 75
rectum, 17
recurrence, 38, 46, 113, 264, 339, 345, 346, 353
red blood cell, 72, 74, 258, 404
red blood cells, 258, 404
redness, 299
reflexes, 14, 19, 170, 242
refractory, 93, 209, 243, 301
regional, 219, 415, 435
registries, 113, 426
registry, 19, 119
regression, 7, 140, 221, 222, 224, 225, 226, 228, 358
regression analysis, 140
regular, 51, 55, 101, 125, 242, 261, 286, 287, 288, 353, 357, 360, 361, 363, 375, 385, 386, 387, 389, 405, 414, 428
regulation, 155, 160, 371
regulations, 168
rehabilitation, 25, 44, 79, 106, 329, 333, 362, 364, 420, 434, 441
reimbursement, 397, 398, 399
reinforcement, 79, 163
reinforcement contingencies, 163
rejection, 104, 126, 133, 153, 156, 159, 251, 263, 268
relapse, 23, 24, 25, 38

relationship, 19, 48, 77, 110, 127, 128, 134, 140, 142, 144, 146, 157, 159, 180, 189, 193, 195, 200, 265, 284, 303, 360, 390, 391, 392, 416
relationships, 6, 68, 73, 75, 79, 102, 103, 104, 106, 123, 126, 129, 133, 141, 143, 144, 154, 155, 159, 160, 161, 179, 182, 184, 258, 260, 285, 287, 289, 351, 352, 353, 363, 390, 404, 412, 413, 414
relatives, 105, 128
relaxation, 17, 182, 214, 239, 241, 359, 360
relevance, 354
reliability, 85, 94, 132, 196, 200, 392
religious beliefs, 160
remission, 23, 38, 111, 209
renal, 70, 71, 76, 78, 100, 107, 194, 236, 248, 250, 252, 253, 255, 256, 257, 258, 259, 260, 261, 262, 263, 264, 265, 266, 267, 268, 269, 308, 309
renal disease, 70, 100, 107, 194, 248, 252, 255, 256, 257, 258, 259, 260, 261, 262, 263, 264, 265, 266, 267, 268
renal dysfunction, 76, 248, 258
renal failure, 236, 250, 257, 263, 269
renal function, 70, 71, 250, 252, 258, 259, 260, 308, 309
renal osteodystrophy, 252, 258
renal replacement therapy, 255, 256, 260, 261
renal scan, 194
renin, 194
repair, 214, 219, 298, 320, 329
replication, 163, 392
repression, 289
reproduction, 39, 281, 289, 322, 345, 422
reproductive organs, 43
resection, 39, 243, 333
resentment, 69
reservation, 31, 181
reservoir, 260
residential, 54, 55, 56, 58, 443
resilience, 158, 163
resistance, 16, 18, 42, 43, 44, 67, 71, 78, 237, 275, 297, 298, 299, 300, 302
resistence, 157
resolution, 206, 216, 217, 219
resources, 100, 104, 105, 115, 125, 151, 160, 161, 174, 222, 265, 266, 275, 278, 364, 387, 389, 391, 413, 416, 417, 421, 424, 426, 427, 428
respirator, 219
respiratory, 4, 14, 15, 16, 52, 58, 60, 61, 85, 91, 100, 204, 205, 214, 216, 218, 219, 222, 228, 231, 232, 238, 239, 242, 276, 278, 376
respiratory disorders, 61
respiratory failure, 15
respiratory problems, 222
respiratory rate, 91

responsibilities, 284, 285, 415, 438
responsiveness, 249
restaurant, 298
restless legs syndrome, 168
retardation, 42, 48, 53, 54, 267, 302, 341, 355
retention, 85, 235, 239, 242, 248, 249, 424
retinoic acid, 295, 299
retinoids, 293, 298, 302
retinopathy, 76
Rett syndrome, 344, 357, 358, 359, 360, 362, 363, 364, 365, 391
rewards, 126
rheumatic, 115
rheumatic heart disease, 115
rheumatoid arthritis, 112, 309
rhythm, 285
rickets, 238, 251
risk behaviors, 27, 190, 274, 280, 381
risk factors, 15, 19, 27, 31, 53, 67, 93, 119, 148, 189, 190, 191, 192, 194, 198, 199, 228, 231, 259, 381, 384, 390, 417
risk profile, 390
risks, 27, 54, 67, 107, 168, 169, 242, 275, 278, 284, 286, 289, 339, 346, 369, 373, 376, 377, 380, 388
risperidone, 169
rofecoxib, 310
rosacea, 295, 299
routines, 256, 260
RTT, 358
rumination, 184
rural, 130, 418, 423
Rutherford, 94

S

safety, 276, 307, 309, 310, 387
salicylates, 301
saline, 206
salt, 207, 248
same-sex friendships, 153
sample, 4, 92, 113, 116, 121, 130, 131, 132, 133, 138, 144, 174, 185, 190, 200, 403, 405, 408, 411
sampling, 264
sarcomas, 24, 26, 31
satisfaction, 27, 31, 124
saturation, 85
savings, 230
scalp, 294, 295
SCD, 71, 72, 73, 74, 76, 79, 403, 404, 405, 406, 408, 409, 410, 411, 412, 413, 414, 415, 416, 420
scheduling, 414
schemas, 107
schizophrenia, 120, 131, 152

scholastic achievement, 25
school activities, 261
school adjustment, 121
school performance, 247, 250, 259
schooling, 229
scientific community, 57, 61
sclerosis, 248, 262, 296
scoliosis, 170, 236, 358, 361, 362, 365, 378
scores, 26, 30, 128, 129, 130, 132, 138, 139, 140, 143, 144, 145, 182, 258, 265, 342, 352, 384, 392
screening programs, 52
scrotum, 295
SDS, 258
search, 6, 146, 308, 310, 357
seasonality, 228
seaweed, 298
sebaceous glands, 294, 299
sebum, 294, 299, 302
secondary education, 25, 415
secondary sexual characteristics, 53
secretion, 14, 16, 38, 42, 43, 44, 46, 47, 48, 301
security, 101, 360
sedation, 85, 398
sedentary, 54, 191, 383, 385, 388, 389, 392
sedentary behavior, 191
sedentary lifestyle, 54, 389
sediment, 248
seeding, 18
segmental glomerulosclerosis, 257
seizure, 14, 112, 168, 380
seizures, 39, 53, 60, 61, 111, 168, 169, 170, 236, 250, 302, 340, 341, 342, 358
self esteem, 29, 73, 182, 193
self-awareness, 284
self-care, 25, 111, 278, 285, 288, 404
self-concept, 127, 385, 391
self-efficacy, 107, 127, 404, 414, 416
self-esteem, 27, 104, 111, 115, 125, 126, 133, 161, 168, 182, 193, 195, 199, 200, 287, 289, 385, 386, 416, 419
self-identity, 6
self-image, 73, 153, 193, 250, 284, 384, 391
self-management, 112, 180, 182, 185, 228, 229, 232, 413
self-report, 130, 132, 196, 389
self-reports, 389
self-worth, 113, 133, 385
senior citizens, 365
sensation, 14, 17, 169, 242, 359, 362, 371, 385
sensation seeking, 385
sensations, 238
sensitivity, 126, 132, 138, 139, 240, 296
sensitization, 228, 232

sensorineural hearing loss, 28
sensory experience, 359
sensory impairments, 370
separation, 101, 115, 127, 299
sepsis, 17, 203, 261
septic arthritis, 312
septicemia, 18
sequelae, 3, 45, 46, 68, 75, 76, 101, 105, 112, 414
series, 27, 240, 354, 400
Sertoli cells, 40
serum, 194, 248, 252, 299, 301, 341, 384
serum transferrin, 341
service provider, 105, 275, 279
severe asthma, 110, 228, 377
severity, 15, 42, 61, 72, 74, 100, 105, 107, 110, 114, 115, 155, 160, 167, 170, 182, 205, 206, 207, 208, 210, 216, 221, 222, 224, 228, 243, 258, 263, 300, 372, 419
sex, 39, 52, 111, 153, 160, 182, 190, 199, 221, 222, 231, 275, 279, 286, 287, 289, 290, 294, 296, 353, 354
sex steroid, 39
sexual abuse, 133, 285, 433
sexual activity, 274, 275, 285, 345
sexual assault, 433
sexual behavior, 285
sexual development, 285
sexual orientation, 286
sexuality, 155, 160, 162, 274, 275, 276, 278, 281, 283, 284, 285, 286, 287, 289, 297, 353, 356
sexually transmitted diseases, 275
shape, 103, 148, 213, 313, 404
sharing, 175, 182
shear, 317
shock, 39, 92
short period, 175, 256, 261
shortage, 400
shortness of breath, 208, 376
short-term, 113, 131, 192, 242, 251, 391
shoulder, 372
shoulders, 69, 71, 175, 295, 358
shy, 175, 414
SIADH, 41
sibling, 117, 133, 144, 155, 158, 159, 352, 385
siblings, 10, 25, 26, 27, 128, 131, 133, 134, 144, 155, 158, 159, 351, 352
sickle cell, 5, 71, 72, 74, 75, 78, 79, 80, 81, 82, 83, 85, 92, 93, 94, 110, 117, 155, 203, 403, 404, 405, 406, 407, 416, 417, 418, 419, 420, 430
sickle cell anemia, 78, 80, 418, 420
side effects, 24, 81, 82, 85, 90, 92, 94, 103, 115, 179, 240, 257, 259, 261, 263, 264, 266, 295, 298, 299, 308, 309

sign, 116, 320, 321, 323, 324, 325, 407
signs, 38, 40, 42, 59, 75, 85, 121, 156, 173, 180, 191, 195, 240, 261, 311, 312, 324, 325, 371
Singapore, 10
singular, 61
sinus, 68, 295
sites, 69, 92, 405, 411
skeleton, 391
skill acquisition, 152
skills, 26, 28, 69, 104, 127, 152, 153, 154, 155, 157, 160, 161, 173, 180, 182, 183, 184, 277, 286, 351, 352, 358, 362, 363, 365, 370, 372, 376, 380, 390, 391, 404, 413, 414, 415, 424, 438
skills training, 415
skin, 29, 100, 242, 243, 294, 295, 296, 298, 299, 301, 302, 303, 308, 353, 372
skin cancer, 29
skin disorders, 299
skin tags, 242
sleep, 6, 168, 169, 192, 208, 213, 259, 352
sleep deprivation, 208
sleep disorders, 169
slipped capital femoral epiphysis, 312, 313, 334
smoke, 113, 160
smokers, 110
smoking, 27, 67, 76, 110, 113, 117, 190, 224, 228, 278, 377
SMR, 377
snoring, 194
social acceptance, 385
social activities, 75, 113
social anxiety, 124
social behavior, 284, 285, 384
social comparison, 182
social competence, 27, 28, 152, 351, 385, 391
social consequences, 6
social context, 169, 285
social environment, 103, 413, 416
social events, 287
social impairment, 71
social isolation, 24, 126, 128, 285, 288, 289, 427
social life, 312, 352, 413
social network, 161, 275
social participation, 167, 170
social phobia, 126
social problems, 24, 116, 132, 139, 140, 145
social relations, 143
social relationships, 143
social services, 413
social situations, 104, 156
social skills, 104, 184, 286, 363
social standing, 153
social stigmatization, 69

social support, 103, 104, 105, 112, 182, 415
social work, 266, 276, 413, 414, 435
social workers, 276, 414, 435
socialization, 30, 69, 168, 170, 353, 387, 389
sociocultural, 174
socioeconomic, 9, 107, 175, 222
socioeconomic status, 9, 222
socioemotional, 184
sociopsychological, 67
sodium, 208, 209, 218, 249, 250, 259, 310
soft drinks, 297
solid tumors, 24
somatic symptoms, 116
somnolence, 28
sores, 17, 277, 369, 372, 373
sounds, 241
spastic, 55, 237
spasticity, 113, 170, 236, 241, 363, 370, 371
spatial, 85, 91, 153
special education, 25, 26, 31, 68, 283, 286
specialisation, 129
specificity, 240
spectrum, 16, 39, 53, 55, 61, 71, 72, 74, 78, 168, 263, 294, 339, 344, 346, 347
speech, 15, 69, 113, 153, 214, 264, 340, 342, 343, 344, 346, 358, 398
speed, 25, 153, 209
sperm, 40, 41, 350
sphincter, 17, 242
spina bifida, xi, 3, 13, 17, 155, 236, 404, 418, 424, 426
spinal cord, 28, 168, 242, 244, 369, 370, 371, 372, 373, 374, 376
spinal cord injury, 168, 242, 369, 370, 371, 372, 373, 374
spinal muscular atrophy, 168
spine, 37, 242, 276, 301, 361
spiritual, 75
spirometry, 205, 208, 209
spleen, 380
splenectomy, 76, 80
splenomegaly, 380
spondyloarthritis, 294
spondylolysis, 379
sporadic, 53
sports, 24, 162, 168, 175, 209, 212, 213, 307, 308, 309, 310, 311, 323, 370, 371, 372, 373, 374, 375, 376, 377, 378, 379, 380, 381, 385, 386, 387, 391, 392, 434
spouse, 159
SPR, 434
sprain, 309, 378
sprains, 372

SPSS, 407, 419
SRD, 259
SSI, 109, 117, 409
stability, 284, 288, 362
stabilize, 206, 207
stages, 7, 29, 66, 75, 127, 154, 158, 181, 192, 216, 250, 255, 265, 267, 273, 278, 349, 350, 358, 360
standard deviation, 85, 258
standards, 229, 236, 237, 307, 399
staphylococcal, 238
Staphylococcus, 14
starvation, 190
statistical analysis, 138
Statistical Package for the Social Sciences, 407, 419
statistics, 85, 129, 142, 190, 407
status of children, 99
steady state, 84
stem cell transplantation, 37
stenosis, 377
stereotype, 427
stereotypes, 195, 276
sterilization, 280
sternum, 214
steroid, 44, 194, 295, 301
Steroid, 295
steroids, 39, 213, 229, 243, 295, 297, 298, 301
stiffness, 327
stigma, 106, 115, 159
stigmatization, 69
stigmatized, 181
stimulus, 249
stock, 277
stoma, 243
stomach, 61, 175, 240, 243, 298
storage, 58, 60, 168
strabismus, 379
strain, 115, 278, 323, 326, 379, 420
strains, 16, 17, 372
strategies, 6, 72, 104, 113, 178, 179, 182, 195, 197, 222, 264, 265, 278, 365, 386, 389, 414, 418
strategy use, 104, 113
stratification, 252
strength, 28, 206, 300, 326, 370, 371, 378, 380, 386, 388, 392
stressful life events, 113, 119, 141
stressors, 6, 10, 112, 142, 159, 265, 266
stretching, 144, 326, 370, 388
stridor, 212, 213
stroke, 15, 19, 61, 72, 73, 76, 79, 80, 168, 189, 360, 404
strokes, 76
structural changes, 206, 216
structuring, 413

students, 107, 125, 131, 190, 221, 223, 224, 225, 229, 230, 389, 390, 393, 408, 409, 418, 435, 437, 438
subacute, 429
subcutaneous injection, 74
subgroups, 317, 341
subjective, 128, 256, 263
subluxation, 317, 321, 323
substance abuse, 116, 125, 128, 435
substance use, 119, 121, 153
substances, 58, 61, 160, 295
success rate, 129, 144, 330
sudden infant death syndrome (SIDS), 59
suffering, 125, 126, 127, 129, 181, 264, 286
sugar, 58, 156, 301
sugars, 157, 387
suicidal, 111, 112, 128, 130, 132, 133, 134, 136, 143, 148
suicidal behavior, 129, 133, 148
suicidal ideation, 111, 112, 129
suicide, 111, 117, 118, 124, 128, 129, 132, 134, 148, 162, 299, 301, 303, 433, 435
suicide attempts, 117
suicide rate, 128
sulfate, 294
summer, 224
sunlight, 54, 295, 387
superiority, 143
supervision, 101, 133, 160, 206, 294, 352, 353, 356, 386
supplemental, 206, 207, 216
supplements, 236, 376
support services, 101
suppression, 44, 54, 241, 252
suppressor, 347
suprachiasmatic, 41
surfactant, 216
Surgeon General, 280, 399, 400, 418
surgeons, 18, 326
Surgeons, 391
surgeries, 311, 312, 330
surgery, 25, 28, 31, 38, 39, 67, 83, 106, 115, 120, 215, 217, 238, 295, 301, 311, 326, 327, 329, 330, 333, 376, 378, 398
surgical, 24, 27, 39, 41, 71, 214, 238, 242, 243, 260, 295, 320, 323, 326, 327, 329, 330, 331, 332, 333, 334, 335, 365, 398, 400
surgical intervention, 326, 365
surgical resection, 24, 39
surprise, 189, 260
surveillance, 230, 256, 307, 354, 424

survival, xi, 3, 7, 13, 15, 16, 19, 23, 24, 26, 27, 30, 36, 72, 106, 158, 206, 247, 248, 255, 260, 262, 263, 404, 426
survival rate, xi, 3, 13, 27, 106, 255, 262
surviving, 73, 351, 404, 424
survivors, 23, 24, 25, 26, 27, 29, 30, 31, 36, 45, 46, 47, 68, 71, 112, 113, 114, 118, 119
susceptibility, 301
swallowing, 14, 16, 235, 239, 398
sweat, 242
sweat chloride test, 242
Sweden, 364, 365
swelling, 67, 70, 71, 248, 308, 379
Switzerland, 116, 146, 162
symbolic, 153
sympathetic, 363, 371
symptom, 60, 82, 93, 129, 130, 140, 196, 240
symptomatic treatment, 312
synovial fluid, 308
synthesis, 58, 66, 71, 72, 152, 308, 345
syringomyelia, 372

T

tachycardia, 237
tachypnea, 71, 236, 237
Taiwan, 52, 55, 438
tandem mass spectrometry, 52
tangible, 105
targets, 194
taste, 169, 359
taxation, 422
Tay-Sachs disease, 60
TBI, 37, 38, 40, 114, 379
teachers, 116, 159, 160, 176, 177, 181, 285, 287, 289, 350, 365, 387, 435
teaching, 157, 434, 435, 437, 441, 443
team members, 412, 414
technological developments, 18
teenagers, 176, 192, 196, 197, 260, 261, 262, 263, 266, 267, 283, 284, 285, 286, 287, 288, 289, 425
teens, 156, 160, 163, 173, 200, 214, 285, 312, 388, 415, 435
teeth, 299, 398
television, 388
temperament, 152
temperature, 74, 371
temporal, 89, 91
tendon, 242
tendons, 308
tension, 261, 363
teratogenic, 169, 299
teratogens, 339

territory, 61
test scores, 26
testicular cancer, 24, 29, 31
testosterone, 40, 41, 296, 301
testosterone levels, 40, 41, 301
testosterone production, 40
tetanus, 376
tetracycline, 295, 298, 299, 300
Texas, 81, 442
textbooks, 438
Thailand, 390
thalassemia, 71, 73, 74, 75, 76, 78, 79, 417, 426
therapeutic change, 129
therapeutic interventions, 24, 25, 70, 333
therapeutics, 35, 94
therapists, 18, 76, 365, 386
thinking, 101, 152, 153, 157, 161, 179, 180, 276, 386
Thomson, 48, 232
thoracic, 361
thorax, 381
thought problems, 116
threat, 23, 24, 133
threatening, 24, 35, 70, 75, 77, 106, 110, 127, 130, 321, 371, 404
threshold, 204, 216, 343
throat, 169, 213
thromboembolic, 68
thrombosis, 67, 68, 70, 71, 77, 78
thrombotic, 66, 67, 68, 70, 76, 78
thymus, 342
thyroid, 24, 29, 38, 41, 42, 44, 46, 47, 53, 54, 76, 240, 353
thyroid cancer, 24, 29
thyroid gland, 38
thyroid releasing hormone, 38
thyroid stimulating hormone, 38
tic disorder, 169
ticks, 426
tics, 169
time consuming, 266, 426
time frame, 131
timing, 107, 183, 209, 425
tissue, 18, 29, 41, 60, 214, 237, 243, 258, 294, 295, 299, 310, 372, 379
title, 284, 429
tobacco, 160, 190, 230, 377
tobacco smoking, 190
toddlers, 101, 327
tolerance, 19, 28, 29, 43, 53, 74, 129, 204, 206, 207, 208, 214, 215, 216, 218, 243, 259, 423
tonsillectomy, 94, 95
topical antibiotics, 295
total body irradiation, 46

total energy, 236
total parenteral nutrition, 239
toxic, 58, 60, 217
toxicity, 24, 25, 29, 30, 39, 40, 41
tracking, 198, 426
trade, 184, 264
trade-off, 184, 264
training, 154, 195, 204, 206, 218, 266, 274, 279, 280, 288, 353, 370, 378, 380, 384, 385, 388, 391, 397, 398, 399, 400, 413, 414, 415, 428, 433, 434, 435, 437, 438
training programs, 288
traits, 126
trajectory, 158, 173, 174, 181
transcripts, 175
transfer, 274, 404, 406, 407, 416, 418, 421, 422, 424, 426, 428, 429, 430
transference, 312
transfusion, 72, 74
transfusions, 73, 75, 80
transition period, 7, 354
transition to adulthood, 26, 418
transitions, 354, 361, 413, 419, 420, 421
translocation, 351
transmembrane, 16, 43
transplant, 16, 25, 248, 251, 253, 256, 258, 260, 261, 262, 263, 264, 265, 268
transplant recipients, 262, 264
transplantation, 37, 46, 47, 60, 72, 247, 248, 251, 252, 253, 255, 256, 257, 262, 263, 264, 267, 268
transport, 43, 58, 278
transportation, 266, 283, 287, 410
trauma, 18, 67, 68, 83, 114, 154, 157, 161, 243, 297, 310, 339, 377, 379
traumatic brain injuries, 238
traumatic brain injury, 114, 120, 167, 168, 170, 376, 379
travel, 260, 423, 428
treatable, 111
trees, 204
tremor, 262, 379
trial, 19, 29, 43, 49, 77, 94, 232, 242, 244, 303, 308, 309, 310, 326, 333, 426
triceps, 237
triggers, 212, 228, 231, 377
triglyceride, 301
triglycerides, 294, 299
triiodothyronine, 38
trisomy, 350, 351
trisomy 21, 350, 351
trochanter, 320, 323
truancy, 116
trust, 101, 196, 354, 360, 423

TSH, 38, 44
tuberous sclerosis, 296
tubular, 248, 250
tumor, 28, 38, 39, 46, 47, 296, 297, 347
tumors, 24, 25, 26, 27, 28, 29, 36, 41, 45, 47, 296, 297
turnover, 249
Twin studies, 128
twins, 147
type 1 diabetes, 117
type 2 diabetes, 53, 61, 100, 117
type 2 diabetes mellitus, 117
type II diabetes, 118, 192
typology, 106
tyrosine, 59

U

U.S. Preventive Services Task Force, 55
UCH, 429
ulcer, 17, 20, 296
ulceration, 20, 239, 299
ulcerative colitis, 114
ultrasonography, 40, 80
ultrasound, 39, 194, 242
uncertainty, 138
unconditional positive regard, 273
undergraduate, 397, 398, 399, 400
undergraduate education, 398
underreported, 74
uniform, 3, 4
uninsured, 5
United Kingdom, 4, 110, 349, 351, 352, 354, 443
univariate, 139, 407
universities, 435
urea, 58
urinary, 14, 17, 20, 85, 238, 262, 340, 371
urinary retention, 85
urinary tract, 14, 17, 20, 238, 262, 371
urinary tract infection, 14, 17, 20, 238, 371
urine, 17, 18, 41, 52, 58, 59, 194, 248, 261
urine catecholamines, 194
urologist, 257, 266
US Department of Health and Human Services, 19, 280, 417

V

vagus nerve, 239
validation, 146, 406
validity, 85, 132, 196
values, 154, 191, 205, 408, 438

variability, 74, 102, 104, 126, 228, 344
variables, 123, 131, 190, 385
variance, 110, 138, 182
variation, 72, 75, 83, 154, 156, 200, 230, 236
varus, 327
vascular disease, 238, 261
vasculature, 204, 216
vasodilation, 208
vasomotor, 371
vaso-occlusion, 82
vasopressin, 41
vegetables, 101, 191
vein, 67, 70, 71, 77, 78, 260
velocity, 28, 38, 39, 48, 241, 249
venous insufficiency, 70
venous pressure, 70
ventilation, 204, 206, 208, 215
ventricular fibrillation, 240
ventricular septal defect, 302
ventriculoperitoneal shunt, 371
vertigo, 299
vessels, 404
vestibular system, 362
veterinary medicine, 67
vibration, 363
victimization, 181, 184
victims, 285, 433
video games, 168
vinblastine, 28, 41
violence, 152, 154, 161
Vioxx, 308, 310
viral infection, 60, 116, 263
virus, 121
virus infection, 121
viscosity, 14
visible, 102, 156, 179, 228, 243, 298
vision, 301, 353, 436
visual images, 155
visual stimuli, 360
visualization, 329
vitamin D, 42, 44, 54, 56, 239, 249, 250
vitamin D deficiency, 42
vitamins, 239
vocational, 6, 25, 26, 79, 154, 350, 353, 404, 405, 413, 415
vocational rehabilitation, 26
vocational training, 353, 413
voice, 157, 213, 214, 405
voiding, 17
volunteerism, 433
vomiting, 24, 59, 60, 85, 89, 90, 92, 103, 237, 238, 239, 250, 371
vulnerability, 127, 147, 158

W

waking, 82, 360, 365
walking, 19, 320, 342, 358, 361, 362, 385, 387, 388
war, 130, 131
waste products, 258, 260
water, 41, 207, 208, 235, 243, 256, 258, 260, 298, 360, 372
weakness, 28, 59, 61, 371, 380
wealth, 124
web, 391
web-based, 391
weight control, 103, 107, 153, 192, 197, 278
weight gain, 42, 43, 44, 103, 114, 191, 192, 196, 238, 277
weight loss, 42, 192, 193, 195, 199, 376
weight management, 197
welfare, 434, 441
wellbeing, 289, 391, 421, 428, 436
well-being, 72, 106, 107, 128, 129, 131, 145, 206, 218, 264, 383, 384, 389, 391, 434
wellness, 280, 281
western countries, 100
western culture, 124, 194
western diet, 259
wheelchair, 276, 277, 362, 370, 371, 372, 374
wheeze, 208, 229, 231, 232
wheezing, 213, 376
white blood cell count, 72
wind, 209
winter, 224, 295, 388
wisdom, 7
withdrawal, 92, 116, 359
women, 67, 77, 107, 124, 146, 147, 148, 195, 273, 274, 275, 276, 277, 278, 279, 280, 281, 286, 288, 303, 345, 353, 362, 390, 408
wool, 228
work activity, 349, 355
workers, 3, 68, 127, 144
working class, 352
working groups, 426
workload, 174, 177, 181
World Health Organization (WHO), 109, 116, 124, 184
worry, 7, 113, 114, 153
wrists, 69
writing, 415

X

X chromosome, 363
X-linked, 66, 340, 345, 357

X-rays, 311

Y

yield, 127, 341, 361
young adults, 24, 30, 31, 41, 68, 70, 78, 94, 109, 112, 118, 119, 191, 219, 262, 284, 285, 293, 302, 312, 335, 385, 404, 405, 406, 412, 413, 415, 416, 419, 420, 422, 424, 429, 430
young women, 125, 273, 274, 275, 276, 277, 278, 279, 280
younger children, 102, 191, 196, 259

Z

zinc, 347